AF752039

INTERVENTION MAPPING

INTERVENTION MAPPING

HEALTH PROMOTION PLANNING, IMPLEMENTATION, AND EVALUATION

Fifth Edition

Maria E. Fernandez
Christine M. Markham
Robert A.C. Ruiter
Rik Crutzen
Andrew E. Springer

JOSSEY-BASS™
A Wiley Brand

Copyright © 2026 by John Wiley & Sons, Inc. All rights reserved, including rights for text and data mining and training of artificial intelligence technologies or similar technologies.

Published by John Wiley & Sons, Inc., Hoboken, New Jersey.

No part of this publication may be reproduced, stored in a retrieval system, or transmitted in any form or by any means, electronic, mechanical, photocopying, recording, scanning, or otherwise, except as permitted under Section 107 or 108 of the 1976 United States Copyright Act, without either the prior written permission of the Publisher, or authorization through payment of the appropriate per-copy fee to the Copyright Clearance Center, Inc., 222 Rosewood Drive, Danvers, MA 01923, (978) 750-8400, fax (978) 750-4470, or on the web at www.copyright.com. Requests to the Publisher for permission should be addressed to the Permissions Department, John Wiley & Sons, Inc., 111 River Street, Hoboken, NJ 07030, (201) 748-6011, fax (201) 748-6008, or online at http://www.wiley.com/go/permission.

The manufacturer's authorized representative according to the EU General Product Safety Regulation is Wiley-VCH GmbH, Boschstr. 12, 69469 Weinheim, Germany, e-mail: Product_Safety@wiley.com.

Trademarks: Wiley and the Wiley logo are trademarks or registered trademarks of John Wiley & Sons, Inc. and/or its affiliates in the United States and other countries and may not be used without written permission. All other trademarks are the property of their respective owners. John Wiley & Sons, Inc. is not associated with any product or vendor mentioned in this book.

Limit of Liability/Disclaimer of Warranty: The contents of this work are intended to further general scientific research, understanding, and discussion only and are not intended and should not be relied upon as recommending or promoting scientific method, diagnosis, or treatment by physicians for any particular patient. In view of ongoing research, equipment modifications, changes in governmental regulations, and the constant flow of information relating to the use of medicines, equipment, and devices, the reader is urged to review and evaluate the information provided in the package insert or instructions for each medicine, equipment, or device for, among other things, any changes in the instructions or indication of usage and for added warnings and precautions. While the publisher and the authors have used their best efforts in preparing this work, including a review of the content of the work, neither the publisher nor the authors make any representations or warranties with respect to the accuracy or completeness of the contents of this work and specifically disclaim all warranties, including without limitation any implied warranties of merchantability or fitness for a particular purpose. No warranty may be created or extended by sales representatives, written sales materials or promotional statements for this work. The fact that an organization, website, or product is referred to in this work as a citation and/or potential source of further information does not mean that the publisher and authors endorse the information or services the organization, website, or product may provide or recommendations it may make. This work is sold with the understanding that the publisher is not engaged in rendering professional services. The advice and strategies contained herein may not be suitable for your situation. You should consult with a specialist where appropriate. Further, readers should be aware that websites listed in this work may have changed or disappeared between when this work was written and when it is read. Neither the publisher nor authors shall be liable for any loss of profit or any other commercial damages, including but not limited to special, incidental, consequential, or other damages.

For general information on our other products and services or for technical support, please contact our Customer Care Department within the United States at (800) 762-2974, outside the United States at (317) 572-3993 or fax (317) 572-4002.

Wiley also publishes its books in a variety of electronic formats. Some content that appears in print may not be available in electronic formats. For more information about Wiley products, visit our web site at www.wiley.com.

Library of Congress Cataloging-in-Publication Data applied for

Hardback ISBN: 9781119774105

Cover Design: Wiley
Cover Image: © oxygen/Getty Images

Set in 10.5/14pt Warnock Pro by Straive, Pondicherry, India

SKY10159991_062326

DEDICATION

This textbook is dedicated to the memory of our esteemed colleagues and co-creators of Intervention Mapping, **L. Kay Bartholomew Eldredge, EdD, MPH (1951–2016),** and **Gerjo Kok, PhD (1948–2025).**

As two of the original authors of *Intervention Mapping,* Kay and Gerjo helped shape a systematic, theory- and evidence-based approach to health promotion that has influenced research and practice worldwide. Their intellectual leadership, unwavering commitment to rigor, and deep belief in the power of thoughtful planning transformed the way we design, implement, and evaluate health interventions.

Beyond their scholarly contributions, they were generous mentors, collaborative partners, and inspiring teachers whose impact lives on through the countless students, practitioners, and communities they guided.

We honor their legacy with gratitude and continue this work in the spirit of their vision.

CONTENTS

FIGURES AND TABLES

Figures

Tables

ACKNOWLEDGMENTS

Our thanks to colleagues who were contributing authors to selected chapters in the Fifth Edition.

Patricia Dolan Mullen, DrPH, MLS, is a Professor Emerita of Health Promotion and Behavioral Sciences, School of Public Health, The University of Texas Health Science Center at Houston and Emerita member of the Center for Health Promotion and Prevention Research. She has been honored as the President's Scholar for Teaching and University of Texas System as a Distinguished Teaching Professor and as a Distinguished Fellow of the Society for Public Health Education. She designed and initiated the School's program evaluation and systematic review courses, and directed long-standing cancer prevention training programs. With Drs. Fernandez and Bartholomew Eldredge, she co-created IM ADAPT, an online decision support tool that uses Intervention Mapping to help practitioners identify, adapt, and evaluate evidence-based interventions. She has served on many expert panels, including the US Community Preventive Services Task Force. Her research interests include promoting the use of evidence-based programs and policy, especially cancer prevention and preconception counseling to avoid tobacco and alcohol during pregnancy. She led Chapter 10 and contributed to Chapter 11.

Melissa Peskin, PhD, is a Distinguished Teaching Professor of Health Promotion and Behavioral Sciences and Epidemiology, Vice Chair and Assistant Dean of Students at the School of Public Health, The University of Texas Health Science Center at Houston. She is an expert in the development, implementation, evaluation, and dissemination of adolescent health promotion interventions. She has led and taught the School's Program Evaluation class for many years and has extensive experience collaborating with community and academic partners to evaluate programs on a broad range of health and training topics. She contributed to Chapter 10.

Casey Durand, PhD, MPH, is a former Assistant Professor in Health Promotion and Behavioral Sciences at the School of Public Health at The University of Texas Health Science Center at Houston. His research interests include obesity prevention and physical activity interventions. He contributed to Chapter 10 on evaluation.

Eunyoung Kang, PhD, is an Assistant Professor in Health Promotion and Behavioral Sciences at the School of Public Health and faculty at the Institute for Implementation Science, The University of Texas Health Science Center at Houston. Her research focuses on the translation of evidence-based interventions for chronic disease and aging into real-world settings. She contributed to Chapter 11 on adaptation and sections of Chapter 9.

Jessica D. Austin, PhD, MPH, is an Assistant Professor of Health Promotion Sciences and a member of the Health Promotion Research Center and Stephenson Cancer Center at The University of Oklahoma Health Sciences Center. She graduated with her PhD from The University of Texas Health Science Center where she completed her tenure as a National Cancer Institute-funded (T32) predoctoral fellow in cancer prevention and control. Dr. Austin's research focuses on developing, adapting, implementing, and evaluating community-centered cancer prevention and control innovations with a focus on reducing health disparities.

Lara Staub Savas, PhD, is an Associate Professor in the Department of Health Promotion and Behavioral Sciences at The University of Texas Health Science Center at Houston (UTHealth Houston) School of Public Health and the Center for Health Promotion and Prevention Research. A behavioral epidemiologist, Dr. Savas specializes in the development, adaptation, and evaluation of theory- and evidence-based health interventions, with particular expertise in applying Intervention Mapping and Implementation Mapping frameworks to guide systematic program planning and dissemination. She leads large-scale, community- and clinic-based cancer prevention initiatives, including a community health worker-delivered breast and cervical cancer screening and HPV vaccination program designed to address structural, social, and behavioral determinants of health among medically underserved women. Her work emphasizes participatory approaches, multilevel intervention design, and implementation strategies to support scale-up and sustainment of evidence-based programs in real-world settings. She has taught and redesigned the Program Evaluation course for over 10 years. She contributed to Chapter 11, including providing the chapter example.

Helen Skouteris, PhD, is the Monash Warwick Professor in Health and Social Care Improvement and Implementation Science (Health and Social Care Unit, School of Public Health and Preventive Medicine). She contributed to sections in Chapter 1.

Sarah Stutterheim, PhD, is an Associate Professor in Health, Medicine and Life Sciences at Maastricht University. She contributed to sections in Chapters 3 and 6.

Harm Veling, PhD, is a Professor at Wageningen University and Research. He contributed to sections in Chapter 3.

Sarah Birken, PhD, is an Associate Professor in the Department of Implementation Science at the Wake Forest School of Medicine. She contributed to sections in Chapter 4.

Gil ten Hoor, PhD, is an Associate Professor at the Faculty of Psychology and Neuroscience (FPN), Maastricht University. He contributed to sections in Chapter 6.

Timothy Walker, PhD, is an Associate Professor in Health Promotion at the UTHealth Houston School of Public Health. He contributed to sections and mini examples in Chapter 9.

Nalini Ranjit, PhD, is an Associate Professor in Health Promotion & Behavioral Sciences at the UTHealth Houston School of Public Health in Austin. She contributed to sections in Chapter 10.

Additional thanks to our colleagues for their excellent work on *Por Nuestros Hijos/For Our Children* and for helping incorporate existing materials into the Intervention Mapping framework for this chapter example.

Lynn Ibekwe-Agunanna, PhD, is an Assistant Professor in the Advancing Implementation & Improvement Science (AIIS) program at The University of Texas Southwestern Medical Center in Dallas, Texas.

Preena Loomba, PhD, is a Postdoctoral Fellow at The University of Texas MD Anderson Cancer Center.

Ileska Valencia-Torres is a Research Coordinator at The University of Texas Health Science Center at Houston, Center for Health Promotion and Prevention Research.

Our thanks to our colleagues who provided support with editing, references, and coordination for the Fifth Edition.

Jeanette Curtain, MPH, is a Graduate Coordinator at the University of Pennsylvania.

Meghan Haffey, DrPH, is a Public Health Program Evaluator for the Defense Health Agency Health Promotion and Wellness Directorate.

Taylor Levy, MS, is a Graduate Research Assistant at The University of Texas Health Science Center at Houston School of Public Health.

Nivedhitha Parthasarathy, PhD, is a Research Associate at The University of Texas at Austin.

Amber Watson, MSPH, is a Research and Implementation Consultant at The University of Texas Health Science Center at Houston, Institute for Implementation Science.

A special thanks to **Julia Shenkman, MPH,** who spearheaded coordination of the book and supplemental materials and provided critical feedback as a student and practitioner.

We gratefully acknowledge the authors of previous editions of *Intervention Mapping*—L. Kay Bartholomew Eldredge Eldredge, Guy Parcel, Gerjo Kok, and Nell Gottlieb—whose leadership in their respective academic positions and foundational contributions continue to shape and inspire this work.

ABOUT THE AUTHORS

Maria E. Fernandez, PhD, is Vice President of Population Health and Implementation Science at The University of Texas Health Science Center at Houston (UTHealth Houston) and the founding Co-Director of the UTHealth Houston Institute for Implementation Science. She also serves as the Lorne Bain Chair of Public Health and Medicine, Professor of Health Promotion and Behavioral Sciences, and Director of the Center for Health Promotion and Prevention Research at the UTHealth Houston School of Public Health, United States of America. Dr. Fernandez has extensive experience conducting community-engaged research to develop, evaluate, implement, and disseminate interventions to improve health and reduce disparities among underserved populations. Her work spans cancer and chronic disease prevention and control, participatory research, and dissemination and implementation science. She has led numerous global, federal, and state-funded studies and has authored more than 250 peer-reviewed publications and several books in these areas.

Christine M. Markham, PhD, is a Professor and Department Chair of Health Promotion and Behavioral Sciences at The University of Texas Health Science Center at Houston School of Public Health and Allan King Professorship in Public Health, United States of America. She has over 30 years' experience in health promotion and behavioral sciences research across multiple health domains, populations, and settings, including determinants studies, intervention development, program evaluation, dissemination and implementation research. With a background in anthropology, she is experienced in qualitative research and mixed-methods studies.

Robert A.C. Ruiter, PhD, is a Professor of Health and Social Psychology at the Department of Work and Social Psychology, Faculty of Psychology and Neuroscience, Maastricht University, the Netherlands. His work integrates psychological theory with a broad range of qualitative and quantitative methods to understand and promote health- and safety-related decision-making and behavior at both individual and collective levels. A central pillar of his scholarship is public health research capacity building, pursued nationally and internationally through the supervision of PhD candidates from the Global South, with a particular focus on Sub-Saharan Africa.

Rik Crutzen, PhD, is a Professor of Behaviour Change & Technology at the Department of Health Promotion, Care and Public Health Research Institute, Maastricht University, the Netherlands. A central theme in his work is the systematic development, implementation, and evaluation of behavior change interventions, with a keen eye on the potential and challenges of using technology in such interventions. He has a strong focus on methodological and theoretical progress, especially to foster understanding of behavior as a crucial first step in intervention development.

Andrew E. Springer, PhD, is an Associate Professor of Health Promotion and Behavioral Sciences at The University of Texas Health Science Center at Houston School of Public Health in Austin, United States of America, who brings over 25 years of experience in the design, implementation, and evaluation of child, adolescent, and community health promotion programs in the United States and Latin America. With a specific interest in socio-environmental influences on health behavior and participatory planning and evaluation methods, he maintains an active community health promotion praxis that includes participation in various community health coalitions, as well as community-engaged research.

ABOUT THE COMPANION WEBSITE

This book is accompanied by a companion website.

www.wiley.com/go/interventionmapping/5e

To access the website materials, click on the link under Related Resources on the book's page on wiley.com. You can also find this by searching www.wiley.com for the ISBN [9781119774105].

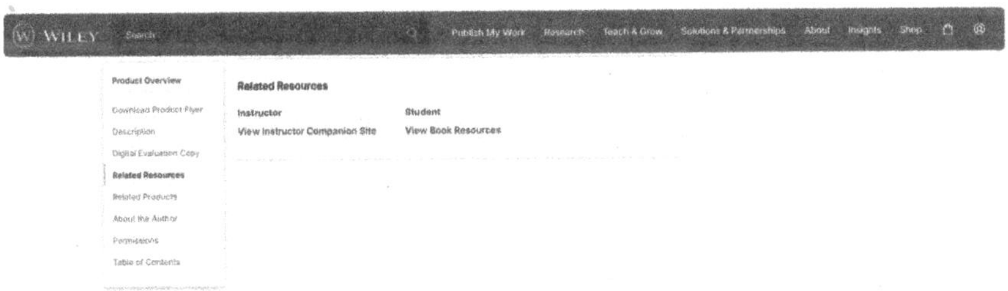

This website includes:

- Instructor's Manual
- Student Assessment Question Bank
- Student Assessment Rubric
- Instructor Slides for Chapters 1-11

PART ONE

OVERVIEW AND FOUNDATIONS

CHAPTER 1

OVERVIEW OF INTERVENTION MAPPING

Intervention Mapping (IM) is a planning approach that uses theory, evidence, and community and partner engagement as foundations for the design and evaluation of multilevel health promotion programs and implementation strategies. IM applies an ecological approach to planning by examining the personal, interpersonal, organizational, community, and societal determinants of health and designing interventions to influence them. In doing so, it ensures that planners address the full spectrum of multilevel influences on behaviors and environmental conditions. The purpose of IM is to provide health promotion program planners with a framework for effective decision-making at each step in the process of intervention design, implementation planning, and evaluation. In this chapter, we present the perspectives underlying IM and a preview of this robust program-planning framework that is used worldwide.

Health promotion is the process of enabling individuals and communities to increase control over and improve their health. It involves creating supportive environments, strengthening community action, developing personal skills, and reorienting health services to address the broader determinants of health—not only individual behavior (World Health, 1986). It has also been defined as "combinations of educational, political, regulatory, and organizational supports for behavior and environmental changes that are conducive to health" (Green & Kreuter, 2005). In this book, we use the terms "program" and "intervention" interchangeably to broadly refer to various types of health promotion interventions. These include more traditional health promotion and education programs (e.g., an eight-course diabetes self-management program), as well as quality improvement initiatives (e.g., improving the delivery of health services), and interventions aimed at policy, systems, and environmental change as part of a community health improvement plan (e.g., The North Karelia Project) (Springer et al., 2024). This book also uses the terms **health educator, health promoter,** and **program planner** interchangeably to mean someone who is planning a health promotion intervention meant to produce health outcomes. Since health promotion program planning often occurs as a team, we also use the term "planning group."

How Intervention Mapping Compares to Other Planning Frameworks

Across the field of health promotion, planning models such as PRECEDE-PROCEED (Green et al., 2022), MAPP (NACCHO, 2023), and others share several core phases: engaging stakeholders, assessing needs and assets, identifying priorities, designing interventions, and planning for implementation and evaluation. This common structure reflects a long-standing consensus about the essential components of systematic health promotion planning. Intervention Mapping (IM) builds from this shared foundation yet offers a deeper level of operational guidance for planners who want to integrate theory, empirical evidence, and community expertise into actionable, multilevel intervention plans. Unlike models that simply describe *what* to do in each phase, IM (through the integration of Core Processes and its step-by-step tasks) provides detailed processes for *how* to carry out intervention design phases in ways that are theory-driven, evidence-informed, culturally responsive, and ecologically aligned.

In this way, IM helps bridge a long-recognized gap in the planning literature: practitioners often understand that theory, empirical evidence, and community engagement are essential, yet lack a practical route for integrating these elements in a systematic and effective way. Knowing where you are (i.e., having identified the health problem, its behavioral and environmental determinants, and the populations most affected) is necessary but not sufficient. Likewise, simply possessing the right tools (theory, epidemiology data, community input) does not guarantee that they will be used well. What planners need is a clear, step-by-step pathway that shows how to apply these tools, in what sequence, and for what purpose. IM provides that route, mapping out the concrete directions that guide planners from problem understanding to the design of a coherent, multilevel intervention with the potential to produce meaningful and lasting improvements in health and quality of life.

IM also advances several innovations that distinguish it from other planning approaches. First, while many models begin with broad population health assessments, IM requires a more focused needs and assets assessment built around a specific health condition, behavior, or environmental influence. This enables planners to move beyond identifying problems toward understanding the behavioral, environmental, and socio-structural determinants that must change to improve health. Second, IM strengthens ecological thinking by guiding planners to specify both individual-level and environmental change objectives, identify environmental agents, and design multilevel strategies aligned with settings and systems. Third, IM integrates a robust set of planning tools including logic models of the problem and of change, matrices that link determinants to performance objectives, and processes for selecting and translating theory-based change methods into practical applications, thus providing more rigorous and transparent planning than most frameworks. Finally, IM embeds equity considerations and community engagement throughout the process. Through the needs and assets assessment and linkage system concepts, planners are guided to identify populations most at risk, activate community assets, and meaningfully engage members of the priority population and local implementers in co-creating feasible and culturally relevant interventions. Together, these features make IM not only consistent with other models in its overall structure but also uniquely powerful in offering planners a clear, detailed, and equitable pathway from problem identification to effective intervention design, implementation, and evaluation.

Theory, Evidence, and New Data

IM is grounded in a set of foundational procedures called the *Core Processes,* which guide planners in systematically using theory, empirical evidence, community insights, and new data to understand and address health and social problems. These Core Processes, composed of posing questions, exploring possible answers, reviewing existing evidence (published literature as well as existing data), identifying theoretical support, determining the need for new data, and assessing the completeness of the information gathered, are used across all steps of IM and ensure that planning decisions are well-reasoned and transparent. Chapter 2 describes each Core Process in detail and illustrates how they function throughout the planning process.

The Core Processes can be particularly helpful for planners using theory for understanding and addressing health problems. We agree with Kurt Lewin's well-known assertion that *nothing is as useful as a good theory* (Hochbaum et al., 1992). Theory is essential in evidence-informed health promotion because it helps explain why behaviors and environmental conditions occur and guides the selection of appropriate methods for change. Scholars have emphasized the need for clearer guidance on how theory can be effectively used to understand and address complex public health and social problems (Fernandez et al., 2019; Glanz et al., 2024; Kok et al., 2017; Ruiter & Crutzen, 2020; ten Hoor et al., 2025). In IM, theory is applied pragmatically: planners draw from multiple theoretical perspectives rather than relying on a single model, which includes applying one or more causal/etiologic theories to understand the problem and change theories to guide solutions.

In addition to theory, empirical evidence plays a central role. In addition to published data, identifying existing evidence from previous (unpublished) studies, evaluations, surveillance systems, and practice-based experience provides critical information about determinants, contextual influences, and strategies that have been effective or ineffective in similar situations. However, theory and existing evidence are not always sufficient. In many cases, planners need new data (often both qualitative and quantitative) to fill gaps, test assumptions, understand context, or explore determinants that have not been adequately examined. In IM, the decision to collect new data is intentional and arises after reviewing the available theory and evidence, consistent with the Core Processes. This ensures that new data collection is targeted, efficient, and justified by the planning questions at hand.

Although community participation is not defined as its own Core Process, it is foundational across all Core Processes and all steps of IM. Community members, implementers, and other stakeholders contribute essential knowledge about local conditions, priorities, feasibility, and acceptability. Community-engaged planning often provides essential tacit knowledge that neither theory nor published evidence alone can provide. Their perspectives help shape the questions planners pose, the way evidence is interpreted, the identification of gaps needing new data, and ultimately the decisions made about intervention design. A later section in this chapter elaborates on the importance of community participation in health promotion planning and its central role in IM.

Through the systematic use of the Core Processes and by integrating theory, existing evidence, new data, and community perspectives, IM strengthens the rigor, completeness, and relevance of planning decisions. This approach ensures that interventions are grounded in a comprehensive understanding of the problem and its context and increases the likelihood that resulting programs will be both effective and feasible in real-world settings.

Ecological Models and Systems Thinking

The social ecological model, an underpinning for IM, has been used extensively in health promotion and is related to and encompassed by systems thinking (Bronfenbrenner, 1989; Bronfenbrenner & Ceci, 1994; Crielaard et al., 2025; McLeroy et al., 1988). In the social ecological model, health is a function of individuals and of the environments in which individuals live, including family, social networks, organizations, communities, and societies (Eriksson et al., 2025; Golden & Wendel, 2020; Springer et al., 2024; Stokols, 1996).

The social ecological paradigm focuses on the interrelationships between individuals (biological, psychological, and behavioral characteristics) and their environments. These environments include physical, social, and cultural aspects that exist across the individual's life domains and social settings. A nested structure of environments allows for multiple influences both within levels and across levels. Throughout the book, there is a focus on identifying and planning interventions that influence *environmental agents* (decision-makers or role actors) at each ecological level: interpersonal (e.g., parents), organizational (e.g., managers of school food services), community (e.g., newspaper editors), or societal (e.g., legislators). Interventions at the various levels focus on agents (individuals or groups, such as boards or committees) in positions to exercise control over aspects of the environment. For example, adolescent uptake of smoking might be influenced by peers and parents at the interpersonal level of the environment and by regulations and access at the social and community levels of the environment. The picture that emerges is a complex web or system of causation as well as a rich context for intervention.

A system consists of interconnected activities, actors, and settings that influence or are influenced by, a particular problem situation (Green, 2006; Leischow & Milstein, 2006). Systems perspectives and approaches can be used to assess the needs and strengths of the population, to understand a health problem and its multilevel and mutually influencing determinants, to select the most effective leverage points to address the problem, and to form a representative group of key actors and interested parties to plan, conduct, implement, and disseminate an intervention. Since interventions are events in systems, other factors within a system can reinforce or dampen the impact of an intervention on the specific behavioral and/or environmental changes being targeted (Douglas & Stamatakis, 2012; Kok et al., 2017).

Systems thinking can also inform implementation planning. For example, Whelan et al. (2023) found that combining systems thinking with implementation science constructs helped build stronger community-based prevention systems. Similarly, Zamantakis et al. (2024) identified key determinants of successful linkage-to-care systems in HIV prevention, emphasizing the role of organizational and interpersonal linkages.

We present, as a beginning point, a template for simple, linear logic models focusing on the presumed cause–effect pathways related to health problems and their solutions articulated from theory and empirical research (Bartholomew Eldredge & Mullen, 2011; Green et al., 2022). However, we encourage the reader to adapt the logic model template to the complexity of the problem being analyzed, and we assume that the intervention, the system activity being targeted, and the proposed outcome are part of a complex multilevel system. An intervention at one environmental level can influence causal factors at multiple levels (Lengnick-Hall et al., 2021; McLeroy et al., 1988).

Participation in Health Promotion Planning

Involving the priority population and interested community partners in the design, implementation, and evaluation of health promotion programs is foundational to the IM process and is rooted in a long history and current practice in the field of health promotion and public health. The right for people to individually and collectively participate in the planning of their health care is a key principle set forth by the *Declaration of Alma Ata,* which originates from the first International Conference on Primary Health Care in 1978 that set forth the goal of "Health for All" (Rifkin, 2018). A decade later, the Institute of Medicine (IOM) published *The Future of Public Health,* which outlined a strategy for improving population health that moved from a sole focus on individual-level medical care to addressing determinants of health based in the community via collective action (IOM, 1988). Subsequent IOM reports further advanced the concept of *intersectoral responsibility for health,* which underscored the importance of community participation, as well as participation from key sectors within a given community (clinical care delivery system, employers and business, the media, and the education sector) (IOM, 2003, 2011).

Involving the priority population and community partners, including potential implementers, in co-creating health promotion interventions brings multiple benefits. First, inclusive community participation helps to ensure that the program focus reflects community concerns and values while also increasing the cultural relevance and potential impact of an intervention (Wallerstein et al., 2018). Broad participation also brings a greater breadth of skills, knowledge, and expertise to a project, and can improve external validity of interventions and evaluation by recognition of the local knowledge of community members and practitioners (Israel et al., 2018; Kok et al., 2017; Springer et al., 2024). Co-creating change with project partners and community partners and stakeholders furthermore allows the planning of interventions within local resource capacity, which holds promise for increasing the sustainability of a given intervention (Hawe, 2015). Evidence-based health promotion interventions may also be more acceptable to communities and potential participants when the research that has produced the evidence does not originate under special circumstances in distant places (Green & Mercer, 2001). Importantly, engaging the priority population and community stakeholders in health promotion planning is based on ethical principles of health promotion practice (Grabowski et al., 2017; Springer et al., 2024). "Nothing about us without us," a quote with a long history that formed the rallying call for the UN Convention on the Rights of Persons with Disabilities, underscores the idea that no policy or program should be decided without the full and direct participation of members of the group(s) affected (see also the section "Ethical Practice of Health Promotion").

To inform a community-engaged approach for health promotion planning, implementation, and evaluation, Community-Based Participatory Research (CBPR) principles provide helpful guidance (Wallerstein et al., 2018) (Box 1.1). In supporting these guiding principles, planners now have access to a growing menu of resources for engaging groups in participatory planning, implementation, and evaluation, including Facilitating Intentional Group Learning (Preskill et al., 2017), Community Tool Box (CCHD),

BOX 1.1. COMMUNITY-BASED PARTICIPATORY RESEARCH PRINCIPLES

- Recognizing a partner community as a unit of identity
- Building upon community strengths and resources
- Facilitating collaborative, equitable decision-making in which partners negotiate desired roles in all project phases and attend to social inequalities
- Fostering colearning among partners
- Balancing knowledge generation with community benefit
- Focusing on ecological perspectives, local problems, and multiple determinants of health
- Developing systems using an iterative process
- Disseminating information, results, and benefits to all partners
- Developing a commitment and long-term process
- Addressing issues of race, ethnicity, racism, and social class, and embodying "cultural humility"

Adapted from Wallerstein et al. (2018).

Liberating Structures (Lipmanowicz & McCandless, 2014), Participatory Learning and Action (Nelson, 2023), and Participatory Methods (Institute of Development Studies, n.d.), among other resources.

Embracing Cultural Humility and Reflexivity as Part of the Planning Group Process

One goal for health promotion planning is developing a perspective of cultural humility, defined as "...a lifelong commitment to self-evaluation and critique, to redressing power imbalances ... and to developing mutually beneficial and non-paternalistic partnerships with communities on behalf of individuals and defined populations" (Tervalon & Murray-García, 1998). Despite ongoing discussion about the use of the terms *cultural humility* versus *cultural competence* within the field of public health, we embrace Greene-Moton and Minkler's (2020) call to move beyond the false choice between these terms to embracing their core purpose as they relate to the:

> ...recognition of the need for public health, medical, social work, and other professionals to reflect on and address our own biases and actively seek to understand and assess the cultural and social realities of the diverse individuals, groups, and communities with whom we and our groups and organizations interact. (Greene-Moton & Minkler, 2020)

In developing cultural humility and in designing more culturally relevant interventions, there is growing emphasis on the importance of practicing *reflexivity* for health promotion practitioners, researchers, and community health improvement teams (Alexander et al., 2020; Aronowitz et al., 2015; Garney et al., 2017). While definitions abound, we embrace a definition of reflexivity as an intentional activity that consists both of an exploration of one's own beliefs, judgements, and practices—which may include one's own social positionality and social and racial biases (Finlay, 1998; Johnson & Duberley, 2003)—as well as examination of the broader social forces that shape health inequities and power imbalances that can unintentionally be perpetuated via the health promotion research and practice process (Alexander et al., 2020; Aronowitz et al., 2015). Below we briefly explore how health promotion practitioners can begin to work toward embracing cultural humility and reflexivity as part of the intervention planning process and also introduce a brief overview of how culture is incorporated into each IM planning step.

Exploring Personal Ethnocentricity

Engaging and involving members of a planning group starts at the onset of the planning process; this principle of inclusivity extends to the personal development of group leaders and group members to help all group participants work both across and within cultures. This personal work involves listening deeply to the people with whom one is working as well as actively exploring one's personal ethnocentrism (Sue, 2003). Locke (1986, 1992) offers the following set of questions, tailored for our field of health promotion, as first steps in developing cultural self-awareness:

- What is my cultural heritage? What was the culture of my parents and grandparents? With what cultural group do I identify?
- What values, beliefs, opinions, and attitudes do I hold that are consistent with the dominant culture? Which are inconsistent? How did I learn these?
- How did I decide to be a health promotion planner and practitioner? What cultural standards were involved in the process? What do I understand to be the relationship between culture and health promotion?
- What unique abilities, aspirations, expectations, and limitations do I have that might influence my relations with culturally diverse individuals?

Through a process of suspending and then observing one's habitual ways of relating to other groups and then observing one's typical ways of seeing and relating to others, a person can move through stages to attain greater cultural awareness, sensitivity, or even humility. The stages may include:

1. Feelings of fear, hostility, defensiveness, and superiority
2. Denial of cultural differences
3. Cultural acceptance and respect
4. Empathy
5. Integration, multiculturalism, and social justice (Bennett, 1993; Rios et al., 1998)

As next steps, one might structure opportunities for *reflexivity* in the planning group to disclose personal backgrounds, including those related to privilege and power (Tervalon & Murray-García, 1998; Wallerstein et al., 2018). Alexander et al. (2020) provide a helpful framework for guiding reflexivity within health promotion practice that is organized by three domains: *reflexivity in action* (e.g., mobilizing knowledge during action), *reflexivity on action* (e.g., exploring ways to improve future action after an action was implemented), and *reflexivity underlying action* (e.g., exploring the power dynamics, cultural values, and other underlying assumptions about the larger systemic change process that can encourage alternative perspectives for action and evaluation). Practical ways to incorporate reflexivity into the planning process may include "pause and reflect" activities that are incorporated in team meetings as part of a *learning agenda* (Nightingale et al., 2018).

Exploring and Working in Another Culture

In addition to becoming aware of one's ethnocentric lens, another prerequisite for planning groups is the ability to identify and embrace the positive aspects of that culture (Airhihenbuwa & Liburd, 2006). The *PEN-3 model* provides a framework for guiding communication about culture and integrating culture into health intervention design (Airhihenbuwa, 1995, 1999; Iwelunmor et al., 2014; Kannan et al., 2009). In this model, the planning group considers three domains of culture:

- *Cultural identity*: Defining the priority population through a consideration of extended families and communities, as well as individuals;
- *Relations and expectations*: Considering aspects of the culture that can affect health and behavior, including perceptions, enablers (community, societal, and structural factors), and nurturers (social support networks such as family, friends, and community);
- *Cultural empowerment*: Building from the cultural beliefs and practices that are positive in relation to the health topic before tackling the practices that may be harmful and have negative health consequences (Airhihenbuwa & Webster, 2004; Iwelunmor et al., 2014).

The Role of Culture in Intervention Planning

A theme that appears in each step of IM is the need to create culturally relevant programs for diverse groups. While there are several important reasons for planners to be able to develop effective programs across cultures, including expanding diversity of populations within countries, globalization, and global health promotion practice, perhaps among the most pressing considerations for culturally relevant health promotion interventions is the critical need to address health disparities that disproportionately affect specific racial and ethnic groups, sexual and gender minority groups, populations of lower socioeconomic position, and other vulnerable populations (Baah et al., 2019; Braveman et al., 2011, 2022; Chu & Leino, 2017; Fernandez et al., 2025; Fiscella et al., 2000; Heim & Kohrt, 2019; Highfield et al., 2015). A recent global report by the World Health Organization underscores the alarming inequities among vulnerable subpopulations in access to quality housing, education, job opportunities, and other social determinants of health that are driving health disparities and shortening lives by decades (WHO, 2025). In the United States, the US Healthy People 2030, like the 2010 and 2020 versions before it, highlights the importance of addressing health disparities in the wake of the COVID-19 pandemic, with eliminating health disparities and addressing the social determinants of health being two of the five overarching goals (NIH, 2019). These disparities and health and social inequities underscore the need for both health promotion planners who bring cultural humility and sensitivity for working with diverse groups and the need for planning approaches that can guide the development of culturally relevant and supportive interventions aimed at reducing disparities and advancing the health of our most vulnerable neighbors.

In developing and implementing interventions aimed at reducing health disparities and advancing health equity, IM provides a helpful framework. As health planners, we first need to be intentional in growing our cultural humility and sensitivity to groups different from our own, as discussed in the section above. Involving the priority population and community partners who know the conditions and challenges experienced by a given population in health promotion planning is a first step toward helping planners become more culturally sensitive while also informing the development of culturally relevant interventions. In IM *Step 1—Needs and Assets Assessment*, we begin with engaging the priority population and other community partners and stakeholders in a planning group, as guided by the linkage system and highlighting the need for both positive group facilitation and participatory planning methods (see Chapter 5). In Step 1, the planner is also guided to consider the roles culture can play in both the causation and the outcomes of health problems, while also highlighting the importance of learning about the community and resources in the community that can be activated for the proposed health promotion intervention.

Importantly, planners complete Step 1 by identifying both program goals and the groups and subgroups most at risk for a given health problem and who merit further intervention and support. Identifying the groups most at risk builds from an equity orientation that is "predicated on the ethical principle of distributive justice; one that requires our decisions regarding the allocation of resources, benefits, and burdens across society be informed by the social conditions of individuals and communities" (Parsons et al., 2021). In *Step 2—Program Outcomes and Objectives,* culture is further explored as an important aspect for defining performance objectives and for understanding a priority population's determinants for engaging in behavior and for engaging environmental agents in implementing environmental change.

Planners are further guided to incorporate culture in *Step 3—Methods and Practical Applications* and *Step 4—Intervention Design and Production.* In Step 3, planners explore theory-based change methods and identify or develop practical applications that align with the priority population, intervention setting, and community of interest—with involvement of the priority population key to informing methods and applications (Chapter 7). In Step 4, planners further incorporate cultural considerations into the production of their intervention via the concepts of *surface and deep culture* (Resnicow et al., 1999), as well as the *mechanisms for increasing cultural relevance* (see Chapter 8). In Step 4, planners are guided to specifically assess cultural relevance of their intervention via processes such as pretesting and pilot-testing.

In *Step 5—Implementation Plan,* culture is further considered via the lens of implementation and involvement of key stakeholders who understand the settings and conditions of the priority population. In *Step 6—Evaluation Plan,* we further consider culture via the audiences for whom the evaluation is being developed, while aiming to advance culturally responsive evaluation approaches that aim to "center" evaluation within the community for which evaluation is being conducted (Kushnier et al., 2023). Lastly and importantly, partnering with underserved communities who experience disproportionate disease or health risk burden holds promise to build community power that can affect change for the advancement of individual and community health and quality of life (Iton et al., 2022).

Ultimately, equity must be a foundational principle in IM, not an afterthought. To achieve meaningful and sustainable change, equity must be embedded intentionally from the earliest stages of program planning and design through to implementation and evaluation. This involves prioritizing the voices and leadership of those with lived experience, especially from historically marginalized communities, and ensuring that diverse perspectives are safely and meaningfully included. Equity-focused IM requires planners to reflect on their own biases, power dynamics, and assumptions, and to use culturally responsive and community-driven approaches. Theories and frameworks that address social determinants of health, structural racism, intersectionality, and post-colonialism provide essential guidance for designing interventions that are just and inclusive.

Effective equity-centered IM also demands multi-sectoral collaboration across health, social care, and education, sectors that are deeply engaged with underserved populations. Strategies such as investing in community-defined evidence, dismantling power structures, and tailoring interventions to local contexts are critical (Gooey et al., 2026). Building capacity through equity-specific education and training, funding community-led initiatives, and improving access to services are practical steps that support equitable outcomes. Efforts to increase explicit guidance for planning that integrates equity perspectives can enhance intervention impact. For example, Intervention Mapping – Equity is the focus of a large program of research led by Monash University in collaboration with the authors of Intervention Mapping among others (O'Connor et al., 2026). The Strengthening implEMentation Practice and Research with Equity (SEMPRE) program is generating new knowledge across theory, methodology, and practice in collaboration with lived experience experts (Griffith et al., 2025). Ultimately, equity must be explicitly planned for, continuously reflected upon, and actively pursued throughout every phase of intervention development and implementation to ensure that programs do not perpetuate existing disparities but instead contribute to transformative, systemic change.

Ethical Practice of Health Promotion

A systematic, thoughtful planning process can provide part of the road map required to establish ethical health promotion practice. Kass (2001) has presented a framework for evaluation of public health programs against standards of ethical integrity as have the American Association of Public Health (APHA, 2019) and the World Health Organization (WHO, 2011). The Society for Public Health Education (SOPHE) has developed specific ethical and professional guidelines for public health educators (CNHEO, 2020) and the International Union for Health Promotion and Education (IUHPE) details ethical values that underpin the health promotion core competencies (Battel-Kirk et al., 2024). Combined, these sources suggest the following guidelines for interventions:

- **Program goals should always be related to the health of the public.** Furthermore, health educators should be proactive in confronting issues that can adversely affect health of persons and communities and should provide services equitably. IM supports this principle by directing planners to focus on health issues and to begin planning with a full appraisal of the health problem and its causes.

- **Interventions should be based on thorough evidence to increase the chance of effectiveness.** IM supports this principle by basing programs on clear evidence of effectiveness. The IM steps help planners systematically consider the following types of evidence: importance, causes (including behavior and environment), and consequences of the health problem; effective approaches to behavioral and environmental change; and useful approaches to implementation.
- **Design and production of interventions should include diverse participation.** As the SOPHE suggested, IM directs planners to involve communities in program development and implementation, consider and accommodate diverse perspectives and values in program development, encourage informed decision-making among individuals, and be transparent in disclosure of all program aspects, including benefits, other outcomes, unexpected consequences, and burdens.
- **Intervention planners should consider the rights of persons and take action to protect them.** Furthermore, public health practitioners are expected to support the worth, dignity, and uniqueness of all people and ground their practice in the ethical principles of respect for autonomy, promotion of social justice, promotion of good, and avoidance of harm. They must address the known and potential burdens of the program, including risks to privacy and confidentiality, liberty, self-determination, and justice. IM suggests that planners consider burdens to participants and minimize them by adopting alternate approaches.

The emphasis on participation helps ensure that communities have input into judgments about appropriate levels of intervention and evaluation burden, as well as an acceptable balance of burden-to-risk based on community values. Members of communities will not necessarily agree on risks and benefits, and a participatory planning process enables disclosure, discussion, consensus, and plans for moving forward through disagreement. Another way that the IM approach helps protect against inequitable burden is the focus on an ecological approach to both problem analysis and intervention. Most problems have contributions from the at-risk group or persons with the problem and from factors and agents in the environment. All significant contributors to the problem should comprise the focus for interventions, and planners should avoid the temptation to blame the victim by burdening the persons with the problem with full responsibility for its solution (Hailu et al., 2024; Tomiyama et al., 2018).

Intervention Mapping Steps

Each step of IM comprises several tasks (Figure 1.1). The completion of the tasks included in a step creates a product that is the guide for the subsequent step. Completion of all steps creates a blueprint for designing,

STEP	TASKS
Step 1 **Needs and Assets Assessment**	• Establish a planning group • Conduct a needs and assets assessment • Describe the context for the intervention including the community, population, and setting • State intervention goals
Step 2 **Intervention Outcomes and Objectives**	• State desired behavioral and environmental outcomes • Specify performance objectives for behavioral and environmental outcomes • Select determinants for behavioral and environmental outcomes • Construct matrices of change objectives
Step 3 **Methods and Practical Applications**	• Generate intervention ideas with the planning group • Choose theory- and evidence-based change methods • Select and design practical applications to deliver change methods
Step 4 **Intervention Design and Production**	• Define intervention structure (themes, components, scope, and sequence) • Plan intervention messages, materials, and activities • Produce intervention materials, activities, and protocols • Pretest, refine, and finalize materials, activities, and protocols
Step 5 **Implementation Mapping**	• Conduct an implementation needs and assets assessment and identify program implementers • Identify implementation performance objectives and determinants to create matrices of change objectives • Choose change methods and design implementation strategies • Produce implementation protocols and materials • Evaluate implementation outcomes
Step 6 **Evaluation Plan**	• Review the logic model of change, matrices, and implementation plan to guide process and effect evaluation • Develop process evaluation questions and identify measures • Develop effect evaluation questions, select a design, and identify measures • Pilot test the intervention and finalize evaluation plan • Plan when and how to report evaluation findings

Evaluation

Implementation

Figure 1.1 Intervention Mapping Steps

implementing, and evaluating an intervention based on a foundation of theoretical, empirical, and community information. Even though IM describes six steps, the process is iterative rather than completely linear. Program developers move back and forth between tasks and steps as they gain new information and perspective. However, the process is also cumulative; planners base each step on the previous steps, and inattention to a step can jeopardize the potential effectiveness of the intervention by compromising the validity of the foundation on which later steps are conducted. Sometimes planners can get carried away by momentum in the process of the planning group and forget a step, or they may perform a step with less-than-optimal rigor. Fortunately, most of the time planners can backtrack and include, repeat, or elaborate on a neglected step.

The six steps of the IM process are the following:

1. Needs and Assets Assessment: Establish a detailed understanding of the health problem, the population at risk, the behavioral and environmental causes, and the determinants of these behavioral and environmental conditions; and assess available resources
2. Intervention Outcomes and Objectives: Describe the behavioral and environmental outcomes, create objectives for changes in the determinants of behavior and environmental causes, and specify the targets of the intervention program
3. Methods and Practical Applications: Identify theory- and evidence-based behavior change methods that influence the determinants and translate these into practical applications that fit the intervention context
4. Intervention Design and Production: Combine the intervention components into a coherent program that uses delivery channels that fit the context
5. Implementation Mapping: Develop implementation strategies to facilitate adoption, implementation, and maintenance of the program
6. Evaluation Plan: Plan both process and outcome evaluation to assess program implementation and efficacy or effectiveness.

Step 1: Needs and Assets Assessment

In Step 1 (Chapter 5), the program planner does the following:

1. Establish a planning group
2. Conduct a needs and assets assessment
3. Describe the context for the intervention, including the community, population, and setting
4. State intervention goals

Before beginning to actually plan an intervention, the planner puts together a team to assess the health problem, behavioral and environmental causes of the problem, and determinants of behavioral and environmental causes. We strongly recommend depicting these relations on a logic model diagram, also called *theory of the problem* and *theory of change* (Chen, 2014; Connell & Kubisch, 1996; Frechtling, 2007; Kirby, 2004; Rossi et al., 2004; Weiss & Coyne, 1997). IM introduces a logic model (theory) of the problem in Step 1 and a logic model (theory) of change in Step 2. Logic models are indispensable guides for program development and evaluation,

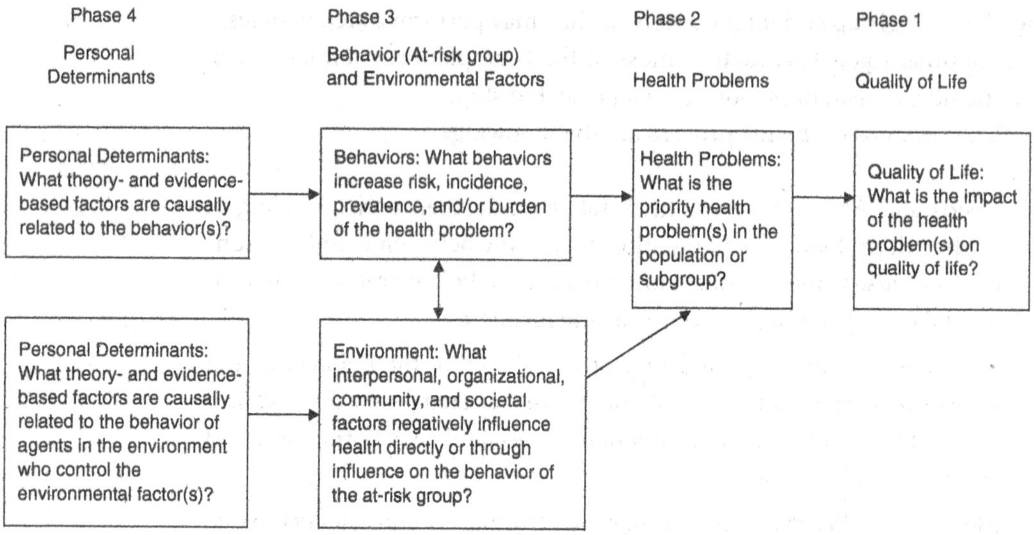

Figure 1.2 Logic Model of the Problem

are an increasingly common requirement in applications to funding agencies, and are taught and supported by the Centers for Disease Control and Prevention as the fundamental framework for program evaluation (ActKnowledge & Aspen Institute Roundtable on Community Change, 2003; CDC 2011; W. K. Kellogg Foundation, 2006, 2010).

We suggest the PRECEDE model as a framework for creating a logic model (theory) of the problem—graphic representations of the causal relations between health problems and their causes (whether demonstrated or hypothesized) (Green et al., 2022). See Figure 1.2. To develop this model beginning with a health problem, the planning team addresses the questions of: What is the problem and who has it? How many people have it or will get it? Moving to the right, in the model, the planner addresses what quality-of-life effects occur because of this health problem. Moving to the left of the health problem, the questions are about causes. What behaviors among the priority population may cause the health problem or make it worse? What environmental factors contribute to the health problem either directly or through behavior? Finally, we address the *why* questions. Why do people in the priority population do the behavior (risk behavior)? Why do people in the environment create the conditions that contribute to the health problem directly or through behavior of the priority population?

In addition to developing the logic model of the problem, an equally important, continuous effort is to understand the character of the community, its members, its strengths, and its knowledge of the health problem and potential solutions. Finally in this step, the planning team sets goals for intervention, including behavioral and environmental change, as well as health and quality-of-life outcomes.

Step 2: Intervention Outcomes and Objectives

In Step 2, the planner completes the following tasks:

1. State desired behavioral and environmental outcomes
2. Specify performance objectives for behavioral and environmental outcomes
3. Select determinants for behavioral and environmental outcomes
4. Construct matrices of change objectives

Step 2 (Chapter 6) specifies who and what will change because of the intervention. A logic model (theory) of change shows what change is needed to prevent, reduce, or manage the health problem, and it depicts the relationship between determinants and behavioral and environmental outcomes that will address the health problem (Figure 1.3). The planner begins this step using the logic model of the problem (Step 1) as a guide. The questions to ask are: What needs to change in the behavior of the priority population (behavioral outcome) or in the environment (environmental outcome)? Then, moving to the right: What impact will these changes have on the health problem? Moving toward the left, the *why* questions become: Why would the priority population make these changes? Why would agents in the environment make these changes? In Step 2, the tasks focus on what needs to change by specifying the program outcomes and objectives. The logic model is expanded at each step and ultimately depicts the proposed mechanisms of action that describe how the intervention is proposed to lead to the health and quality of life outcomes.

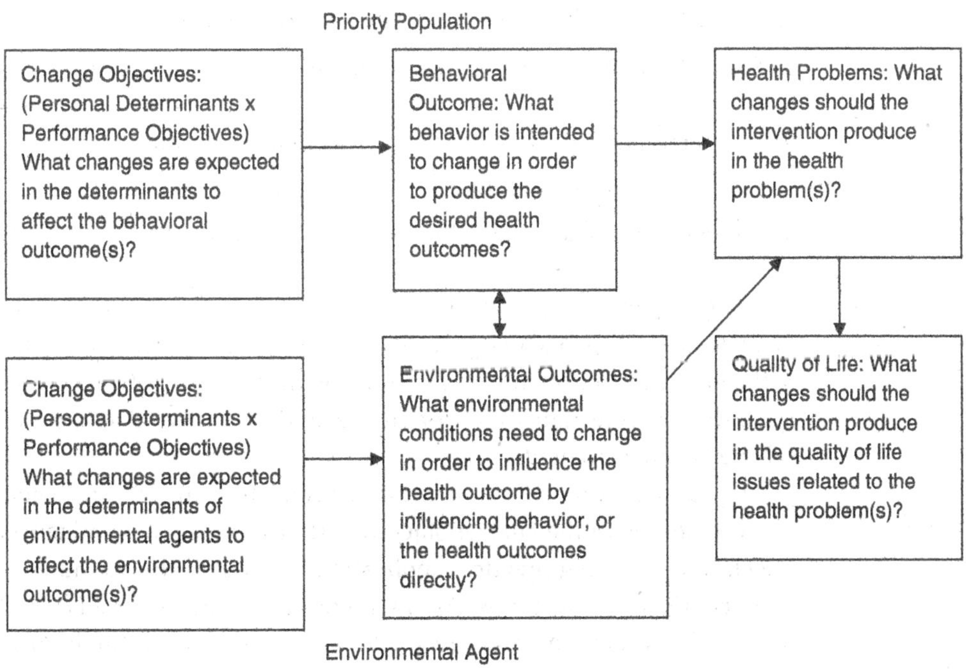

Figure 1.3 Logic Model of Change

Once the planning team has identified the health-promoting behaviors, environmental conditions, and their determinants, the next task in Step 2 is to develop matrices of change objectives. Performance objectives are the description of the specific behaviors that the at-risk group or the environmental agents have to perform to achieve the desired change. The change objectives are created by combining determinants and performance objectives (asking what has to change in the determinant in order to accomplish the performance objective). Change objectives then inform the rest of the design including the selection of theory- and evidence-based change methods and program content. The matrices represent detailed changes at relevant ecological levels (individual, interpersonal, organizational, community, or societal) and are the most immediate targets of an intervention.

To develop performance objectives for environmental outcomes, planners identify roles of environmental agents at each relevant ecological level. For example, superintendents, principals, and teachers may have roles for school environmental change. Statements of what must change at each ecological level and who must make the change are more specific intervention foci than are traditional program goals and objectives. For example, in a program to increase fruit and vegetable consumption by children in elementary school, matrices would be created for both the child and the food service personnel. The food service matrix might contain more than one role: for example, the manager's purchasing practices; the dietitian's menu development, and the cooks' food preparation. When Step 2 is completed, planners can think explicitly about the intervention in Step 3.

Step 3: Methods and Practical Applications

In Step 3 (Chapter 7), the planner completes the following tasks:

1. Generate intervention ideas with the planning group
2. Choose theory- and evidence-based change methods
3. Select and design practical applications to deliver change methods

In this step, the planning team works from the logic model of change and matrices (Step 2) to design a coherent, deliverable intervention. In Step 3, the logic model of change is expanded with the *how* of change by identifying the theoretical methods for change and the practical applications of selected change methods.

Designing the intervention means first matching theory- and evidence-based methods to the change objectives they are meant to influence and selecting or devising practical applications to deliver the methods to the various priority populations. An intervention change method is a defined process by which theories postulate and empirical research provides evidence for how change may occur. Whereas a method is a theory-based technique to influence determinants, an application is a way of organizing, operationalizing, and delivering the intervention methods. Examples include a meeting with community members (application) to encourage community participation (change method), role model stories (application) for modeling (change method), and signing a public pledge (application) for commitment (change method). The planning team will strategize practical applications that will reach the priority population and that the population will find acceptable. For example, a planning group might want an intervention that influences parents' outcome expectations regarding human papillomavirus (HPV) vaccination so that they get the vaccination for their children. Change methods might include cultural similarity, modeling, verbal persuasion, and anticipated regret. One application for all of these methods could be a videotaped testimonial by parents who have made the decision to have their children vaccinated for HPV and can model positive aspects of their decision.

Once the planning group has a basic plan of methods and applications, it will be able to describe intervention themes, components, scope, and sequence. All of these tasks are done with the full planning group, but perhaps it is particularly important to listen carefully to practical program ideas from community members who may implement the intervention or participate in it. Also, throughout these tasks, reference to the matrices is important to ensure that the final applications will address the change objectives adequately.

Step 4: Intervention Design and Production

In Step 4 (Chapter 8), the planner completes the following tasks:

1. Define intervention structure (themes, components, scope, and sequence)
2. Plan intervention messages, materials, and activities
3. Produce intervention materials, activities, and protocols
4. Pretest, refine, and finalize materials, activities, and protocols

The products in this step are all of the support materials needed in an intervention. This step gives specific guidance for designing communications that convey the intent and form of the intervention as planned in Step 3. It also describes pretesting and pilot testing of applications, activities, materials, and messages before they are finally produced. The most common scenario for producing a new intervention is that most of the needed materials will have to be developed de novo. Nevertheless, some materials may be available and can be adapted to address change objectives, methods, and applications. Only after completing IM Steps 1–4 can a planner adequately evaluate whether existing materials fit the program objectives.

Step 5: Implementation Mapping

In Step 5 (Chapter 9), the planner completes the following tasks:

1. Conduct an implementation needs and assets assessment and identify program implementers
2. Identify implementation performance objectives and determinants to create matrices of change objectives
3. Choose change methods and design implementation strategies
4. Produce implementation protocols and materials
5. Evaluate implementation outcomes

The purpose of this step is to design a plan to promote program implementation, beginning with conducting an implementation needs assessment and identifying implementers through to evaluating implementation outcomes (Figure 1.4). Although Figure 1.4 presents the five tasks of Implementation Mapping in a linear sequence, they are, like all IM steps, iterative in practice.

In cases where Step 5 (Implementation Mapping) is used to plan initial implementation of an intervention developed using IM, consideration of implementation actually begins in Step 1 (needs assessment), and then continues in this step. To design the implementation strategies, the planning team will develop new matrices (distinct from those in Step 2) in that these matrices address performance objectives and determinants of program adoption, implementation, and maintenance. Linking of each performance objective with a determinant produces a change objective to promote program use. The team then matches change methods and applications to these objectives to develop theory-informed plans for program adoption, implementation, and maintenance.

In this step, the planning team would ask, "Who is responsible for program adoption, implementation, and/or maintenance?"; "What specific

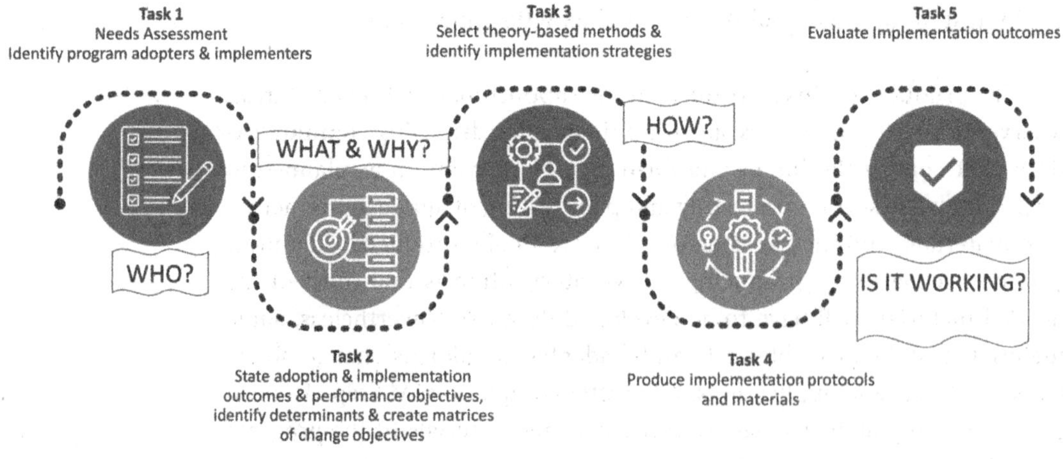

Figure 1.4 Implementation Mapping Tasks

performance (implementation actions or tasks) would be necessary at each stage?"; and "What would motivate performance?"

The planner then uses theory and evidence to define the adoption, implementation, and maintenance performance objectives (implementation tasks) and the factors influencing implementation (determinants). The product for Step 5 is a detailed plan for accomplishing program use by influencing behavior of individuals or groups who will make decisions about adopting and using the program.

Step 6: Evaluation Plan

In Step 6 (Chapter 10), the planner completes the following tasks:

1. Review the logic model of change, matrices, and implementation plan to guide process and effect evaluation
2. Develop process evaluation questions and identify measures
3. Develop effect evaluation questions, select a design, and identify measures
4. Pilot test the intervention and finalize evaluation plan
5. Plan when and how to report evaluation findings

An evaluation plan is actually begun in the needs assessment (Step 1) and is developed throughout each step. In the process of IM, planners make decisions about goals to change behavior, environment, health and quality of life, change objectives, change methods, applications, and implementation. The decisions, although informed by theory and evidence from research, still may not be optimal or may even be completely wrong. Through effect and process evaluation, planners can determine the impact of the intervention and can begin to understand the influence of decisions that were made at each planning step (Grant et al., 2013; Patton, 2008, 2012; Rossi et al., 2004; Steckler & Linnan, 2002; Windsor et al., 2003).

To evaluate the effect of an intervention, researchers analyze the change in health and quality-of-life problems, behavior and environment, and their determinants. Optimally, planners have defined these factors in a measurable way during the preceding steps. Effect evaluation may show positive, negative, or mixed effects or show no effect at all. Planners want to understand the reasons behind the effects that were achieved, regardless of what those effects were. They need to know more about the process and the changes in intermediate variables. They ask such questions as the following: "Were the behaviors and determinants well specified?" "Were change methods well matched to influence determinants?" "Were practical applications appropriate to deliver the change methods and did they reach the populations?" and "Was the implementation complete and appropriate?"

Beyond Traditional Health Promotion

Although IM originated as a health promotion planning framework, it has also been applied successfully to design interventions outside the traditional health promotion domain, particularly within social care, early childhood education, and organizational change. For example, Skouteris and colleagues in Australia used IM to guide the development of programs in early childhood education and care (ECEC) settings aimed at strengthening children's social and emotional development, educator–family engagement, and pedagogical practices (O'Connor et al., 2018). These programs sit squarely within the education and social-care sectors, not health behavior change (O'Connor et al., 2018).

IM has also been used to develop trauma-informed organizational change initiatives in ECEC systems, a social-care application that focuses on improving organizational climate, staff practice, and systemic responsiveness to childhood trauma, rather than promoting specific health behaviors (Sun et al., 2024). These examples demonstrate IM's flexibility for structuring interventions in settings where the primary goals are educational, developmental, or organizational, not health-focused.

It is also important to note that many applications of IM arise through the use of Implementation Mapping, which is Step 5 of Intervention Mapping. Implementation Mapping extends IM into the design of multilevel implementation strategies, often for system or workforce change. Although many examples occur in health systems, several involve organizational behavior change, professional practice, and structural redesign rather than health promotion per se. For instance, Durks et al. (2017) conducted a systematic review showing that IM has been used to plan interventions focused on organizational practice change and professional behaviors such as modifying workplace routines, decision-making, and implementation processes (Durks et al., 2017). These applications illustrate IM's usefulness for designing organizational and systems-level change interventions, which can extend beyond classic health behavior outcomes.

Navigating the Book

The process of IM is essentially unchanged from the fourth edition text. However, we have rearranged the presentation of some aspects of the process. We also have tried to simplify some explanations and discard terms that have caused confusion.

Organization of the Book

The book has two sections. The first section, overview and foundations (first four chapters) provides foundational content critical for program planning. It includes an introductory chapter, an overview of Core Processes for using theory and empirical evidence in practice, and two chapters that are reviews of theories often used in health education and promotion. Chapter 3 provides an overview of behavior-oriented theories, and Chapter 4 provides an overview of environment-oriented theories. The next six chapters explain the IM steps and include a case study example using For Our Children/Por Nuestros Hijos, an intervention to improve HPV vaccine uptake that runs at the end of each chapter. The final chapter explains how to use IM ADAPT, or Intervention Mapping for Adaptation, for evidence-based interventions in new populations and settings.

Changes from the Previous Editions

Although Core Processes were described in previous versions of this book, we felt that it would be valuable for the reader to have a chapter dedicated to these processes. Chapter 2, therefore, focuses on how and when to use community engagement, evidence, theories, and new research to plan health promotion interventions and refers to available tools that are useful when applying Core Processes in various steps of IM.

No major structural changes were made to the behavioral and environmental theory chapters; however, content has been streamlined and updated with more recent literature. The chapters continue to cover largely the same theories at both the individual and environmental levels, but with enhanced support from contemporary sources.

In building from previous versions, enhancements to Step 1 include: further highlighting of the key planning processes, methods, and tools as well as participatory processes for implementing Step 1; further emphasis on assessing assets as part of the Step 1 tasks as well as guidance for conducting an assets assessment (Step 1-Task 2); additional description for defining one's community of interest as well as the inclusion of an organizing table for describing the context for the intervention, including the community, population, and setting (Step 1-Task 3); and updated examples.

Step 2 enhancements include additional guidance on "doing the flip"—using findings from Step 1's logic model of the problem to identify important, changeable behaviors and environmental outcomes based on priority populations and settings. It clarifies distinctions between environmental agents (responsible for overseeing outcomes) and program implementers (responsible for delivering interventions in Step 5), provides real-world multilevel environmental examples, and expands matrices of change objectives with a broader range of determinants. The chapter reinforces the importance of validating performance objectives prior to intervention development and introduces a new process, Confidence Interval-Based Estimation of Relevance (CIBER), to help select determinants for behavior change.

For Step 3, content remains largely unchanged, reflecting the stability of the core tasks associated with Step 3. However, one structural adjustment has been made: the previous Task 3.1 has been relocated to Step 4, returning to its placement in earlier editions of Intervention Mapping, where we believe it is more appropriately situated.

In comparison to earlier versions, more attention in Step 4 is paid to the first task of defining intervention structure. This is a crucial point of departure for describing the intervention and when there is contact with each group of intervention participants. A participatory approach has always been fundamental to IM and in this new version we describe in more detail how this relates to approaches such as co-creation, human-centered design, and agile methods. Finally, the process of pretesting, refining and finalizing materials, activities, and protocols is described in a more structured way.

Step 5 of IM, now called Implementation Mapping, has changed to better accommodate the use of the process during initial planning of an intervention (and, in Step 5, its implementation strategies) as well as for planning strategies for existing evidenced based interventions. The field of implementation science has evolved substantially since the last edition of the book as has the uptake of Implementation Mapping for planning implementation strategies following the publication of an article describing the process by the IM authors and other colleagues (Fernandez et al., 2019). The process was adopted by many implementation scientists globally providing excellent examples of how Step 5 can be used even beyond the initial IM planning process. While the essential process has not changed, the tasks have changed slightly (again to ensure that the entire process of planning implementation strategies is included even in cases when the other steps have not been used). The comparison of the tasks from the previous Step 5 version and the version presented in this new edition are in Table 1.1.

The fifth edition of Step 6 emphasizes the integration between program evaluation and program planning by framing the logic model of change, matrices, and implementation plan as the critical foundation for both process and effect evaluation. The updated edition introduces sequential tasks that link each stage of evaluation directly to the program's design and implementation plan. Methodologically, this version broadens its scope with a more expansive description of process evaluation methods

Table 1.1 Changes to Step 5 Tasks

Intervention Mapping, 4th Edition (Bartholomew Eldredge et al., 2016)	Implementation Mapping Process (Fernandez et al., 2019)
Task 1. Identify potential program implementers	Task 1. Conduct a needs and assets assessment and identify adopters and implementers
Task 2. State outcomes and performance objectives for program use	Task 2. Identify adoption and implementation outcomes, performance objectives, and determinants; create matrices of change
Task 3. Construct matrices of change objectives for program use	Task 3. Choose theoretical methods; select or create implementation strategies
Task 4. Design implementation interventions	Task 4. Produce implementation protocols and materials
	Task 5. Evaluate implementation outcomes

and a more comprehensive description of evaluation designs, including comparison group designs, natural experiments, and regression discontinuity studies, and features more robust measurement approaches including mixed methods and cost assessments. It also refines effect evaluation planning by highlighting further considerations for design selection, unit of assignment, and external validity.

Chapter 11, Intervention Mapping for Adaptation (IM ADAPT) has been updated substantially. First, the adaptation tasks are refined through more explicit labeling of tasks and subtasks to align consistently with the latest IM ADAPT framework. We more clearly incorporate Task 2 for situations in which an EBI has already been selected. In addition, several IM ADAPT steps are expanded to explicitly include the use of EBI Mapping (Walker et al., 2022), Implementation Mapping (Fernandez et al., 2019), and more detailed evaluation-related subtasks. We also expanded content related to adaptation decision-making, including the discussion of the types and timing of adaptations, key adaptation challenges, and adaptation at multiple levels. The background section of the chapter has been substantially updated as have the sections on perspectives of cross-cutting topics such as adaptation and health equity.

Important Repeating Concepts in the Book

Throughout the book, several key concepts are repeated in different contexts. These are planning matrices, iterative planning, logic models, and evaluation.

Matrices as a Foundation for Intervention Planning

In IM, matrices that combine performance objectives with their determinants are the basis for program development. They are used in both planning a program (Step 2) and planning its implementation (Step 5). If a change method or practical application used in an intervention is not intended to change the objectives in the matrices, then either it does not belong in the program or the matrix is not adequate and should be revisited.

Planning as an Iterative Process

To describe program development, we have laid out a series of steps. This orderly presentation may suggest to the reader that every step is completed only once and in a rigid order. This is not the case. Each step provides the basis for the next; each step also generates new information that may suggest revision or embellishment of a previous step. With increasing ideas about the program, knowledge about the intended beneficiaries, community participation, and research and theory, a planner often needs to revisit and fine-tune a previous step. In addition to the process of revisiting prior steps, some processes are repeated in many of the steps. For example, using the Core Processes to access relevant theory and evidence, planning evaluation, involving stakeholders, and thinking about implementation all begin in the needs assessment and continue in each step. Also, each step provides information for generating an evaluation plan.

Logic Models

We described the use of logic models above in the descriptions of Steps 1 and 2. In the process of IM, the planner will build a logic model of the health problem causation in Step 1 and begin a logic model of change in Step 2. In Step 3, the planner will add change methods to the logic model of change. These are the only logic models that are necessary components of IM. However, in addition to the logic model that is pieced together as intervention development progresses, we present a number of models to help clarify relations among concepts, such as theoretical constructs (Chapters 3 and 4). We also use other graphic devices that do not imply causal relations, such as Figure 1.1, a depiction of the steps involved in IM. When a figure is a logic model, that is, implies causal relations, we clearly label it as such.

Program Evaluation

Program evaluation begins with a thorough description of the program to be evaluated and its proposed causal pathways for change. This description is accomplished step-by-step in IM. First, in the needs assessment, the planner begins to formulate goals for intervention outcomes. These become part of the plan for evaluating effects (Chapter 10). In Step 2, the planner specifies desired changes in behavior and environment as well as their determinants, which again become further outcomes for evaluating effects. Steps 3, 4, and 5 guide the specification of program components and implementation plans that link closely to process evaluation. Step 4 also contains discussion of pretesting and pilot testing or formative evaluation of the program.

Planning with Limited Resources

Finally, we encourage health promotion planners to use IM regardless of the time or resources available. We point this out because we often hear people say that IM is not practical for use in the "real world." We have also seen people belabor the importance of following the IM steps sequentially and to the "letter of the law" at the cost of losing constituent buy-in. To avoid these pitfalls, the planning group's health promotion practitioner often works behind the scenes to draft end products for each IM step, for example, the matrices of change objectives. This can take an afternoon, a weekend, or a month, depending on the time available. Other time- and resource-saving strategies include using a rapid assessment approach to complete the needs assessment in Step 1, or having longer workshop-type meetings so that planning groups do not forget what has been accomplished between meetings. Above all, simply posing the key questions for each IM step, for example, "Why do adolescents have sexual intercourse without using condoms?" will result in a more well-defined program based in theory and evidence and will increase the potential for effective behavioral and environmental change.

Summary

IM is a series of steps, tasks, and processes to help health promotion and health education planners develop theory- and evidence-based health promotion programs and interventions. Well-designed and effective interventions should be guided by theory and informed by empirical evidence regarding the targets for change. For example, a meta-analysis of physical activity interventions in breast cancer survivors found that larger effect sizes are achieved when interventions are based on theory (Bluethmann et al., 2017). However, no one theoretical model completely predicts or explains health behaviors or environmental changes (Bartholomew Eldredge & Mullen, 2011; Rimer, 2002). Therefore, a system is needed to help intervention developers choose useful theories and integrate relevant constructs from multiple theories to describe health problems and develop health promotion and health education solutions (Fernandez et al., 2019; Springer et al., 2024; ten Hoor et al., 2025). IM ensures that theoretical models and empirical evidence guide planners in two areas:

- The identification of determinants of behavioral and environmental causes related to a health problem
- The selection of the most appropriate change methods and applications to address the identified determinants to achieve changes in behavioral and environmental outcomes related to a health problem

IM has been used to develop many health promotion programs and interventions, and Table 1.2 presents some examples. IM is also being used to further the description of intervention characteristics and to deconstruct why interventions were effective or not; that is, clarifying the mechanisms of interventions and their implementation strategies (Durks et al., 2017; Fernandez et al., 2019; Walker et al., 2022). Further, IM is being used to help health promoters find and adapt evidence-based interventions (see Chapter 11; Highfield et al., 2015) and to evaluate the quality of planning that has been used to create interventions (Kok et al., 2016), and others have used IM as a checklist to evaluate the quality of program planning of existing programs (Fassier et al., 2019; Lamort-Bouché et al., 2018; Stutterheim et al., 2025).

Table 1.2 Programs Developed Using Intervention Mapping

Topic	Intervention Title	References
Adolescent Reproductive Health	Project Community-Embedded Reproductive Health Care for Adolescents (CERCA)	Decat et al. (2013)
Alcohol Abuse Prevention	What Do You Drink mHealth Intervention	van Keulen et al. (2022)
Alcohol Abuse Prevention	Preventing alcohol abuse in middle school-aged children	de Visser et al. (2020)
Asthma Self-Management	Management and Interventions for Asthma (MIA) Project	Lakhanpaul et al. (2020)
Breast Cancer Screening & Chemotherapy	Increase Breast Cancer Screening & Chemotherapy Adherence	Sacca et al. (2020)
Breast and Cervical Cancer Screening	*Salud en Mis Manos*	Savas et al. (2023)
Breast Cancer—Medication Adherence	Medication Self-Management for Breast Cancer Survivors	Moon et al. (2021)
Breastfeeding	Promotion of Breastfeeding among Infants with Asthma	Mesters et al. (2018)
Blood Pressure Management	Intervention for Prevention of High Blood Pressure	Guzman-Tordecilla et al. (2022)
Cancer	Interventions for Cancer	Lamort-Bouché et al. (2018)
Cardiovascular Disease Prevention	Community-engaged Cardiovascular Disease Prevention Intervention	Kang et al. (2025)
Childhood Obesity Prevention	Interdisciplinary Theory- and Evidence-Based Intervention to Prevent Childhood Obesity	ten Hoor et al. (2017)
Childhood Obesity Prevention	Hoosier Sport Intervention	Major et al. (2024)
Childhood Obesity Prevention	Niño Sano Adulto Sano	Zacarías et al. (2019)
Chronic Disease	Chronic Disease Supportive Work Environment via Occupational Physicians	Bosma et al. (2020)
Chronic Disease Management	MyGoals	Kang and Foster (2023)
Chronic Disease Management	Health Promotion for Chronic Conditions among Adults	Herbert et al. (2025)
Chronic Disease Management for Stroke Survivors	The Stroke Coach	Sakakibara et al. (2017)
Chronic Musculoskeletal Conditions	Coach2Move	Thackeray et al. (2022)
Colorectal Cancer Screening	Salud por la Vida	Serra et al. (2017)
Colorectal Cancer Screening	CRC Screening Intervention in Egypt	Nawwar et al. (2022)
COVID-19 Vaccination	Virtual Immersive Communication Training on Recommending Immunization COVID-19	Real et al. (2025)
Dementia	STAYING ACTIVE (STAYing well and active—scheduliNg meaninGful and enjoyAble aCTIvities to promote Vitality and wEll-being in mild dementia)	Orgeta et al. (2022)
Diabetes Distress	Platform 0	Halliday et al. (2021)
Diabetes Self-Management	Powerful Together with Diabetes	Vissenberg et al. (2017)
Diabetic Retinopathy	Kilimanjaro Diabetic Programme	Hall et al. (2022)
Doctor Prescribing	Multicomponent Intervention to Improve Antibiotic and NSAID Prescribing	Reese et al. (2023)
Doctor Prescribing	Multicomponent Intervention to Improve Antibiotic and NSAID Prescribing	Shegog and Begley (2017)
Fruit and Vegetable Promotion	Increase Fruit, Vegetable, and Water Intake among Mothers and Teachers of Infants	Mérida Rios et al. (2019)

Table 1.2 *(Continued)*

Topic	Intervention Title	References
Depression	Intervention for Depressive Symptoms in Nursing Home Residents	van Venrooij et al. (2019)
EMS Activation for Stroke	HOBIT: school-based stroke awareness program	Volevach et al. (2025)
Healthy Lifestyle Promotion	Prescribe Vida Saludable	Sanz-Guinea et al. (2017)
Hepatitis B Screening	HBV Screening Programme Aimed at Turkish Immigrants	van Der Veen et al. (2012)
HIV Care	Medical-legal partnership for organizations providing HIV care	Muñoz-Laboy et al. (2025)
HIV Prevention	HIV Linkage Intervention	Ravicz et al. (2022)
HIV Prevention	Reducing HIV/AIDS Transmission	Chen et al. (2024)
HIV Prevention	HIV Risk Reduction Program	Li et al. (2020)
HIV Stigma	Reducing the Risk of HIV/AIDS Transmission	Stutterheim et al. (2025)
HPV Vaccination	Interactive Web-based Tailored Intervention Promoting HPV-Vaccination Acceptability	Pot et al. (2018)
HPV Vaccination	Parent-Centered HPV Vaccination Intervention	Rodriguez et al. (2018)
HPV Vaccination	Provider-Centered HPV Vaccination Intervention	Austin et al. (2020)
Low Back Pain	Decision Support System–Based Smartphone App (selfBACK)	Svendsen et al. (2022)
Liver Cirrhosis	Liver Education About Pain	Rogal et al. (2022)
Mammography Screening	Implementation Intervention to Increase Mammography Among Low Income Women	Highfield et al. (2018)
Medical Communication Skills	Communication Skills Training Programme for Specialists With Patients With Medically Unexplained Physical Symptoms	Weiland et al. (2013)
Medication Adherence	Adherence to Adjuvant Endocrine Therapy among Breast Cancer Survivors	Labonté et al. (2020)
Mental Health	Psychosocial service to support youth experiencing mental illness	Savaglio et al. (2025)
Movement	GOAL-Intervention	van Grootel et al. (2023)
Neonatal Clinical Trial Recruitment	Better Research Interactions for Every Family (BRIEF) Intervention	Weiss et al. (2025)
Occupational Health	Return to Work (RTW) Intervention	Varela-Mato et al. (2023)
Pain Management	Chronic Pain Treatment & Management in Breast Cancer Survivors	Slaghmuylder et al. (2023)
Parent–Child Communication	What Should We Tell the Children About Relationships and Sex?	Newby et al. (2011)
Physical Activity	Physical Activity Routines After Stroke (PARAS)	Moore et al. (2022)
Physical Activity	MOVE12	Barene et al. (2025)
Physical Activity	ParticipACTION	Flood et al. (2023)
Physical Activity	Physical Activity Intervention for Physically-Disabled Individuals	Krops et al. (2018)
Physical Activity	Physical Activity Post Cervical Cancer Treatment	Millet et al. (2022)
Pre-Adolescent Health	The CIrCLE of Life Initiative	Arthur et al. (2020)
Return-to-Work	Return-to-work Intervention for Cancer Survivors	Fassier et al. (2018)
Sexual Harassment Prevention	Benzies & Batchies; Boys interventions	de Lijster et al. (2019)

(continued)

Table 1.2 *(Continued)*

Topic	Intervention Title	References
Sex Education	A comprehensive and gender-transformative sex education program in Latin America	Torres-Cortés et al. (2024)
Smoking Cessation	Tobacco Cessation Intervention	Domlyn et al. (2022)
Smoking Prevention	Media literacy-based smoking prevention program (MLSP)	Kim (2021)
STI Testing	Self-sampling STI/HIV Testing	Leenen et al. (2021)
Stroke Prevention	Emergency Medical Services Activation for Stroke	Volevach et al. (2024)
Sun Protection	Improve Adherence of Sun Protection	Walburn et al. (2019)
Teen Dating Violence Prevention	Me & You: Building Healthy Relationships	Peskin et al. (2018)
Work Safety	Occupational Risk Prevention and Health Promotion	Bakhuys Roozeboom et al. (2021)
Worksite Wellness	Physical Activity RCT Intervention	Sun et al. (2020)

Even though IM has not been directly compared to other processes for developing interventions, planners of the referenced projects and others considering guidance for intervention development think that the systematic process has been useful and flexible and that continued use will strengthen future program development (Bartholomew Eldredge & Mullen, 2011; Springer et al., 2024).

Discussion Questions and Learning Activities

1. Why is it important to apply a systematic approach to the development of health promotion programs? What are the risks if a systematic approach is not used for health promotion program development?
2. Explain what is meant by ecological and systems approaches to intervention development. Give examples of how factors at different ecological levels can have an impact on health.
3. Discuss why it is important for health promotion programs to go beyond a focus only on behavior change of individuals at risk for a health problem and instead also address environmental influences.
4. Using tobacco control as an example, describe the types of interventions that have been used at the individual, organizational, community, and societal levels.
5. Access the website for Evidence-Based Cancer Control Programs (EBCCP) at https://ebccp.cancercontrol.cancer.gov/index.do (National Cancer Institute, 2024) and select three different health promotion/prevention intervention programs to review. Determine which ecological level the program is addressing for change, and describe how the intervention will make a change to improve health or prevent a health problem.

References

ActKnowledge & Aspen Institute Roundtable on Community Change. (2003). *Making sense: Reviewing program design with theory of change.* Retrieved from https://www.theoryofchange.org/pdf/making_sense.pdf

Airhihenbuwa, C. O. (1995). *Health and culture: Beyond the Western paradigm.* Sage.

Airhihenbuwa, C. O. (1999). Of culture and multiverse: Renouncing '93the universal truth'94 in health. *Journal of Health Education, 30*(5), 267–273.

Airhihenbuwa, C. O., & Liburd, L. (2006). Eliminating health disparities in the African American population: The interface of culture, gender, and power. *Health Education & Behavior, 33*(4), 488–501. doi:10.1177/1090198106287731

Airhihenbuwa, C. O., & Webster, J. D. (2004). Culture and African contexts of HIV/AIDS prevention, care and support. *SAHARA J: Journal of Social Aspects of HIV/AIDS Research Alliance, 1*(1), 4–13.

Alexander, S. A., Jones, C. M., Tremblay, M. C., Beaudet, N., Hulvej Rod, M., & Wright, M. T. (2020). Reflexivity in health promotion: A typology for training. *Health promotion practice, 21*(4), 499–509.

American Public Health Organization (APHA) (2019). Public health code of ethics. https://www.apha.org/about-apha/apha-code-of-ethics

Aronowitz, R., Deener, A., Keene, D., Schnittker, J., & Tach, L. (2015). Cultural reflexivity in health research and practice. *American Journal of Public Health, 105*, S403–S408. doi:10.2105/AJPH.2015.302551

Arthur, K., Christofides, N., & Nelson, G. (2020). Development of a pre-adolescent inter-generational intervention to address HIV and obesity using intervention mapping. *Health Education Journal, 79*(8), 932–947. doi:10.1177/0017896920937042

Austin, J. D., Rodriguez, S. A., Savas, L. S., Megdal, T., Ramondetta, L., & Fernandez, M. E. (2020). Using intervention mapping to develop a provider intervention to increase HPV vaccination in a federally qualified health center. *Frontiers in Public Health, 8*, 530596. doi:10.3389/fpubh2020.503596. eCollection 2020

Baah, F. O., Teitelman, A. M., & Riegel, B. (2019). Marginalization: Conceptualizing patient vulnerabilities in the framework of social determinants of health—An integrative review. *Nursing Inquiry, 26*(1). doi:10.1111/nin.1226

Bakhuys Roozeboom, M. C., Wiezer, N. M., Boot, C. R. L., Bongers, P. M., & Schelvis, R. M. C. (2021). Use of intervention mapping for occupational risk prevention and health promotion: A systematic review of literature. *International Journal of Environmental Research and Public Health, 18*(1775). doi:10.3390/ijerph18041775

Barene, S., Johansen, P. F., Tjomsland, H. E., Ølberg, R. I., & Thurston, M. (2025). Applying intervention mapping to develop a program for promoting short physical activity breaks during class time in upper secondary schools: The MOVE12 protocol study. *Frontiers in Sports and Active Living, 6*. doi:10.3389/fspor.2024.1460373

Bartholomew Eldredge, L. K., & Mullen, P. D. (2011). Five roles for using theory and evidence in the design and testing of behavior change interventions. *Journal of Public Health Dentistry, 71*(s1), S20–S33. doi:10.1111/j.1752-7325.2011.00223.x

Bartholomew Eldredge, L. K., Markham, C. M., Ruiter, R. A. C., Fernández, M. E., Kok, G., & Parcel, G. S. (2016). *Planning health promotion programs: An intervention mapping approach* (4th ed.). Jossey-Bass.

Battel-Kirk, B., Dempsey, C., Harte, P., & Barry, M.M. (2024). The IUHPE core competencies framework for health promotion (Short version). https://iuhpe.org/wp-content/uploads/2025/08/Core-HP-Competencies-Framework_IUHPE_Sept2024_June2025.pdf

Bennett, M. J. (1993). Towards ethnorelativism: A developmental model of intercultural sensitivity. In R. Paige (Ed.), *Education for the intercultural experience* (pp. 21–71). Intercultural Press.

Bluethmann, S. M., Bartholomew, L. K., Murphy, C. C., & Vernon, S. W. (2017). Use of theory in behavior change interventions: An analysis of programs to increase physical activity in posttreatment breast cancer survivors. *Health Education & Behavior, 44*, 245–253. doi:10.1177/1090198116647712

Bosma, A. R., Boot, C. R. L., Schaafsma, F. G., Kok, G., & Anema, J. R. (2020). Development of an intervention to create a supportive work environment for employees with chronic conditions: An intervention mapping approach. *Journal of Occupational Rehabilitation, 30*(4), 624–634. doi:10.1007/s10926-020-09885-z

Braveman, P., Egerter, S., & Williams, D. R. (2011). The social determinants of health: Coming of age. *Annual Review of Public Health, 32*, 381–398.

Braveman, P. A., Arkin, E., Proctor, D., Kauh, T., & Holm, N. (2022). Systemic and structural racism: Definitions, examples, health damages, and approaches to dismantling. *Health Affairs, 41*(2), 171–178. doi:10.1377/hlthaff.2021

Bronfenbrenner, U. (1989). Ecological systems theory. In R. Vasta (Ed.), *Annals of child development* (Vol. 6, pp. 187–249). Jessica Kingsley Publishers.

Bronfenbrenner, U., & Ceci, S. (1994). Nature-nurture reconceptualized in developmental perspective: A bioecological model. *Psychological Review, 101*, 568–586.

Center for Community Health and Development (CCHD). *Developing an organizational structure for the initiative. Community Tool Box.* https://ctb.ku.edu/en/table-of-contents/structure/organizational-structure

Centers for Disease Control and Prevention (CDC). (2011). *Introduction to program evaluation for public health programs: Evaluating appropriate antibiotic use programs. A self-study guide.* Office of the Director. Office of Strategy and Innovation. Retrieved from https://stacks.cdc.gov/view/cdc/26245

Chen, H. T. (2014). *Practical program evaluation: Theory-driven evaluation and the integrated evaluation perspective* (2nd ed.). Sage.

Chen, J., Liu, W., Chen, J., & Ma, C. (2024). Reducing the risk of HIV/AIDS transmission using intervention mapping: A systematic review. *AIDS Care, 36*(12), 1838–1851. doi:10.1080/09540121.2024.2390062

Chu, J., & Leino, A. (2017). Advancement in the maturing science of cultural adaptations of evidence-based interventions. *Journal of Consulting and Clinical Psychology, 85*(1), 45–47. doi:10.1037/ccp0000145

Coalition for National Health Education Organizations (CNHEO) (2020). *Code of ethics for the health education profession.* https://www.sophe.org/ethics/

Connell, J. P., & Kubisch, A. C. (1996). Applying a theories of change approach to the evaluation of comprehensive community initiatives: Progress, prospects, and problems. In K. Fulbright-Anderson, A. C. Kubisch, & J. P. Connell (Eds.), *New approaches to evaluating community initiatives: Theory, measurement, and analysis* (Vol. 2, pp. 15–44). The Aspen Institute.

Crielaard, L., Nicolaou, M., Brown, A. D., Dijkstra, S. C., Ter Ellen, F., Elsenburg, L. K., Luna Pinzon, A., Waterlander, W. E., & Stronks, K. (2025). Systems approaches in public health: Beyond mapping the causes. *The International Journal of Behavioral Nutrition and Physical Activity, 22*(74). doi:10.1186/s12966-025-01766-z

de Lijster, G. P. A., Kok, G., & Kocken, P. L. (2019). Preventing adolescent sexual harassment: Evaluating the planning process in two school-based interventions using the Intervention Mapping framework. *BMC Public Health, 19*(1), 1455. doi:10.1186/s12889-019-7808-8

de Visser, R. O., Graber, R., Abraham, C., Hart, A., & Memon, A. (2020). Resilience-based alcohol education: Developing an intervention, evaluating feasibility and barriers to implementation using mixed-methods. *Health Education Research, 35*(2), 123–133. doi:10.1093/her/cyaa006

Decat, P., Nelson, E., De Meyer, S., Jaruseviciene, L., Orozco, M., Segura, Z., Gorter, A., Vega, B., Cordova, K., Maes, L., Temmerman, M., Leye, E., & Degomme, O. (2013). Community embedded reproductive health interventions for adolescents in Latin America: Development and evaluation of a complex multi-centre intervention. *BMC Public Health, 13*, Article 31. doi:10.1186/1471-2458-13-31

Domlyn, A. M., Crowder, C., Eisenson, H., Pollak, K. I., Davis, J. M., Calhoun, P. S., & Wilson, S. M. (2022). Implementation mapping for tobacco cessation in a federally qualified health center. *Frontiers in Public Health*, 10. doi:10.3389/fpubh.2022.908646

Douglas, A. L., & Stamatakis, K. A. (2012). Systems science methods in public health: Dynamics, networks, and agents. *Annual Review Public Health, 33*, 357–376. doi:10.1146/annurev-publhealth-031210-101222

Durks, D., Fernandez-Llimos, F., Hossain, L. N., Franco-Trigo, L., Benrimoj, S. I., & Sabater-Hernández, D. (2017). Use of intervention mapping to enhance health care professional practice: A systematic review. *Health Education & Behavior: The Official Publication of the Society for Public Health Education, 44*, 524–535. doi:10.1177/1090198117709885

Eriksson, M., Sundberg, L. R., Santosa, A., Lindgren, H., Ng, N., & Lindvall, K. (2025). Health behavioural change: The influence of social-ecological factors and health identity. *International Journal of Qualitative Studies on Health and Well-Being, 20*(2458309). doi:10.1080/17482631.2025.2458309

Fassier, J. B., Lamort-Bouché, M., Broc, G., Guittard, L., Péron, J., Rouat, S., Carretier, J., Fervers, B., Letrilliart, L., & Sarnin, P. (2018). Developing a return to work intervention for breast cancer survivors with the intervention mapping protocol: Challenges and opportunities of the needs assessment. *Frontiers in Public Health, 6*. doi:10.3389/fpubh.2018.00035

Fassier, J. B., Sarnin, P., Rouat, S., Peron, J., Kok, G., Letrilliart, L., & Lamort-Bouche, M. (2019). Interventions developed with the intervention mapping protocol in work disability prevention: A systematic review of the literature. *Journal of Occupational Rehabilitation, 29*, 11–24. doi:10.1007/s10926-018-9776-8

Fernandez, M., ten Hoor, G., van Lieshout, S., Rodriguez, S., Beidas, R., Parcel, G., Ruiter, R., Markham, C., & Kok, G. (2019). Implementation mapping: Using intervention mapping to develop implementation strategies. *Frontiers in Public Health, 7*(June), 1–15. doi:10.3389/fpubh.2019.00158

Fernandez, M. E., Baumann, A. A., & Beg, S. S. (2025). Cultural adaptations of interventions. In T. A. R. N. Schneiderman, A. F. Abraído-Lanza, T. W. Smith, N. B. Anderson, M. H. Antoni, & F. J. Penedo (Eds.), *APA handbook of health psychology, Vol. 3. Health psychology and public health* (pp. 127–153). American Psychological Association.

Fernandez, M. E., Ruiter, R. A. C., Markham, C. M., & Kok, G. (2019). Intervention mapping: Theory- and evidence-based health promotion program planning: Perspective and examples. *Frontiers in Public Health, 7*(209). doi:10.3389/fpubh.2019.00209

Finlay, L. (1998). Reflexivity: An essential component for all research? *British Journal of Occupational Therapy, 61*(10), 453–456. doi:10.1177/030802269806101005

Fiscella, K., Franks, P., Gold, M. R., & Clancy, C. M. (2000). Inequality in quality: Addressing socioeconomic, racial, and ethnic disparities in health care. *JAMA, 283*(19), 2579–2584. doi:10.1001/jama.283.19.2579

Flood, S. M., Thompson, B., Faulkner, G., Vanderloo, L. M., Blackett, B., Dolf, M., Latimer-Cheung, A. E., Duggan, M., Di Sebastiano, K. M., Lane, K. N., Brouwers, M. C., McKenna, J., Chulak-Bozzer, T., Fuller, D., Ruissen, G. R., Sturrock, S. L., & Tomasone, J. R. (2023). Development of a ParticipACTION app-based intervention for improving postsecondary students' 24-hour movement guideline behaviors: Protocol for the application of intervention mapping. *JMIR Research Protocols, 12*. doi:10.2196/39977

Frechtling, J. A. (2007). *Logic modeling methods in program evaluation*. Jossey-Bass.

Garney, W. R., Wendel, M., McLeroy, K., Alaniz, A., Cunningham, G., Castle, B., Ingram, M., & Burdine, J. (2017). Using a community health development framework to increase community capacity: A multiple case study. *Family & Community Health, 40*(1).

Glanz, K., Rimer, B. K., & Viswanath, K. (2024). *Health behavior: Theory, research, and practice*, 6th ed. Jossey-Bass.

Golden, T. L., & Wendel, M. L. (2020). Public health's next step in advancing equity: Re-evaluating epistemological assumptions to move social determinants from theory to practice. *Frontiers in Public Health, 8*. doi:10.3389/fpubh.2020.00131

Gooey, M., Morris, H., Madill, R., Walsh-Bailey, C., Griffiths, A., Savaglio, M., Blewitt, C., O'Connor, A., Holton, S., Khalesi, H., Grage-Moore, S., Fernandez, M., Ezeanolue, E. E., Metz, A., Baumann, A., & Skouteris, H., Promoting equity for children and adolescents through implementation processes in health and social care: A scoping review. *Systematic Reviews*. in press.

Grabowski, D., Aagaard-Hansen, J., Willaing, I., & Jensen, B. B. (2017). Principled promotion of health: Implementing five guiding health promotion principles for research-based prevention and management of diabetes. *Societies, 7*(2), 10.

Grant, A., Treweek, S., Dreischulte, T., Foy, R., & Guthrie, B. (2013). Process evaluations for cluster-randomised trials of complex interventions: A proposed framework for design and reporting. *Trials, 14,* Article 15. doi:10.1186/1745-6215-14-15

Green, L., Gielen, A., Peterson, D., Kreuter, M., & Ottoson, J. (2022). *Health program planning, implementation, and evaluation.* Johns Hopkins University Press.

Green, L. W. (2006). Public health asks of systems science: To advance our evidence-based practice, can you help us get more practice-based evidence? *American Journal of Public Health, 96*(3), 406–409. doi:10.2105/AJPH.2005.066035

Green, L. W., & Kreuter, M. W. (2005). *Health program planning: An educational and ecological approach.* McGraw Hill.

Green, L. W., & Mercer, S. L. (2001). Can public health researchers and agencies reconcile the push from funding bodies and the pull from communities? *American Journal of Public Health, 91*(12), 1926–1929. doi:10.2105/ajph.91.12.1926

Greene-Moton, E., & Minkler, M. (2020). Cultural competence or cultural humility? Moving beyond the debate. *Health Promotion Practice, 21*(1), 142–145. doi:10.1177/1524839919884912

Griffiths, A., Madill, R., Martawidjaja, P., Moss, T., Kelly, B., Whitehouse, C., McCall, J., Hakimi, S.,Dawson, N., Galvin, E., Gunatillaka, N., Putt, M., Bowden, M., Rakic, S., & Skouteris, H. (2025). *Authentic Inclusion of Lived Experience Experts in Health and Social Care Research.* The Health and Social Care Unit, Monash University. Available at: https://shorturl.at/SQVUv

Guzman-Tordecilla, D. N., Lucumi, D., & Peña, M. (2022). Using an intervention mapping approach to develop a program for preventing high blood pressure in a marginalized Afro-Colombian population: A community-based participatory research. *Journal of Prevention, 43,* 209–224. doi:10.1007/s10935-022-00668-1

Hailu, H., Skouteris, H., Incollingo Rodriguez, A. C., & Hill, B. (2024). SWIPE: A conceptual, multi-perspective model for understanding and informing interventions for weight stigma in preconception, pregnancy, and postpartum. *Health Psychology Review, 18,* 681–697. doi:10.1080/17437199.2024.2333801

Hall, C. E., Hall, A. B., & Mallya, J. (2022). Establishing a screening programme for diabetic retinopathy in Kilimanjaro Region, Tanzania using intervention mapping. *Eye,* 17–24. doi:10.1038/s41433-022-02001-w

Halliday, J. A., Speight, J., Russell-Green, S., Eric, O., Hagger, V., Morris, A., & Hendrieckx, C. (2021). Developing a novel diabetes distress e-learning program for diabetes educators: An intervention mapping approach. *Translational Behavioral Medicine, 11,* 1264–1273.

Hawe, P. (2015). Lessons from complex interventions to improve health. *Annual Review of Public Health, 36*(1), 307–323. doi:10.1146/annurev-publhealth-031912-114421

Heim, E., & Kohrt, B. A. (2019). Cultural adaptation of scalable psychological interventions: A new conceptual framework. *Clinical Psychology in Europe, 1*(4), 1–22. doi:10.32872/

Herbert, T., Malone, M., Rhind, N., & Cooper, K. (2025). Intervention mapping in the development of health promotion interventions for adults with chronic conditions: A scoping review. *JBI Evidence Synthesis, 23,* 2236–2291. doi:10.11124/JBIES-24-00201

Highfield, L., Hartman, M. A., Mullen, P. D., Rodriguez, S. A., Fernandez, M. E., & Bartholomew, K. (2015). Intervention mapping to adapt evidence-based interventions for use in practice: Increasing mammography among African American women. *BioMed Research International*. doi:10.1155/2015/160103

Highfield, L., Valerio, M. A., Fernandez, M. E., & Eldridge-Bartholomew, L. K. (2018). Development of an implementation intervention using intervention mapping to increase mammography among low income women. *Frontiers in Public Health*, *6*(300). doi:10.3389/fpubh.2018.00300

Hochbaum, G. M., Sorenson, J. R., & Lorig, K. (1992). Theory in health education practice. *Health Education & Behavior*, *19*(3), 295–313. doi:10.1177/109019819201900303

Institute of Development Studies (n.d.). *Participatory methods*. https://www.participatorymethods.org/

Institute of Medicine (IOM) (1988). *The future of public health*. National Academies Press.

Institute of Medicine (IOM) (2003). *The future of the public's health in the 21st century*. National Academies Press.

Institute of Medicine (IOM) (2011). *For the public's health: The role of measurement in action and accountability*. National Academies Press.

Israel, B., Schulz, A., Parker, E., Becker, A., Allen III, A., Guzman, R., & Lichtenstein, R. (2018). Critical issues in developing and following CBPR principles. In *Community-based participatory research for health: Advancing social and health equity* (3rd ed.). Jossey-Bass.

Iton, A., Ross, R. K., & Tamber, P. S. (2022). Building community power to dismantle policy-based structural inequity in population health. *Health Affairs*, *41*(12), 1763–1771. doi:10.1377/hlthaff.2022.00540

Iwelunmor, J., Newsome, V., & Airhihenbuwa, C. O. (2014). Framing the impact of culture on health: A systematic review of the PEN-3 cultural model and its application in public health research and interventions. *Ethnicity & Health*, *19*(1), 20–46. doi:10.1080/13557858.2013.857768

Johnson, P., & Duberley, J. (2003). Reflexivity in management research. *Journal of Management Studies*, *40*, 1279–1303. doi:10.1111/1467-6486.00380

Kang, B., Chin, L., Camacho-Rivera, M., Garza, M., de Jesús Espinosa, T., Cong, X., Fraser, M., Boutjdir, M., & Ramos, S. R. (2025). Intervention mapping for systematic development of a community-engaged CVD prevention intervention in ethnic and racial sexual minority men with HIV. *Front Public Health*, *13*, 1529152. doi:10.3389/fpubh.2025.1529152

Kang, E., & Foster, E. R. (2023). Development of a goal setting and goal management system: Intervention mapping. *Frontiers in Rehabilitation Sciences*, *4*, 1274191. doi:10.3389/fresc.2023.1274191

Kannan, S., Webster, D., Sparks, A., Acker, C. M., E., G.-M., Tropiano, E., & Turner, T. (2009). Using a cultural framework to assess the nutrition influences in relation to birth outcomes among African American women of childbearing age: Application of the PEN-3 theoretical model. *Health Promotion Practice*, *10*(3), 349–358. doi:10.1177/1524839907301406

Kass, N. E. (2001). An ethics framework for public health. *American Journal of Public Health*, *91*(11), 1776–1782.

Kim, S. (2021). Using intervention mapping to develop a media literacy-based smoking prevention program for female adolescents. *International Journal of*

Environmental Research and Public Health, 18(12). doi:10.3390/ijerph18126305

Kirby, D. (2004). *BDI logic models: A useful tool for designing, strengthening, and evaluating programs to reduce adolescent sexual risk-taking, pregnancy, HIV, and other STDs.* ETR Associates. Retrieved from http://www.etr.org/recapp/documents/BDILOGICMODEL20030924.pdf

Kok, G., Gottlieb, N. H., Peters, G.-J. Y., Mullen, P. D., Parcel, G. S., Ruiter, R. A. C., Fernández, M. E., Markham, C., & Bartholomew, L. K. (2016). A taxonomy of behaviour change methods: An Intervention Mapping approach. *Health Psychology Review, 10*(3), 297–312. doi:10.1080/17437199.2015.1077155

Kok, G., Peters, L. W. H., & Ruiter, R. A. C. (2017). Planning theory- and evidence-based behavior change interventions: A conceptual review of the intervention mapping protocol. *Psicologia, reflexao e critica : revista semestral do Departamento de Psicologia da UFRG, 30*(19). doi:10.1186/s41155-017-0072-x

Krops, L. A., Dekker, R., Geertzen, J. H. B., & Dijkstra, P. U. (2018). Development of an intervention to stimulate physical activity in hard-to-reach physically disabled people and design of a pilot implementation: An intervention mapping approach. *BMJ Open, 8*(3). doi:10.1136/bmjopen-2017-020934

Kushnier, L., Nadin, S., Hill, M. E., Taylor, M., Jun, S., Mushquash, C. J., Puinean, G., & Gokiert, R. (2023). Culturally responsive evaluation: A scoping review of the evaluation literature. *Evaluation and Program Planning, 100.* doi:10.1016/j.evalprogplan.2023.102322

Labonté, M., Guillaumie, L., Dionne, A., Dorval, M., Nabi, H., Lemieux, J., Provencher, L., & Lauzier, S. (2020). Development of a community pharmacy-based intervention to enhance adherence to adjuvant endocrine therapy among breast cancer survivors guided by the Intervention Mapping approach. *Research in Social and Administrative Pharmacy, 16*(12), 1724–1736. doi:10.1016/j.sapharm.2020.02.004

Lakhanpaul, M., Culley, L., Robertson, N., Alexander, E. C., Bird, D., Hudson, N., Johal, N., McFeeters, M., Hamlyn-Williams, C., Manikam, L., Boo, Y. Y., Lakhanpaul, M., & Johnson, M. R. D. (2020). A structured collaborative approach to intervention design using a modified intervention mapping approach: A case study using the Management and Interventions for Asthma (MIA) project for South Asian children. *BMC Medical Research Methodology, 20*(271). doi:10.1186/s12874-020-01148-y

Lamort-Bouché, M., Sarnin, P., & Kok, G. (2018). Interventions developed with the Intervention Mapping protocol in the field of cancer: A systematic review. *Psycho-Oncology, 27,* 1138–1149. doi:10.1002/pon.4611

Leenen, J., Hoebe, C. J. P. A., Bos, A. E. R., Wolffs, P. F. G., van Loo, I. H. M., de Wit, J. B. F., Jonas, K. J., & Dukers-Muijrers, N. H. T. M. (2021). Systematic development of an intervention to promote self-sampling for HIV and sexually transmitted infections for men who have sex with men: An intervention mapping approach. *Frontiers in Reproductive Health, 3.* doi:10.3389/frph.2021.634032

Leischow, S. J., & Milstein, B. (2006). Systems thinking and modeling for public health practice. *American Journal of Public Health, 96*(3), 403–405. doi:10.2105/ajph.2005.082842

Lengnick-Hall, R., Stadnick, N. A., & Dickson, K. S. (2021). Forms and functions of bridging factors: specifying the dynamic links between outer and inner contexts during implementation and sustainment. *Implementation Science, 16*(34). doi:10.1186/s13012-021-01099-y

Li, D. H., Moskowitz, D. A., Macapagal, K., Saber, R., & Mustanski, B. (2020). Using intervention mapping to developmentally adapt an online HIV risk reduction program for adolescent men who have sex with men. *Prevention Science: The Official Journal of the Society for Prevention Research, 21*(7), 885–897. doi:10.1007/s11121-020-01148-w

Lipmanowicz, H., & McCandless, K. (2014). *The surprising power of liberating structures: Simple rules to unleash a culture of innovation.* Liberating Structures Press. http://www.liberatingstructures.com/

Locke, D. C. (1986). Cross-cultural counseling issues. In A. J. Palmo, W. J. Weikel, & D. P. Borsos (Eds.), *Foundation of mental health counseling.* Charles C. Thomas.

Locke, D. C. (1992). *Increasing multicultural understanding: A comprehensive model.* Sage.

Major, M. G., Watkins, J. M., Goss, J. M., Craig, D. W., Waggoner, Z., Martinez Kercher, V. M., & Kercher, K. A. (2024). Intervention mapping for refining a sport-based public health intervention in rural schools. *International Journal of Environmental Research and Public Health, 21*(12). doi:10.3390/ijerph21121557

McLeroy, K. R., Bibeau, D., Steckler, A., & Glanz, K. (1988). An ecological perspective on health promotion programs. *Health Education Quarterly, 15,* 351–377. doi:10.1177/109019818801500401

Mérida Rios, L., Serrano, M. M., Aguilar, A. J., Chacón, L. B., Rueda Neria, C. M., & Monreal, L. A. (2019). Promoting fruit, vegetable and simple water consumption among mothers and teachers of preschool children: An intervention mapping initiative. *Evaluation and Program Planning, 76.* doi:10.1016/j.evalprogplan.2019.101675

Mesters, I., Gijsbers, B., & Bartholomew, L. K. (2018). Promoting sustained breastfeeding of infants at risk for asthma: Explaining the "active ingredients" of an effective program using intervention mapping. *Frontiers in Public Health, 6.* doi:10.3389/fpubh.2018.00087

Millet, N., McDermott, H. J., Moss, E. L., Edwardson, C. L., & Munir, F. (2022). Increasing physical activity levels following treatment for cervical cancer: An intervention mapping approach. *Journal of Cancer Survivorship, 16*(3), 650–658. doi:10.1007/s11764-021-01058-y

Moon, Z., Moss-Morris, R., Hunter, M. S., & Hughes, L. D. (2021). Development of a self-management intervention to improve tamoxifen adherence in breast cancer survivors using an Intervention Mapping framework. *Supportive Care in Cancer: Official Journal of the Multinational Association of Supportive Care in Cancer, 29,* 3329–3338. doi:10.1007/s00520-020-05850-x

Moore, S. A., Flynn, D., Price, C. I. M., & Avery, L. (2022). Using intervention mapping to develop and facilitate implementation of a multifaceted behavioural intervention targeting physical activity and sedentary behaviour in stroke survivors: Physical activity routines after stroke (PARAS): Intervention development study. *Health Psychology and Behavioral Medicine, 10*(1), 439–466. doi:10.1080/21642850.2022.2066534

Muñoz-Laboy, M., French, A., Davison, R., Morton, S. J., Arnold, E. A., Rudolph, A. E., Jones, R. M., Fernandez, M. I., & Martinez, O. (2025). Adapting and applying intervention mapping to integrate medical-legal partnership into organizations providing HIV care: An implementation methodology study. *Frontiers in Health Services, 5*. doi:10.3389/frhs.2025.1435663

National Association of County and City Health Officials (NACCHO). (2023). *Mobilizing for action through planning & partnerships: MAPP 2.0.* National Association of County and City Health Officials.

National Cancer Institute. (2024). *Transforming research into community and clinical practice.* https://ebccp.cancercontrol.cancer.gov/index.do

Nawwar, A., Brand Bateman, L., Khamess, S., Fouad, M. N., Arafat, W. O., Abdelmonem, S. E., Bae, S., Rogers, L. Q., Hansen, B., Falkner, K., Abdeltawab, K. M., Aboismail, E., El Kholy, A., & Scarinci, I. (2022). Using intervention mapping to develop a theory-based intervention to promote colorectal cancer screening in Egypt. *Asian Pacific Journal of Cancer Prevention: APJCP, 23*, 1975–1981. doi:10.31557/APJCP.2022.23.6.1975

Nelson, T. (2023). Participatory Learning and Action. In: J.M. Okoko, S. Tunison, & K.D. Walker (Eds.), *Varieties of Qualitative Research Methods.* Springer Texts in Education. Springer, Cham. https://doi.org/10.1007/978-3-031-04394-9_56

Newby, K., Bayley, J., & Wallace, L. M. (2011). What should we tell the children about relationships and sex? Development of a program for parents using intervention mapping. *Health Promotion Practice, 12*(2), 209–228. doi:10.1177/1524839909341028

Nightingale, D. S., Fudge, K., & Schupmann, W. (2018). *Evidence toolkit for learning agendas.* Urban Institute. https://www.urban.org/sites/default/files/publication/97406/evidence_toolkit_learning_agendas_2.pdf

National Institutes of Health (NIH) (2019). *Appendix E, Healthy People Framework.* National Academies Press (US). https://www.ncbi.nlm.nih.gov/books/NBK552645/

O'Connor, A., Blewitt, C., Gooey, M., Griffiths, A., Madill, R., Melder, A., Morris, H., Rakic, S., Boothby, C., Cameron, L., Cunningham, H., Davis, M., Davies, S., Fernandez, M., Greenaway, S., Higgins, C., Ho, P., Hooper, N., Ibrhaim, A., Kearney, S., Kutin, J., Leembruggen, M., May, C., Perri, S., Kurzeme, A., Halfpenny, N., Veale, H., & Skouteris, H. Equity in intervention design: A workshop report and recommendations for intervention planners. *Global Implementation Research and Applications.* in press.

O'Connor, A., Blewitt, C., Nolan, A., & Skouteris, H. (2018). Using Intervention Mapping for child development and wellbeing programs in early childhood education and care settings. *Evaluation and Program Planning, 68*, 57–63. doi:10.1016/j.evalprogplan.2018.02.011

Orgeta, V., Palpatzis, E., See, Y. N., Tuijt, R., Verdaguer, E. S., & Leung, P. (2022). Development of a psychological intervention to promote meaningful activity in people living with mild dementia: An intervention mapping approach. *Gerontologist, 62*(4), 629–641. doi:10.1093/geront/gnab047

Parsons, A., Unaka, N. I., Stewart, C., Foster, J., Perez, V., Yayah Jones, N.-H., Khan, R., Beck, A. F., & Riley, C. (2021). Seven practices for pursuing equity through learning health systems: Notes from the field. *Learning Health Systems, 5*, e10279.

Patton, M. Q. (2008). *Utilization-focused evaluation* (4th ed.). Sage Publications.

Patton, M. Q. (2012). *Essentials of utilization-focused evaluation.* Sage Publications.

Peskin, M. F., Markham, C. M., Gabay, E. K., Shegog, R., Cuccaro, P. M., Temple, J. R., Hernandez, B., Thiel, M., & Emery, S. T. (2018). Using intervention mapping to develop "Me & You: Building Healthy Relationships," a healthy relationship intervention for early middle school students. In D. A. Wolfe & J. R. Temple (Eds.), *Adolescent dating violence* (pp. 467–501). Academic Press.

Pot, M., Ruiter, R. A. C., Paulussen, T. W. G. M., Heuvelink, A., de Melker, H. E., van Vliet, H. J. A., & van Keulen, H. M. (2018). Systematically developing a web-based tailored intervention promoting hpv-vaccination acceptability among mothers of invited girls using intervention mapping. *Frontiers in Public Health*, *6*(226). doi:10.3389/fpubh.2018.00226

Preskill, H., Gutierrez, E., & Mack, K. (2017). *Facilitating intentional group learning: A practical guide to 21 learning activities.* FSG. http://www.fsg.org/tools-and-resources/facilitatingintentional-group-learning

Ravicz, M., Muhongayire, B., Kamagaju, S., Klabbers, R. E., Faustin, Z., Kambugu, A., Bassett, I., & O'Laughlin, K. (2022). Using intervention mapping methodology to design an HIV linkage intervention in a refugee settlement in rural Uganda. *AIDS Care*, *34*(4), 446–458. doi:10.1080/09540121.2021.1900532

Real, F. J., Meisman, A., Wijesooriya, J., Crosby, L. E., & Rosen, B. L. (2025). Using intervention mapping to develop a virtual reality intervention to support covid-19 vaccination among black families. *Journal of Medical Extended Reality, 2*. doi:10.1177/29941520251377072

Reese, T. J., Mixon, A. S., Matheny, M. E., Flatt, C. N., Rubenstein, M., Han, J. H., Wrenn, J., Dagostino, C., Bonnet, K., Anders, S., Schlundt, D., & Ward, M. J. (2023). Using intervention mapping to design and implement a multicomponent intervention to improve antibiotic and NSAID prescribing. *Translational Behavioral Medicine: Practice, Policy, Research*, *13*(12), 928–943. doi:10.1093/tbm/ibad063

Resnicow, K., Baranowski, T., Ahluwalia, J. S., & Braithwaite, R. L. (1999). Cultural sensitivity in public health: Defined and demystified. Ethnicity & Disease, 9(1), 10–21.

Rifkin, S. B. (2018). Alma Ata after 40 years: Primary Health Care and Health for All—from consensus to complexity. *BMJ Global Health*, *3*(Suppl 3), e001188. doi:10.1136/bmjgh-2018-001188

Rimer, B. K. (2002). Perspectives on intrapersonal theories of health behavior. In K. Glanz, B. K. Rimer, & F. M. Lewis (Eds.), *Health behavior and health education: Theory, research, and practice* (Vol. 3, pp. 144–159). Jossey-Bass.

Rios, R. A., McDaniel, J. E., & Stowell, J. P. (1998). Pursuing the possibilities of passion: The affective domain of multicultural education. In M. Dillworth (Ed.), *Being responsive to cultural differences: How teachers learn* (pp. 160–181). Corwin Press.

Rodriguez, S. A., Roncancio, A. M., Savas, L. S., Lopez, D. M., Vernon, S. W., & Fernandez, M. E. (2018). Using intervention mapping to develop and adapt two educational interventions for parents to increase HPV vaccination among Hispanic adolescents. *Frontiers in Public Health*, *6*, 164.

Rogal, S. S., Hansen, L., Patel, A., Ufere, N. N., Verma, M., Woodrell, C. D., & Kanwal, F. (2022). AASLD Practice Guidance: Palliative care and symptom-based management in decompensated cirrhosis. *Hepatology*, *76*(3), 819–853. doi:10.1002/hep.32378

Rossi, P. H., Freeman, H. E., & Lipsey, M. W. (2004). *Evaluation: A systematic approach* (7th ed.). Sage Publications.

Ruiter, R. A. C., & Crutzen, R. (2020). Core processes: How to use evidence, theories, and research in planning behavior change interventions. *Frontiers in Public Health, 8*(247). doi:10.3389/fpubh.2020.00247

Sacca, L., Markham, C., & Fares, J. (2020). Using intervention mapping to develop health education and health policy components to increase breast cancer screening and chemotherapy adherence among Syrian and Iraqi refugee women in Beirut, Lebanon. *Frontiers in Public Health, 8*(101). doi:10.3389/fpubh.2020.00101

Sakakibara, B. M., Lear, S. A., Barr, S. I., Benavente, O., Goldsmith, C. H., Silverberg, N. D., Yao, J., & Eng, J. J. (2017). Development of a chronic disease management program for stroke survivors using intervention mapping: The stroke coach. *Archives of Physical Medicine and Rehabilitation, 98*(1195–1202). doi:10.1016/j.apmr.2017.01.019

Sanz-Guinea, A., Espinosa, M., Grandes, G., Á., l. S., Catalina Martínez, C., Haizea Pombo, H., Bully, P., & Cortada, J. (2017). Efficiency of "Prescribe Vida Saludable", a health promotion innovation: Pilot phase. *Gaceta Sanitaria, 31*(5), 404–409.

Savaglio, M., Yap, M. B. H., Mitchell, G., O'Connor, M., Vincent, A., & Skouteris, H. (2025). Using intervention mapping to co-design a psychosocial service with youth experiencing mental illness. *Evaluation and Program Planning, 108*, 102513. doi:10.1016/j.evalprogplan.2024.102513

Savas, L. S., Loomba, P., Shegog, R., Alaniz, A., Costa, C., Adlparvar, E., Allicock, M. A., Chenier, R., Goetz, M., Markham, C. M., & Fernandez, M. E. (2023). Using implementation mapping to increase uptake and use of Salud en Mis Manos: A breast and cervical cancer screening and HPV vaccination intervention for Latinas. *Frontiers in Public Health, 11*. doi:10.3389/fpubh.2023.966553

Serra, Y. A., Colón-López, V., Savas, L. S., Vernon, S. W., Fernández-Espada, N., Vélez, C., Ayala, A., & Fernández, M. E. (2017). Using intervention mapping to develop health education components to increase colorectal cancer screening in Puerto Rico. *Frontiers in Public Health, 5*(324). doi:10.3389/fpubh.2017.00324

Shegog, R., & Begley, C. E. (2017). Clinic-based mobile health decision support to enhance adult epilepsy self-management: An intervention mapping approach. *Frontiers in Public Health, 5*(256). doi:10.3389/fpubh.2017.00256

Slaghmuylder, Y., Pype, P., Van Hecke, A., & Lauwerier, E. (2023). Development of an intervention aimed at the prevention and treatment of chronic pain in breast cancer survivors: An intervention mapping approach. *Patient Education & Counseling, 108*. doi:10.1016/j.pec.2022.107618

Springer, A., Barroso, C., Rabl, A., & van den Berg, A. (2024). Planning health promotion and disease prevention programs and interventions. In J. Coreil (Ed.), *Social and behavioral foundations of public health* (3rd ed.). SAGE

Steckler, A., & Linnan, L. A. (Eds.). (2002). *Process evaluation for public health interventions and research*. Jossey-Bass.

Stokols, D. (1996). Translating social ecological theory into guidelines for community health promotion. *American Journal of Health Promotion, 10*(4), 282–298.

Stutterheim, S. E., van der Kooij, Y. L., Crutzen, R., Ruiter, R. A. C., Bos, A. E. R., & Kok, G. (2025). Intervention mapping as a guide to developing, implementing, and evaluating stigma reduction interventions. *Stigma and Health, 10,* 13–20. doi:10.1037/sah0000445

Sue, D. W. (2003). *Overcoming our racism.* Jossey-Bass.

Sun, Y., Bowden, M., Cameron, L., Skouteris, H., & Blewitt, C. (2024). Understanding the need and opportunity for a trauma-informed early childhood organisations (TIO) program using intervention mapping. *Australasian Journal of Early Childhood, 49*(2), 169–184. doi:10.1177/18369391241250103

Sun, Y., Wang, A., Yu, S., Hagger, M. S., Chen, X., Fong, S. S. M., Zhang, C., Huang, W. Y., Baker, J. S., Dutheil, F., & Gao, Y. (2020). A blended intervention to promote physical activity, health and work productivity among office employees using intervention mapping: A study protocol for a cluster-randomized controlled trial. *BMC Public Health, 20*(1). doi:10.1186/s12889-020-09128-z

Svendsen, M. J., Sandal, L. F., Kjær, P., Nicholl, B. I., Cooper, K., Mair, F., Hartvigsen, J., Stochkendahl, M. J., Søgaard, K., Mork, P. J., & Rasmussen, C. (2022). Using intervention mapping to develop a decision support system-based smartphone app (selfBACK) to support self-management of nonspecific low back pain: Development and usability study. *Journal of Medical Internet Research, 24*(1), e26555. doi:10.2196/26555

ten Hoor, G. A., Markham, C. M., Fernandez, M. E., & Ruiter, R. A. C. (2025). Intervention mapping: Planning health promotion programs. In *The Sage handbook of health psychology: Issues, debates and applications of health psychology* (Vol. 3, Chapter 6). Sage Publications Ltd. https://bookshelf.vitalsource.com/reader/books/9781529679526

ten Hoor, G. A., Plasqui, G., Schols, A. M. W. J., & Kok, G. (2017). Development, implementation, and evaluation of an interdisciplinary theory- and evidence-based intervention to prevent childhood obesity: Theoretical and methodological lessons learned. *Frontiers in Public Health, 5*(352). doi:10.3389/fpubh.2017.00352

Tervalon, M., & Murray-García, J. (1998). Cultural humility versus cultural competence: A critical distinction in defining physician training outcomes in multicultural education. *Journal of Health Care for the Poor and Underserved, 9*(2), 117–125. doi:10.1353/hpu.2010.0233

Thackeray, A., Waring, J., Hoogeboom, T. J., Nijhuis-van Der Sanden, M. W., Hess, R., Fritz, J. M., & Fernandez, M. E. (2022). Implementing a Dutch therapy intervention into a US health system: Selecting strategies using implementation mapping. *Frontiers in Public Health, 10,* 908484.

Tomiyama, A., Carr, D., & Granberg, E. (2018). How and why weight stigma drives the obesity 'epidemic' and harms health. *BMC Medicine, 16*(123). doi:10.1186/s12916-018-1116-5

Torres-Cortés, B., Leiva, L., Canenguez, K. M., & Greaves, L. (2024). Promoting equity in adolescent health in Latin America: Designing a comprehensive Sex education program using Intervention Mapping. A mixed methods study. *Frontiers in Reproductive Health, 6,* 1447016. doi:10.3389/frph.2024.1447016

van Der Veen, Y. J. J., van Empelen, P., & Richardus, J. H. (2012). Development of a culturally tailored Internet intervention promoting hepatitis B screening in the Turkish community in the Netherlands. *Health Promotion International, 27*(3), 342–355. doi:10.1093/heapro/dar044 van Grootel, J. W. M., Bor, P., Veenhof, C., & Valkenet, K. (2023). Development of a goal-directed movement intervention (GOAL) using a movement sensor for hospitalized patients: An intervention mapping approach. *Clinical Rehabilitation. 38*(2):251–262.

van Keulen, H., Voogt, C., Kleinjan, M., Kramer, J., Andree, R., & van Empelen, P. (2022). Development of a dynamically tailored mHealth intervention (what do you drink) to reduce excessive drinking among Dutch lower-educated students: User-centered design approach. *JMIR Formative Research, 6*. doi:10.2196/36969

van Venrooij, I., Spijker, J., Westerhof, G. J., Leontjevas, R., & Gerritsen, D. L. (2019). Applying intervention mapping to improve the applicability of precious memories, an intervention for depressive symptoms in nursing home residents. *International Journal of Environmental Research and Public Health, 16*(5163). doi:10.3390/ijerph16245163

Varela-Mato, V., Blake, H., Yarker, J., Godfree, K., Daly, G., Hassard, J., & Munir, F. (2023). Using intervention mapping to develop evidence-based toolkits that support workers on long-term sick leave and their managers. *BMC Health Services Research, 23*(1), 1–14.

Vissenberg, C., Nierkens, V., Uitewaal, P. J. M., Middelkoop, B. J. C., Nijpels, G., & Stronks, K. (2017). Development of the social network-based intervention "Powerful Together with Diabetes" using intervention mapping. *Frontiers in Public Health, 5*(334). doi:10.3389/fpubh.2017.00334

Volevach, E., Maršálková, H., & Mikulik, R. (2025). Enhancing stroke response in school children: Efficacy of the HOBIT program - a cluster randomized trial. *Preventive Medicine Reports, 53*, 103049. doi:10.1016/j.pmedr.2025.103049

Volevach, E., Schneider, F., Maršálková, H., & Mikulik, R. (2024). The use of intervention mapping to guide the development of a school-based intervention to improve emergency medical services activation for stroke. *BMC Public Health, 24*(1), 3322. doi:10.1186/s12889-024-20809-x

W. K. Kellogg Foundation (2006). *W. K. Kellogg Foundation logic model development guide* (Vol. 2015). W.K. Kellogg Foundation.

W. K. Kellogg Foundation (2010). *W.K. Kellogg Foundation evaluation handbook* (Vol. 2015). W.K. Kellogg Foundation.

Walburn, J., Norton, S., Sarkany, R., Sainsbury, K., Araújo-Soares, V., Morgan, M., Canfield, M., Foster, L., Heydenreich, J., McCrone, P., Mander, A., Sniehotta, F. F., Wulf, H. C., & Weinman, J. (2019). Evaluation of a personalised adherence intervention to improve photoprotection in adults with Xeroderma Pigmentosum (XP): Protocol for the trial of XPAND. *BMJ Open, 9*(7), e028577. doi:10.1136/bmjopen-2018-028577

Walker, T. J., Foster, M., Szeszulski, J., Craig, D. W., Mullen, P. D., & Fernández, M. E. (2022). Evidence-based intervention (EBI) mapping: A systematic approach to understanding the components and logic of EBIs. *BMC Public Health, 22*(1), 1300. doi:10.1186/s12889-022-13692-x

Wallerstein, N., Duran, B., Oetzel, J., & Minkler, M. (Eds.) (2018). *Community-based participatory research for health: Advancing social and health equity*, 3rd ed. Jossey-Bass.

Weiland, A., Blankenstein, A. H., Willems, M. H. A., Van Saase, J. L. C. M., Van der Molen, H. T., Van Dulmen, A. M., & Arends, L. R. (2013). Post-graduate education for medical specialists focused on patients with medically unexplained physical symptoms; Development of a communication skills training programme. *Patient Education and Counseling, 92*(3), 355–360. doi:10.1016/j.pec.2013.06.027

Weiss, B. D., & Coyne, C. (1997). Communicating with patients who cannot read. *New England Journal of Medicine, 337*(4), 272–274. doi:10.1056/nejm199707243370411

Weiss, E. M., Duenas, D. M., Kelsh, A., Gray, M. M., Oslin, E., McNeil, D., Juul, S. E., & Kraft, S. A. (2025). Piloting the better research interactions for every family (BRIEF) researcher intervention to support recruitment for a neonatal clinical trial: Parent experience and infant enrollment. *Journal of Perinatology, 45*(6), 773–789. doi:10.1038/s41372-025-02245-w

Whelan, J., Fraser, P., Bolton, K. A., Love, P., Strugnell, C., Boelsen-Robinson, T., Blake, M. R., Martin, E., Allender, S., & Bell, C. (2023). Combining systems thinking approaches and implementation science constructs within community-based prevention: A systematic review. *Health Research Policy and Systems, 21*(1), 85. doi:10.1186/s12961-023-01023-4

World Health Organization (WHO) (2011). *Standards and operational guidance for ethics review of health-related research with human participants.* https://www.who.int/publications/i/item/9789241502948.

World Health Organization (WHO) (2025). *World report on social determinants of health equity, 2025.* https://www.who.int/teams/social-determinants-of-health/equity-and-health/world-report-on-social-determinants-of-health-equity

Windsor, R., Clark, N., Boyd, N. R., & Goodman, R. M. (2003). *Evaluation of health promotion, health education and disease prevention programs* (Vol. 3). McGraw-Hill.

World Health Organization (1986). Ottawa charter for health promotion. *Health Promotion International, 1*, iii–iv.

Zacarías, G., Shamah-Levy, T., Elton-Puente, E., Garbus, P., & García, O. P. (2019). Development of an intervention program to prevent childhood obesity targeted to Mexican mothers of school-aged children using intervention mapping and social cognitive theory. *Evaluation and Program Planning, 74*, 27–37.

Zamantakis, A., Merle, J. L., Queiroz, A. A., Zapata, J. P., Deskins, J., Pachicano, A. M., Mongrella, M., Li, D., Benbow, N., Gallo, C., Smith, J. D., & Mustanski, B. (2024). Innovation and implementation determinants of HIV testing and linkage-to-care in the U.S.: A systematic review. *Implementation Science Communications, 5*(1), 111. doi:10.1186/s43058-024-00638-0

CHAPTER 2

CORE PROCESSES: A GUIDE TO USING COMMUNITY ENGAGEMENT, EVIDENCE, THEORIES, AND RESEARCH TO PLAN HEALTH PROMOTION INTERVENTIONS

Overview

This chapter focuses on how and when to use community engagement, evidence, theories, and new research to plan health promotion interventions and refers to available tools that are useful when applying Core Processes in various steps of Intervention Mapping. In the context of Intervention Mapping, Core Processes are a set of foundational procedures that, collectively, inform answers to questions raised in each step of Intervention Mapping in a systematic way. Understanding a health problem, its causes, potential solutions, or approaches for addressing it, can be complex and time-consuming; sometimes planners do not persevere through the challenges. Consequently, understanding can be incomplete; thus, attempts to solve it are faulty. Using Core Processes minimizes the likelihood of an incomplete understanding of a health problem and the selection of ineffective solutions by planners. Although Core Processes are described within the context of Intervention Mapping, they were originally described by Veen in 1985 and can be applied in any planning framework and in each step of program planning from problem analysis to intervention design and program implementation and evaluation (see Chapter 1 for an overview).

Intervention Mapping emphasizes the use of *Core Processes,* described below because too often planners (regardless of whether they use Intervention Mapping) claim to have engaged community members and other interested parties, reviewed literature, applied theories, and collected data but, in fact, have done this incompletely and selectively. Community engagement, reviewing existing literature, applying appropriate theories, and collecting additional research data are fundamental in different phases/steps of planning frameworks, but it is often unclear to planners exactly how and when they should use these processes for analyzing and solving problems (Buunk & Van Vugt, 2013; Ruiter et al., 2013). Therefore, we describe *how* to use *Core Processes,* and provide examples of their application in the Intervention Mapping steps. The six Core Processes (defined by Ruiter & Crutzen, 2020) are as follows:

- Core Process 1: Pose questions
- Core Process 2: Explore possible answers by engaging community members and other interested parties
- Core Process 3: Review evidence from previous research
- Core Process 4: Find theoretical support using the topic, concepts, and general theories approaches
- Core Process 5: Identify and address the need for new research with community members and other interested parties
- Core Process 6: Complete and assess the list of possible answers

The Core Processes should be followed in the order presented above. It would be imprudent for planners to begin exploring possible answers (Core Process 2) without first clearly articulating what question needs to be answered (Core Process 1). Similarly, it is unwise to start by finding theories aimed at explaining behavior (Core Process 4) before reviewing available evidence on determinants related to a specific behavior of interest (Core Process 3). Progressing through these processes can be done in various ways, at varying intensities – ranging from a few meetings to a comprehensive effort lasting several months or even years. In instances when only limited time is available among planners, it is better to address all Core Processes – even briefly – rather than focusing on just one or two processes (e.g., only using theory or jumping straight into research). This is because each of these Core Processes provides information from a unique type of source providing different (and sometimes unique) "ways of knowing" that are iterative in nature. So, their findings build upon each other.

Core Process 1: Pose Questions

The first Core Process, which is rooted in Freire's method of teaching that emphasizes critical thinking, is *posing questions* (Freire, 1970). Early on in intervention planning, questions are often asked as a means of analyzing possible causes of the health problem (e.g., what are important risk behaviors?). In later steps of Intervention Mapping, questions concern, for example, determinants of behavior and environmental conditions, and adoption and implementation outcomes.

It is crucial that the planning group is on the same page regarding *which* question needs to be answered and at *what moment* (e.g., problem analysis in Step 1, identifying determinants in Step 2, selecting change methods in Step 3), before beginning any of the other Core Processes. Lack of clarity about the questions that have to be answered creates confusion and unorganized discussions and can limit progress as planners proceed to the subsequent Core Processes.

Throughout this book, we present crucial questions that need to be answered in each Intervention Mapping step. For example, in Step 1, to facilitate a more complete understanding of the problem, planners may ask, "What behaviors and environmental factors are related to the problem?" In Step 2, they may ask, "What do the people have to do to perform the health promoting behavior?" to identify performance objectives. Core Process 1 – formulating and structuring effective questions – is essential and helps guide the remaining Core Processes.

Core Process 2: Explore Possible Answers

Exploring possible answers by engaging community members and other interested parties can be done in various ways. Brainstorming with the planning group, which contains members of both the community and other interested parties, is a commonly used method to explore answers. Brainstorming is a creative process that primarily involves free association with the aim of generating as many answers as possible, in response to a specific question (Svihla, 2021). Planning group members will likely already possess significant preexisting knowledge about the topic of interest (e.g., this can be based on experiences of community members and other interested parties or expertise regarding a health problem or related behaviors among the planning group members). The brainstorming process should facilitate the sharing of this knowledge. For example, to understand multiple concurrent sexual partnerships among adolescents in Uganda, we engaged in brainstorming sessions with adolescents themselves, community leaders and policy makers, and other experts (e.g., behavioral scientists, health promotion practitioners). Adolescents brought up the issue of transactional sex, which was then further explored when reviewing the literature. Brainstorming answers is often an illuminating, engaging, and productive element of the Intervention Mapping process (at various stages). Nevertheless, after the initial brainstorming session, planners may choose to disregard answers that are poorly supported in the literature. Similarly, it is important to avoid getting stuck on a single answer too soon. In fact, during the initial brainstorming stage, the planning group should avoid evaluating or even commenting on ideas and instead, freely generate as many ideas as possible. This notion aligns with Linus Pauling's adage that "The best way to have a good idea is to have lots of ideas."

In formulating provisional answers to questions, applied behavioral scientists typically draw on theoretical and empirical knowledge, whether consciously or not. Doing so is unavoidable at this stage; however, the brainstorming should be as open as possible and should not be limited to data- or theory-informed answers. It is crucial to embrace the lived experiences of community members and other interested parties. Participation is a crucial perspective in the Intervention Mapping approach, and community engagement is expected to live up to the idea of "Nothing about us without us." Only at a later stage are empirical findings and theoretical support incorporated – to avoid haphazard decisions based on a brainstorm only. For these reasons, the brainstorming process should allow for – and in fact encourage – engagement with community members and other interested parties.

There are several ways to structure brainstorming sessions, depending on the composition of the attendee group, and the specific questions that are targeted. For example, in the development of an intervention aimed at increasing condom use for 16–24-years-olds who access chlamydia self-sampling websites, we organized a workshop to design intervention strategies (in Step 3 of Intervention Mapping) (Newby et al., 2019). The workshop engaged these youth in generating ideas for targeting the change objectives related to five different performance objectives. Attendees were encouraged to think openly about intervention strategies that might help achieve the performance objectives. A large wall display was presented at the workshop which included images representing each of the five performance objectives (e.g., obtaining condoms, discussing condom use with a partner). Attendees were split into groups, with each group generating ideas for positively impacting one of the performance objectives that were represented on the wall chart. Each group was provided with a variety of materials (e.g., colored pens and highlighters, paper, sticky notes, and Blu Tack) to inspire and support creativity. Each group was also provided with a description of the performance objective they were assigned to think about and discuss, along with questions that directed the group to focus on the related change objectives. All groups were encouraged to formulate a list of novel ideas (e.g., intervention strategies) that could potentially impact the performance objectives.

Group brainstorming is a popular ideation method, but outcomes vary greatly as the method depends on individuals working collectively to generate ideas. So, group dynamics determine the extent to which the method is successful. Previous work shows how interaction designers use techniques from theatrical improvization, or improv, to enhance group interactions while collaborating and improve engagement (Gerber, 2009). Improvization activities serve to reinforce the rules of brainstorming, such as withholding judgment, building on the ideas of others, and generating a large quantity of ideas. Brainstorming can lead to multiple answers and ideas, and there is no reason to favor one of those over another. In other words, brainstorming does not lead to final answers. It is crucial, however, to do this before the next Core Process of reviewing evidence as it might guide the search for evidence (e.g., see the earlier example of transactional sex in the project on multiple concurrent sexual partnerships among adolescents in Uganda).

Core Process 3: Review Evidence

The purpose of this Core Process is to support or refute provisional answers to the questions, which the planning group has already posed and explored answers to together with members of the community and other interested parties, with empirical evidence. In addition to academic journals, it is recommended to also explore "gray" literature, such as websites and registries (see Chapter 5 for an overview). We suggest that planners start the process by searching for existing reviews. There are many sources available in the burgeoning field of systematic reviews and evidence-based health promotion that are worthwhile to consult before looking for individual studies. When appraising available reviews, or conducting a new one (see Peters, 2014 for basic how-to guidance), planners should understand the nature of the numerator (what studies are used in the evidence summary) in relation to the denominator (what studies were conducted or reported), and be aware of the variation that exists in the quality of evidence. Of course, the latter also applies when assessing individual studies (Peters, 2014).

A principle of evidence-based medicine is that a hierarchy of evidence exists (Murad et al., 2016). At the lower end of the evidence pyramid are *individual studies* with various designs and at the very top, *systematic reviews* and *meta-analyses*. More recently, a plea has been made to remove systematic reviews from the top of the pyramid and instead use them as a lens through which other types of studies should be seen (i.e., appraised and applied in the context to which they are applied) (Murad et al., 2016). So, when planning health promotion interventions, it is not the case that systematic reviews provide more valuable evidence than individual studies. Different types of studies provide different types of evidence relevant to the context. For example, a systematic review might provide an overview of determinants of, and interventions for, pro-environmental behaviors in organizations in general, whereas an individual qualitative study might provide more in-depth insight into determinants of pro-environmental work-related travel behavior among Dutch office workers specifically (Lo et al., 2012). Similarly, from the gray literature, information from reports of community needs assessments that include interviews and observation across a range of individuals, and interested parties can provide a broad, multilevel understanding of factors influencing behavioral, health, and/or environmental outcomes. When reviewing evidence, effect sizes derived from quantitative studies (either reviews or individual studies) indicate association strength between, for example, determinants and a specific behavior (Rosenthal, 1996). This provides information about the importance of, in this example, determinants, which is useful in the final Core Process when completing and assessing the list of possible answers.

Sometimes evidence regarding a well-defined question may be scarce. For example, there might be limited evidence available when trying to answer the question: "What factors predict cervical cancer screening in young women in Ghana?" In that case, the search can be broadened by looking for (1) studies in populations that are somewhat similar (e.g., sharing demographic and cultural characteristics) to young women in Ghana (e.g., young women in other West African countries) or (2) studies about similar behaviors (e.g., other cancer screening-related behaviors). Before a decision is made to rely on theories that by definition are general in nature, it is important to first review evidence, even when that evidence is about participant groups or settings that are somewhat different from those in a specific project.

Core Process 4: Find Theoretical Support

This Core Process involves finding a theory that supports answers to the planning question. The purpose is to make the provisional list of answers to the planning question as extensive as possible before conducting new research (Core Process 5). Theories can be defined as formal and abstract statements about a selected aspect of reality (Kok & Ruiter, 2014). As a consequence of their very nature, theories are always a reduction of reality. This is not a shortcoming, but rather a definition, which is important to keep in mind when using theory in addressing problems (e.g., a specific health problem). Criteria for success of an intervention are formulated in terms of problem reduction (e.g., less people suffering from a specific health problem), with contributions to theory seen as a useful by-product. While Intervention Mapping is a robust framework that allows for the testing of theoretical principles, it is first and foremost a practical and pragmatic framework that allows incorporation of a range of theoretical perspectives with the overall goal of making a positive impact in terms of reducing a real-life health problem.

Real-life problems are – by definition – complex; otherwise, they would already have been solved without the need to involve health promoters or the design of complex interventions. It follows, then, that a multi-theory approach is likely required (see Chapter 1) to understand and solve real-life problems. From this perspective, applying theory to real-life problems can be likened to completing a jigsaw puzzle with various theories fitting together to provide a more complete explanation or answer to a planning question than applying a single theory (Peters & Crutzen, 2017). In a problem-driven context, all theories, theoretical models, and concepts are potentially useful within the parameters that the theory describes (Buunk & Van Vugt, 2013). For example, the Reasoned Action Approach is a theory about reasoned behavior (Fishbein & Ajzen, 2010). Of course, not all behavior is reasoned and this theory does not make claims about other types of behavior (e.g., impulsive behavior). So, it cannot explain all possible variances in all possible behaviors. However, this is not a reason to reject this theory, but instead, an important parameter is to only apply it to reasoned behavior. Moreover, there are common and unique elements regarding each theory (Noar, 2005). Within the Reasoned Action Approach, for example, beliefs ultimately lead to behavior. However, behaving in a certain way also affects the beliefs that people hold. This reciprocal influence between beliefs and behaviors is the focus of the cognitive dissonance theory (Festinger, 1957). Limiting the pool of candidate theories too soon may lead to inadequate answers or, worse, it may lead to conclusions being drawn that are counterproductive. There are three approaches to finding theories: the topic, concept, and general theories approaches; these should be utilized in combination but also in that order.

Topic Approach

First, the planning group should look for and examine the theoretical concepts and frameworks (if any) that were used to design the reported empirical studies and/or explain the findings. The planning group should then assess these theories through the lens of their *utility in providing additional answers to the formulated question.* For example, a literature review might have resulted in identifying a meta-analysis on the psychosocial determinants of condom use in heterosexual populations (Sheeran et al., 1999). In the introduction and discussion sections, there are references to different psychosocial theories of (health) behavior such as the Health Belief Model, the Theory of Planned Behavior, and the Aids Risk Reduction Model (Catania et al., 1994; Monta'flo & Kasprzyk, 2015; Skinner et al., 2015). By studying these theories in detail, additional answers can be added to the list of potential explanations that are supported by theories of human behavior. The purpose is to make the provisional list of answers to the planning question as extensive as possible before conducting new research (Core Process 5).

Concept Approach

Second, the planning group should examine concepts that are generated during the second Core Process, when exploring possible answers, for example, by engaging community members and other interested parties. It is likely that these concepts are initially stated in lay terms, but it might be advantageous to relabel them with their theoretical labels. For example, a lack of confidence could also be labeled as the theoretical construct of self-efficacy. There is potentially more information that can be garnered when examining theories that include this theoretical construct in comparison to the simple lay concept. One person cannot be familiar with all potentially useful theories; this is why it is advisable to include in the planning group individuals from various disciplines and why expertise in behavior change (e.g., an applied psychologist) is always required. It is also worth noting that reading comprehensive overviews of theories may aid this process (see Chapters 3 and 4).

General Theories Approach

Third, the planning group may consider alternative frameworks that have not been accessed through the other two approaches but which could provide valuable information for further extending and refining the list of explanations. For example, dual-process models of human behavior that differentiate between impulsive or automatic decision-making and more reasoned routes of planning or theories of self-regulation and self-management may be informative (Mann et al., 2013; Strack & Deutsch, 2004). The general theories approach should be seen as a last resort in a problem-driven context. When there is tension between generalizability and utility of theories, utility should be given preference given the applied nature of the problem-driven context (Head & Noar, 2014).

A theory that is helpful in making one planning decision (e.g., during needs assessment) might not be very helpful for making another planning decision (e.g., during intervention design). Table 2.1 presents examples of types of theories that might be applied to various questions that arise during

Table 2.1 Examples of Theories for Intervention Mapping Steps and Questions

Intervention Mapping Step	Decision (Sample Question)	Examples of Theories
Step 1	Needs assessment (What quality-of-life issues are related to [a specific] health problem?)	Quality-of-life theories
Step 2	Behaviors (What behaviors benefit [a specific] health outcome?) Environmental conditions (What agents control health-promoting environmental conditions?) Personal determinants (What factors influence the health-promoting behavior?)	Self-regulatory theories Power theories Expectancy-value theories
Step 3	Change methods and practical applications (What strategies have been shown to influence [specific] determinants and behavior?)	Persuasive communication theories
Step 4	Messages (What factors have been shown to influence comprehension and retention of messages?)	Theories of information processing
Step 5	Implementation (What factors have been shown to influence implementation of similar interventions?)	Diffusion theories Dissemination and implementation models

the planning process. For example, in a project to understand factors influencing multiple concurrent sexual partnerships among adolescents in Uganda, the planning group started by using the topic approach (Nalukwago et al., 2018). Six theories identified from previous empirical studies included: Theories of Reasoned Action and Planned Behavior, Health Belief Model, Social Cognitive Theory, Social Exchange Theory, Social Ecological Model, and Social Norms Theory. In the concept approach, the ideas generated from brainstorming and reviewing evidence were grouped and relabeled using these six theories. Labels such as attitude, perceived susceptibility beliefs, self-efficacy, and social/subjective norms were drawn from the aforementioned theories. Using the general theories approach, we reviewed theories that helped us to understand why some adolescents engage in multiple concurrent sexual partnerships. We explored alternative theoretical frameworks that were not identified at the topic and concept approach steps, but were deemed relevant for the problem at hand. Two alternative theoretical frameworks explored included the Self-Regulation Theory and the Extended Parallel Process Model. The latter was not only helpful to understand the problem, but also helped us understand why many existing interventions in Uganda that attempted to use a risk-messaging approach were found to be unsuccessful: they tended to focus on fear while limiting focus on efficacy. Chapters 3 and 4 provide a more in-depth explanation of various theories and how to apply them in Intervention Mapping.

Core Process 5: Identify and Address the Need for New Research

The planning group should complete the previously described Core Processes before conducting new research. Please note that "new" research concerns both primary data collection as well as secondary data analyses. A very practical reason is that conducting this work requires a great deal of resources (in terms of time, expertise, and money). More importantly, before conducting new research, all available evidence and insights should be considered. In fact, progressing through the previously described Core Processes will likely result in better research; if new research needs to be conducted, then it should be clear what types of questions should be asked, and addressed, in that research. For example, the planning group may want to know whether certain theoretical constructs that look promising are actually explanatory in relation to their population or behavior of interest. Additionally, through community engagement activities across earlier core processes, answers to posed questions may not have been corroborated by existing literature; yet, they were strongly held opinions and or experiences shared by members of the priority population or other key actors. Findings from community engagement processes, promising theoretical constructs, or inconclusive findings from the evidence review could then be the focus of new research.

Often, health promotion planners use a combination of qualitative and quantitative methods to explore the questions of interest in their population (Bryman, 2006; De Vries et al., 1992; Morgan, 2007). For example, for a question regarding determinants, planners first search the available theoretical and empirical literature on the cause of the behavior or environmental condition of interest to find theories and data. They might then use a qualitative method (e.g., focus group discussions, one-on-one interviews) to learn about the population's beliefs regarding determinants of their behavior followed by a quantitative study (such as a structured questionnaire with questions that are based on the results of the qualitative phase) to establish the relevance of these determinants. In some situations, qualitative methods are used later in the research process to better understand the findings from a quantitative method. Contrary to the belief of some, quantitative methods are not, by definition, better than qualitative methods (or the other way around), but serve a different purpose or provide a different (and unique) type of evidence. Besides commonly used qualitative methods such as focus group discussions and one-on-one interviews, there are other methods that more actively engage community members and other interested parties. For example, in a project about health inequalities among the most vulnerable populations in the post-conflict-affected Eastern part of the Democratic Republic of Congo, both community walks and community-engaged mapping were used. A community walk is a data collection method where researchers walk through a neighborhood of interest to map out and collect information about that neighborhood's resources and dynamics, for the purpose of community organizing and development. It provides a first-hand view of the community, its people, and its assets. During community-engaged mapping, community members are formed into small, breakout groups that allow them to collectively discuss and map their communities. The purpose is to identify strengths and assets within the community, resources that they access outside of the community, and areas that can be improved to become assets (Chapter 5 provides more details on needs and asset assessment).

When using quantitative methods, more specifically a structured questionnaire with questions about determinants, an approach to establish the relevance of determinants when planning a health promotion intervention exists. Confidence Interval-Based Estimation of Relevance (CIBER) is an approach based on the visualization of confidence intervals for the mean scores of determinants and correlations with behavior for all determinants simultaneously. This visualization facilitates comparison, which is necessary when making selections (see Crutzen & Peters, 2020 for how-to guidance). Assessing the correlations of determinants with behavior is important: those determinants that are not associated with behavior will often be the least likely candidates to intervene upon. The mean scores on determinants are important because these are indicative of where there is room for improvement (e.g., whether participants already hold certain desirable beliefs or not).

We have illustrated this approach by means of a case study on the determinants of using a high dose of ecstasy (Crutzen et al., 2017). This case study demonstrated, for example, that users of ecstasy are already convinced that using a high dose of ecstasy is much worse for their health. So, messages about dangers to their health would only reinforce what participants are already convinced about. However, regret after using a high dose of ecstasy is associated with the outcome of interest and participants score around the middle of the scale in terms of how much they would regret this. This combination of being associated with the outcome of interest and scoring on the middle of the scale makes regret a highly relevant target to intervene upon. In this example, feelings of regret could be reinforced (Chapter 7 provides an overview of change methods) and are a more important target than convincing people that using a high dose of ecstasy is bad for their health.

Core Process 6: Complete and Assess the List of Possible Answers

After completing the first five Core Processes, the planning team and community partners are ready to summarize and complete its provisional list of answers to the planning question into a working list for which the evidence is sufficient. The planners will judge their answers for relevance and changeability. Relevance is about, for example, the strength of the evidence for the relationship between the determinant and the behavior (e.g., using CIBER in Step 2), the extent to which various environmental agents contribute to the health problem (in Step 1), or the appropriateness of change methods for targeting certain determinants (in Step 3). Changeability refers to the strength of the evidence suggesting that the proposed change can be realized by a health promotion intervention. The latter criterion requires planners, for example, to consider that some determinants may be changed by interventions directed at the individual, and other determinants possibly changed by interventions directed at environmental agents. Whenever possible, judgments regarding changeability should be based on evidence from the research literature (Ashford et al., 2010). However, when data regarding changeability are scarce, such judgments have to rely on a theoretical or conceptual basis. Behavior change expertise is then needed to make judgments regarding changeability.

Transitioning from a working list of answers to a planning question to a final list requires making decisions about what to focus on for a particular effort and what to de-emphasize. The key reason is that resources are finite. The decisions during this selection process will have an impact on the quantity and quality of intervention content that can be developed and delivered. The latter is especially relevant if there are additional costs per participant (e.g., delivering a health promotion intervention in a face-to-face setting with a health professional). However, even when the additional costs per participant are relatively low (e.g., when using a digital intervention), there are still limits in terms of the amount of intervention content to which participants can be exposed. Although intervention content can be delivered in multiple sessions over a longer period of time, this might lead to increased levels of dropout, which also limits exposure to intervention content (Rutherford et al., 2013).

After completing Core Process 6, the planning group will have enough information to finalize a list of answers. At this point, it can be useful to tie everything together in one visualization, which is known as a logic model (Earp & Ennett, 1991). There is a tool available to do exactly that: the acyclic behavior change diagram (ABCD) (Metz et al., 2022). ABCD consists of two components: (1) The diagram – a visual representation of the most important structural and causal assumptions underlying a health promotion intervention. This diagram is generated based on (2) the ABCD-matrix. This matrix is a table with several columns, with each row representing one causal-structural chain. Using this tool – which is helpful during the planning process, – also provides insight into the rationale of the intervention, and fosters replicability of health promotion interventions.

Summary

Chapter 2 presents Core Processes - a set of foundational procedures that, collectively, inform answers to questions raised in each step of Intervention Mapping in a systematic way. The chapter focuses on how and when to use community engagement, evidence, theories, and new research to plan health promotion interventions and refers to available tools that are useful when doing so.

Progressing through these processes can be done in various ways, at varying intensities. In instances when only limited time is available among planners, it is better to address all Core Processes –even briefly– rather than focusing on just one or two (e.g., only using theory or jumping straight into research).

It is crucial that the planning group is on the same page regarding which question needs to be answered and at what moment (e.g., problem analysis in Step 1, identifying determinants in Step 2, selecting change methods in Step 3) before beginning any of the other Core Processes. Intervention Mapping provides guidance by means of posing the questions that need to be answered in each step.

Discussion Questions and Learning Activities

1. What are the six Core Processes?
2. Why do Core Processes need to be followed in a specific order?
3. Why is it crucial to engage with community members and other interested parties?

4. What is the role of different types of studies when reviewing evidence?
5. Why is a multi-theory approach needed in a problem-driven context?
6. What are different approaches to find theoretical support?
7. When is it necessary to conduct additional research?

References

Ashford, S., Edmunds, J., & French, D. P. (2010). What is the best way to change self-efficacy to promote lifestyle and recreational physical activity? A systematic review with meta-analysis. *British Journal of Health Psychology, 15*, 265–288.

Bryman, A. (2006). Integrating quantitative and qualitative research: How is it done? *Qualitative Research, 6*, 97–113.

Buunk, A. P., & Van Vugt, M. (2013). *Applying social psychology: From problems to solutions* (2nd ed.). Sage.

Catania, J. A., Coates, T. J., & Kegeles, S. (1994). A test of the AIDS risk reduction model: Psychosocial correlates of condom use in the AMEN cohort survey. *Health Psychology, 13*, 548–555.

Crutzen, R., & Peters, G.-J. Y. (2020). *The book of behavior change* (1th ed.). doi: 10.5281/zenodo.3570967

Crutzen, R., Cyr, D., Taylor, S. E., Lim, E., & Ruiter, R. A. C. (2017). Self-Reevaluation and Anticipated Regret Did Not Change Attitude, Nor Perceived Distance in an Online Context [Original Research]. *Frontiers in Psychology, 7*. doi: 10.3389/fpsyg.2016.02038

De Vries, H., Weijts, W., Dijkstra, M., & Kok, G. (1992). The utilization of qualitative and quantitative data for health education program planning, implementation, and evaluation: A spiral approach. *Health Education & Behavior, 19*, 101–115.

Earp, J. A., & Ennett, S. T. (1991). Conceptual models for health education research and practice. *Health Education Research, 6*, 163–171.

Festinger, L. (1957). *A theory of cognitive dissonance*. Stanford University Press.

Fishbein, M., & Ajzen, I. (2010). *Predicting and changing behavior: The reasoned action approach*. Taylor & Francis Group.

Freire, P. (1970). *Pedagogy of the oppressed*. Herder and Herder.

Gerber, E. (2009). Using improvisation to enhance the effectiveness of brainstorming. *CHI '09: Proceedings of the SIGCHI Conference on Human Factors in Computing Systems*, 97–104.

Head, K. J., & Noar, S. M. (2014). Facilitating progress in health behaviour theory development and modification: The reasoned action approach as a case study. *Health Psychology Review, 8*, 34–52.

Kok, G., & Ruiter, R. A. C. (2014). Who has the authority to change a theory? Everyone! A commentary on Head and Noar. *Health Psychology Review, 8*, 61–64.

Lo, S. H., Peters, G. J. Y., & Kok, G. (2012). A review of determinants of and interventions for proenvironmental behaviors in organizations. *Journal of Applied Social Psychology, 42*, 2933–2967.

Mann, T., De Ridder, D., & Fujita, K. (2013). Self-regulation of health behavior: Social psychological approaches to goal setting and goal striving. *Health Psychology, 32*, 487–498.

Metz, G., Peters, G.-J. Y., & Crutzen, R. (2022). Acyclic behavior change diagrams: A tool to report and analyze interventions. *Health Psychology and Behavioral Medicine, 10*(1), 1216–1228.

Monta'flo, D. E., & Kasprzyk, D. (2015). Theory of Reasoned Action, Theory of Planned Behavior, and the Integrated Behavioral Model. In K. Glanz, B. K. Rimer, & K. Viswanath (Eds.), *Health behavior: Theory, research, and practice* (Vol. 5th, pp. 168–222). Jossey-Bass.

Morgan, D. L. (2007). Paradigms lost and pragmatism regained: Methodological implications of combining qualitative and quantitative methods. *Journal of Mixed Methods Research, 1*, 48–76.

Murad, M. H., Asi, N., Alsawas, M., & Alahbad, F. (2016). New evidence pyramid. *BMJ. Evidence-Based Medicine, 21*, 125–127.

Nalukwago, J., Alaii, J., Van den Borne, B., Bukuluki, P. M., & Crutzen, R. (2018). Application of core processes for understanding multiple concurrent sexual partnerships among adolescents in Uganda. *Frontiers in Public Health, 6*, 371.

Newby, K., Crutzen, R., Brown, K., Bailey, J., Saunders, J., Szczepura, A., Hunt, J., Alston, T., Sadiq, S. T., & Das, S. (2019). An intervention to increase condom use among users of chlamydia self-sampling websites (Wrapped): Intervention mapping and think-aloud study. *JMIR Formative Research, 3*, e11242.

Noar, S. M. (2005). A health educator's guide to theories of health behavior. *International Quarterly of Community Health Education, 24*, 75–92.

Peters, G.-J. Y. (2014). A practical guide to effective behavior change: How to identify what to change in the first place. *The European Health Psychologist, 16*, 142–155.

Peters, G.-J. Y., & Crutzen, R. (2017). Pragmatic nihilism: How a theory of nothing can help health psychology progress. *Health Psychology Review, 11*, 103–121.

Rosenthal, J. A. (1996). Qualitative descriptors of strength of association and effect size. *Journal of Social Service Research, 21*, 37–59.

Ruiter, R., & Crutzen, R. (2020). Core processes: How to use evidence, theories, and research in planning behavior change interventions. *Frontiers in Public Health, 8*(June), 1–8. doi: 10.3389/fpubh.2020.00247

Ruiter, R. A. C., Massar, K., Van Vugt, M., & Kok, G. (2013). Applying social psychology to understanding social problems. In A. G. de Zavala & A. Cichocka (Eds.), *Social psychology of social problems: The intergroup context* (pp. 337–362). Palgrave MacMillan.

Rutherford, B. R., Cooper, T. M., Persaud, A., Brown, P. J., Sneed, J. R., & Roose, S. P. (2013). Less is more in antidepressant clinical trials: A meta-analysis of the effect of visit frequency on treatment response and dropout. *Journal of Clinical Psychiatry, 74*, 703–715.

Sheeran, P., Abraham, C., & Orbell, S. (1999). Psychosocial correlates of heterosexual condom use. *Psychological Bulletin, 125*, 90–132.

Skinner, C. S., Tiro, J., & Champion, V. L. (2015). The health belief model. In K. Glanz, B. K. Rimer, & K. Viswanath (Eds.), *Health behavior and health education: Theory, research, and practice* (5th ed., pp. 131–167). Jossey-Bass.

Strack, F., & Deutsch, R. (2004). Reflective and impulsive determinants of social behavior. *Personality and Social Psychology Review, 8*, 220–247.

Svihla, V. (2021). Generating ideas. In J. K. McDonald & R. E. West (Eds.), *Design for learning: Principles, processes, and praxis*. BYU Open Textbook Network. https://open.byu.edu/id/generating_ideas

CHAPTER 3

BEHAVIORAL THEORIES USED IN HEALTH PROMOTION

Overview

The purpose of Chapters 3 and 4 is to describe some of the prominent theories for understanding health education and promotion-related problems and guiding the design of health promotion programs. Both chapters describe theories that can help predict or explain health-related behavior, including the social and physical environments related to the behavior and the environmental conditions that affect health directly. In this chapter, we review theories that help explain or change the health-related behavior of the at-risk or target population as well as the behavior of individuals who are responsible for conditions in the environment that affect health.

In Chapters 3 and 4 we provide brief reviews of selected theories to give the reader an overview of the use of theories in understanding and changing behavior at the individual and higher-order ecological levels. The overviews of theories in the chapters provide a basis for understanding them. Nevertheless, we recommend that planners delve further into theories by consulting the references provided and searching for applications of the theory using the topic and concept approach described in the Core Processes (see Chapter 2).

An understanding of theoretical frameworks and constructs applicable to health promotion can broaden the planner's ability to complete the planning tasks. Table 3.1 presents some uses of theory in health promotion planning and examples of theories for each use.

Moreover, theories often link different ecological levels. For example, Social Cognitive Theory (Luszczynska & Schwarzer, 2020) includes determinants from the social and physical environments, and the Theory of Planned Behavior (and other approaches to explain reasoned behavior) has a person's perception of the normative expectations of others (in the environment) as a key

Table 3.1 Examples of When to Use Theory in Intervention Planning

Task	Examples
Describing the at-risk and target group members	Stage theories Diffusion of Innovations Theory Stakeholder theory
Understanding the risk and health-promoting behaviors	Theories of self-regulation Self-Determination Theory Diffusion of Innovations Theory
Understanding the risky and health-promoting environmental conditions	Social Cognitive Theory Theories of social support Organizational development theories
Describing possible determinants of both health-promoting and healthful behavior and environments	Reasoned Action Approach Social Cognitive Theory Health Belief Model Diffusion of Innovations Theory
Finding methods to promote change in the determinants, behavior, and environmental conditions	Communication-persuasion matrix Goal-Setting Theory Social Cognitive Theory
Identifying relevant program adopters, implementers, and maintainers, describing determinants of program adoption and implementation, and identifying methods for promoting program use	Diffusion of Innovations Theory Reasoned Action Approach Interactive systems framework Consolidated Framework for Implementation Research

predictor of behavior (Ajzen & Schmidt, 2020; Fishbein & Ajzen, 2010). In addition, many theories are potentially applicable to all ecological levels. The Theory of Planned Behavior, for example, is often applied to individual health behavior (Godin & Kok, 1996) but can be applied to explain the behavior of environmental agents, such as politicians or clinicians (Flynn et al., 1998; Gottlieb et al., 2003;) and program implementers as well (Paulussen et al., 1995; Williams, 2015). Also, some theories are primarily explanatory (e.g., Protection Motivation Theory); some are primarily about methods of change (e.g., Goal-Setting Theory); and others have elements of both types (e.g., Social Cognitive Theory). Explanatory theories suggest what needs to change; theories of change ideally tell how to change it. In practice, the jump from objectives about what to change to methods for creating change may sometimes be difficult. If applicable, in the current chapter, we first present the theory's contribution to understanding behavior and then its contribution to change.

We start by arguing for the importance of an ecological understanding of health problems and their solutions. We encourage planners to refrain from approaches that use single theories when developing multilevel programs and instead use a variety of theories to enhance their practice. We also encourage planners to consider the cultural relevance of theories and understand that different theories share common constructs. The remaining part of this chapter covers major behavior-oriented theories used in health promotion, in which understanding and changing human behavior at the individual level are the processes of interest. In Chapter 4, the focus is on environment-oriented theories, in which understanding and changing environmental conditions for health at higher-order ecological levels are the major processes of interest.

Eclectic Use of Theory

Several authors have described the limitations of current theories, including how they have been used in epidemiological research and intervention design (Head & Noar, 2014; Moore & Evans, 2017; Resnicow & Page, 2008; Resnicow & Vaughan, 2006; Sniehotta et al., 2014). Others have argued that increasing the sophistication of our models and measurement will show the usefulness of our current behavioral theories (Ajzen, 2015; Baranowski, 2006; Brug, 2006; Kok & Ruiter, 2014). Theories of human behavior and environmental change provide a basis for understanding and predicting behavior change and designing interventions. However, we encourage planners to break away from their habitual single-theory approaches and use a variety of theories to enhance their practice. One theory will never explain all aspects of real-life problems; multitheory approaches encourage the planner to consider the complexity of health problems and multilevel interventions (Schaalma & Kok, 2009; Ruiter & Crutzen, 2020; see also Chapter 2).

The use of various theories when planning behavior change allows planners to focus on different aspects of the behavior or the behavior change. Some theories are especially relevant for identifying the determinants of behavior (e.g., Reasoned Action Approach, Dual-Systems Models); others are more useful in choosing and applying behavior change methods (e.g., Social Cognitive Theory, Goal-Setting Theory). The unique skill of the well-trained behavioral scientist is to identify useful theories to address relevant elements of a given problem (Buunk et al., 2021; Crosby & Noar, 2010; Ruiter & Crutzen, 2020), which emphasizes the requisite of including behavioral scientists and their unique expertise in an intervention planning team (Kok, 2014).

Multilevel Interventions

Intervention Mapping acknowledges that human behaviors happen within complex ecological systems. Research continues to recognize the environmental influences that shape opportunities for health and healthy living. For example, longitudinal research shows that one's 'place of residence' may be more important than one's genetic code for predicting health outcomes (Chetty et al., 2016). The National Institute on Minority Health and Health Disparities has developed a research framework that reflects a variety of domains and levels of influence on health outcomes and encourages the consideration of such influences in identifying and addressing health disparities (see Table 3.2).

Table 3.2 The National Institute on Minority Health and Health Disparities Research Framework

		Levels of Influence[a]			
		Individual	**Interpersonal**	**Community**	**Societal**
Domains of Influence *(Over the Lifecourse)*	**Biological**	Biological Vulnerability and Mechanisms	Caregiver–child interaction Family Microbiome	Community Illness Exposure Herd Immunity	Sanitation Immunization Pathogen Exposure
	Behavioral	Health Behaviors Coping Strategies	Family Functioning School/Work Functioning	Community Functioning	Policies and Laws
	Physical/Built Environment	Personal Environment	Household Environment School/Work Environment	Community Environment Community Resources	Societal Structure
	Sociocultural Environment	Sociodemographics Limited English Cultural Identity Response to Discrimination	Social Networks Family/Peer Norms Interpersonal Discrimination	Community Norms Local Structural Discrimination	Social Norms Societal Structural Discrimination
	Health Care System	Insurance Coverage Health Literacy Treatment Preferences	Patient–Clinician Relationship Medical Decision-Making	Availability of Services Safety Net Services	Quality of Care Health Care Policies
Health Outcomes		**Individual Health**	**Family/Organizational Health**	**Community Health**	**Population Health**

[a] Health Disparity Populations: Racial and Ethnic Minority Groups (defined by OMB Directive 15), People with Lower Socioeconomic Status, Underserved Rural Communities, Sexual and Gender Minority Groups, People with Disabilities
Other Fundamental Characteristics: Sex and Gender, Disability, Geographic Region / U.S. Department of Health and Human Services / Public domain.

Individuals live and work in many different kinds of environments at the interpersonal, organizational, community, and societal levels (Kok et al., 2008). Changing people's health behaviors therefore also involves changing the relevant environmental conditions where people live, learn, work, pray, and play (CDC, 2022). These settings are often not under the control of the individual but are shaped by agents or decision makers (e.g., a line manager). Thus, changing an environmental condition for health purposes means changing the behavior of the *environmental agent.* Environmental agents might be addressed with individual-level behavior change methods or, if they belong to a decision-making body such as a board of education or city council, be addressed with organizational change or community development methods (discussed in Chapter 4) (Kok, 2014; Kok et al., 2015; Ruiter et al., 2020).

Intervention Mapping incorporates both individual- and environmental-level change to affect factors influencing health from multiple levels within an ecological system. Not only should health promotors understand a health problem, including behavioral causes, environmental conditions, and their determinants, but they should also make an informed choice of the appropriate ecological level(s) of intervention, including the relevant theories that can help understand how the environment influences behaviors (or health outcomes directly) and how to create change in that setting.

Health promoters need to look at the determinants of the behavior of the target population as well as the agents who influence the environmental conditions and of those who bring the program to the targeted population by adopting and using the program (see Chapter 9). Figure 3.1 depicts the determinants of behaviors of individuals at the individual and environmental levels. Using a nutrition example, it illustrates the various influences on the behavior of individuals, environmental agents, and program users at different ecological levels to increase understanding of the determinants and inform future interventions.

At the individual level, the planner might ask: What influences the individual to eat more fruits and vegetables? At higher ecological levels, the question might be: What influences the environmental agent to change

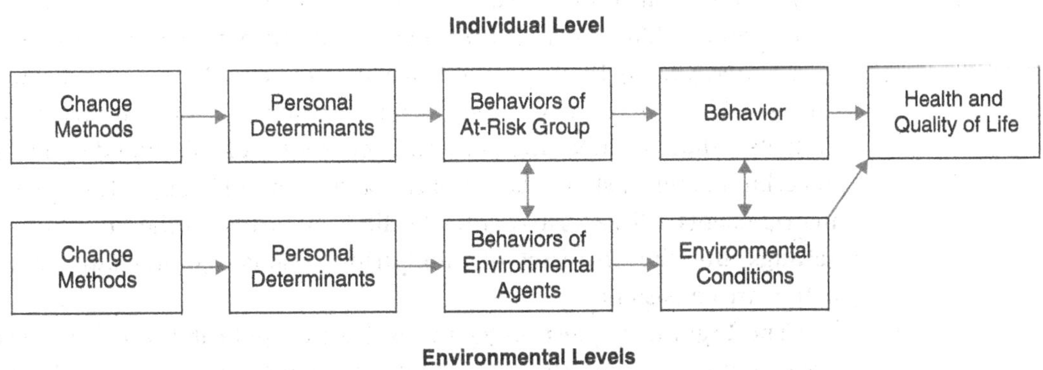

Figure 3.1 Logic Model for Methods, Determinants, Behaviors, Environmental Conditions, and Health

environmental conditions that will facilitate the consumption of more fruits and vegetables? Why, for example, do the decision-making agents at various levels buy fruits and vegetables for the home, purchase or modify healthful foods for the school cafeteria, develop feature articles in the regional newspaper about how families are changing the way they eat for health and well-being, or pass legislation subsidizing healthful school meals for low-income children? As with individual health behavior, personal determinants and environmental conditions influence the agent's decision-making. At higher-order levels, however, complexity increases and different factors come into play. For example, decisions related to environmental changes are often made by individuals within groups, such as school boards or legislatures. Emergent processes unique to each level constrain the behavior of these agents, act within roles (e.g., school principal, medical director, health care provider) with certain expectations and responsibilities, and may be influenced by organizational level factors or social influence (see Chapter 4).

Figure 3.1 presents a logic model for the relationships among theory- and evidence-based change methods, personal determinants, environmental conditions, behaviors, and health. As planners ask the questions pertinent to each step in the model, theories will be one source for answers as planners search for the personal determinants and environmental conditions that influence both beneficiaries' and agents' behavior. Finally, they identify change methods and practical applications that may influence these determinants.

Cultural Relevance of Theories

With respect to applying theories across cultures, our position is that theories are descriptions of processes that can be generalized across cultural groups. However, the weight of different constructs in a theory may vary across cultures in the same way it varies over subpopulations. For example, researchers have used the constructs in the Health Belief Model (HBM) to describe health behavior in various cultures, even though the relative importance of the variables may differ from culture to culture (Champion & Skinner, 2008). Likewise, self-efficacy expectations may vary across groups for a specific behavior and yet still predict behavior change. The role models used in interventions—a surface structure variable—should reflect the cultural background of the intended audience, but modeling should be a useful change method in any culture. Self-management of diseases may also take different forms in different cultural settings, but the processes of monitoring, evaluating, and moving to action are consistent.

The argument questioning the universal applicability of theories across cultures, especially among individuals impacted by social determinants of health, stems from the recognition of the profound influence of cultural context and social factors on health behaviors and outcomes. While theories may offer general frameworks, their application across diverse cultural contexts warrants scrutiny. However, finding specific elements that are not part of a general theory does not in itself invalidate the usefulness of the theory (see also Fishbein, 2000). The challenge is in determining the content and application of selected theories through systematic analyses among intervention groups and not in deciding whether the use of theory in general is advantageous or having specific theories for specific contexts (Ajzen, 2015; Kok & Ruiter, 2014). Examples of such systematic analyses are belief elicitation studies to learn about the outcome expectations that inform people's attitude toward recommended action (Fishbein & Ajzen, 2010) and learning about the context-specific application of theoretical principles underlying change methods.

Questioning the universal applicability of theories across cultures, particularly among populations affected by social determinants of health, highlights the need for culturally relevant and context-specific approaches to health promotion and intervention. By acknowledging the diversity of human experiences and addressing the complex interplay of cultural and social factors, we can develop more effective programs to improve health equity and outcomes for all.

Theories and Common Constructs

Many of the theories we discuss in this chapter and Chapter 4 have similar constructs but use different names for them. Some attempts to come to an agreement regarding important theoretical constructs across theories include the 2001 initiative in which five major behavioral science theorists (Albert Bandura, Marshall Becker, Martin Fishbein, Frederick Kanter, and Harry Triandis) agreed on a set of eight variables as key personal determinants of behavior (Committee on Communication for Behavior Change in the 21st Century: Improving the Health of Diverse Populations, 2002; Fishbein et al., 2001).

1. The person has formed a strong positive intention (or made a commitment) to perform the behavior.
2. No environmental constraints make it difficult for the behavior to occur (barriers).
3. The person has the skills necessary to perform the behavior.
4. The person believes that the advantages of performing the behavior outweigh the disadvantages (attitude).
5. The person perceives more social (normative) pressure to perform the behavior than not to do so.
6. The person perceives that performing the behavior is more consistent than inconsistent with his or her own self-image (personal norms, personal standards).

7. The person's emotional reaction to performing the behavior is more positive than negative.
8. The person perceives that he or she has the capability to perform the behavior under a number of different circumstances (perceived self-efficacy, perceived behavioral control).

The five theorists saw the first three constructs as necessary and sufficient to determine behavior and the remaining five as influencing the strength and direction of behavioral intention. Many of these variables have different names in different theories (see Noar & Zimmerman, 2005; Sheeran et al., 2016). When we discuss a theory, we point out similar or related constructs from other theories.

Overview of Behavioral Theories

Learning Theories

Learning theory is the foundation of most behavioral science theories. Learning refers to any enduring change in the way an organism responds based on its experience (Kazdin, 2012; Robbins et al., 2001). Learning theories assume that experiences shape behavior and that learning is adaptive. Two major learning theory perspectives are classical conditioning and operant conditioning (McSweeney & Murphy, 2014).

Classical Conditioning

Classical, or Pavlovian, conditioning is the learning of an association between a biologically relevant (appetitive or aversive), unconditioned stimulus (US), and a neutral, conditioned stimulus (CS) (Gottlieb & Begej, 2014). A US produces an unconditioned response (UR), which is a response that does not have to be learned (e.g., pleasure as a result of drinking coffee). A conditioned response (CR) is a learned response that follows the CS (e.g., time) when people learned to associate the CS with the US (e.g., drinking coffee).

Attitudes toward a stimulus (CS) may become more positive or negative when that stimulus is spatiotemporally paired with an appetitive or aversive stimulus, or evaluative conditioning. For example, women with high body concern completed a conditioning procedure in which pictures of their own bodies (CS) were selectively linked to positive social feedback: smiling faces (US) (Martijn et al., 2010). The result was an increase in body satisfaction, compared with a control group not learning this specific CS–US association.

Operant Conditioning

Like classical conditioning, operant conditioning is a form of associative learning in which a behavioral act becomes associated with its outcome:

reward or punishment resulting in more or less frequent occurrence of the behavior (Murphy & Lupfer, 2014). Receiving a stimulus that is rewarding (e.g., a valued gift) is positive reinforcement and makes a behavior more likely to occur, whereas the removal of an aversive stimulus (e.g., silencing a loud noise) is called negative reinforcement. Punishment, on the other hand, decreases the probability that a behavior will recur either through the application of an unpleasant stimulus (positive punishment) or the removal of a pleasant stimulus (negative punishment).

People learn to discriminate between situations that lead to reinforcement or not and between behaviors that are reinforced immediately vs. delayed (Robbins et al., 2001). People with weak cognitive control will prefer a smaller immediate reward (tasty food) over a large, delayed reward (good health). Therefore, change methods might include helping people develop self-control and skills to follow through with a behavior change. This training should preferably start early in life, as the ability or tendency to delay gratification in early childhood is associated with better life and health outcomes in adolescence and adulthood. The effect of delayed gratification on future behavioral outcomes is particularly strong under conditions where children grow up in supportive home and school environments in which future-oriented decision-making is valued (Michaelson & Munakata, 2020).

Reinforcement

The reinforcing effects of positive feelings form the basis for social cognitive theories such as the Theory of Planned Behavior and Social Cognitive Theory. The basic assumption is that the *perception of* the environmental stimulus rather than the stimulus itself is crucial to learning (Conner & Norman, 2015). Perceptions of environmental stimuli include, for instance, negative and positive evaluations of behavioral outcomes (outcome expectations) and the feasibility of a behavior in a given context (self-efficacy expectations) (Bandura, 1986; Luszczynska & Schwarzer, 2020).

Reinforcement is an effective method to induce changes in various determinants and behavior. Kazdin (2012) suggests that in a behavior modification program, punishment should be avoided because it may result in negative side effects, such as escaping or avoiding the source. Bandura (1986) distinguished among three types of directly applied reinforcement:

Social Reinforcement: Praise from other people

Vicarious Reinforcement: Observation of reinforcement of another

Self-Reinforcement: Giving oneself a reward

Another relevant aspect of learning theory is that people learn behaviors through positive reinforcement, but only slowly learn to inhibit the learned associations through lack of reinforcement (Robbins et al., 2001). Experiencing that an unhealthy behavior sometimes has negative consequences may not have much influence as long as these behaviors sometimes lead to positive reinforcement (e.g., the relaxation pleasure of smoking). Indeed, that is why stopping unhealthy behavior is so difficult (Bouton, 2014).

The association between behavior and its consequences can be weakened but not unlearned (Bouton, 2014). A more effective approach is to learn new associations between recommended behavior and positive outcomes, for example through evaluative conditioning (Martijn et al., 2010) or direct experience (Maibach & Cotton, 1995). Modeling, as a form of indirect experience, is also powerful, especially if it is clear that the model's behavior resulted in a lower risk (negative reinforcement) and improved health or other positive attributes (positive reinforcement).

Repeated Exposure

Learning also occurs in forms other than responses to reinforcing stimuli. For example, people become more positive about stimuli to which they are repeatedly exposed, even if they are not consciously aware of the process. This mere exposure effect is believed to be limited to stimuli to which a person has a relatively neutral attitude at the start (Zajonc, 1980, 2001). Thus, one method to change people's attitudes in a positive direction is to expose them repeatedly to the new behavior or object. For instance, educators could show condoms repeatedly in classroom HIV-prevention education, and parents and teachers could expose children repeatedly to new foods (Nekitsing et al., 2018).

Social or vicarious learning comes from observing and imitating others' behavior. Albert Bandura (1965, 1969) demonstrated observational learning through observation of a role model. The effect of observing people perform the recommended behavior successfully may be stronger when the social model is liked and respected and if the model's behavior is positively reinforced (Bandura, 1977). Many health promotion campaigns have applied observational learning, such as the "This Girl Can" campaign in the United Kingdom, a nationwide intervention to get women and girls moving, regardless of shape, size, and ability (Sport England, 2015). Also, most professional skills training programs and self-management programs include a social learning component either through life role models in self-help groups and work settings or through symbolic models in videos or narratives, mostly targeting change in self-efficacy and outcome beliefs (Luszczynska & Schwarzer, 2020).

Information Processing Theories

Conventional wisdom has long held that giving people information helps them change their behavior and thereby solve health and social problems. However, knowledge alone does not generally lead directly to behavior change; successful communication is a prerequisite for any message that aims for change (McGuire, 1985). A program cannot achieve its goals if the audience is not exposed to or does not understand the message. Successful communication therefore is essential when applying behavior change methods (see Chapter 7).

Ensuring that people acquire knowledge is not always an easy task. Theories of Information Processing, such as Semantic Network Theory (Kintsch & van Dijk, 1978) and Mental Model Theory (Mayer, 1989), provide several concepts that suggest methods for successfully conveying information. Health promoters can incorporate evidence-based principles of information processing to improve the presentation and coherence of textual material to enhance message comprehension (Kools et al., 2004).

Theories of Information Processing are concerned with how information is perceived, stored, and retrieved. Drawing from the Gestalt school of psychology (Koffka, 1935), these theories suggest that the senses perceive information in the context of what people already know. For instance, someone who sees only eyes and a forehead will tend to perceive a face in order to complete the expected pattern. Theorists in perception, learning, and cognition suggest that people use their short-term or "working" memory to complete the pattern.

Working memory is a small "working space," and its effectiveness can be increased by a method called chunking (Garrison et al., 2001; Smith, 2008). A chunk combines smaller pieces of information that have strong associations with one another to create one meaningful unit (Gobet et al., 2001). Chunking is typically employed by expert decision makers (as compared with novices). For example, Dutch chess master and psychologist Adriaan de Groot (1946/1978, as cited in Gobet et al., 2001), introduced chunking to explain the enhanced ability of expert chess players to recall briefly presented positions from a tournament game. Other illustrations of chunking identify relevant sub-behaviors (referred to as performance objectives in Chapter 6) such as "Stop, drop, and roll" for burn prevention and "Stop, look, and listen" for traffic safety.

Text Comprehension

When readers try to comprehend a text, they encode the incoming information by linking concepts to the knowledge they already have (see also Chapter 8). The encoding (comprehension) of a text can take place on a textbase level (memory) and on a situation model level (learning) (Kintsch, 1994; van Dijk & Kintsch, 1983). Textbase comprehension refers to a relatively superficial form of understanding; readers will be able to memorize the text from long-term memory rather literally, without necessarily having a thorough understanding of its content. In contrast, readers who have formed a situation model representation of a text have elaborated on the information by actively integrating it with their prior knowledge. Based on this more extensive representation of the information in the text, learning takes place, and readers will be able to generalize the acquired knowledge to other situations. The use of imagery, the encoding of pictures with concepts to be stored in long-term memory, also improves memory and learning (Wright, 2012). Kools et al. (2006) show that graphic organizers, a graphic representation that conveys important relations between concepts in the text and thus helps in activating relevant knowledge networks, could improve the learning of health education materials substantially.

Elaboration

To enhance learning and memory, learners must add meaning to the material presented to them—they must elaborate. Learners are particularly likely to elaborate if they have the ability to process information (e.g., sufficient time) and are motivated to do so (e.g., message relevance). Elaboration is effective if it helps tie the information together so that it can be consolidated into more durable and stronger memory representations (Bayliss et al., 2015). Methods to encourage effective elaboration include group discussion and rehearsal of information. Contributing to a discussion can increase later recall of its content (Van Blankenstein et al., 2011), and rehearsal of information may help make the information more salient for people (Smith, 2008). Hamilton and Ghatala (1994) related rehearsal to the ancient Greek method of *loci*, in which orators mentally attached parts of long speeches to landmarks on well-known travel routes. One might imagine a patient educator helping a learner memorize a long self-care process by attaching the steps in the procedure to one's daily route. Verbal images or analogies are also helpful for encoding information to long-term memory (cf. Foer, 2011).

Cues

People retrieve information from memory more easily when the memory is a strong one, and they make stronger memories when encoding requires effort as in processes of elaboration and rehearsal. Health promoters can provide cues to help people retrieve relevant information that can influence their decision-making or behavior. For a cue to be effective, it should be present at both the time of encoding and retrieval. For example, for teens who are learning to negotiate condom use, the cues present during learning and practice, such as what the partner says and the situation or setting, should be as similar as possible, for instance through role play, to what teens will encounter when they try to apply the steps of negotiation in the real world (Evans et al., 1991; Godden & Baddeley, 1975; Tulving & Thomson, 1973). Cues work best when people systematically select and provide their own cues and among individuals with high (as opposed to low) working memory capacity (Unsworth et al., 2013).

In the context of health promotion, cues can come in various forms and from different sources, including environmental cues, social cues, and internal cues. Environmental cues are external stimuli in the physical or social environment that prompt individuals to engage in certain health behaviors. For example, seeing signage promoting physical activity in a park may serve as a cue for individuals to exercise. Social cues arise from social interactions, norms, or expectations within a person's social network. For instance, observing friends or family members engaging in healthy behaviors, such as quitting smoking or wearing sunscreen, can serve as powerful cues for individuals to adopt similar behaviors. Internal cues originate from within the individual, such as physical sensations, emotions, or cognitive processes. For example, experiencing symptoms of illness can prompt individuals to seek medical attention or engage in self-care behaviors. In health promotion efforts, leveraging cues effectively can help nudge individuals toward adopting healthier behaviors. By strategically designing environments, messages, and interventions to incorporate cues that encourage desired health behaviors, health promoters can facilitate positive behavior change and promote population health.

Theories of Persuasive Communication

Theories of persuasive communication are applicable to any behavior that can be influenced by communication. Persuasive communication typically aims to change attitudes by making appeals to logic and reasoning.

Communication-Persuasion Matrix

A longstanding theory for attitude and behavior change is McGuire's (1985, 2001) Communication-Persuasion Matrix (CPM). The model outlines seven steps of effective persuasion with four communication variables in a matrix. The first steps posit that successful communication should result in the receiver's attention and comprehension. The subsequent steps refer to the receiver's changes in attitudes, social influences, self-efficacy, and behavior, while the last step refers to the maintenance of the behavior change. Choices related to the communication variables (i.e., message content, program audience, communication channels, and message source) depend on the step that is addressed. For instance, statements by famous sports heroes may attract a lot of attention but may have negative effects on self-efficacy if the individual cannot match the skills or capacities of the person delivering the message. According to the CPM, every method that uses communication must go through all the steps for successful communication in order to be effective. Pretesting of educational materials should also apply these steps and in practice, most of them do (US Department of Health and Human Services, Office of Cancer Communications, National Cancer Institute, 2002).

Cultural Similarity

The CPM may be applied to analyze the role of cultural factors in health communication. Kreuter and McClure (2004) addressed message source, context, and communication channel because these aspects are modifiable by communication developers. Cultural similarity between source and receivers leads to greater message recall and favorable attitudes, especially among receivers who identify strongly with the cultural group. With respect to message content, using the preferred language of the intervention group enhances receptivity. Using deep structures such as social-cultural characteristics leads to a more favorable processing of the message. Different cultural groups use different media based on variable needs and contexts for their sense of community, cohesiveness, and culturally relevant information. For example, culturally tailored information on sexual health for minority youth in disadvantaged neighborhoods might use online communities, or "digital neighborhoods," that provide culturally tailored information (Stevens et al., 2016, 2017).

When individuals perceive a cultural affinity or similarity with the source of a message, they are more likely to recall the message and develop favorable attitudes toward it. This is especially pronounced among receivers who strongly identify with their cultural group, as they are more attuned to messages that resonate with their cultural values, beliefs, and norms. Numerous studies have demonstrated the impact of cultural similarity on message recall and attitudes across various domains, including health communication. For instance, a study by Kim et al. (2016) showed that Asian American participants exhibited more positive attitudes toward health messages when they were culturally tailored to align with their cultural identity.

Elaboration Likelihood Model

The basic idea of the Elaboration Likelihood Model (ELM) is that people differ in their ability and motivation for thoughtful information processing. Petty and Cacioppo (1986a, 1986b) explained two ways of processing information: central and peripheral. Central processing occurs when a person carefully considers a message and compares it with other messages and beliefs. Peripheral processing occurs when a person merely acts in response to cues such as communicator attractiveness, mood, and number of arguments rather than the perceived strength of the argumentation.

Similar message characteristics might have different effects depending on the processing route (Chaiken, 1980; Petty & Wegener, 1998). For example, the use of a sports hero as a role model may have a positive effect when receivers process the message through the peripheral route but a negative effect when they follow the central route and realize that their behavioral capabilities are different from those of the sports hero. The same variable, source credibility, may also influence motivation and ability to think, thus shifting people from the peripheral route to the central route or vice versa.

Research findings suggest that thoughtful (elaborate) information processing relates to stronger persistence of attitude change, resistance to counterpersuasion, and consistency between attitude and behavior (Sheeran et al., 2005). Health educators should thus promote thoughtful information processing as much as possible. The ELM suggests three ways to do this: making the message personally relevant, unexpected, and repeated; allowing self-pacing, environments without distractions, and the use of language that people easily understand; and instructing recipients to process the message carefully (Petty & Wegener, 1998). When the intervention group has the time and the behavioral capability, health promoters can use active learning to promote central information processing—for example, making individuals search for answers to questions they pose or using digital quizzes in classroom settings.

Persuasive Arguments

One of the most widely used intervention methods for attitude change is the presentation of arguments in a persuasive message. Dual process models (Eagly & Chaiken, 1993; Petty & Cacioppo, 1986a, b) predict that high-quality arguments are effective only when the receivers process the message through the central route. A higher number of arguments does not ensure quality and, in fact, may negatively affect attitude change (Petty & Wegener, 1998). A greater number of arguments may be convincing for people who process the information through the peripheral route, but they will be less convincing for people who process through the central route. Empirical studies have identified the following characteristics that determine argument strength, that is, their effectiveness in changing people's attitude after careful processing (Kok, 2021; Petty and Wegener, 1998; Vinokur & Burnstein, 1978):

- Expectancy Value: People like outcomes that are likely and desirable and avoid outcomes that are unlikely and undesirable.
- Causal Explanations: A causal explanation will convince receivers of the likelihood of the outcome.
- Functionality: Arguments that match the way people look at the world are more convincing.
- Importance: The relevance of outcomes determines the argument's effectiveness.
- Novelty: An unfamiliar or unique argument has more impact than a familiar argument.

Health promoters may use carefully crafted persuasive arguments at the individual level to encourage people to adopt healthful behaviors, and they may use them to influence agents at higher ecological levels. For example, viewing a television broadcast on the health consequences to children from environmental tobacco smoke may influence a mother to declare her home smoke-free. Seeing other legislators receive media attention for promoting a healthy policy may lead legislators to vote for health legislation. The receivers must both expect positive health outcomes and value the outcomes for persuasion to be effective. For example, a city council must be persuaded that fluoridation prevents dental caries (the outcome expectation) and that this is something to value because of its effect on children's health (the outcome expectancy).

Theories of Health Behavior

Historically, a number of theories have focused directly on health and risk-related behavior (Conner & Norman, 2015; Hagger et al., 2020a). Most of these models are based on psychological expectancy theory, which hypothesizes that human behavior depends mainly on the value individuals place on a particular goal and their estimate of the likelihood that a specific action will achieve that goal. With respect to health, the components are typically the desire to avoid illness or to get well and the belief that a specific behavior will prevent or reduce illness and promote health.

Health Belief Model

HBM has been widely used across a range of health-related contexts (Orbell et al., 2020). The original HBM comprises the following four psychological constructs (Janz & Becker, 1984): perceived susceptibility, perceived severity, perceived benefits, and perceived barriers. Individuals decide to engage in a health action based on their perceptions of personal susceptibility to, and the severity of, a particular condition balanced against perceived benefits and barriers ascribed to taking the action. This decision-making is triggered by a cue to action, which may be internal (e.g., symptoms of a disease) or external (e.g., a health education message).

Although an impressive body of research findings has linked HBM dimensions to health actions other factors that were not originally part of the model have been incorporated to strengthen its explanatory value. These additions include recognizing that perceptions of barriers and benefits are not always health-related (Ajzen, 1988) and the impact of social influences and behavioral control/self-efficacy (Conner & Norman, 2015; Fishbein & Ajzen, 2010). Later applications of the model have incorporated self-efficacy specifically and the role of social influences more generally (Orbell et al., 2020). For recent examples of applications of the HBM to the Covid-19 pandemic, see Mirzaei et al. (2021) and Rukchart et al. (2024)

Protection Motivation Theory

Protection Motivation Theory (PMT) includes the same basic ingredients as the HBM (Orbell et al., 2020; Ruiter et al., 2001), but focuses on mediating cognitive processes (threat appraisal and coping appraisal) that, together, promote responses to the threat. Threat appraisal includes assessments of threat seriousness and personal susceptibility, whereas coping appraisal involves assessments of the effectiveness of potential responses (response efficacy) and one's ability to undertake these successfully (self-efficacy). Together, these appraisals generate protection motivation that is measured as an intention to adopt the protective recommendations (Rogers, 1983). PMT incorporates two additional constructs: rewards or reinforcement associated with maladaptive responses (e.g., smoking and relaxation) and costs or punishment associated with adaptive responses (e.g., not smoking and gaining weight). PMT has been extensively tested (de Hoog et al., 2007; Floyd et al., 2000; Milne et al., 2002). Although the relationship of response efficacy and especially self-efficacy with protection motivation is strong, the relationship of susceptibility and severity is relatively weak (Ruiter et al., 2001, 2014).

Extended Parallel Process Model

Witte (1992) proposed the Extended Parallel Process Model (EPPM) and presented evidence supporting hypotheses generated by EPPM (Witte et al., 2001). As in PMT, EPPM suggests that when people perceive a threat, they initially evaluate a recommended action based on its expected effectiveness and feasibility. If they think the recommended action is effective and feasible, then they formulate intentions to perform the action. However, if they think the recommended action is ineffective or impossible, then the continuing perception of threat causes fear arousal. At this point, they may use fear control processes, such as denial and avoidance coping, resulting in maladaptive responses aimed at controlling unpleasant affective responses rather than approaching the presented health threat (Ruiter et al., 2014; Witte et al., 2001).

Fear Appeal Theory

Fear arousal—vividly showing people the negative health consequences of life-endangering behaviors—has been suggested as a method to raise awareness of risk behavior. Using fear appeals may be intuitively appealing to health educators and policy makers, and research on fear-arousing communication has a long tradition in social psychology and public health education (Peters et al., 2014). The perception of threat, as a result of subjective appraisals of personal susceptibility and severity, motivates an individual to action; however, the type of action taken depends on both outcome expectations and self-efficacy expectations (Peters et al., 2013). For instance, smokers may become afraid of cancer when they recognize their own susceptibility to cancer and the severity of the disease, but they may stop smoking only when they are convinced that quitting is effective in preventing cancer (response efficacy or outcome expectation) and when they feel confident that they are able to quit (self-efficacy). In this example, low self-efficacy may be the most important barrier to quitting for most smokers. What happens when people are afraid but are not convinced of the effectiveness of the alternative behavior or of their own self-efficacy? Most data suggest that under those conditions, the resulting behavior may be defensive, in essence, oriented toward avoidance of the health-threatening message rather than health-promoting action, especially when the threat is highly personally relevant (Kessels et al., 2010; Kok et al., 2018; Ruiter et al., 2014). In situations in which people are aware of their risk but lack self-efficacy for engaging in a health-promoting alternative, messages should focus on improving self-efficacy (Peters et al., 2013; Ruiter et al., 2014).

Rather than emphasizing the detrimental consequences of unhealthy behavior, health messages may also be framed in terms of the beneficial consequences of healthy behavior. For example, "Getting a Pap test every year may enable you to live longer" (gain frame) may be more effective than a loss frame focusing on risk (de Hoog et al., 2007). A large body of literature has investigated which type of message frame is more effective under which circumstances, however, the evidence for the effects of different frames is weak and inconsistent (O'Keefe & Jensen, 2006, 2007, 2009; van't Riet et al., 2014). Given this inconsistency, Werrij et al. (2012) recommend using a gain frame because such messages are more easily processed by the receiver.

Self-Affirmation Theory

Self-Affirmation Theory has been applied to make people less defensive in the face of threatening health messages (Epton et al., 2015; Harris et al., 2007; Schüz et al., 2013; Sherman et al., 2000; Sweeney & Moyer, 2015). It suggests that threatening information indeed may motivate health-promoting actions, but may also cause defensive reactions because these messages, at least in part, threaten people's self-integrity. Therefore, affirming a person's self-integrity by acts that manifest one's moral or adaptive adequacy, even in domains of self-perception that are unrelated to the health threat, would increase the acceptance of the risk information and motivate engagement with the healthy behavior (Harris et al., 2020). Empirical evidence suggests that self-affirmation increases sensitivity to the self-relevance of health information (Falk et al., 2015; Griffin & Harris, 2011; Kessels et al., 2016), such as a writing exercise in which people record as many of their desirable characteristics as they can think of (Brown et al., 2019; Manke et al., 2021; Zhu & Yzer, 2019). Interestingly, self-affirmation can also be adaptive in contexts that involve self-control (Churchill et al., 2018; Fox et al., 2017) or applied in fields other than health (Cohen & Sherman, 2014; Easterbrook et al., 2021).

Unrealistic Optimism and Risk Communication

One relevant factor in deciding not to act is that people systematically underestimate their own risk, a condition that risk-perception theorists call unrealistic optimism: People think they are less at risk than comparable others (Chapin, 2014; Harris et al., 2008; Shepperd et al., 2013). The main reasons for unrealistic optimism are that people underestimate what techniques others undertake to protect themselves and that they have stereotypes of people who run high risks. To illustrate, adolescents may refrain from condom use because they think that other adolescents have multiple partners whereas they have regular partners, and they think that only adolescents who often change partners are at risk of contracting HIV. Health educators can help make each person's risks clear by making comparisons to an absolute and a normative standard (the risks of others), preferably using undeniable feedback. They should also indicate that risk is a matter of risk behavior rather than of the risk groups to which the person belongs.

There are various methods to effectively communicate risks (Holtgrave et al., 1995). Health educators can, for example, compare risks on the same dimensions (dread, control, catastrophic potential, equity, and novelty) or compare risks with similar dimensional profiles. However, sometimes people become angry when a risk over which they have no control, such as air pollution, is compared to a risk over which they do have control, such as smoking (Visschers et al., 2007). Visschers et al. (2009) summarized the empirical evidence on the effects of risk communication, especially probability information. Their recommendations include the following:

1. Use the same denominator in probability information throughout the risk message.
2. Use step-by-step probability descriptions that are easy to understand and are likely to result in adequate risk estimates.
3. Be careful about presenting relative risk reduction, as this may be mistaken for absolute risk reduction.
4. Take the context of the risk communication into account (setting, frame, and severity).
5. Present both numerical and verbal probability information in a risk message.
6. Use graphs to present probability of harm.

When trying to increase perceived susceptibility for sexually transmitted infections (STIs), scenario-based risk information was the most effective method, especially when people generated their own scenarios and when multiple risk scenarios were provided. When people find it very difficult to imagine the risk situation, scenario information is ignored (Mevissen et al., 2009, 2012). Communicating risk seems to induce defensive reactions (van't Riet & Ruiter, 2013). It is therefore advisable to pilot test messages carefully before using them on a large scale. Personalized probability-based risk information is promising, especially in combination with behavioral recommendations and information tailored to motivation and skills.

Theories of Reasoned Action

The Theory of Reasoned Action (TRA) (Fishbein & Ajzen, 1975), subsequently extended into the Theory of Planned Behavior (TPB) (Ajzen, 1988), has been integrated with other theories of behavior to produce the Integrated

Behavioral Model (IBM) (Fishbein et al., 2001). Further refinement led to recasting the theory as the Reasoned Action Approach (RAA) (Fishbein & Ajzen, 2010), a more parsimonious formulation than the IBM. All of these theories focus primarily on determinants of behavior and can be seen as expectancy-value theories. Although they do not propose specific methods for behavior change, these theories help us understand the constructs (i.e., determinants) that need to be targeted for behavior change (Fishbein & Ajzen, 2010). Research using these theories has almost solely focused on the TPB (Ajzen & Schmidt, 2020).

Theory of Planned Behavior

The TPB has successfully been applied to understand many types of health and other behaviors, such as blood donation (Bagot et al., 2015), helmet use (Brijs et al., 2014), and energy conservation (Abrahamse & Steg, 2011). The TPB postulates that intention, the most important determinant of behavior, is in turn influenced by three constructs: attitude, subjective norms, and perceived behavioral control (Ajzen, 1988; Fishbein & Ajzen, 2010).

Icek Ajzen defines attitude as "the individual's positive or negative evaluation of performing the particular behavior of interest" (Ajzen, 1988, p. 117). The attitude toward a behavior is informed by salient beliefs about that behavior. Each behavioral belief links the behavior to a certain outcome or to an attribute (e.g., "Going on a low-fat diet reduces my blood pressure"). Beliefs are weighed by the evaluations of those outcomes ("Reducing my blood pressure is very good for me"). The aggregate of beliefs and evaluations is theorized to produce a negative or positive attitude toward the behavior (Ajzen & Schmidt, 2020).

Subjective norms (perceived social expectations) are a function of the beliefs that specific groups or individuals (social referents) approve or disapprove of performing a specific behavior and how important that opinion is to them. Beliefs about specific social referents, such as "my partner thinks..." or "my mother thinks..." are termed normative beliefs. Some authors distinguish between social expectations and social pressure, describing the latter as a much stronger influence (de Vries et al., 1995).

Perceived behavioral control (Ajzen, 1988), or self-efficacy (Bandura, 1986), refers to the subjective probability that a person is capable of executing a certain course of action (e.g., "For me to go on a low-fat diet would be [easy versus difficult]"). Related factors can be internal resources such as skills and abilities or external resources and barriers such as time, money, and social support. Ajzen (1988) described perceived behavioral control as influencing behavior through intention, whereas actual behavioral control moderates the intention-behavior relationship. More recently, perceived behavioral control is given a more central role in the model, thus moderating the effects of attitude and subjective norms on intention (Ajzen & Schmidt, 2020).

Interventions using TPB target the behavioral, normative, and control beliefs underlying the determinants of attitude, subjective norm, and perceived behavioral control, respectively. This requires the identification of those beliefs that are important in shaping behavior and also are amenable to change. The CIBER approach (Crutzen et al., 2017) is helpful in this regard (see Chapter 2). The first step, however, is garnering a set of potentially relevant beliefs through elicitation procedures in samples of the target population, typically through the use of qualitative research methods including individual interviews and focus group techniques (Fishbein & Ajzen, 2010). This is then followed by quantitative (often survey) research to determine the relevant contribution of the beliefs in predicting behavioral intention through attitude, subjective norm, and perceived behavioral control. This latter evidence is largely of correlational nature not suggesting though that causal relationships cannot be implied. In a meta-analysis of experimental studies manipulating attitude, subjective norm, and perceived behavioral control/self-efficacy, Sheeran and colleagues showed that changes in attitudinal, normative, and control evaluations with regard to specific behavior resulted in medium-sized changes in measures of intention and small to medium-sized changes in behavior (Sheeran et al., 2016).

Although most often applied at the individual level, the TPB can be applied to other ecological levels as well. For example, investigators used the TPB to examine the voting intentions of state legislators in North Carolina, Vermont, and Texas (Flynn et al., 1998; Gottlieb et al., 2003). Legislators' general attitudes and norms concerning cigarette tax increases were predictive of their intentions to vote for a cigarette tax.

The TPB has also been used to plan the implementation of innovative health education programs. For example, differences in beliefs, perceived social expectations, and self-efficacy were associated with teachers' adoption and implementation of an HIV-prevention program (Paulussen et al., 1994, 1995; Schutte et al., 2014). Diffusion of the innovation was associated with the social influence of colleagues through professional networks, adoption with outcome expectations, and implementation with self-efficacy expectations and moral opinions on sexuality. Surprisingly, knowledge of the effectiveness of the program had no influence on teachers' implementation decisions.

Additional TPB Variables

Some authors have suggested determinants in addition to the three that are currently in the TPB, such as personal moral norms regarding whether they themselves think they should or should not perform a certain behavior (Godin et al., 1997). Personal moral norms related to condom use, for example, are measured as "I personally think I should always use a condom." Another suggested addition is anticipated regret: having people imagine how they would feel after they behaved in a risky way contrary to their own intentions (Koch, 2014). Anticipated regret and other anticipated feelings and emotions (e.g., shame or positive affect) are different from anticipatory affective feelings, as postulated by the risk-as-feelings hypothesis (Loewenstein et al., 2001). Whereas anticipated affective feelings are part of the expected outcomes of behavior in the future, anticipatory affective feelings, such as worry, fear, dread, or anxiety, result directly from thinking about risks and uncertainties. Studies by Janssen and colleagues suggest that affective risk beliefs (i.e., reported feelings about a risk) are more strongly related to health behavior than cognitive risk beliefs (i.e., reported thoughts about a risk; Janssen et al., 2011, 2012, 2014). In general, however, Fishbein and Ajzen have argued that these and other suggested additional variables do not meet the criteria that the variable should consistently add variance to the explanation of intention and action across a wide variety of behaviors (see Fishbein & Ajzen, 2010, p. 282)

Integrated Behavioral Model

The IBM was developed in response to the recognition that different models to explain and predict behavior use similar concepts. An integration of these models can help reduce redundancy across theories while addressing the shortcomings of individual theories (Hagger, 2009). IBM states that behavior is determined in a two-step process in which certain variables determine intention and then another set determines behavior. The two-step idea is also reflected in other theories such as the Information-Motivation-Behavioral Skills model (IMB) (Fisher et al., 2006), Social Cognitive Theory (see Social Cognitive Theory section) (Kelderet al., 2015), as well as the so-called stage models such as the Trans Theoretical Model (DiClemente & Graydon, 2020), the Precaution-Adoption Process Model (PAPM) (Weinstein, 1988), or the I-Change model (de Vries, 2017) that assume that behavior change moves along phases including a premotivational (or awareness), motivational, and post-motivational (or volitional or action) stage (see Stage Models of Behavior Change section).

Reasoned Action Approach

In their book on the Reasoned Action Approach, Fishbein and Ajzen (2010) explained that after their early collaboration on explaining reasoned behavior (not to be confused with rational behavior), both authors independently developed new theoretical ideas and later discovered that those ideas were comparable, resulting in the RAA. Fishbein and Ajzen selected constructs for the new model very carefully, referring back to the discussion in the empirical literature and intended for the RAA to succeed the TPB, although Ajzen in his latest overview seemed to have reverted to the TPB (Ajzen & Schmidt, 2020). In the RAA, behavior is determined by intention, as far as people have actual control over their behavior. Actual control is determined by environmental factors and skills to deal with these factors. Intention is determined by attitude, perceived norm, and perceived behavioral control, which in turn are all determined by salient beliefs (behavioral beliefs, normative beliefs, and control beliefs). Compared with the TPB, the RAA includes the affective part of attitude next to the instrumental component of attitude, the descriptive norm about what others do along with the injunctive norm about what others approve of to form the perceived norm, self-efficacy along with perceived behavioral control to highlight both perceptions of control and confidence in assessing feasibility of the behavior, and environmental constraints to further explain the often reported intention-behavior gap (Webb & Sheeran, 2006).

Changing Intention and Behavior

In the reasoned approach to behavior change, there is a distinction between goals (e.g., avoiding HIV infection), behaviors (e.g., condom use), intentions, and beliefs (Fishbein & Ajzen, 2010). Change is seen as a planned process in three phases: eliciting the relevant beliefs that underlie attitude, perceived norm, and perceived behavioral control/self-efficacy; changing intention by changing these factors; and changing behavior by influencing intentions and increasing skills or decreasing environmental constraints. The basic idea behind selecting any potential change method is that the salient beliefs are the initial focus and therefore measurement of beliefs is important (for a practical guide, see Peters, 2014).

In a project to design an intervention to get people who are about to turn 50 to obtain a colonoscopy, pilot work identified the following four primary beliefs as targets for the intervention (Fishbein & Ajzen, 2010, p. 345):

- My getting a colonoscopy in the next two months would be embarrassing (attitude).
- My getting a colonoscopy in the next two months would be painful (attitude).
- My doctor thinks I should get a colonoscopy in the next two months (perceived norm).
- My health insurance won't cover my getting a colonoscopy in the next two months (perceived control).

Based on these beliefs, Fishbein and Ajzen (2010) suggested that, whatever intervention method one chooses, the essential message should be: "Your getting a colonoscopy in the next two months will be neither embarrassing nor painful, it is recommended by your doctor, and there are ways to have the cost of a colonoscopy paid for even if you don't have health insurance." The message should be formulated at the personal level and should be truthful.

Witte (1995) suggested organizing the results of a determinants analysis into a list of relevant categories (e.g., beliefs, social influences, self-efficacy, and values) and then deciding which determinants need to be changed, which need to be reinforced, and which need to be introduced. For example, in a program for HIV prevention in Hispanic men, the men's belief that condoms were unclean needed to be *changed*; the importance of family values needed to be *reinforced*; and the belief that condoms could prevent HIV infection needed to be *introduced*. Varol et al. (2021) conducted a qualitative and quantitative study to elicit relevant beliefs underlying adherence to COVID-19 guidelines among undergraduate students. They then selected those determinants that showed room for improvement and described how these determinants served as targets for specific behavior change methods to enhance adherence behavior (ten Hoor et al., 2021; Varol et al., 2021a, 2021b, 2022).

Shifting Perceived Norms

The perceived norm is a special case of social influence: the impact of others on people's perceptions and behaviors (Forsyth, 2014). The TPB focuses on the perceived expectations of others, whereas Social Cognitive Theory focuses on vicarious learning or modeling, the observation of the behavior of others, and the RAA combines both types of norms referred to as the injunctive norm and descriptive norm, respectively (Fishbein & Ajzen, 2010). There are several ways to influence the perceived norms in the TPB and RAA. The most obvious way is making peer expectations or peer behaviors visible, provided these norms are supportive of the health-promoting behavior (Mollen et al., 2010). If not, building resistance to social pressure to engage in risk behavior is advised. Resistance to social pressure, for instance, can be seen as a skill. Therefore, methods for changing social influences and for improving self-efficacy are sometimes the same, relating both to self-efficacy and skills. How can we teach people to resist social pressure? A summary of the literature (McGuire, 1985) suggested five methods: training refusal skills, modeling resistance, committing to earlier intention and behavior, relating intended behavior to values, and executing a psychological inoculation against pressure.

Theories of Goal-Directed Behavior

A central tenet of theories of goal-directed behavior is that people hold personal goals that represent desired states or outcomes to be achieved or avoided (Gollwitzer, 1999). Goals are reference points against which people compare current states or outcomes. Theorists distinguish two aspects of goals, goal content and goal process (Locke & Latham, 2019).

For goals to be useful in achieving behavioral change, they must be salient and shielded from other potentially conflicting goals (Stroebe et al., 2013). For instance, Stroebe et al. (2008) described the food intake of dieters as characterized by two conflicting and incompatible goals, eating enjoyment and weight control. Dieters would have to make major efforts to shield their weight control goal against the chronic stimulation of eating enjoyment.

Goal processes follow a sequence: (1) establishment, (2) planning, (3) striving and monitoring, and (4) attainment, revision, and persistence (Austin

& Vancouver, 1996). Gollwitzer (1993) described the sequence as wishing, planning, acting, and evaluating. Theories of goal-directed behavior suggest that successful behavioral changes are the result of these goal-striving processes (not necessarily in a fixed order). In addition, people engage in a series of subgoals in order to attain the overall health goal (see Chapter 6 on formulating performance objectives).

A goal should be behaviorally specific, measurable, and observable (Epton & Armitage, 2020). Goals should therefore be stated in terms of behavior (e.g., exercise behavior and food intake) instead of health outcomes (Strecher et al., 1995). Setting a challenging goal, a goal that is feasible though somewhat difficult, leads to better performance than setting an easy goal or simply urging people to do their best (Locke & Latham, 2019). The positive effect of difficult goals occurs only if a person accepts the challenge, has sufficient goal commitment, experience, and self-efficacy, and experiences few personal and situational constraints. In situations that maximally challenge people's abilities, goal setting is more effective when the task is not too complex. In that case, the health promoter can help the client set subgoals (e.g., not to quit smoking permanently but first to abstain for one week and then set a new goal; Brown & Latham, 2002) including the use of attribution strategies that relate failures to external, unstable, and controllable causes (Epton & Armitage, 2020). Another method is to focus on learning goals—that is, a goal to acquire the requisite skills—as opposed to performance goals (Seijts & Latham, 2005; Seijts et al., 2004).

Goal-Setting Theory

Goal-setting theory describes a method for behavior change involving an action sequence, as described above (Austin & Vancouver, 1996; Locke & Latham, 1990). Goal setting leads to better performance because people with goals exert themselves to a greater extent, persevere in their tasks, concentrate more, and develop strategies for carrying out the behavior (Latham & Locke, 2007; Locke & Latham, 1990, 2002, 2019). Goal-setting theory thus helps close what is referred to as "the intention-behavior gap," which arises because people with positive intentions to act often fail to perform the behavior (Sheeran, 2002). For example, de Bruin et al. (2012) studied HIV medication adherence and found that when patients monitored goal progress by keeping track of medication intake, identified discrepancies with their goal, and developed concrete action plans to manage the discrepancies, the intention-behavior relationship was strengthened (de Bruin et al., 2012).

Implementation Intentions

Gollwitzer (1999) distinguishes between goal intentions and implementation intentions. Goal intentions ("I intend to pursue X," as in the TPB) result in a commitment to realize a desire. Implementation intentions ("I intend to initiate behavior X when conditions Y are met") connect goal-directed behavior with an anticipated situation (Sheeran et al., 2005). By forming implementation intentions, people pass the control of the behavior over to the environment (Gollwitzer, 1999). Situations and means are turned into cues to action that are hard to forget, ignore, or miss. For example, when the goal is to effectively regulate one's emotions when going for a mammography, an implementation intention may look like: "As soon as I feel concerned about attending my appointment, then I will ignore that feeling and tell myself this is perfectly understandable." It appears that forming an implementation intention is a conscious cognitive act that has automatic consequences.

Several studies have supported the usefulness of implementation intentions for behavior change (Hagger et al., 2016; Keller et al., 2019). Based on a meta-analysis of 94 studies, Gollwitzer and Sheeran (2006) concluded that forming an implementation intention influences whether people achieve their goals. If-then planning facilitated goal striving no matter what self-regulatory problem was at hand. Forming implementation intentions may also help in goal shielding, in that people can identify cues that may result in relapse and describe adequate responses in advance of exposure (Achtziger et al., 2008).

In a critical empirical and theoretical review, Sniehotta (2009) argued that implementation intentions are most effective in changing behavior if the situational cue is frequent and the behavior appears exclusively in this situation. For many health promotion behaviors, however, the behavior appears in various kinds of situations and not always frequently. Sniehotta (2009) distinguished between action plans that describe goal intention and coping plans that describe how a person will overcome obstacles; interventions that involve both action and coping planning seem to be more efficacious (Kwasnicka et al., 2013; Rhodes et al., 2020).

Theories of Automatic Behavior, Impulsive Behavior, and Habits

Human behavior is largely directed toward attaining goals. These goals can be triggered by cues that are present in physical and social environments (e.g., a safety sign to warn people of the potential risk of falling). Environmental cues trigger behavioral responses that are instrumental in attaining goals. Cues are particularly effective if they are associated with the goal rather than simply predicting the instrumental response needed for goal attainment, and if the goal has high personal value (Qin et al., 2021).

Much of health promotion research and theory is based on the assumption that people are consciously and systematically processing information to interpret their world and to plan and engage in courses of action. In contrast, social psychologists argue that most of our moment-to-moment psychological life occurs through nonconscious means following a learning process in which environmental cues become associated with goal-relevant behavior (Chartrand & Bargh, 1999; Custers & Aarts, 2010;

Hassin et al., 2005). Take the case of priming, in which people are exposed to a stimulus—often subconsciously—and later their actions are congruent with the stimulus. For example, in one series of studies, participants were invited to a behavioral laboratory and seated either in a cubicle that contained a hidden bucket with lukewarm water mixed with citrus-scented all-purpose cleaner or in a cubicle in which no scent was diffused. Participants previously exposed to the cleaning scent showed greater cognitive access to cleaning-related words and activities in experimental tasks than those assigned to the control condition (Holland et al., 2005).

Goal-directed behavior may start consciously but may become automatic over time, as in habit formation such as driving a car (Verplanken, 2018). Automatic behavior, as Chartrand and Bargh (1999) pointed out, is a necessity for living. If all life's simple decisions and actions involved deliberate thought, people would simply not have enough time and resources for the demands of daily life. Because a large part of behavior is conducted on automatic pilot, people are, for instance, able to do two things at the same time (driving and talking to your passenger).

Attitudes can also be activated automatically, without a person's being aware (Fazio, 2001). Exposure to an attitude object, such as a cockroach or baby, may evoke a negative or positive automatic evaluative reaction that subsequently influences how a person categorizes objects or people (e.g., dirty, lovely). When a person later encounters members of the category, the related knowledge and attitudes may be activated and influence behavioral responses. A good example of this is stereotyping, in which people assign a person to a group, access knowledge about that group, and then enact prejudice and discrimination toward the person (Devine, 1989).

Impulsive Behavior: Dual-Systems Models

Dual-systems models explain social cognitions and behavior as a joint function of two interconnected mental faculties that operate according to different principles. The Reflective-Impulsive Model (RIM) is an example of dual-systems models (Deutsch & Strack, 2006, 2020; Strack & Deutsch, 2004). The RIM distinguishes between a reflective system and an impulsive system. The impulsive system directs behavior by linking perceptual stimuli to behavior based on previously learned associations of pleasure or pain (feelings). With the reflective system, on the other hand, people act based on judgments, decisions, and intentions (cognitions). Together, these two systems result in behavior. The impulsive system is always active, while the reflective system acts on intentions.

Often, health-promoting behavior entails a conflict between feeling and knowing, between the impulsive system and the reflective system. For example, a person may have an urge to smoke even while having an awareness of the negative consequences of smoking. People with strong preferences for snack foods and low inhibitory capacity are more susceptible to the temptations of palatable foods, eat more, and are more often overweight and obese

(Nederkoorn et al., 2010). In the case of conflicting systems, interventions must help people suppress impulses or seek distractions.

Interventions aimed at changing impulsive behavior make use of evaluative conditioning and avoidance training to reduce the hedonic appeal of tempting stimuli (Houben et al., 2010 Wiers et al., 2011), or they may involve making a commitment in which a person pledges in front of others to perform the healthful behavior (Ajzen et al., 2009; Conn et al., 2002).

A dual-systems approach may also explain why adolescents and young adults take more risks than younger or older individuals. Research in developmental neuroscience suggests a temporal gap between puberty, which impels adolescents toward thrill-seeking, and the slow maturation of the cognitive control system that regulates these impulses (Crone & Dahl, 2012). This temporal gap makes adolescence a time of heightened vulnerability for risky behavior in which perceived benefits of risk-taking outweigh perceived risks (Blankenstein et al., 2021). Interventions such as preventing teens from driving in the presence of other teens to reduce crash rates are based on this view (Chein et al., 2011; Ross et al., 2015).

Value-Based Model of Self-Control

An alternative to dual-systems models is the value-based choice model of self-control (Berkman et al., 2017; Berkman, 2018). In this model, self-control is conceptualized as a specific instance of decision-making instead of a battle between conflicting impulses. Self-control is conceptualized as a choice between alternatives, such as, for instance, scrolling through Instagram or studying for an exam. People's difficulty with resisting temptations stems from an information integration process where some types of information, such as the pleasure of reading Instagram posts, are integrated more quickly into the decision-making process than information regarding the positive consequences of acquiring knowledge. When people choose without time to consider all relevant information they may select the most attractive choice in the moment, but one that does not fit long-term (health) goals.

According to the value-based model, the relative attractiveness of different options at the moment is the most proximal determinant of behavior. To promote healthy over unhealthy behaviors, then, it is important that healthy options are considered more attractive than alternative unhealthy options at the moment a choice is made. This may be accomplished by prompts or just-in-time adaptive interventions that point people's attention to the positive aspects of healthy behaviors and the negative aspects of unhealthy behaviors. Furthermore, conditioning or cognitive training can be applied to achieve these goals (Veling et al., 2022).

Training Executive Function

Approaches to impulse control fall within the larger category of executive function, that is, the application of cognitive skills to help plan and implement tasks and to regulate emotions. One method to help people keep their impulses in check is inhibitory control, a top-down mental control that people use when going on automatic pilot or relying on instinct or intuition would be ill-advised, insufficient, or impossible (Diamond, 2013, p. 136). Executive functions involve working memory and cognitive flexibility (e.g., thinking outside the box). Stress, lack of sleep, and loneliness negatively influence executive function (Diamond, 2013).

Executive functions can be trained and improved with practice. For example, executive function in children has been improved by computerized training, interactive games, and martial arts (Diamond & Lee, 2011). The evidence for other approaches, such as aerobics, mindfulness, and yoga, is less strong (Diamond, 2013). In clinical settings, interventions to strengthen response inhibition and working memory have been successful in reducing unhealthy drinking and eating behaviors (Wiers et al., 2013). For all these approaches, the parameters for effectiveness are that the task has to be challenging and that substantial repetition is required (Hofmann et al., 2008). There is also evidence that executive training can change people's evaluations of and preferences for temptations such as food items, smartphone applications, and smoking cues (Chen et al., 2016; Johannes et al., 2021; Najberg et al., 2021; Scholten et al., 2019; Tzavella & Chambers, 2023). For example, participants may consistently respond to some products (e.g., healthy food items) and inhibit responses to other products (e.g., unhealthy food items) depending on the presentation of a go or no-go cue (Veling et al., 2022).

Habits

Habits are a special case of automatic behavior. "Habits are learned sequences of acts that have become automatic responses to specific cues and are functional in obtaining certain goals or end-states" (Verplanken & Aarts, 1999, p. 104). The most prominent characteristics of habits are that they are efficient and occur without much awareness. Habits predict behaviors, especially when individuals repeatedly perform the behaviors and when the habit is strong (Orbell et al., 2020). Habits overrule intentions when the representation of the habitual behavior can be easily accessed from memory (Danner et al., 2008). For example, when people have an intention to eat healthy foods but have a habit of eating fatty foods, their eating pattern will often be unhealthy.

Habits are difficult to change, and they are not particularly influenced by information for two reasons (Verplanken & Aarts, 1999). First, information influences attitude and intentions, but these do not change behavior when they have to compete with a strong habit. Second, people with strong habits are usually not very interested in new information. Therefore, forming new habits may be the best method to change old habits. Wood and Neal (2007) listed possible interventions for habit change. People can break habits after exposure to relevant contextual cues by actively inhibiting the cued response, or people can try to alter or disrupt the exposure to relevant contextual cues. An example of cue altering is to use smaller sizes of plates, spoons, and glasses to reduce the amounts of food and drink that people consume (Sobal & Wansink, 2007). However, individuals' efforts to control habit cueing are only as strong as their self-control resources. Wood and Neal (2007) expected the most success when changes in context occurred naturally as a function of life events, such as changing jobs or moving to a new home, and suggested that interventions to break habits should be directed to people when they are best able to respond. Support for the habit discontinuity hypothesis was found in a study among 800 households in the United Kingdom (Verplanken & Roy, 2016) that showed results only in those households that had moved house in the previous three months.

Nudging

A nudge is a simple change in the presentation of alternatives that makes the desired behavior the easy, automatic, or default choice (Thaler & Sunstein, 2008). The nudge approach advocates libertarian paternalism; it respects freedom of choice (libertarian) but suggests sensible choices (paternalistic) (de Ridder, 2014). Applying nudges requires that health promoters respect the autonomy of the decision maker by encouraging freedom of choice and a sense of awareness and by making the healthy choice easy and attractive. Examples of nudging include increasing the distance to unhealthy food in a buffet spread (Maas et al., 2012) and using floor markers to encourage people to use stairs instead of elevators (van Nieuw-Amerongen et al., 2009). Another useful type of nudge is to make the "opt-in" decision the default one when promoting a voluntary health action such as getting an influenza vaccination shot among health workers (Lehmann et al., 2016). However, such approaches can backfire if participants feel disrespected in their sense of autonomous decision-making. Furthermore, the complexity of health behavior change makes it often necessary to integrate nudging in a broader set of interventions and measures at the individual and environmental levels (van Rookhuijzen & de Vet, 2021)

Stage Theories

Stage theories suggest that people in different stages of behavior change need different methods to help them move through the stages and ultimately change (Weinstein, 1988). People who have decided not to act are a particularly difficult group because they may be well-informed but reject information that challenges their decision. Of various stage models proposed, the Transtheoretical Model of Behavior Change (TTM) (DiClemente & Graydon, 2020; Prochaska & DiClemente, 1982) and the Precaution-Adoption Process Model (PAPM) (Weinstein, 1988; Weinstein et al., 2008) are the most prominent ones. Both models propose stages of change and processes of change and have been used by health promoters to tailor change methods to stages (Prochaska et al., 2015). Researchers have used these models to describe the cessation of addictive behaviors and to predict uptake of health-promoting behaviors.

The TTM describes behavior change in five stages: precontemplation, contemplation, preparation, action, and maintenance. The processes of change include consciousness raising, dramatic relief, environmental reevaluation, self-reevaluation, self-liberation, helping relationships, counterconditioning, contingency management, and stimulus control (DiClemente & Graydon, 2020). Armitage (2009) concluded that critical evaluations of the TTM focus too much on the stages and ignore other aspects of the theory, such as the processes of change. Brug and colleagues (2005) suggested that distinguishing only between two larger stages of motivation is well supported, in essence, precontemplation, contemplation, and preparation on the one hand and action, maintenance, and termination on the other. A more general distinction between two stages of change—motivational stage and volitional stage—receives more empirical support (Gollwitzer, 1999; Keller et al., 2020). Brug and colleagues (2005) added that longer-term behavioral changes need interventions that go beyond health messages to incorporate methods for changing environmental conditions, but few applications of TTM have incorporated environmental determinants.

The PAPM pays more attention to the issue of awareness of the risk and to the difficulty of reaching high-resistant groups compared to the TTM (Weinstein, 1988; Weinstein et al., 2008). The PAPM incorporates determinants and methods for change that other health promotion theories, especially Social Cognitive Theory, support (Bandura, 1997), but can be criticized for the same reasons as the TTM with regard to the idea of stage transitions in the process of behavior change.

Attribution Theory and Relapse Prevention

Attribution theory describes the impact of the way people attribute the outcomes of behavior on their future cognition and behavior (Weiner, 1986). When experiencing successes or failures people have a tendency to look for causes, especially when the events or outcomes are negative and unexpected. Whether people perceive a cause as internal or external, stable or unstable, and controllable or uncontrollable, will influence how people experience different emotions and their motivation to continue or discontinue a behavior that led to the outcome (Weiner, 2018).

Stability is the relevant dimension for the understanding of success expectations for health behavior change. A person attributing a failure to a stable cause (e.g., ability) will have a lower expectancy of success for performing the same task again, as compared with somebody who attributes a failure to an unstable cause (e.g., bad luck). In the case of success, this effect is reversed. Furthermore, attribution theory suggests that lower success expectancy leads to less adaptive task behavior; people will invest less energy in the task at hand. Hospers et al. (1990) found that the success of participants in a weight-reduction program was positively related to the participants' self-efficacy at the start of the program. Self-efficacy was inversely related to the stability of attributions for earlier failures, and both relationships were independent of the number of failures.

One method for changing attributions to improve self-efficacy is attributional retraining, or reattribution (Kok et al., 1992). The health educator or counselor tries to help people reinterpret previous failures in terms of unstable attributions ("You were in a very difficult situation there") and previous successes in terms of stable attributions ("You are the type of person who has been able to stay off cigarettes during your whole pregnancy").

Attributional retraining is often used in attempts to prevent relapse (Marlatt & Donovan, 2005). Relapses are caused when a person lapses in a high-risk situation due to a lack of coping resources. Self-efficacy expectations and perceived skills are relevant not only for new behavior but also for the maintenance of behavior changes. Relapse prevention theory describes the process of lapses, attributions, self-efficacy estimations, coping, craving, emotional states, and successes and failures in maintaining the behavior change. The major distinction between success and failure in a relapse situation is the presence or absence of a coping response in situations that invite or pressure people to take up their risk behavior again (Marlatt & Donovan, 2005). For instance, a worker who has quit smoking goes to the coffee shop, where colleagues are smoking. If the worker has an adequate coping response, she will be more likely to maintain her health-promoting behavior and may develop an even higher estimation of self-efficacy. However, if she does not have an adequate coping response, she may lapse into her earlier risk behavior and experience a sense of failure.

To help people prevent relapse, attribution theory suggests a series of primarily face-to-face or group methods that involve helping the person identify high-risk situations, plan coping responses, and practice the responses until they become automatic (Marlatt & Donovan, 2005). It also suggests reattribution training for incidental lapses so that the at-risk person attributes failure to an unstable and controllable cause.

Theories of Self-Regulation

Self-regulatory concepts explain how individuals adjust their own behavior to achieve a desired outcome (de Ridder et al., 2020; Hofmann et al., 2020; Mann et al., 2013). Creer (2000) argued that self-management, the term used more often in the health domain, and self-regulation, the term used in psychology (Baumeister & Vohs, 2004), refer to the same phenomenon. Self-management is an active, iterative process of observing oneself, making judgments based on observation (as opposed to judgments based on habit, fear, or tradition), setting a goal, choosing strategies, reacting appropriately in light of one's goal, and revising one's strategy accordingly (Clark, 2003). Rothman et al. (2004) have extended the self-management stages to include continuation, maintenance, and habit formation. They also pointed out that the determinants for change and the methods to promote change vary over these stages, comparable to other stage models.

Interventions Based on Self-Regulation

Self-regulatory theory is useful for designating health-promoting behaviors for the self-management of chronic disease. For example, in a family-oriented pediatric asthma self-management program, Bartholomew et al. (2000a) conceptualized both asthma-specific skills (e.g., taking control medications) and self-regulatory skills (e.g., monitoring for symptoms of asthma). Shegog et al. (2013) also used self-regulation models among other theories to develop the Management Information Decision-Support Epilepsy Tool (MINDSET), a tablet-based program to provide real-time self-management decision support to patients living with epilepsy. Another excellent example of interventions based on self-management is the use of monitoring tools in programs to promote therapy adherence with HIV-positive patients (de Bruin et al., 2010, 2017). In general, literature syntheses show positive effects of self-management interventions across different domains of chronic health including type 2 diabetes, blood pressure control, asthma, and depression, with particular interest in eHealth interventions and the use of smartphone applications (Aminuddin et al., 2021; Coorey et al., 2018; Firth et al., 2017; Hodkinson et al., 2020; Odgers-Jewell et al., 2017; Shaw et al., 2020; Sua et al., 2020).

Self-Determination Theory

Self-Determination Theory (SDT) examines the degree to which an individual's behavior is self-motivated or self-determined. SDT studies individual, social, and cultural factors that affect the impetus to act in a particular way in given situations and how in turn personal well-being is affected (Ryan & Deci, 2017). This theory differentiates motivation between individuals who act from a sense of personal commitment toward certain behaviors (autonomous motivation) and those whose behavior is driven by fear or pressure from external sources (controlled motivation), and posits that the two types lie on a continuum of perceived locus of causality. With autonomous motivation, individuals engage in behaviors for interest, enjoyment, satisfaction, or to achieve outcomes that are important to them, whereas with controlled motivations, others' wants and needs are placed above the individual's own needs (Ng et al., 2012). Interventions based on SDT have successfully increased autonomous motivation to achieve positive effects on health (Ntoumanis et al., 2021). A wide range of behavior change methods have been used but no conclusions can be drawn yet on what (combinations of) methods are effective in strengthening autonomous motivation (Hagger et al., 2020b; Reeve & Cheon, 2020; Teixeira et al., 2020).

SDT posits that the three basic needs at the core of human motivation are autonomy (versus control), competence, and relatedness (Deci & Ryan, 2002; Ryan & Deci, 2000). Autonomy requires an environment that enables freedom, agency, initiative, and control over decision-making without burden from external pressures (Ryan & Deci, 2006). Autonomy has been shown to be an important predictor of health-promoting behaviors, as it determines whether decisions and beliefs are internalized and therefore will be sustained in the long term (Ng et al., 2012; Ryan & Deci, 2006). Similar to self-efficacy, competence forms the foundation for self-esteem and self-confidence and involves feelings of being effective in ongoing interactions with one's external environment. Finally, relatedness can be defined as feeling connected to a partner, feeling secure, and having a sense of belonging to a community. When these three needs are met, motivation, well-being, and mental health are enhanced, thus people may feel more efficacious to protect their physical health (Milyavskaya & Koestner, 2011; Ntoumanis et al., 2021; Weinstein & Ryan, 2011). The resulting behavior can be said to be self-determined and is more likely to be continued.

Motivational Interviewing

Motivational Interviewing (MI) is a counseling approach that originated in clinical psychology but has been proven effective also in motivating behavior change in the context of public health (Magill et al., 2018; Pace et al., 2017), with a particular focus on strengthening therapy adherence and motivating people to start treatment (Lawrence et al., 2017; Suire et al., 2021; Zomahoun et al., 2016). MI recognizes that people have different levels of readiness to change and often have ambivalent feelings and emotions about potential change-related decisions. MI works together with clients by helping them develop intrinsic motivation, think about how change may happen, deal with difficulties along the way, and align specific behavior change with personal values (Miller & Rollnick, 2013). MI originated in clinical practice without guidance from an underlying theoretical framework (Miller & Rose, 2009), but empirical evidence is garnered to support MI with theory (Berman et al., 2020). Because of the conceptual overlap in regard to processes of internalization and needs satisfaction, SDT and MI have been linked. An integration of the two frameworks may provide theorists and practitioners with a good, practical theory for both understanding and changing health behavior (Patrick & Williams, 2012; Rutten et al., 2014; Vansteenkiste & Sheldon, 2006).

Social Cognitive Theory

Albert Bandura (1986) developed Social Cognitive Theory (SCT) as an interpersonal theory that covers both determinants of behavior and methods for behavior change (Bandura, 1997; Kelder et al., 2015; Luszczynska & Schwarzer, 2020). SCT explains human behavior as a model of reciprocal determinism in which behavioral, cognitive, and other personal factors interact with environmental events to determine behavior (Bandura, 1986). Major concepts in the model include outcome expectations, outcome expectancies, self-efficacy, behavioral capability, perceived behavior of others, and the social environment.

Outcome Expectations, Self-Efficacy, and Behavioral Capability

An outcome expectation is a person's judgment of the likely consequence of a behavior (e.g., "When I use a condom consistently, I will prevent sexually transmitted infections"). Outcome expectancies, on the other hand, are the values that individuals place on a certain outcome (e.g. "Preventing sexually transmitted infections is something I value") (Kelder et al., 2015). Outcome expectations are comparable to behavioral beliefs and outcome expectancies are comparable to evaluations in the TPB or RAA.

Self-efficacy has been previously defined and is illustrated by perceptions such as "I am confident that I can use a condom consistently." According to Bandura (1986), judgments of one's ability to perform a behavior greatly influence expected outcomes. When a person is in a situation in which outcome expectations are positive and strong but self-efficacy for that behavior is low, a situation of avoidance or denial may occur, and the person is unlikely to attempt the behavior (Bandura, 1986). The concept of behavioral capability, on the other hand, assumes that someone must know about and be able to perform the behavior (necessary skills). Health promotion programs should go beyond simply providing knowledge and develop behavioral capability, which is closer to actual performance. The development of behavioral capability is the result of the individual's training, intellectual capacity, and learning style.

Observational Learning and Environment

According to SCT, most human behavior is learned through observation of models (vicarious learning). By observing others, a person can form rules for behavior and on future occasions, this coded information can serve as a guide for action. Four constituent processes govern modeling (Bandura, 1986):

- Attention to and perception of the relevant aspects of modeled activities (including characteristics of the observer and the model).
- Retention and representation of learned knowledge and remembering.
- Production of appropriate action.
- Motivation as a result of observed positive incentives and reinforcement.

When providing models to encourage the learning of certain behaviors, the health educator should find a role model from the community or at-risk group with whom participants are likely to identify. The model should represent coping behavior (e.g., "I tried to quit smoking several times and was not successful. Then I tried again ... Now I have been off cigarettes for ...") rather than mastery (e.g., "I just threw my pack away, and that was it"). Learners should be able to observe models being reinforced for their behavior (e.g., being congratulated by friends for staying off cigarettes or having a partner say how fresh the ex-smoker smells).

In addition to focusing on individuals, planners should focus on creating environments that facilitate health-promoting change. The social environment includes family members, peers, and neighbors, while the physical environment includes the availability of certain foods, indoor and outdoor air quality, restrictions for smoking, and so on. All learning has to be facilitated by the provision of means to take action or to reduce barriers (Bandura, 1986; Mullen & DiClemente, 1992; Mullen et al., 1985). For instance, a program that targets improvement in drug users' self-efficacy for using clean needles must also facilitate access to clean needles. Keeping the concept of reciprocal determinism in mind will help planners avoid the common pitfall of underusing the environment.

SCT and Behavior Change

SCT integrates determinants of behavior with methods for behavior change (Clark & Zimmerman, 2014; Luszczynska & Schwarzer, 2020; Stacey et al., 2014). All SCT interventions are based on active learning that promotes performance during the learning process. Perceived behavior of others is not only a determinant of behavior but also a very effective method for behavior change through modeling. Reinforcement is a general method of SCT and may be external (such as receiving money) or internal (such as doing something that one perceives as right). Modeling, in which a person experiences vicarious reinforcement, is a special case of reinforcement. A person may experience vicarious reinforcement by observing a model receiving reinforcement. Self-efficacy and behavioral capability may be improved through the following (Bandura, 1997):

- Enactive mastery experiences (enabling the person to succeed in attainable but increasingly challenging performances of desired behaviors).
- Vicarious experiences (showing the person that others like that person can do it, including detailed demonstrations of the small steps taken in the attainment of a complex objective).
- Verbal persuasion (telling the person that he or she can do it, strong encouragement can boost confidence enough to induce the first efforts toward behavior change).
- Improving physical and emotional states (making sure people are well rested and relaxed before attempting a new behavior).

Relevance, tailoring, and individualization have all been shown to be effective basic methods in health education interventions, and they can be traced to a number of theories, especially SCT. Adapting the program to the knowledge, beliefs, circumstances, and prior experience of the learner, as assessed by pretesting or other means, can increase relevance. Computer programs enable one to tailor interventions to measured characteristics of the individual, such as beliefs, attitude, and self-efficacy (Peels et al., 2013; Portnoy et al., 2008). Tailoring the message to the salient beliefs of the intervention group increases people's motivation and ability to process the message carefully, thereby increasing the chance of persistent changes in attitudes and behavior (Kessels et al., 2011; Ruiter et al., 2006). Tailoring effectiveness may be further increased if tailored support is delivered at the exact time of need, referred to as Just-in-Time Adaptive Intervention (JITAI) (Wang & Miller, 2020).

Individualization can involve the provision of opportunities for learners to have personal questions answered or instructions paced according to their individual progress, or it may include the ability to offer instruction that is geared to the specific needs and disease characteristics of the target group. For example, the Watch, Discover, Think, and Act asthma computer application individualizes instruction to each child's asthma triggers and symptoms based on information the child enters (Bartholomew et al., 2000a, 2000b).

Theories of Stigma

Stigmatization is a socially and culturally constructed process by which a person is labeled as different and then devalued, resulting in status loss and discrimination (Link & Phelan, 2014; Pescosolido & Martin, 2015). As such, stigmatization reproduces social inequalities and is perpetuated by the exercise of social, economic, and political power (Hatzenbuehler et al., 2013; Herek, 2014; Link & Phelan, 2014; Phelan et al., 2014; Pryor & Bos, 2015). Accordingly, Phelan et al., 2008 have delineated three functions of stigmatization: to keep people "down" through domination or exploitation, to keep people "in" through norm enforcement, and to keep people "out" as a form of disease avoidance. Stigmatization takes many forms (e.g., avoidance, blame, exclusion) and is prevalent across a number of identities and conditions including, but not limited to, sexual orientation, gender identity, substance use, mental illness, HIV, leprosy, and physical and intellectual disabilities (Stutterheim & Ratcliffe, 2021).

Understanding Stigma: The Theory

According to Bos et al., 2013, there are four types of stigma: public stigma, self-stigma, structural stigma, and stigma-by-association. Public stigma represents people's cognitive, affective, and behavioral reactions (i.e., discrimination or enacted stigma) to people with a stigmatized identity or condition, and manifests on an interpersonal level. Self-stigma is the anticipation (i.e., anticipated stigma) and internalization (i.e., internalized stigma) of society's negative beliefs about the stigmatized identity or condition and occurs on an intrapersonal level. Structural or institutional stigma is the legitimatization and perpetuation of a stigma by society's institutions and ideological systems through, for example, policy and legislation, and occurs at the organizational, institutional, or societal levels. Lastly, stigma-by-association entails social and psychological reactions to people associated with a stigmatized person (e.g., family and friends) as well as the impact of being connected to a person with a stigmatized identity or condition, and can be considered analogous to courtesy stigma (Goffman, 1963). The four types of stigma are interrelated in that public stigma underlies the other three types; the consensual understanding that an identity or condition is devalued (public stigma) leads to anticipated negative reactions and the internalization of society's negative beliefs in people with a stigmatized identity or condition (self-stigma) and/or their associates (stigma-by-association).

From a social cognitive perspective, the process of stigmatization comprises thoughts in the form of stereotypes, emotional reactions in the form of prejudice, and behavior in the form of discrimination. Determinants can thus be ascertained by looking at the beliefs embedded in stereotypes. For example, Dijker & Koomen, 2003 outlined three features of stigma (seriousness, responsibility, and negative valence of behavioral cause) and their impact on emotions (anxiety, [lack of] pity, and irritation) that can contribute to stigmatization. Bos et al. (2008) later adapted this model and applied it to HIV. They claimed that four features of, or beliefs about, HIV lead to emotions that, in turn, yield stigmatization. The four features are contagiousness, seriousness, personal responsibility, and norm-violating behavior, and the posited emotions are fear, anger, and (lack of) pity. When HIV is believed to be highly contagious and very severe, when people with HIV are considered personally responsible for acquiring HIV, and when HIV is associated with behaviors that violate the norms of the majority, stigmatization is highly likely (Stutterheim et al., 2012).

Changing Stigma: Stigma Reduction

There is a broad evidence base supporting a number of public stigma reduction strategies that target those who stigmatize, including interpersonal contact (Allport, 1954; Corrigan et al., 2012; Dickstein et al., 2010; Doley et al., 2017; Maunder & White, 2019; Morgan et al., 2018), empathy induction (Batson et al., 2002), and perspective taking (Todd et al., 2012). These have the capacity to change stereotypes and negative emotional responses to people with a stigmatized identity. Conscious repression of stereotypes is not advised (Paluck & Green, 2009) and interpersonal contact is considered most effective (Corrigan et al., 2015; Griffiths et al., 2014). Additionally, other methods for attitude change can be used to reduce negative affect toward stigmatized people.

For those who experience stigmatization, strategies for reducing self-stigma include planning coping responses (Dobson et al., 2019; Mittal et al., 2012; White Hughto et al., 2015), improving psychological flexibility via Acceptance and Commitment Therapy (Livingston et al., 2012; Masuda et al., 2012), providing counseling or support (Sommerland et al., 2017), and building skills and resilience (Mittal et al., 2012; Pantelic et al., 2019). Many of these strategies lean heavily on psycho-education and/or techniques from cognitive behavioral therapy to debunk myths about the stigmatized condition and to prevent or overcome the internalization of negative beliefs (i.e., public stigma) about people with a given stigmatized identity or condition (Stutterheim et al., 2025).

To change structural stigma, environmental-level theories can be applied to change policy and legislation. This can be applied on various levels such as within organizations or communities or in the context of broader society and governments. Examples of structural change methods that are relevant for structural stigma reduction include media advocacy, agenda setting, timing to coincide with policy windows, and creating and enforcing laws and regulations (Stutterheim et al., 2025).

Diffusion of Innovations Theory

An innovation is an idea, practice, or product that is new to the adopter, which may be an individual or an organization (Brownson et al., 2015). Healthy behavior such as physical activity, cessation of smoking, and use of contraceptives may be innovations for individuals while programs to encourage these behaviors may be innovations in an organization. For example, patient self-management programs may be an innovation in an organization because they change the power relationship between patients and providers.

Everett Rogers's Diffusion of Innovations Theory (DIT) is useful for health promotion because it describes decision-making not only of individuals but also of change agents and program implementers. The DIT can be applied to any new behavior, but in the context of Intervention Mapping, the main focus is on diffusion of a (new) health promotion program. Implementers may be compared to agents in the environment, and the Intervention Mapping steps guide planners to develop a separate intervention for implementation (see Schutte et al., 2014; Chapter 9).

Diffusion is conceptualized as happening in phases; in health promotion programs these are usually dissemination, adoption, implementation, and maintenance (Wiecha et al., 2004).

- Dissemination is the planned strategy to make a program or innovation more widely available.
- Adoption refers to the uptake and commitment to initiate the program or innovation.
- Implementation includes active planned efforts to implement an innovation within a defined setting.
- Maintenance, sustainability, and institutionalization occur with continuance and routinization of the innovation.

Characteristics of Adopters and Innovations

Classic diffusion theory has dealt with the characteristics of both adopters and innovations. Adopters can be segmented into innovators, early adopters, early majority, late majority, and laggards, based on the point in time at which they adopt the innovation. Rogers (2003) proposed that the adoption process follows a normal, bell-shaped distribution that places majority adopters within one standard deviation on either side of the mean, early adopters and laggards two standard deviations away, and innovators three standard deviations away. Innovators are considered venturesome, early adopters are opinion leaders, the early majority are deliberators, the late majority are skeptical, and the laggards are traditional.

Innovations are often communicated through two different channels: media and interpersonal communication. Initially, media increase awareness of the innovation; as people hear about the innovation and begin to adopt it, they talk with others about their interests and experiences. The interpersonal channel thus becomes more important as more members of the population adopt the innovation. More potent outreach and incentives are needed for late adopters and laggards. Thus, for intervention planning, it is important to understand the adopter category of interest (Green et al., 1991; Rogers, 2003).

SCT provides explanations of the psychological mechanisms by which diffusion occurs (Bandura, 1997). For implementers to adopt, implement, and maintain a new program, they must be aware of the program, hold positive outcome expectations and expectancies for it, and have sufficient self-efficacy and behavioral capability for both adoption and implementation. Teachers adopting a new sex education program, for example, must know the program is available, see the benefits of the program for themselves, find the program practical and easy to use, and believe that others appreciate and support their use of the program (Schutte et al., 2014).

Also important to consider are the characteristics of the innovations themselves (Brownson et al., 2015; Rogers, 2003). Some of these characteristics include the following:

- Relative advantage of the innovation compared with what is being used.
- Compatibility with the intended users' current behavior.
- Complexity.
- Observability of the results.
- Impact on social relations.
- Reversibility in case of discontinuation.
- Communicability.
- Required time.
- Risk and uncertainty.
- Required commitment.
- Ability to be modified.

Each of these characteristics of innovation must be considered as either a predictor of or a barrier to adoption and implementation, both in innovation design and in the creation of an intervention to aid diffusion.

DIT suggests methods and applications for achieving objectives (Rogers, 2003). Communication within the community about the innovation is essential for the diffusion process; the health promoter will want to stimulate communication and mobilize social support for the innovation. One effective method to speed this process is the use of mass media to communicate the stories of people who have been successful in adopting the new behavior. These early adopters then serve as role models for the early majority in the intervention community, and then the early majority serve as models for the late majority (see McAlister et al., 1995; van Empelen et al., 2003). Chapter 9 elaborates on the role of planning for dissemination, adoption, implementation, and maintenance of health promotion programs as part of Step 5 in Intervention Mapping.

Summary

The purpose of this chapter is to identify individual-oriented theories and models that are useful for planning health promotion interventions, including three theories at the interpersonal level. We first present learning theories, then theories of information processing; theories of persuasive communication; theories of health behavior; theories of reasoned action; goal-setting theory; theories of automatic, impulsive, and habitual behavior; stage theories; attribution theory and relapse prevention; and theories of self-regulation. Finally, we present SCT, theories of stigma and discrimination, and DIT. Each theory is summarized in terms of its contribution to problem analysis and intervention development.

Discussion Questions and Learning Activities

1. Describe what is meant by an eclectic, or problem-focused, approach to theory, and explain why this approach is useful in planning health promotion programs.
2. Select a theory that explains behavior at the individual level and describe how the theory could be used to understand or predict behavior at the organizational, community, or societal levels.
3. Describe eight variables that are considered important determinants of behavior across five different theories. Which variables are considered necessary and sufficient to explain behavior?
4. Describe a method from SCT that can be used to improve self-efficacy for changing a behavior.
5. Sometimes health promotion campaigns use sports heroes as role models to influence people to practice a health behavior (such as eating

fruits and vegetables) or not to do a health risk behavior (such as not using drugs). Use SCT to explain why sports heroes may not be the best role models to influence a change in health-related behavior for most community members.

6. When considering the ELM, give examples of what that theory says about effective ways to stimulate central processing of information.
7. List ways to reduce stigma. How much evidence is there for each of these methods?

References

Abrahamse, W., & Steg, L. (2011). Factors related to household energy use and intention to reduce it: The role of psychological and socio-demographic variables. *Human Ecology Review, 18*(1), 30–40.

Achtziger, A., Gollwitzer, P. M., & Sheeran, P. (2008). Implementation intentions and shielding goal striving from unwanted thoughts and feelings. *Personality and Social Psychology Bulletin, 34*(3), 381–393.

Ajzen, I. (1988). *Attitudes, personality and behavior*. Chicago, IL: Dorsey Press.

Ajzen, I. (2015). The theory of planned behaviour is alive and well, and not ready to retire: A commentary on Sniehotta, Presseau, and Araújo-Soares. *Health Psychology Review, 9*(2), 131–137. doi:10.1080/17437199.2014.883474

Ajzen, I., & Schmidt, P. (2020). Changing behavior using the theory of planned behavior. In M. S. Hagger, L. D. Cameron, K. Hamilton, N. Hankonen, & T. Lintunen (Eds.), *The handbook of behavior change* (pp. 17–31). Cambridge University Press. doi:10.1017/9781108677318

Ajzen, I., Czasch, C., & Flood, M. G. (2009). From intentions to behavior: Implementation intention, commitment, and conscientiousness. *Journal of Applied Social Psychology, 39*(6), 1356–1372.

Allport, G. W. (1954). *The nature of prejudice*. Addison-Wesley.

Aminuddin, H. B., Jiao, N., Jiang, Y., Hong, J., & Wang, W. (2021). Effectiveness of smartphone-based self-management interventions on self-efficacy, self-care activities, health-related quality of life and clinical outcomes in patients with type 2 diabetes: A systematic review and meta-analysis. *International Journal of Nursing Studies, 116*. doi:10.1016/j.ijnurstu.2019.02.003

Armitage, C. J. (2009). Is there utility in the transtheoretical model? *British Journal of Health Psychology, 14*(Pt 2), 195–210.

Austin, J. T., & Vancouver, J. B. (1996). Goal constructs in psychology: Structure, process, and content. *Psychological Bulletin, 120*(3), 338–375.

Bagot, K. L., Masser, B. M., & White, K. M. (2015). Using an extended theory of planned behavior to predict a change in the type of blood product donated. *Annals of Behavioral Medicine, 49*(4), 510–521.

Bandura, A. (1965). Influence of models' reinforcement contingencies on the acquisition of imitative responses. *Journal of Personality and Social Psychology, 1*(6), 589.

Bandura, A. (1969). Social-learning theory of identificatory processes. In D. A. Goslin (Ed.), *Handbook of socialization theory and research* (pp. 213–262). Chicago, IL: Rand McNally.

Bandura, A. (1986). *Social foundations of thought and action: A social cognitive theory*. Englewood Cliffs, NJ: Prentice Hall.

Bandura, A. (1997). *Self-efficacy: The exercise of control*. New York, NY: W.H. Freeman.

Baranowski, T. (2006). Crisis and chaos in behavioral nutrition and physical activity. *International Journal of Behavioral Nutrition and Physical Activity, 3*, 27.

Bartholomew, L., Gold, R., Parcel, G., Czyzewski, D., Sockrider, M., Fernández, M., ... Swank, P. (2000a). Watch, discover, think, and act: Evaluation of computer-assisted instruction to improve asthma self-management in inner-city children. *Patient Education and Counseling, 39*(2), 269–280.

Bartholomew, L., Shegog, R., Parcel, G., Gold, R., Fernández, M., Czyzewski, D., ... Berlin, N. (2000b). Watch, discover, think, and act: A model for patient education program development. *Patient Education and Counseling, 39*(2), 253–268.

Batson, C. D., Chang, J., Orr, R., & Rowland, J. (2002). Empathy, attitudes, and action: Can feeling for a member of a stigmatized group motivate one to help the group? *Personality and Social Psychology Bulletin, 28*(12), 1656–1666. doi:10.1177/014616702237647

Baumeister, R. F., & Vohs, K. D. (Eds.). (2004). *Handbook of self-regulation: Research, theory, and applications*. New York, NY: Guilford Press.

Bayliss, D. M., Bogdanovs, J., & Jarrold, C. (2015). Consolidating working memory: Distinguishing the effects of consolidation, rehearsal and attentional refreshing in a working memory span task. *Journal of Memory and Language, 81*, 34–50.

Berkman, E. T. (2018). Value-based choice: An integrative, neuroscience-informed model of health goals. *Psychology & Health, 33*(1), 40–57. doi:10.1080/08870446.2017.1316847

Berkman, E. T., Hutcherson, C. A., Livingston, J. L., Kahn, L. E., & Inzlicht, M. (2017). Self-control as value-based choice. *Current Directions in Psychological Science, 26*(5), 422–428. doi:10.1177/0963721417704394

Berman, A. H., Beckman, M., & Lindqvist, H. (2020). Motivational interviewing interventions. In M. S. Hagger, L. D. Cameron, K. Hamilton, N. Hankonen, & T. Lintunen (Eds.), *The handbook of behavior change*. Cambridge University Press. doi:10.1017/9781108677318

van Blankenstein, F. M., Dolmans, D. H. J. M., van der Vleuten, C. P. M., & Schmidt, H. G. (2011). Which cognitive processes support learning during small-group discussion? The role of providing explanations and listening to others. *Instructional Science, 39*, 189–204.

Blankenstein, N. E., van Hoorn, J., Dekkers, T. J., Popma, A., Jansen, B. R. J., Weber, E., Pollak, Y., Figner, B. C., Crone, E. A., Huizenga, H. M., & van Duijvenvoorde, A. C. K. (2024). Adolescent risk-taking likelihood, risk perceptions, and benefit perceptions across domains. *Personality and Individual Differences, 231*. doi:10.1016/j.paid.2024.112806

Bos, A. E. R., Schaalma, H. P., & Pryor, J. B. (2008). Reducing AIDS-related stigma in developing countries: The importance of theory- and evidence-based interventions. *Psychology Health and Medicine, 13*(4), 450–460. doi:10.1080/13548500701687171

Bos, A. E. R., Pryor, J. B., Reeder, G. D., & Stutterheim, S. E. (2013). Stigma: Advances in theory and research. *Basic and Applied Social Psychology, 35*(1), 1–9. doi:10.1080/01973533.2012.746147

Bouton, M. E. (2014). Why behavior change is difficult to sustain. *Preventive Medicine, 68*, 29–36. doi:10.1016/j.ypmed.2014.06.010

Brijs, K., Brijs, T., Sann, S., Trinh, T. A., Wets, G., & Ruiter, R. A. C. (2014). Psychological determinants of motorcycle helmet use among young adults in Cambodia. *Transportation Research Part F: Traffic Psychology and Behaviour, 26*(Pt A), 273–290.

Brown, T. C., & Latham, G. P. (2002). The effects of behavioural outcome goals, learning goals, and urging people to "do their best" on an individual's teamwork behaviour in a group problem-solving task. *Canadian Journal of Behavioural Science, 34*(4), 276–285.

Brown, S. D., Fotuhi, O., Grijalva, C. S., Tsai, A.-L., Quesenberry, C. P., Jr., Ritchie, J. L., Cohen, G. L., & Ferrara, A. (2019). A randomized study of values affirmation to promote interest in diabetes prevention among women with a history of gestational diabetes. *Medical Care, 57*(7), 528–535. doi:10.1097/MLR.0000000000001133

Brownson, R., Glanz, K., Tabak, R., & Stamatakis, K. (2015). Implementation, dissemination, and diffusion of public health interventions. In K. Glanz, B. K. Rimer, & K. Viswanath (Eds.), *Health behavior: Theory, research, and practice* (5th ed., pp. 544–592). San Francisco, CA: Jossey-Bass.

Brug, J. (2006). Order is needed to promote linear or quantum changes in nutrition and physical activity behaviors: A reaction to "A chaotic view of behavior change" by Resnicow and Vaughan. *The International Journal of Behavioral Nutrition and Physical Activity, 3*, 29.

Brug, J., Conner, M., Harré, N., Kremers, S., McKellar, S., & Whitelaw, S. (2005). The transtheoretical model and stages of change: A critique: Observations by five commentators on the paper by Adams, J. &White, M. (2004)). Why don't stage-based activity promotion interventions work? *Health Education Research, 20*(2), 244–258.

de Bruin, M., Hospers, H. J., van Breukelen, G. J., Kok, G., Koevoets, W. M., & Prins, J. M. (2010). Electronic monitoring-based counseling to enhance adherence among HIV-infected patients: A randomized controlled trial. *Health Psychology, 29*(4), 421.

de Bruin, M., Sheeran, P., Kok, G., Hiemstra, A., Prins, J. M., Hospers, H. J., & van Breukelen, G. J. (2012). Self-regulatory processes mediate the intention-behavior relation for adherence and exercise behaviors. *Health Psychology, 31*(6), 695–703.

de Bruin, M., Oberjé, E. J. M., Viechtbauer, W., Nobel, H.-E., Hiligsmann, M., van Nieuwkoop, C., Veenstra, J., Pijnappel, F. J., Kroon, F. P., van Zonneveld, L., Groeneveld, P. H. P., van Broekhuizen, M., Evers, S. M. A. A., & Prins, J. M. (2017). Effectiveness and cost-effectiveness of a nurse-delivered intervention to improve adherence to treatment for HIV: A pragmatic, multicentre, open-label, randomised clinical trial. *The Lancet Infectious Diseases, 17*(6). doi:10.1016/S1473-3099(16)30534-5

Buunk, A. B., Dijkstra, P., & van Vugt, M. (2021). *Applying social psychology: From problems to solutions* (3rd ed.). SAGE Publications Ltd.

CDC. (2022). Social determinants of health. Retrieved May 17, 2023, from https://www.cdc.gov/about/sdoh/index.html.

Chaiken, S. (1980). Heuristic versus systematic information processing and the use of source versus message cues in persuasion. *Journal of Personality and Social Psychology, 39*(5), 752–766. doi:10.1037/0022-3514.39.5.752

Champion, V. L., & Skinner, C. S. (2008). The health belief model. In K. Glanz, B. K. Rimer, & K. Viswanath (Eds.), *Health behavior and health education: Theory, research, and practice* (4th ed., pp. 45–65). San Francisco, CA: Jossey-Bass.

Chapin, J. (2014). Adolescents and cyber bullying: The precaution adoption process model. *Education and Information Technologies, 19*, 719.

Chartrand, T. L., & Bargh, J. A. (1999). The chameleon effect: The perception–behavior link and social interaction. *Journal of Personality and Social Psychology, 76*(6), 893–910.

Chein, J., Albert, D., O'Brien, L., Uckert, K., & Steinberg, L. (2011). Peers increase adolescent risk taking by enhancing activity in the brain's reward circuitry. *Developmental Science, 14*(2), F1–F10.

Chen, Z., Veling, H., Dijksterhuis, A., & Holland, R. W. (2016). How does not responding to appetitive stimuli cause devaluation: Evaluative conditioning or response inhibition? *Journal of Experimental Psychology: General, 145*(12), 1687–1701. doi:10.1037/xge0000236

Chetty, R., Hendren, N., & Katz, L. F. (2016). The effects of exposure to better neighborhoods on children: New evidence from the moving to opportunity experiment. *American Economic Review, 106*(4), 855–902. doi:10.1257/aer.20150572

Churchill, S., Jessop, D. C., Green, R., & Harris, P. R. (2018). Self-affirmation improves self-control over snacking among participants low in eating self-efficacy. *Appetite, 123*, 264–268. doi:/10.1016/j.appet.2017.12.028

Clark, N. M. (2003). Management of chronic disease by patients. *Annual Review of Public Health, 24*(1), 289–313.

Clark, N. M., & Zimmerman, B. J. (2014). A social cognitive view of self-regulated learning about health. *Health Education & Behavior, 41*(5), 485–491.

Cohen, G. L., & Sherman, D. K. (2014). The psychology of change: Self-affirmation and social psychological intervention. *Annual Review of Psychology, 65*, 333–371.

Committee on Communication for Behavior Change in the 21st Century: Improving the Health of Diverse Populations (2002). *Speaking of health: Assessing health communication strategies for diverse populations.* Washington, DC: National Academies Press.

Conn, V. S., Valentine, J. C., & Cooper, H. M. (2002). Interventions to increase physical activity among aging adults: A meta-analysis. *Annals of Behavioral Medicine, 24*(3), 190–200.

Conner, M., & Norman, P. (2015). *Predicting and changing health behaviour: Research and practice with social cognition models.* In P. N. Mark Conner (Ed.) (3rd ed.). Open University Press (McGraw Hill Education).

Coorey, G. M., Neubeck, L., Mulley, J., & Redfern, J. (2018). Effectiveness, acceptability and usefulness of mobile applications for cardiovascular disease self-management: Systematic review with meta-synthesis of quantitative and qualitative data. *European Journal of Preventive Cardiology, 25*(5). doi:10.1177/2047487317750913

Corrigan, P. W., Morris, S. B., Michaels, P. J., Rafacz, J. D., & Rüsch, N. (2012). Challenging the public stigma of mental illness: A meta-analysis of outcome studies. *Psychiatric Services, 63*(10). doi:10.1176/appi.ps.201100529

Corrigan, P., Michaels, P. J., & Morris, S. (2015). Do the effects of antistigma programs persist over time? Findings from a meta-analysis. *Psychiatric Services, 66*(5). doi:10.1176/appi.ps.201400291

Creer, T. L. (2000). Self-management of chronic illness. In M. Boekaerts, P. R. Pintrich, & M. Zeidner (Eds.), *Handbook of self-regulation* (pp. 601–629). San Diego, CA: Academic Press.

Crone, E. A., & Dahl, R. E. (2012). Understanding adolescence as a period of social–affective engagement and goal flexibility. *Nature Reviews Neuroscience, 13*(9), 636–650.

Crosby, R., & Noar, S. M. (2010). Theory development in health promotion: Are we there yet? *Journal of Behavioral Medicine, 33*(4), 259–263.

Crutzen, R., Peters, G. J. Y., & Noijen, J. (2017). Using confidence interval-based estimation of relevance to select social-Cognitive determinants for behavior change interventions. *Frontiers in Public Health, 5*(JUL), 1–9. doi:10.3389/fpubh.2017.00165

Custers, R., & Aarts, H. (2010). The unconscious will: How the pursuit of goals operates outside of conscious awareness. *Science, 329*(5987), 47–50.

Danner, U. N., Aarts, H., & de Vries, N. K. (2008). Habit vs. intention in the prediction of future behaviour: The role of frequency, context stability and mental accessibility of past behaviour. *British Journal of Social Psychology, 47*(Pt 2), 245–265.

Deci, E. L., & Ryan, R. M. (Eds.). (2002). *Handbook of self-determination research.* Rochester, NY: University of Rochester Press.

Deutsch, R., & Strack, F. (2006). Duality models in social psychology: From dual processes to interacting systems. *Psychological Inquiry, 17*(3), 166–172.

Deutsch, R., & Strack, F. (2020). Changing behavior using the reflective-impulsive model. In M. S. Hagger, L. D. Cameron, K. Hamilton, N. Hankonen, & T. Lintunen (Eds.), *The handbook of behavior change* (pp. 164–177). Cambridge University Press.

Devine, P. G. (1989). Stereotypes and prejudice: Their automatic and controlled components. *Journal of Personality and Social Psychology, 56*, 5–18.

Diamond, A. (2013). Executive functions. *Annual Review of Psychology, 64*, 135–168.

Diamond, A., & Lee, K. (2011). Interventions shown to aid executive function development in children 4 to 12 years old. *Science, 333*(6045), 959–964.

Dickstein, B. D., Vogt, D. S., Handa, S., & Litz, B. T. (2010). Targeting self-stigma in returning military personnel and veterans: A review of intervention strategies. *Military Psychology, 22*(2). doi:10.1080/08995600903417399

DiClemente, C. C., & Graydon, M. M. (2020). Changing behavior using the transtheoretical model. In M. S. Hagger, L. D. Cameron, K. Hamilton, N. Hankonen, & T. Lintunen (Eds.), *The handbook of behavior change* (pp. 136–149). Cambridge University Press. doi:10.1017/9781108677318

van Dijk, T. A., & Kintsch, W. (1983). *Strategies of discourse comprehension.* San Diego, CA: Academic Press.

Dijker, A. J., & Koomen, W. (2003). Extending Weiner's attribution-emotion model of stigmatization of ill persons. *Basic and Applied Social Psychology, 25*(1), 51–68. doi:10.1207/S15324834BASP2501_4

Dobson, K. S., Szeto, A., & Knaak, S. (2019). The working mind: A meta-analysis of a workplace mental health and stigma reduction program. *The Canadian Journal of Psychiatry, 64*(1_suppl). doi:10.1177/0706743719842559

Doley, J. R., Hart, L. M., Stukas, A. A., Petrovic, K., Bouguettaya, A., & Paxton, S. J. (2017). Interventions to reduce the stigma of eating disorders: A systematic review and meta-analysis. *International Journal of Eating Disorders, 50*(3). doi:10.1002/eat.22691

Eagly, A. H., & Chaiken, S. (1993). *The psychology of attitudes.* Harcourt Brace Jovanovich.

Easterbrook, M. J., Harris, P. R., & Sherman, D. K. (2021). Self-affirmation theory in educational contexts: Exploring whether, when, why and how self-affirmation interventions are effective at reducing educational inequalities. *Journal of Social Issues, 77*(3), 683–701.

van Empelen, P., Kok, G., van Kesteren, N. M. C., van den Borne, B., Bos, A. E. R., & Schaalma, H. P. (2003). Effective methods to change sex-risk among drug users: A review of psychosocial interventions. *Social Science & Medicine, 57*(9), 1593–1608.

England, S. (2015). This girl can. https://www.thisgirlcan.co.uk/. Accessed August 19, 2025.

Epton, T., & Armitage, C. J. (2020). Goal setting interventions. In M. S. Hagger, L. D. Cameron, K. Hamilton, N. Hankonen, & T. Lintunen (Eds.), *The handbook of behavior change* (pp. 554–571). Cambridge University Press. 10.1017/9781108677318

Epton, T., Harris, P. R., Kane, R., van Koningsbruggen, G. M., & Sheeran, P. (2015). The impact of self-affirmation on health-behavior change: A meta-analysis. *Health Psychology, 34*(3), 187–196. doi:10.1037/hea0000116

Evans, R., Getz, J., & Raines, B. (1991). *Theory-guided models on prevention of AIDS in adolescents.* San Francisco, CA: Paper presented at the Science Weekend of the American Psychological Association.

Falk, E. B., O'Donnell, M. B., Cascio, C. N., Tinney, F., Kang, Y., Lieberman, M. D., Taylor, S. E., An, L., Resnicow, K., & Strecher, V. J. (2015). Self-affirmation alters the brain's response to health messages and subsequent behavior change. *Proceedings of the National Academy of Sciences, 201500247.* doi:10.1073/pnas.1500247112

Fazio, R. H. (2001). On the automatic activation of associated evaluations: An overview. *Cognition & Emotion, 15*(2), 115–141.

Firth, J., Torous, J., Nicholas, J., Carney, R., Pratap, A., Rosenbaum, S., & Sarris, J. (2017). The efficacy of smartphone-based mental health interventions for depressive symptoms: A meta-analysis of randomized controlled trials. *World Psychiatry, 16*(3). doi:10.1002/wps.20472

Fishbein, M. (2000). The role of theory in HIV prevention. *AIDS Care, 12*(3), 273–278.

Fishbein, M., & Ajzen, I. (1975). *Belief, attitude, intention and behavior: An introduction to theory and research.* Reading, MA: Addison Wesley.

Fishbein, M., & Ajzen, I. (2010). *Predicting and changing behaviour: The reasoned action approach*. New York, NY: Psychology Press.

Fishbein, M., Triandis, H. C., Kanfer, F. H., Becker, M., Middlestadt, S. E., & Eichler, A. (2001). Factors influencing behavior and behavior change. In A. S. Baum, T. A. Revenson, & J. E. Singer (Eds.), *Handbook of health psychology* (pp. 1–17). Mahwah, NJ: Lawrence Erlbaum.

Fisher, J. D., Fisher, W. A., Amico, K. R., & Harman, J. J. (2006). An information-motivation-behavioral skills model of adherence to antiretroviral therapy. *Health Psychology, 25*(4), 462–473.

Floyd, D. L., Prentice-Dunn, S., & Rogers, R. W. (2000). A meta-analysis of research on protection motivation theory. *Journal of Applied Social Psychology, 30*(2), 407–429.

Flynn, B. S., Goldstein, A. O., Solomon, L. J., Bauman, K. E., Gottlieb, N. H., Cohen, J. E., ... Dana, G. S. (1998). Predictors of state legislators' intentions to vote for cigarette tax increases. *Preventive Medicine, 27*(2), 157–165.

Foer, J. (2011). *Moonwalking with Einstein: The art and science of remembering everything*. New York, NY: Penguin.

Forsyth, D. R. (2014). *Group dynamics* (6th ed.). Belmont, CA: Wadsworth Cengage Learning.

Fox, K. J., Harris, P. R., & Jessop, D. C. (2017). Experimentally manipulated self-affirmation promotes reduced alcohol consumption in response to narrative information. *Annals of Behavioral Medicine, 51*(6), 931–935. doi:10.1007/s12160-017-9912-2

Garrison, D. R., Anderson, T., & Archer, W. (2001). Critical thinking, cognitive presence, and computer conferencing in distance education. *American Journal of Distance Education, 15*, 7–23.

Gobet, F., Lane, P. C., Croker, S., Cheng, P. C., Jones, G., Oliver, I., & Pine, J. M. (2001). Chunking mechanisms in human learning. *Trends in Cognitive Sciences, 5*(6), 236–243.

Godden, D. R., & Baddeley, A. D. (1975). Context-dependent memory in two natural environments: On land and underwater. *British Journal of Psychology, 66*(3), 325–331.

Godin, G., & Kok, G. (1996). The theory of planned behavior: A review of its applications to health-related behaviors. *American Journal of Health Promotion, 11*(2), 87–98.

Godin, G., Fortin, C., Michaud, F., Bradet, R., & Kok, G. (1997). Use of condoms: Intention and behaviour of adolescents living in juvenile rehabilitation centres. *Health Education Research, 12*(3), 289–300.

Goffman, I. (1963). *Stigma: Notes on the management of spoiled identity*. Prentice-Hall.

Gollwitzer, P. M. (1993). Goal achievement: The role of intentions. *European Review of Social Psychology, 4*, 141–185.

Gollwitzer, P. M. (1999). Implementation intentions: Strong effects of simple plans. *American Psychologist, 54*(7), 493–503.

Gollwitzer, P. M., & Sheeran, P. (2006). Implementation intentions and goal achievement: A meta-analysis of effects and processes. *Advances in Experimental Social Psychology, 38*, 69–119.

Gottlieb, D. A., & Begej, E. L. (2014). Principles of Pavlovian conditioning: Description, content, function. In F. K. McSweeney & E. S. Murphy (Eds.), *The Wiley Blackwell handbook of operant and classical conditioning* (pp. 3–26). Chichester, United Kingdom: John Wiley & Sons.

Gottlieb, N. H., Goldstein, A. O., Flynn, B. S., Cohen, E. J., Bauman, K. E., Solomon, L. J., ... McMorris, L. E. (2003). State legislators' beliefs about legislation that restricts youth access to tobacco products. *Health Education & Behavior, 30*(2), 209–224.

Green, L. W., Gottlieb, N., & Parcel, G. (1991). Diffusion theory extended and applied. In W. B. Ward & F. M. Lewis (Eds.), *Advances in health education and promotion* (Vol. 3, pp. 91–117). Philadelphia, PA: Jessica Kingsley.

Griffin, D. W., & Harris, P. R. (2011). Calibrating the response to health warnings: Limiting both overreaction and underreaction with self-affirmation. *Psychological Science, 22*(5), 572–578.

Griffiths, K. M., Carron-Arthur, B., Parsons, A., & Reid, R. (2014). Effectiveness of programs for reducing the stigma associated with mental disorders. A meta-analysis of randomized controlled trials. *World Psychiatry, 13*(2). doi:10.1002/wps.20129

Hagger, M. S. (2009). Theoretical integration in health psychology: Unifying ideas and complementary explanations. *British Journal of Health Psychology, 14*(Pt 2), 189–194. doi:10.1348/135910708X397034

Hagger, M. S., Luszczynska, A., de Wit, J., Benyamini, Y., Burkert, S., Chamberland, P.-E., ... Gollwitzer, P. M. (2016). Implementation intention and planning interventions in health psychology: Recommendations from the synergy expert group for research and practice. *Psychology & Health, 31*(7). doi:10.1080/08870446.2016.1146719

Hagger, M. S., Cameron, L. D., Hamilton, K., Hankonen, N., & Lintunen, T. (Eds.). (2020a). *The handbook of behavior change*. Cambridge University Press. doi:10.1017/9781108677318

Hagger, M. S., Hankonen, N., Chatzisarantis, N. L. D., & Ryan, R. M. (2020b). Changing behavior using self-determination theory. In M. S. Hagger, L. D. Cameron, K. Hamilton, N. Hankonen, & T. Lintunen (Eds.), *The handbook of behavior change* (pp. 104–119). Cambridge University Press. doi:10.1017/9781108677318

Hamilton, R. J., & Ghatala, E. (1994). *Learning and instruction*. New York, NY: McGraw-Hill.

Harris, P. R., Mayle, K., Mabbott, L., & Napper, L. (2007). Self-affirmation reduces smokers' defensiveness to graphic on-pack cigarette warning labels. *Health Psychology, 26*(4), 437.

Harris, P. R., Griffin, D. W., & Murray, S. (2008). Testing the limits of optimistic bias: Event and person moderators in a multilevel framework. *Journal of Personality and Social Psychology, 95*(5), 1225–1237.

Harris, P. R., Jessop, D. C., & Harris, P. S. (2020). Self-affirmation and health. In S. B. Gulliver & L. M. Cohen (Eds.), *The Wiley encyclopedia of health psychology* (pp. 587–595). John Wiley & Sons, Ltd. doi:10.1002/9781119057840.ch109

Hassin, R. R., Uleman, J. S., & Bargh, J. A. (Eds.). (2005). *The new unconscious*. New York, NY: Oxford University Press.

Hatzenbuehler, M. L., Phelan, J. C., & Link, B. G. (2013). Stigma as a fundamental cause of population health inequalities. *American Journal of Public Health, 103*(5). doi:10.2105/AJPH.2012.301069

Head, K. J., & Noar, S. M. (2014). Facilitating progress in health behaviour theory development and modification: The reasoned action approach as a case study. *Health Psychology Review, 8*(1), 34–52.

Herek, G. M. (2014). HIV-related stigma. In P. W. Corrigan (Ed.), *The stigma of disease and disability* (pp. 121–138). American Psychological Association.

Hodkinson, A., Bower, P., Grigoroglou, C., Zghebi, S. S., Pinnock, H., Kontopantelis, E., & Panagioti, M. (2020). Self-management interventions to reduce healthcare use and improve quality of life among patients with asthma: Systematic review and network meta-analysis. *BMJ*. doi:10.1136/bmj.m2521

Hofmann, W., Friese, M., & Wiers, R. (2008). Impulsive versus reflective influences on health behavior: A theoretical framework and empirical review. *Health Psychology Review, 2*(2), 111–137. doi:10.1080/17437190802617668

Hofmann, W., Dohle, S., & Diel, K. (2020). Changing behavior using self-control theory. In M. S. Hagger, L. D. Cameron, K. Hamilton, N. Hankonen, & T. Lintunen (Eds.), *The handbook of behavior change* (pp. 150–163). Cambridge University Press. doi:10.1017/9781108677318

Holland, R. W., Hendriks, M., & Aarts, H. (2005). Smells like clean spirit. Nonconscious effects of scent on cognition and behavior. *Psychological Science, 16*(9), 689–693.

Holtgrave, D. R., Tinsley, B. J., & Kay, L. S. (1995). Encouraging risk reduction: A decision-making approach to message design. In E. Maibach & R. L. Parrott (Eds.), *Designing health messages: Approaches from communication theory and public health practice* (pp. 24–40). Thousand Oaks, CA: Sage.

de Hoog, N., Stroebe, W., & de Wit, J. B. (2007). The impact of vulnerability to and severity of a health risk on processing and acceptance of fear-arousing communications: A meta-analysis. *Review of General Psychology, 11*(3), 258–285.

ten Hoor, G. A., Varol, T., Mesters, I., Schneider, F., Kok, G., & Ruiter, R. A. C. (2023). Just-in-time, but still planned: Lessons learned from speeding up the development and implementation of an intervention to promote COVID-19 vaccination in university students. *Health Promotion Practice, 24*(5), 921–931. doi:10.1177/15248399221095077

Hospers, H. J., Kok, G., & Strecher, V. J. (1990). Attributions for previous failures and subsequent outcomes in a weight reduction program. *Health Education Quarterly, 17*(4), 409–415.

Houben, K., Havermans, R. C., & Wiers, R. W. (2010). Learning to dislike alcohol: Conditioning negative implicit attitudes toward alcohol and its effect on drinking behavior. *Psychopharmacology, 211*(1), 79–86. doi:10.1007/s00213-010-1872-1

Janssen, E., van Osch, L., de Vries, H., & Lechner, L. (2011). Measuring risk perceptions of skin cancer: Reliability and validity of different operationalizations. *British Journal of Health Psychology, 16*(Pt 1), 92–112.

Janssen, E., van Osch, L., Lechner, L., Candel, M., & de Vries, H. (2012). Thinking versus feeling: Differentiating between cognitive and affective components of perceived cancer risk. *Psychology & Health, 27*(7), 767–783.

Janssen, E., Waters, E. A., van Osch, L., Lechner, L., & de Vries, H. (2014). The importance of affectively-laden beliefs about health risks: The case of tobacco use and sun protection. *Journal of Behavioral Medicine, 37*(1), 11–21.

Janz, N. K., & Becker, M. H. (1984). The health belief model: A decade later. *Health Education Quarterly, 11*(1), 1–47.

Johannes, N., Buijzen, M., & Veling, H. (2021). Beyond inhibitory control training: Inactions and actions influence smartphone app use through changes in explicit liking. *Journal of Experimental Psychology: General, 150*(3), 431–445. doi:10.1037/xge0000888

Kazdin, A. E. (2012). *Behavior modification in applied settings* (7th ed.). Long Grove, IL: Waveland Press.

Kelder, S., Hoelscher, D., & Perry, C. L. (2015). How individuals, environments, and health behaviour interact: Social cognitive theory. In K. Glanz, B. K. Rimer, & K. Viswanath (Eds.), *Health behavior: Theory, research, and practice* (5th ed., pp. 285–325). San Francisco, CA: Jossey-Bass.

Keller, L., Bieleke, M., & Gollwitzer, P. M. (2019). Mindset theory of action phases and if-then planning. In K. Sassenberg & M. L. W. Vliek (Eds.), *Social psychology in action* (pp. 23–37). Springer International Publishing. doi:10.1007/978-3-030-13788-5_2

Keller, L., Gollwitzer, P. M., & Sheeran, P. (2020). Changing behavior using the model of action phases. In M. S. Hagger, L. D. Cameron, K. Hamilton, N. Hankonen, & T. Lintunen (Eds.), *The handbook of behavior change* (pp. 77–88). Cambridge University Press. doi:10.1017/9781108677318

Kessels, L. T. E., Ruiter, R. A. C., & Jansma, B. M. (2010). Increased attention but more efficient disengagement: Neuroscientific evidence for defensive processing of threatening health information. *Health Psychology, 29*, 346–354.

Kessels, L. T. E., Ruiter, R. A. C., Brug, J., & Jansma, B. M. (2011). The effects of tailored and threatening nutrition information on message attention. Evidence from an event-related potential study. *Appetite, 56*(1). doi:10.1016/j.appet.2010.11.139

Kessels, L. T., Harris, P. R., Ruiter, R. A., & Klein, W. M. (2016). Attentional effects of self-affirmation in response to graphic antismoking images. *Health Psychology: Official Journal of the Division of Health Psychology, American Psychological Association, 35*(8). doi:10.1037/hea0000366

Kim, M., Popova, L., & Halvorson, K. (2016). The role of culture and media in promoting cancer screening among korean americans: A review of the literature. *Journal of Community Health, 41*(1), 198–213. doi:10.1007/s10900-015-0083-5

Kintsch, W. (1994). Text comprehension, memory, and learning. *American Psychologist, 49*(4), 294–303.

Kintsch, W., & van Dijk, T. A. (1978). Toward a model of text comprehension and production. *Psychological Review, 85*(5), 363–394.

Koch, E. J. (2014). How does anticipated regret influence health and safety decisions? A literature review. *Basic and Applied Social Psychology, 36*(5), 397–412.

Koffka, K. (1935). *Principles of Gestalt psychology*. New York, NY: Harcourt Brace.

Kok, G. (2014). A practical guide to effective behavior change: How to apply theory- and evidence-based behavior change methods in an intervention. *European Health Psychologist, 16*(5), 156–170.

Kok, G. (2021). Novelty as a parameter for using arguments in persuasive communication. *Health Psychology Bulletin, 5*(1), 12. doi:10.5334/hpb.13

Kok, G., & Ruiter, R. A. C. (2014). Who has the authority to change a theory? Everyone! A commentary on Head and Noar. *Health Psychology Review, 8*(1), 61–64.

Kok, G., den Boer, D. J., de Vries, H., Gerards, F., Hospers, H. J., & Mudde, A. N. (1992). Self-efficacy and attribution theory in health education. In R. Schwarzer (Ed.), *Self-efficacy: Thought control of action* (pp. 245–262). New York, NY: Taylor & Francis.

Kok, G., Gottlieb, N. H., Commers, M., & Smerecnik, C. (2008). The ecological approach in health promotion programs: A decade later. *American Journal of Health Promotion, 22*(6), 437–442.

Kok, G., Zijlstra, F. R. H., & Ruiter, R. A. C. (2015). Changing environmental conditions impacting health: A focus on organizations. In R. J. Burke & A. M. Richardsen (Eds.), *Corporate wellness programs: Linking employee and organizational health* (pp. 28–58). Cheltenham, United Kingdom: Edward Elgar.

Kok, G., Peters, G. J. Y., Kessels, L. T. E., ten Hoor, G. A., & Ruiter, R. A. C. (2018). Ignoring theory and misinterpreting evidence: The false belief in fear appeals. *Health Psychology Review, 12*(2), 111–125. doi:10.1080/17437199.2017.1415767

Kools, M., Ruiter, R. A. C., van de Wiel, M. W., & Kok, G. (2004). Increasing readers' comprehension of health education brochures: A qualitative study into how professional writers make texts coherent. *Health Education & Behavior, 31*(6), 720–740.

Kools, M., van de Wiel, M. W., Ruiter, R. A. C., Crüts, A., & Kok, G. (2006). The effect of graphic organizers on subjective and objective comprehension of a health education text. *Health Education & Behavior, 33*(6), 760–772.

Kreuter, M. W., & McClure, S. M. (2004). The role of culture in health communication. *Annual Review of Public Health, 25*, 439–455.

Kwasnicka, D., Presseau, J., White, M., & Sniehotta, F. F. (2013). Does planning how to cope with anticipated barriers facilitate health-related behaviour change? A systematic review. *Health Psychology Review, 7*(2), 129–145.

Latham, G. P., & Locke, E. A. (2007). New developments in and directions for goal-setting research. *European Psychologist, 12*(4), 290–300.

Lawrence, P., Fulbrook, P., Somerset, S., & Schulz, P. (2017). Motivational interviewing to enhance treatment attendance in mental health settings: A systematic review and meta-analysis. *Journal of Psychiatric and Mental Health Nursing, 24*(9–10). doi:10.1111/jpm.12420

Lehmann, B. A., Chapman, G. B., Franssen, F. M. E., Kok, G., & Ruiter, R. A. C. (2016). Changing the default to promote influenza vaccination among health care workers. *Vaccine, 34*(11). doi:10.1016/j.vaccine.2016.01.046

Link, B. G., & Phelan, J. (2014). Stigma power. *Social Science & Medicine, 103*. doi:10.1016/j.socscimed.2013.07.035

Livingston, J. D., Milne, T., Fang, M. L., & Amari, E. (2012). The effectiveness of interventions for reducing stigma related to substance use disorders: A systematic review. *Addiction, 107*(1). doi:10.1111/j.1360-0443.2011.03601.x

Locke, E. A., & Latham, G. P. (1990). *A theory of goal setting & task performance.* Englewood Cliffs, NJ: Prentice Hall.

Locke, E. A., & Latham, G. P. (2002). Building a practically useful theory of goal setting and task motivation: A 35-year odyssey. *American Psychologist, 57*(9), 705–717.

Locke, E. A., & Latham, G. P. (2019). The development of goal setting theory: A half century retrospective. *Motivation Science, 5*(2). doi:10.1037/mot0000127

Loewenstein, G. F., Weber, E. U., Hsee, C. K., & Welch, N. (2001). Risk as feelings. *Psychological Bulletin, 127*(2), 267–286.

Luszczynska, A., & Schwarzer, R. (2020). Changing behavior using social cognitive theory. In M. S. Hagger, L. D. Cameron, K. Hamilton, N. Hankonen, & T. Lintunen (Eds.), *The handbook of behavior change* (pp. 32–45). Cambridge University Press. doi:10.1017/9781108677318

Maas, J., de Ridder, D. T., de Vet, E., & de Wit, J. B. (2012). Do distant foods decrease intake? The effect of food accessibility on consumption. *Psychology & Health, 27*(S2), 59–73.

Magill, M., Apodaca, T. R., Borsari, B., Gaume, J., Hoadley, A., Gordon, R. E. F., Tonigan, J. S., & Moyers, T. (2018). A meta-analysis of motivational interviewing process: Technical, relational, and conditional process models of change HHS public access. *Journal of Consulting and Clinical Psychology, 86*(2), 140–157. doi:10.1037/ccp0000250

Maibach, E. W., & Cotton, D. (1995). Moving people to behavior change: A staged social cognitive approach to message design. In E. W. Maibach & R. L. Parrott (Eds.), *Designing health messages: Approaches from communication theory and public health practice* (pp. 41–64). Thousand Oaks, CA: Sage.

Manke, K. J., Brady, S. T., Baker, M. D., & Cohen, G. L. (2021). Affirmation on the go: A proof-of-concept for text message delivery of values affirmation in education. *Journal of Social Issues*. doi:10.1111/josi.12435

Mann, T., de Ridder, D., & Fujita, K. (2013). Self-regulation of health behavior: Social psychological approaches to goal setting and goal striving. *Health Psychology, 32*(5), 487–498.

Marlatt, G. A., & Donovan, D. M. (Eds.). (2005). *Relapse prevention: Maintenance strategies in the treatment of addictive behaviors* (2nd ed.). New York, NY: Guilford Press.

Martijn, C., Vanderlinden, M., Roefs, A., Huijding, J., & Jansen, A. (2010). Increasing body satisfaction of body concerned women through evaluative conditioning using social stimuli. *Health Psychology, 29*(5), 514–520. doi:10.1037/a0020770

Masuda, A., Hill, M. L., Morgan, J., & Cohen, L. L. (2012). A psychological flexibility-based intervention for modulating the impact of stigma and prejudice: A descriptive review of empirical evidence. *Psychology, Society, & Education, 4*(2), 211–223. http://psye.org/articulos/Masuda.pdf

Maunder, R. D., & White, F. A. (2019). Intergroup contact and mental health stigma: A comparative effectiveness meta-analysis. *Clinical Psychology Review, 72*. doi:10.1016/j.cpr.2019.101749

Mayer, R. E. (1989). Models for understanding. *Review of Educational Research, 59*, 43–64.

McAlister, A. L., Fernandez-Esquer, M. E., Ramirez, A. G., Trevino, F., Gallion, K. J., Villarreal, R., ... Zhang, Q. (1995). Community level cancer control in a Texas barrio: Part II—Base-line and preliminary outcome findings. *Journal of the National Cancer Institute Monographs, 18*, 123–126.

McGuire, W. J. (1985). Attitudes and attitude change. In G. Lindzey & E. Aronson (Eds.), *Handbook of social psychology* (3rd ed., Vol. 2, pp. 233–346), Special fields and applications. New York, NY: Random House.

McGuire, W. J. (2001). Input and output variables currently promising for constructing persuasive communications. In R. E. Rice & C. K. Atkin (Eds.), *Public communication campaigns* (3rd ed., pp. 22–48). Thousand Oaks, CA: Sage.

McSweeney, F. K., & Murphy, E. S. (Eds.). (2014). *The Wiley Blackwell handbook of operant and classical conditioning.* Chichester, United Kingdom: John Wiley & Sons.

Mevissen, F. E., Meertens, R. M., Ruiter, R. A. C., Feenstra, H., & Schaalma, H. P. (2009). HIV/STI risk communication: The effects of scenario-based risk information and frequency-based risk information on perceived susceptibility to chlamydia and HIV. *Journal of Health Psychology, 14*(1), 78–87.

Mevissen, F. E., Meertens, R. M., Ruiter, R. A. C., & Schaalma, H. P. (2012). Bedtime stories: The effects of self-constructed risk scenarios on imaginability and perceived susceptibility to sexually transmitted infections. *Psychology & Health, 27*(9), 1036–1047.

Michaelson, L. E., & Munakata, Y. (2020). Same data set, different conclusions: Preschool delay of gratification predicts later behavioral outcomes in a preregistered study. *Psychological Science, 31*(2), 193–201. doi:10.1177/0956797619896270

Miller, W. R., & Rollnick, S. (2013). *Motivational interviewing: Helping people change* (3rd ed.). Guilford Press.

Miller, W. R., & Rose, G. S. (2009). Toward a theory of motivational interviewing. *American Psychologist, 64*(6), 527–537.

Milyavskaya, M., & Koestner, R. (2011). Psychological needs, motivation, and well-being: A test of Self-Determination Theory across multiple domains. *Personality and Individual Differences, 50*(3), 387–391.

Mirzaei, A., Kazembeigi, F., Kakaei, H., Jalilian, M., Mazloomi, S., & Nourmoradi, H. (2021). Application of health belief model to predict COVID-19-preventive behaviors among a sample of Iranian adult population. *Journal of Education and Health Promotion, 27*(10), 69. doi:10.4103/jehp.jehp_747_20. PMID: 34084816; PMCID: PMC8057168

de Ridder, D. (2014). Nudging for beginners: A shortlist of issues in urgent needs research. *The European Health Psychologist, 16*(1), 1–6.

de Ridder, D., Gillebaart, M., & Friese, M. (2020). Self-control interventions. In M. S. Hagger, L. D. Cameron, K. Hamilton, N. Hankonen, & T. Lintunen (Eds.), *The handbook of behavior change* (pp. 586–598). Cambridge University Press. doi:10.1017/9781108677318

de Vries, H. (2017). An integrated approach for understanding health behavior; the I-change model as an example. *Psychology and Behavioral Science International Journal, 2*(2). doi:10.19080/PBSIJ.2017.02.555585

de Vries, H., Backbier, E., Kok, G., & Djikstra, M. (1995). The impact of social influences in the context of attitude, self-efficacy, intention, and previous behavior as predictors of smoking onset. *Journal of Applied Social Psychology, 25*(3), 237–257.

Mittal, D., Sullivan, G., Chekuri, L., Allee, E., & Corrigan, P. W. (2012). Empirical studies of self-stigma reduction strategies: A critical review of the literature. *Psychiatric Services, 63*(10). 10.1176/appi.ps.201100459

Mollen, S., Ruiter, R. A. C., & Kok, G. (2010). Current issues and new directions in psychology and health: What are the oughts? The adverse effects of using social norms in health communication. *Psychology & Health, 25*(3), 265–270.

Moore, G. F., & Evans, R. E. (2017). What theory, for whom and in which context? Reflections on the application of theory in the development and evaluation of complex population health interventions. *SSM-Population Health, 3,* 132–135. doi:10.1016/j.ssmph.2016.12.005

Morgan, A. J., Reavley, N. J., Ross, A., Too, L. S., & Jorm, A. F. (2018). Interventions to reduce stigma towards people with severe mental illness: Systematic review and meta-analysis. *Journal of Psychiatric Research, 103.* doi:10.1016/j.jpsychires.2018.05.017

Mullen, P. D., & DiClemente, C. C. (1992). Sustaining women's smoking cessation postpartum. Paper presented at the 8th World Conference on Tobacco or Health, Buenos Aires, Argentina.

Mullen, P. D., Green, L. W., & Persinger, G. S. (1985). Clinical trials of patient education for chronic conditions: A comparative meta-analysis of intervention types. *Preventive Medicine, 14*(6), 753–781.

Murphy, E. S., & Lupfer, G. J. (2014). Basic principles of operant conditioning. In F. K. McSweeney & E. S. Murphy (Eds.), *The Wiley Blackwell handbook of operant and classical conditioning* (pp. 167–194). Chichester, United Kingdom: John Wiley & Sons.

Najberg, H., Rigamonti, M., Mouthon, M., & Spierer, L. (2021). Modifying food items valuation and weight with gamified executive control training. *Royal Society Open Science, 8*(5), 191288. doi:10.1098/rsos.191288

Nederkoorn, C., Houben, K., Hofmann, W., Roefs, A., & Jansen, A. (2010). Control yourself or just eat what you like? Weight gain over a year is predicted by an interactive effect of response inhibition and implicit preference for snack foods. *Health Psychology, 29*(4), 389–393.

Nekitsing, C., Hetherington, M. M., & Blundell-Birtill, P. (2018). Developing healthy food preferences in preschool children through taste exposure, sensory learning, and nutrition education. *Current Obesity Reports, 7*(1), 60–67. doi:10.1007/s13679-018-0297-8

Ng, J. Y. Y., Ntoumanis, N., Thøgersen-Ntoumani, C., Deci, E. L., Ryan, R. M., Duda, J. L., & Williams, G. C. (2012). Self-determination theory applied to health contexts a meta-analysis. *Perspectives on Psychological Science, 7*(4), 325–340.

Noar, S. M., & Zimmerman, R. S. (2005). Health behavior theory and cumulative knowledge regarding health behaviors: Are we moving in the right direction? *Health Education Research, 20*(3), 275–290.

Ntoumanis, N., Ng, J. Y. Y., Prestwich, A., Quested, E., Hancox, J. E., Thøgersen-Ntoumani, C., Deci, E. L., Ryan, R. M., Lonsdale, C., & Williams, G. C. (2021). A meta-analysis of self-determination theory-informed intervention studies in the health domain: Effects on motivation, health behavior, physical, and psychological health. *Health Psychology Review, 15*(2). doi:10.1080/17437199.2020.1718529

Odgers-Jewell, K., Ball, L. E., Kelly, J. T., Isenring, E. A., Reidlinger, D. P., & Thomas, R. (2017). Effectiveness of group-based self-management education for individuals with Type 2 diabetes: A systematic review with meta-analyses and meta-regression. *Diabetic Medicine, 34*(8). doi:10.1111/dme.13340

O'Keefe, D. J., & Jensen, J. D. (2006). The advantages of compliance or the disadvantages of noncompliance? A meta-analytic review of the relative persuasive effectiveness of gain-framed and loss-framed messages. *Communication Yearbook, 30*, 1–43.

O'Keefe, D. J., & Jensen, J. D. (2007). The relative persuasiveness of gain-framed loss-framed messages for encouraging disease prevention behaviors: A meta-analytic review. *Journal of Health Communication, 12*(7), 623–644.

O'Keefe, D. J., & Jensen, J. D. (2009). The relative persuasiveness of gain-framed and loss-framed messages for encouraging disease detection behaviors: A meta-analytic review. *Journal of Communication, 59*(2), 296–316.

Orbell, S., Zahid, H., & Henderson, C. J. (2020). Changing behavior using the health belief model and protection motivation theory. In M. S. Hagger, L. D. Cameron, K. Hamilton, N. Hankonen, & T. Lintunen (Eds.), *The handbook of behavior change* (pp. 46–59). Cambridge University Press. doi:10.1017/9781108677318

Pace, B. T., Dembe, A., Soma, C. S., Baldwin, S. A., Atkins, D. C., & Imel, Z. E. (2017). A multivariate meta-analysis of motivational interviewing process and outcome. *Psychology of Addictive Behaviors, 31*(5), 524–533. doi:10.1037/adb0000280

Paluck, E. L., & Green, D. P. (2009). Prejudice reduction: What works? A review and assessment of research and practice. *Annual Review of Psychology, 60*(1). doi:10.1146/annurev.psych.60.110707.163607

Pantelic, M., Steinert, J. I., Park, J., Mellors, S., & Murau, F. (2019). 'Management of a spoiled identity': Systematic review of interventions to address self-stigma among people living with and affected by HIV. *BMJ Global Health, 4*(2). 10.1136/bmjgh-2018-001285

Patrick, H., & Williams, G. C. (2012). Self-determination theory: Its application to health behavior and complementarity with motivational interviewing. *International Journal of Behavioral Nutrition and Physical Activity, 9*, 18.

Paulussen, T., Kok, G., & Schaalma, H. (1994). Antecedents to adoption of classroom-based AIDS education in secondary schools. *Health Education Research, 9*(4), 485–496.

Paulussen, T., Kok, G., Schaalma, H., & Parcel, G. S. (1995). Diffusion of AIDS curricula among Dutch secondary school teachers. *Health Education Quarterly, 22*(2), 227–243.

Peels, D. A., de Vries, H., Bolman, C., Golsteijn, R. H., van Stralen, M. M., Mudde, A. N., & Lechner, L. (2013). Differences in the use and appreciation of a web-based or printed computer-tailored physical activity intervention for people aged over 50 years. *Health Education Research, 28*(4), 715–731.

Pescosolido, B. A., & Martin, J. K. (2015). The stigma complex. *Annual Review of Sociology, 41*(1). doi:10.1146/annurev-soc-071312-145702

Peters, G.-J. Y. (2014). A practical guide to effective behavior change: How to identify what to change in the first place. *European Health Psychologist, 16*(5), 142–155.

Peters, G. J. Y., Ruiter, R. A. C., & Kok, G. (2013). Threatening communication: A critical re-analysis and a revised meta-analytic test of fear appeal theory. *Health Psychology Review, 7*(sup1), S8–S31. doi:10.1080/17437199.2012.703527

Petty, R. E., & Cacioppo, J. T. (1986a). *Communication and persuasion: Central and peripheral routes to attitude change.* New York, NY: Springer.

Petty, R. E., & Cacioppo, J. T. (1986b). The elaboration likelihood model of persuasion. In L. Berkowitz (Ed.), *Advances in experimental social psychology* (Vol. 19, pp. 123–205). San Diego, CA: Academic Press.

Petty, R. E., & Wegener, D. T. (1998). Attitude change: Multiple roles for persuasive variables. In D. T. Gilbert, S. T. Fiske, & G. Lindzey (Eds.), *The handbook of social psychology* (4th ed., pp. 323–390). Boston, MA: McGraw-Hill.

Phelan, J. C., Link, B. G., & Dovidio, J. F. (2008). Stigma and prejudice: One animal or two? *Social Science & Medicine, 67*(3). doi:10.1016/j.socscimed.2008.03.022

Phelan, J. C., Lucas, J. W., Ridgeway, C. L., & Taylor, C. J. (2014). Stigma, status, and population health. *Social Science & Medicine, 103*. doi:10.1016/j.socscimed.2013.10.004

Portnoy, D. B., Scott-Sheldon, L. A. J., Johnson, B. T., & Carey, M. P. (2008). Computer-delivered interventions for health promotion and behavioral risk reduction: A meta-analysis of 75 randomized controlled trials, 1988–2007. *Preventive Medicine, 47*(1), 3–16.

Prochaska, J. O., & DiClemente, C. C. (1982). Transtheoretical therapy: Toward a more integrative model of change. *Psychotherapy: Theory, Research & Practice, 19*(3). doi:10.1037/h0088437

Prochaska, J. O., Redding, C. A., & Evers, K. E. (2015). The transtheoretical model of stages of change. In K. Glanz, B. K. Rimer, & K. Viswanath (Eds.), *Health behavior: Theory, research, and practice* (5th ed., pp. 168–222). San Francisco, CA: Jossey-Bass.

Pryor, J. B., & Bos, A. E. R. (2015). Stigma: Implications for helping behavior. In D. A. Schroeder & W. G. Graziano (Eds.), *The Oxford handbook of prosocial behavior* (pp. 433–455). Oxford University Press.

Qin, K., Marien, H., Custers, R., & Aarts, H. (2021). Environmental control of human goal pursuit: Investigating cue-based forced responses in a Pavlovian-to-instrumental transfer paradigm. *Motivation Science*. doi:10.1037/mot0000219

Reeve, J., & Cheon, S. H. (2020). Autonomy-supportive interventions. In M. S. Hagger, L. Cameron, K. Hamilton, N. Hankonen, & T. Lintunen (Eds.), *The handbook of behavior change* (pp. 510–522). Cambridge University Press.

Resnicow, K., & Page, S. E. (2008). Embracing chaos and complexity: A quantum change for public health. *American Journal of Public Health, 98*(8), 1382–1389.

Resnicow, K., & Vaughan, R. (2006). A chaotic view of behavior change: A quantum leap for health promotion. *International Journal of Behavioral Nutrition and Physical Activity, 3*(1), 25.

Rhodes, R. E., Grant, S., & de Bruijn, G.-J. (2020). Planning and implementation intention interventions. In M. S. Hagger, L. D. Cameron, K. Hamilton, N. Hankonen, & T. Lintunen (Eds.), *The handbook of behavior change* (pp. 572–585). Cambridge University Press. doi:10.1017/9781108677318

van 't Riet, J., & Ruiter, R. A. C. (2013). Defensive reactions to health-promoting information: An overview and implications for future research. *Health Psychology Review, 7*(SUPPL1). doi:10.1080/17437199.2011.606782

van 't Riet, J., Cox, A. D., Cox, D., Zimet, G. D., De Bruijn, G., Van den Putte, B., ... Ruiter, R. A. C. (2014). Does perceived risk influence the effects of message framing? A new investigation of a widely held notion. *Psychology & Health, 29*(8), 933–949.

Robbins, S. J., Schwartz, B., & Wasserman, E. A. (2001). *Psychology of learning and behavior* (5th ed.). New York, NY: W. W. Norton.

Rogers, E. M. (2003). *Diffusion of innovations* (5th ed.). New York, NY: Free Press.

Rogers, R. (1983). Cognitive and physiological processes in fear-based attitude change: A revised theory of protection motivation. In J. T. Cacioppa & R. E. Petty (Eds.), *Social psychophysiology: A sourcebook* (pp. 153–176). New York, NY: Guilford Press.

Ross, V., Jongen, E., Brijs, T., Ruiter, R., Brijs, K., & Wets, G. (2015). The relation between cognitive control and risky driving in young novice drivers. *Applied Neuropsychology. Adult, 22*(1), 61–72. doi:10.1080/23279095.2013.838958

Rothman, A. J., Baldwin, A. S., & Hertel, A. W. (2004). Self-regulation and behavior change. In R. F. Baumeister & K. D. Vohs (Eds.), *Handbook of self-regulation: Research, theory, and applications* (pp. 130–148). New York, NY: Guilford Press.

Ruiter, R. A. C., Abraham, C., & Kok, G. (2001). Scary warnings and rational precautions: A review of the psychology of fear appeals. *Psychology and Health, 16*(6), 613–630. doi:10.1080/08870440108405863

Ruiter, R. A. C., & Crutzen, R. (2020). Core processes: How to use evidence, theories, and research in planning behavior change interventions. *Frontiers in Public Health, 8*(June), 1–8. doi:10.3389/fpubh.2020.00247

Ruiter, R. A. C., Crutzen, R., de Leeuw, E., & Kok, G. (2020). Changing behavior using theories at the interpersonal, organizational, community, and societal levels. In M. S. Hagger, L. D. Cameron, K. Hamilton, N. Hankonen, & T. Lintunen (Eds.), *The handbook of behavior change* (pp. 251–266). Cambridge University Press. doi:10.1017/9781108677318

Ruiter, R. A. C., Kessels, L. T. E., Jansma, B. M., & Brug, J. (2006). Increased attention for computer-tailored health communications: An event-related potential study. *Health Psychology, 25*(3). doi:10.1037/0278-6133.25.3.300

Ruiter, R. A. C., Kessels, L. T. E., Peters, G.-J. Y., & Kok, G. (2014). Sixty years of fear appeal research: Current state of the evidence. *International Journal of Psychology, 49*(2), 63–70.

Rukchart, N., Hnuploy, K., Eltaybani, S., Sonlom, K., Chutipattana, N., Le, C. N., Khammaneechan, P., Jongjit, W., & Supaviboolas, S. (2024). Prevalence and determinants of COVID-19 vaccine acceptance among vulnerable populations in Thailand: An application of the health belief model. *Heliyon, 10*(4), e26043. doi:10.1016/j.heliyon.2024.e26043

Rutten, G. M., Meis, J. J. M., Hendriks, M. R. C., Hamers, F. J. M., Veenhof, C., & Kremers, S. P. J. (2014). The contribution of lifestyle coaching of overweight patients in primary care to more autonomous motivation for physical activity and healthy dietary behaviour: Results of a longitudinal study. *International Journal of Behavioral Nutrition and Physical Activity, 11*, 86.

Ryan, R. M., & Deci, E. L. (2000). Self-Determination Theory and the facilitation of intrinsic motivation, social development, and well-being. *American Psychologist, 55*, 68–78.

Ryan, R. M., & Deci, E. L. (2006). Self-regulation and the problem of human autonomy: Does psychology need choice, self-determination, and will? *Journal of Personality, 74*(6), 1557–1586.

Ryan, R. M., & Deci, E. L. (2017). *Self-determination theory: Basic psychological needs in motivation, development and wellness*. Guilford Press.

Schaalma, H., & Kok, G. (2009). Decoding health education interventions: The times are a changin'. *Psychology and Health, 24*(1), 5–9.

Scheier, M. F., & Carver, C. S. (2003). Goals and confidence as self-regulatory elements underlying health and illness behavior. In L. D. Cameron & H. Leventhal (Eds.), *The self-regulation of health and illness behavior* (pp. 17–41). New York, NY: Routledge.

Scholten, H., Granic, I., Chen, Z., Veling, H., & Luijten, M. (2019). Do smokers devaluate smoking cues after go/no-go training? *Psychology & Health, 34*(5), 609–625. doi:10.1080/08870446.2018.1554184

Schutte, L., Meertens, R. M., Mevissen, F. E., Schaalma, H., Meijer, S., & Kok, G. (2014). Long live love. The implementation of a school-based sex-education program in the Netherlands. *Health Education Research, 29*(4), 583–597.

Schüz, N., Schüz, B., & Eid, M. (2013). When risk communication backfires: Randomized controlled trial on self-affirmation and reactance to personalized risk feedback in high-risk individuals. *Health Psychology, 32*(5), 561–570.

Seijts, G. H., & Latham, G. P. (2005). Learning versus performance goals: When should each be used? *Academy of Management Executive, 19*(1), 124–131.

Seijts, G. H., Latham, G. P., Tasa, K., & Latham, B. W. (2004). Goal setting and goal orientation: An integration of two different yet related literatures. *Academy of Management Journal, 47*(2), 227–239.

Shaw, G., Whelan, M. E., Armitage, L. C., Roberts, N., & Farmer, A. J. (2020). Are COPD self-management mobile applications effective? A systematic review and meta-analysis. *npj Primary Care Respiratory Medicine, 30*(1). doi:10.1038/s41533-020-0167-1

Sheeran, P. (2002). Intention–behavior relations: A conceptual and empirical review. In W. Stroebe & M. Hewstone (Eds.), *European review of social psychology* (Vol. 12, pp. 1–36). Chichester, United Kingdom: John Wiley & Sons.

Sheeran, P., Maki, A., Montanaro, E., Avishai-Yitshak, A., Bryan, A., Klein, W. M. P., Miles, E., & Rothman, A. J. (2016). The impact of changing attitudes, norms, and self-efficacy on health-related intentions and behavior: A meta-analysis. *Health Psychology, 35*(11), 1178–1188. doi:10.1037/hea0000387

Sheeran, P., Milne, S., Webb, T. L., & Gollwitzer, P. M. (2005). Implementation intentions and health behaviour. In M. Conner & P. Norman (Eds.), *Predicting health behaviour* (2nd ed., pp. 276–323). London, United Kingdom: Open University Press.

Shegog, R., Begley, C. E., Harding, A., Dubinsky, S., Goldsmith, C., Hope, O., & Newmark, M. (2013). Description and feasibility of MINDSET: A clinic decision aid for epilepsy self-management. *Epilepsy & Behavior, 29*(3), 527–536.

Shepperd, J. A., Klein, W. M., Waters, E. A., & Weinstein, N. D. (2013). Taking stock of unrealistic optimism. *Perspectives on Psychological Science, 8*(4), 395–411.

Sherman, D. A., Nelson, L. D., & Steele, C. M. (2000). Do messages about health risks threaten the self? Increasing the acceptance of threatening health messages via self-affirmation. *Personality and Social Psychology Bulletin, 26*(9), 1046–1058.

Smith, R. M. (2008). *Conquering the content: A step-by-step guide to online course design*. San Francisco, CA: Jossey-Bass.

Sniehotta, F. F. (2009). Towards a theory of intentional behaviour change: Plans, planning, and self-regulation. *British Journal of Health Psychology, 14*(Pt 2), 261–273.

Sniehotta, F. F., Presseau, J., & Araújo-Soares, V. (2014). Time to retire the theory of planned behaviour. *Health Psychology Review, 8*(1), 1–7.

Sobal, J., & Wansink, B. (2007). Kitchenscapes, tablescapes, platescapes, and foodscapes: Influences of microscale built environments on food intake. *Environment and Behavior, 39*(1), 124–142.

Sommerland, N., Wouters, E., Mitchell, E. M. H., Ngicho, M., Redwood, L., Masquillier, C., van Hoorn, R., van den Hof, S., & van Rie, A. (2017). Evidence-based interventions to reduce tuberculosis stigma: A systematic review. *The International Journal of Tuberculosis and Lung Disease, 21*(11). doi:10.5588/ijtld.16.0788

Stacey, F. G., James, E. L., Chapman, K., Courneya, K. S., & Lubans, D. R. (2014). A systematic review and meta-analysis of social cognitive theory-based physical activity and/or nutrition behavior change interventions for cancer survivors. *Journal of Cancer Survivorship, 9*(2), 305–338.

Stevens, R., Dunaev, J., Malven, E., Bleakley, A., & Hull, S. (2016). Social media in the sexual lives of African American and Latino youth: Challenges and opportunities in the digital neighborhood. *Media and Communication, 4*(3), 60–70. doi:10.17645/mac.v4i3.524

Stevens, R., Gilliard-Matthews, S., Dunaev, J., Todhunter-Reid, A., Brawner, B., & Stewart, J. (2017). Social media use and sexual risk reduction behavior among minority youth. *Nursing Research, 66*(5), 368–377. doi:10.1097/NNR.0000000000000237

Strack, F., & Deutsch, R. (2004). Reflective and impulsive determinants of social behavior. *Personality and Social Psychology Review, 8*(3), 220–247.

Strecher, V. J., Seijts, G. H., Kok, G. J., Latham, G. P., Glasgow, R., DeVellis, B., ... Bulger, D. W. (1995). Goal setting as a strategy for health behavior change. *Health Education Quarterly, 22*(2), 190–200.

Stroebe, W., Mensink, W., Aarts, H., Schut, H., & Kruglanski, A. W. (2008). Why dieters fail: Testing the goal conflict model of eating. *Journal of Experimental Social Psychology, 44*, 26–36.

Stroebe, W., Van Koningsbruggen, G. M., Papies, E. K., & Aarts, H. (2013). Why most dieters fail but some succeed: A goal conflict model of eating behavior. *Psychological Review, 120*(1), 110–118.

Stutterheim, S. E., Bos, A. E. R., van Kesteren, N. M. C., Shiripinda, I., Pryor, J. B., de Bruin, M., & Schaalma, H. P. (2012). Beliefs contributing to HIV-related stigma in African and Afro-Caribbean communities in the Netherlands. *Journal of Community & Applied Social Psychology, 22*, 470–484. doi:10.1002/casp.1129

Stutterheim, S. E., & Ratcliffe, S. E. (2021). Understanding and addressing stigma through qualitative research: Four reasons why we need qualitative studies. *Stigma and Health, 6*(1), 8–19. doi:10.1037/sah0000283

Stutterheim, S. E., van der Kooij, Y. L., Crutzen, R., Ruiter, R. A. C., Bos, A. E. R., & Kok, G. (2025). Intervention mapping as a guide to developing, implementing, and evaluating stigma reduction interventions. *Stigma and Health, 10*(1), 3–20. doi:10.1037/sah0000445

Sua, Y. S., Jiang, Y., Thompson, D. R., & Wang, W. (2020). Effectiveness of mobile phone-based self-management interventions for medication adherence and change in blood pressure in patients with coronary heart disease: A systematic review and meta-analysis. *European Journal of Cardiovascular Nursing, 19*(3). doi:10.1177/1474515119895678

Suire, K. B., Kavookjian, J., Feiss, R., & Wadsworth, D. D. (2021). Motivational interviewing for weight management among women: A meta-analysis and systematic review of RCTs. *International Journal of Behavioral Medicine, 28*(4). doi:10.1007/s12529-020-09934-0

Sweeney, A. M., & Moyer, A. (2015). Self-affirmation and responses to health messages: A meta-analysis on intentions and behavior. *Health Psychology, 34*(2), 149–159. doi:10.1037/hea0000110

Teixeira, P. J., Marques, M. M., Silva, M. N., Brunet, J., Duda, J. L., Haerens, L., ... Hagger, M. S. (2020). A classification of motivation and behavior change techniques used in self-determination theory-based interventions in health contexts. *Motivation Science, 6*(4). doi:10.1037/mot0000172

Thaler, R. H., & Sunstein, C. R. (2008). *Nudge: Improving decisions about health, wealth, and happiness.* New Haven, CT: Yale University Press.

Todd, A. R., Galinsky, A. D., & Bodenhausen, G. V. (2012). Perspective taking undermines stereotype maintenance processes: Evidence from social memory, behavior explanation, and information solicitation. *Social Cognition, 30*(1). doi:10.1521/soco.2012.30.1.94

Tulving, E., & Thomson, D. M. (1973). Encoding specificity and retrieval processes in episodic memory. *Psychological Review, 80*(5), 352–373.

Tzavella, L., & Chambers, C. D. (2023). Explicit and implicit devaluation effects of food-specific response inhibition training. *Journal of Cognition, 6*(1), 10. doi:10.5334/joc.256

U.S. Department of Health and Human Services, Office of Cancer Communications, National Cancer Institute (2002). *Making health communication programs work: A planner's guide.* Bethesda, MD: U.S. Department of Health and Human Services.

Unsworth, N., Brewer, G. A., & Spillers, G. J. (2013). Working memory capacity and retrieval from long-term memory: The role of controlled search. *Memory & Cognition, 41*(2), 242–254.

van Nieuw-Amerongen, M., Kremers, S. P. J., de Vries, N. M., & Kok, G. (2009). The use of prompts, increased accessibility, visibility, and aesthetics of the stairwell to promote stair use in a university building. *Environment and Behavior, 43*(1), 131–139.

van Rookhuijzen, M., & de Vet, E. (2021). Nudging healthy eating in Dutch sports canteens: A multi-method case study. *Public Health Nutrition, 24*(2). doi:10.1017/S1368980020002013

Vansteenkiste, M., & Sheldon, K. M. (2006). There's nothing more practical than a good theory: Integrating motivational interviewing and self-determination theory. *British Journal of Clinical Psychology, 45*(Pt 1), 63–82.

Varol, T., Crutzen, R., Schneider, F., Mesters, I., Ruiter, R. A. C., Kok, G., & ten Hoor, G. A. (2021a). Selection of determinants of students' adherence to COVID-19 guidelines and translation into a brief intervention. *Acta Psychologica, 219,* 103400. doi:10.1016/j.actpsy.2021.103400

Varol, T., Schneider, F., Mesters, I., Crutzen, R., Ruiter, R. A. C., Kok, G., & ten Hoor, G. (2021b). University students' adherence to the COVID-19-guidelines: A qualitative study on facilitators and barriers. *Health Psychology Bulletin, 5*(1). doi:10.5334/hpb.32

Veling, H., Becker, D., Liu, H., Quandt, J., & Holland, R. W. (2022). How go/no-go training changes behavior: A value-based decision-making perspective. *Current Opinion in Behavioral Sciences, 47,* 101206. doi:10.1016/j.cobeha.2022.101206

Verplanken, B. (Ed.). (2018). *The psychology of habit.* Springer International Publishing. doi:10.1007/978-3-319-97529-0

Verplanken, B., & Aarts, H. (1999). Habit, attitude, and planned behaviour: Is habit an empty construct or an interesting case of goal-directed automaticity? *European Review of Social Psychology, 10,* 101–134.

Verplanken, B., & Roy, D. (2016). Empowering interventions to promote sustainable lifestyles: Testing the habit discontinuity hypothesis in a field experiment. *Journal of Environmental Psychology, 45.* doi:10.1016/j.jenvp.2015.11.008

Vinokur, A., & Burnstein, E. (1978). Novel argumentation and attitude change: The case of polarization following group discussion. *European Journal of Social Psychology, 8*(3), 335–348. doi:10.1002/ejsp.2420080306

Visschers, V. H. M., Meertens, R. M., Passchier, W. F., & de Vries, N. K. (2007). How does the general public evaluate risk information? The impact of associations with other risks. *Risk Analysis, 27*(3), 715–727.

Visschers, V. H. M., Meertens, R. M., Passchier, W. W. F., & de Vries, N. N. K. (2009). Probability information in risk communication: A review of the research literature. *Risk Analysis, 29*(2), 267–287.

Wang, L., & Miller, L. C. (2020). Just-in-the-moment adaptive interventions (JITAI): A meta-analytical review. *Health Communication, 35*(12). doi:10.1080/10410236.2019.1652388

Webb, T. L., & Sheeran, P. (2006). Does changing behavioral intentions engender behavior change? A meta-analysis of the experimental evidence. *Psychological Bulletin, 132*(2), 249–268.

Weiner, B. (1986). *An attributional theory of motivation and emotion.* New York, NY: Springer-Verlag.

Weiner, B. (2018). The legacy of an attribution approach to motivation and emotion: A no-crisis zone. *Motivation Science, 4*(1). doi:10.1037/mot0000082

Weinstein, N., & Ryan, R. M. (2011). A self-determination theory approach to understanding stress incursion and responses. *Stress and Health, 27*(1), 4–17.

Weinstein, N. D. (1988). The precaution adoption process. *Health Psychology, 7*(4), 355–386.

Weinstein, N. D., Sandman, P. M., & Blalock, S. J. (2008). The precaution adoption process model. In K. Glanz, B. K. Rimer, & K. Viswanath (Eds.), *Health behavior and health education: Theory, research, and practice* (4th ed., pp. 123–165). San Francisco, CA: Jossey-Bass.

Werrij, M. Q., Ruiter, R. A. C., Riet, J. V. T., & de Vries, H. (2012). Message framing. In C. Abraham & M. Kools (Eds.), *Writing health communication: An evidence-based guide* (pp. 134–143). London, United Kingdom: Sage.

White Hughto, J. M., Reisner, S. L., & Pachankis, J. E. (2015). Transgender stigma and health: A critical review of stigma determinants, mechanisms, and interventions. *Social Science & Medicine, 147.* doi:10.1016/j.socscimed.2015.11.010

Wiecha, J. L., El Ayadi, A. M., Fuemmeler, B. F., Carter, J. E., Handler, S., Johnson, S., ... Gortmaker, S. L. (2004). Diffusion of an integrated health education program in an urban school system: Planet health. *Journal of Pediatric Psychology, 29*(6), 467–474.

Wiers, R. W., Gladwin, T. E., Hofmann, W., Salemink, E., & Ridderinkhof, K. R. (2013). Cognitive bias modification and cognitive control training in addiction and related psychopathology: Mechanisms, clinical perspectives, and ways forward. *Clinical Psychological Science, 1*, 192–212.

Wiers, R. W., Eberl, C., Rinck, M., Becker, E. S., & Lindenmeyer, J. (2011). Retraining automatic action tendencies changes alcoholic patients' approach bias for alcohol and improves treatment outcome. *Psychological Science, 22*(4). doi:10.1177/0956797611400615

Witte, K. (1992). Putting the fear back into fear appeals: The extended parallel process model. *Communication Monographs, 59*(4), 329–349.

Witte, K. (1995). Fishing for success: Using the persuasive health message framework to generate effective campaign messages. In E. Maibach & R. L. Parrott (Eds.), *Designing health messages: Approaches from communication theory and public health practice* (pp. 145–166). Thousand Oaks, CA: Sage.

Witte, K., Meyer, G., & Martell, D. (2001). *Effective health risk messages: A step-by-step guide*. Thousand Oaks, CA: Sage.

Wood, W., & Neal, D. T. (2007). A new look at habits and the habit-goal interface. *Psychological Review, 114*(4), 843–863.

Wright, P. (2012). Using graphics effectively in text. In C. Abraham & M. Kools (Eds.), *Writing health communication: An evidence-based guide* (pp. 62–82). London, United Kingdom: Sage.

Zajonc, R. B. (1980). Feeling and thinking: Preferences need no inferences. *American Psychologist, 35*(2), 151.

Zajonc, R. B. (2001). Mere exposure: A gateway to the subliminal. *Current Directions in Psychological Science, 10*(6), 224–228.

Zhu, X., & Yzer, M. (2019). Testing a brief scale format self-affirmation induction for use in health communication research and practice. *Communication Methods and Measures, 13*(3), 178–197. doi:10.1080/19312458.2019.1572084

Zomahoun, H. T. V., Guénette, L., Grégoire, J.-P., Lauzier, S., Lawani, A. M., Ferdynus, C., Huiart, L., & Moisan, J. (2016). Effectiveness of motivational interviewing interventions on medication adherence in adults with chronic diseases: A systematic review and meta-analysis. *International Journal of Epidemiology, dyw273*. doi:10.1093/ije/dyw273

CHAPTER 4

ENVIRONMENTAL-LEVEL THEORIES

Background

As we discussed in the previous chapters, the individual is embedded within social networks, organizations, community, and society; and each lower level is embedded within higher levels. A facilitating environment that makes the health-promoting behavior the easiest behavior to perform is critical for changing the behavior of the priority population. Examples of facilitating environmental conditions include social and cultural influences (such as social support, organizational climate) and economic and political influences (such as affordable access to resources, price policies, and health regulations). Barriers to achieving desired outcomes are often structural, such as lack of health insurance, inconvenient clinic hours, lack of transportation, easy access to high-fat cafeteria foods, high cost of healthy foods, intense advertising of cigarettes and alcohol, and unsafe neighborhoods for outdoor activities.

The purpose of this chapter is to explore and describe theories that are useful for guiding change in environmental conditions to support healthy behavior. Typically these theories describe methods that instigate change at the group or collective level. Examples are the use of organizational change theory to install new work procedures of employees, community organization theories to strengthen access to local health care services, or theories of public policy to put health promotion at the forefront in processes of legislation. We first describe perspectives to orient readers to dynamics that influence environmental conditions. We then discuss how to describe and select environmental conditions to be changed, and then we suggest how to change these conditions. The theories are organized by ecological level: interpersonal, organizational, community, and societal (see Figure 4.1). Notably, we present theories that may be useful in identifying factors

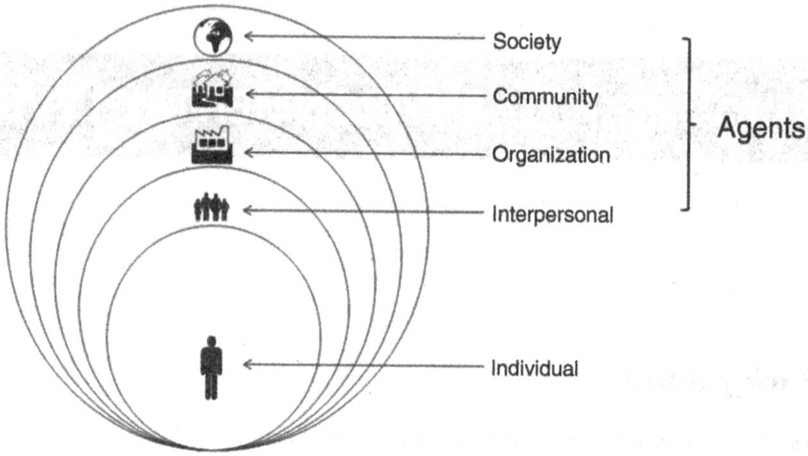

Figure 4.1 Socio-ecological Approach

"outside the individual" that influence health and behavior change and that can guide intervention planning. While we explore a range of environmental theories in this chapter, explaining specific environmental phenomena may require seeking familiarity with theories not described in this book. Examples of the use of theory at the environmental level to promote health can also be found elsewhere (Kok et al., 2015; Ruiter et al., 2020; Salmon et al., 2020).

The Logic of Changing Environmental Conditions

In this chapter, we discuss our logic model for the relations between behavior change methods, determinants, agents, environmental conditions, and health and how decision-makers can exercise their role and power in influencing behavior and environmental change at different ecological levels.

Working to influence change at multiple ecological levels can create synergy across levels to produce and sustain changes in environmental conditions. Environmental conditions influence health either directly or indirectly through behavior (Marteau et al., 2020). The accessibility of hiking and bicycling trails, for example, is a community-level condition that may facilitate physical activity and thus promote health. The presence of toxic particles in the air acts directly on health. Human agents can also influence the existence or intensity of environmental conditions at lower ecological levels. For example, a city council allocates money to build hiking and bicycling trails, and a higher governmental authority may authorize money for use by cities to build such trails. Members of city councils and legislators are environmental agents in this case that operate at the collective level, and their respective behaviors are proposing and voting to allocate funds targeting the same environmental condition.

Theories from both Chapters 3 and 4 are needed as the health promoter plans for change in environmental conditions. Once the agents and their behaviors have been identified, the planner can select determinants and methods to change them according to the logic of Chapter 7. In Chapter 3, we presented theoretical constructs that described personal determinants for behavior and theoretical methods to change specific determinants. These constructs and methods can be applied to behavior of both the priority population and the environmental agent. For example, positive outcome expectations may influence a legislator to vote to allocate funds ("If I vote to allocate funds for trails, people in my district will have more opportunities to exercise and this might increase my popularity") as well as to influence the priority population to jog ("If I jog, I will reduce my level of stress"). Similarly, persuasive communication is a method to influence the outcome expectations of both the population at risk and the environmental agents, the joggers and the legislators.

However, we realize that the perspective of working through environmental agents does not fully capture the process of collective action—how behaviors occur as part of a collective (such as a legislative body, workplace, or social network) or how these collectives are systems in their own right with their own regulatory processes. In a collective, the whole is greater than the sum of its parts. Clearly, a single legislator's vote does not lead to passage of a law. Lawmaking is a complex process. For example, in the United States, a powerful Speaker of the House sometimes assigns the bills to committees in which they will die; key committee chairs schedule hostile hearings; senators make compromise deals in the construction of bills; opposition party members add fatal amendments; and political party leaders bring their legislators' votes in line.

Furthermore, collective conditions are often sustained without agents' direct influence; organizations tend toward inertia, sustaining conditions regardless of their potential harms. For example, electronic health record programming has been found to contribute to urologists' persistent use of computed tomography (CT) imaging despite its limited detection of malignancies and its exposure of patients to high doses of harmful radiation (Skaggs et al., 2021).

While multilevel interventions are increasingly applied in practice, their usage remains limited, and research on them is still relatively scarce (Sallis, 2018). Glenn and colleagues evaluated the effectiveness of a mutilevel, multi-component, system-level intervention to improve HPV vaccination rates among adolescents in eight clinics (Glenn et al., 2022). The intervention was associated with modest improvements in HPV vaccine initiation across gender groups, while completion rate was higher only among boys. Garland et al. (2024) describe the development of IPACT (Intervention to Promote Autonomy and Competence in Transition-aged Youth): a multilevel (adolescent, caregiver, provider), multimodal (interactive skill-building sessions, educational materials, videos) intervention to address gaps in all three groups simultaneously and achieve a successful transition into the adult care system for those adolescents and young adults with special health care needs. They do indicate that rigorous evaluation will be necessary to demonstrate its potential.

In 2020, the United States National Cancer Institute initiated the Multilevel Intervention Training Institute with the goal of educating scholars in conducting multilevel intervention research. In this chapter, we describe interpersonal, organizational, community, and social change methods that rely on the power and authority vested in organizations, associations of citizens, and government. You can also refer Chapter 7, which describes Step 3 of Intervention Mapping and provides examples of change methods and practical applications aimed at addressing collective action at higher ecological levels. For example, a health promotion intervention might influence the behavior of the priority population directly or indirectly. A legislature may pass a law limiting minors' access to e-cigarettes or force a company to go smoke-free; or a social network may be leveraged to support a first-time mother in quitting smoking. Alternatively, a legislature might pass a law that companies must reduce emissions of pollutants, which, in turn, influences the environment of the priority population.

When health promotion planners seek to address these upper ecological levels, they often find general methods for community organization and organizational development, but they may find little guidance on ways to engage in the process. Through an analysis of interviews with health promotion researchers and professionals in the United States and the Netherlands, Kok et al. (2012) discovered that these higher-level methods are sometimes bundles of lower-level methods. For example, advocacy includes the methods of persuasion, raising awareness, informing, social comparison, networking, participation, and media exposure. In other cases, higher-level methods operate independently of lower-level methods. For example, systems change within a healthcare organization sometimes includes methods that act directly on environmental levels such as modifying information technology and redesigning workflow.

Looking at Healthy Environments as Outcomes

Intervention Mapping considers environmental conditions as they relate to health outcomes directly or impact health through the behavior of the priority group. Others have looked at creating potentially healthier environments as a desired outcome, irrespective of individual health outcomes. Since the 1986 Ottawa Charter for Health Promotion (World Health Organization et al., 1986), the World Health Organization has focused on the healthy settings approach. Adopting a settings-based approach to health promotion involves focusing on the environments where people live, work, and play, making these settings the focus of investigation and intervention, alongside addressing the needs and capacities of individuals within those settings (Poland et al., 2009). The settings approach is rooted in social ecology and systems thinking (Dooris, 2009, 2013). For example, a healthy city could be characterized as one that has health-promoting policy and characteristics across all sectors (such as a large greenbelt, low population density, recreation facilities, and low unemployment). In addition, a healthy city has explicit political commitment at the highest levels to promote health and investment in formal and informal networking and cooperation to enhance equity and build individual and social competence to deal with issues of importance to the community (de Leeuw, Tsouros, et al., 2014).

A healthy worksite setting would have healthy policies, a health-promoting culture, commitments to self-knowledge and development, respect for individual differences, jobs that foster responsibility and autonomy, safe and healthy working spaces, and equitable salaries and promotion opportunities. Health-promoting workplaces balance a focus on customer expectations and organizational targets with a focus on employees' skills and health (Kok et al., 2014; Marenus et al., 2023; van der Put et al., 2023). A healthy school would have a coherent, sequential health and physical education curriculum, teacher training, and an ethos that supports student and staff well-being. It would also have health-promoting policies and practices, including those of nutrition and food services, comprehensive health services, counseling, social services, and school–community partnerships, all established with the principles of democracy and equity (Bartelink et al., 2022; Vennegoor et al., 2023a, 2023b).

General Theories

This section provides an overview of perspectives to orient readers to overarching properties of general environmental conditions: systems thinking and how systems influence health and behavior ("Systems Theory") and consideration of power for influencing systems change ("Power Theory") (Cranley et al., 2019; Dori et al., 2019).

Systems Theory

We begin our discussion of general theories at environmental levels with a description of systems theory. There are many branches of systems theory, including general systems theory, complexity science, nonlinear dynamics, cybernetics, computational simulation, game theory, and ecology. All share the systems thinking focus on understanding how things work. In the domain of public health, where the complexity of health problems is generally high and decision-making contexts continuously change, systems thinking implies that healthy action can only be attained if there is simultaneous action that addresses the totality of personal and external factors that promote healthy behaviors. Such "whole system" or "complex adaptive system thinking" approaches require a coordinated and integrated effort that involves policy actors and key partners from inside and outside of public health including local governments, private partners and public institutions, and stimulates multilevel action and cross-sectoral working. Furthermore, it should have the capacity to respond to changes in a continuously evolving structure of complex relationships among personal, social, physical, and policy factors (Hawe, 2015a, 2015b; Hawe et al., 2009).

Systems thinking bridges theory and practice and provides an analytic strategy both to address understanding complex systems and to intervene on them (Grabowski et al., 2023). In this regard, it is both a theory of the problem and a theory of change. Systems theory suggests that individuals, organizations, communities, and societies are inextricably linked; these linkages have important implications for health promotion. In line with systems thinking, interventions are conceptualized as events in systems, and factors at various levels (also those not directly targeted by an intervention) can reinforce or dampen the impact of an intervention. This stressed the need to focus on the interrelationships between individuals and their environments.

Complex Adaptive Systems

Through the lens of systems theory, human behavior is a product of lower level complex adaptive systems (CASs) involving the brain, nervous system, and other biological systems and embedded within other, higher level CASs (such as dyads, groups, organizations, communities, and societies). CASs demonstrate a number of key characteristics (Bartelink et al., 2023; Lambe et al., 2020; Luna Pinzon et al., 2022; Ruiter et al., 2020):

- Agents, including people and human processes, have the capacity to exchange information with their environment and adjust their behavior accordingly. Diversity of agents increases the likelihood of novel behavior and is necessary for the sustainability of CASs.
- Agents interact and exchange information, creating connections among all agents in the system. Although agents interact locally and no single agent knows the pattern as a whole, global patterns and complexity result as information is spread through the system.
- Interactions are nonlinear; small "causes" can have large effects, and vice versa; large "causes" can have small effects.
- Because of sensitivity to initial conditions, small differences in initial conditions can lead to exponential differences in future conditions.
- CASs are self-organizing as people mutually adjust their behaviors to meet changing internal and external environmental demands. They adapt and evolve over time as spontaneous patterns emerge at the macro level from collective interactions of independent agents at the micro level.
- CASs are open systems, and agents interact with the environment beyond the system's boundaries so that the CAS and systems around it or in which it is embedded coevolve.

Structure, meaning, resources, and power relations have been described as key to understanding social systems, be they groups, organizations, communities, or societies. Structure includes agents, their activities, and their relationships. People act based on the meanings that actions or issues have for them and create meaning through interactions with others via an interpretive process that is highly dependent on context. Agents bring resources to the system, and whether they possess or need resources influences power relationships within the system. In the next section, we will discuss power as an emergent aspect of human interactions.

As we will see throughout this chapter, the health promoter addresses structure, meaning, resources, and power in designing system change efforts. Foster-Fishman et al. (2007) distinguished deep and apparent, that is, visible elements of a system. Norms, including attitudes, values, and beliefs, are deep elements of a system and are often found to be root causes of system problems. Regulatory processes—such as policies and procedures, available resources, and dominant operations, especially power and decision-making processes and structures—are apparent elements and are key to change. These elements are interdependent, emerging from interaction and meaning making among system members.

Systems theory is used to define and address all levels of the environment as interrelated social systems. Agents at each level can engage in activities to change the system to facilitate health. Influences of these agents' behavior at environmental levels can include norms, regulatory processes, and resources, whereas methods address social change broadly and include dialogue, planning, organizing, evaluation, and feedback. While integrating many aspects of complexity in logic models may be possible, it also runs the risk of producing artifacts that become equally complex instead of equipping intervention planners with decision-making tools to estimate the effects of interventions (Keshavarz Mohammadi et al., 2024). Mkhitaryan (2023) and Mkhitaryan et al. (2020) demonstrate how a hybrid approach of Fuzzy Cognitive Maps and machine learning may support various aspects of complexity in intervention design.

Theories of Power

Power theories are applicable to all environmental levels, and agents at each level with power are able to exert their influence to make changes at environmental levels. Power has been defined as the probability that an individual or group will determine what another individual or group will do even if it is contrary to the latter's interests (Orum, 1988). Sociologist Max Weber (Weber, 1974) defined three sources of power: authority, charisma, and legitimacy. Social psychologists have studied power as an emergent property of relationships.

A social psychological analysis suggests that each ecological level has different power structures and methods for social change. In small groups, social influence occurs through interaction and leadership. The leadership might be shared by members of the group, given over voluntarily to an individual leader by the group, or vested in an individual from a higher authority. At the organizational level, organizational change comes through the power of authority, which is determined by the hierarchical structure or who is above whom in the organizational chart. Alternatively, change can arise from informal power, such as an individual's charisma, satisfaction with a person's previous leadership activities, or legitimacy from being elected as a chairperson or inheriting a position in a family business. At the community and societal levels, power is "the social capacity to make binding decisions that have major consequences over the directions in which a society moves" (Orum, 1988).

Turner (2005) has developed the three-process theory of power that views power as an emergent quality of human social relationships. In this theory, power is the capacity to exert one's will through other people—that is, using either persuasion or control to get people to do something they are not interested in doing. Control in turn is subdivided into authority, in which group norms have given someone the right to control, or coercion, the attempt to control others against their will. Persuasion, authority, and coercion are the chief mechanisms for obtaining power, both individually and as a group. Group identity can unify people so that they gain the power of collective action to act as a coordinated body. Social change occurs when a subordinate group develops a distinct identity and its own goals and beliefs and can challenge the power of the dominant group.

Wallerstein et al. (2015) have distinguished between the concepts of **power with** and **power over**. They suggest that community building and capacity building are models of **power with**, whereas empowerment-oriented social action is a model of challenging **power over**. These two types of community organization strengthen community engagement, community organization, and community building.

Using Power to Create Change at Environmental Levels

Power is the key to creating change at the higher ecological levels. Health promotion planners can bring power to play in several ways: They can identify the agent who has the power to carry out the desired change, choose the change method that is most effective given the position and form of power the agent holds and the form of power the health promotor holds. If the health promoter represents a powerful organization, they will have more power relative to the agent than one from a small community agency. If the health promoter has moral power, that will increase the likelihood of getting the agent to carry out the action, or the health promoter can select another actor (based on their having more power) to influence a change agent at a higher level. For example, the health promoter gets a major donor to influence a legislator to act.

However, Friel et al. (2021) argue that expecting rapid progress in reducing health inequities is unrealistic. They emphasize that the persistent power imbalances within policy processes, coupled with the prevailing neoliberal emphasis on market forces, deregulation, and individualism in contemporary political systems, make the pursuit of health equity through a comprehensive policy agenda addressing social determinants of health "a power-saturated long game." Popay et al. (2021) are less pessimistic and more pragmatic. They outline three key imperatives for health-promoting interventions to effectively enhance equity. First, it is essential to understand the pathways linking empowerment to health equity and the factors driving the depoliticization of contemporary empowerment practices. Second, there is a need to revisit the original concept of empowerment processes, which support communities—whether defined by place or shared interests—in building the capabilities required to exercise collective control over decisions and actions in pursuit of social justice. Third, it is crucial to understand and actively engage with power dynamics within community settings. To facilitate these shifts, they propose two complementary frameworks: the Emancipatory Power Framework and the Limiting Power Framework. Together, these frameworks address and mitigate negative forms of power that hinder the development and exercise of a community's collective capabilities to enhance health equity.

In conclusion, health promoters must be conscious of the unintended negative effects of power in their work with communities, which can reinforce the status quo and lead to oppression of some groups by others. But, agents at each ecological level with power are able to exert their influence to make changes at environmental levels. The determinants of an agent's power include authority, charisma, legitimacy, expertise, group norms, and group identity. Methods for changing the behavior of others and the collective conditions include persuasion, social networking, coalition building, community organizing, and agenda setting.

Empowerment Theories

Within public health, empowerment has been defined as a "social action process for people to gain mastery over their lives and the lives of their communities" (Wallerstein et al., 2015). Empowerment is a multilevel process, focusing on the individual, organizational, and community levels (Commers et al., 2007). Empowerment can be viewed as an outcome as well as a process (Zimmerman, 2000). Empowerment as a process describes how to enable people to take power; empowerment as an outcome refers to the consequences of this process. An empowering process may result in empowerment as an outcome and may also result in other desired outcomes, such as improvement of health, safer neighborhoods, relocation of resources, or policy change. For example, Aiyer et al. (2015) describe how strengthening social relationships among residents, promoting trust and social capital, and undertaking collective actions, thus empowering residents to build strong social and institutional connections, can foster busy streets and thus encourage positive social interactions, reduce crime, and enhance overall health and safety.

Zimmerman (2000) compared empowering processes and empowered outcomes at the individual, organizational, and community levels (Table 4.1). Each level influences and is influenced by empowerment at the

Table 4.1 A Comparison of Empowering Processes and Empowered Outcomes Across Levels of Analysis

Level of Analysis	Process (Empowering)	Outcome (Empowered)
Individual	Learning decision-making skills Managing resources Working with others	Sense of control Critical awareness Participatory behavior
Organizational	Opportunities to participate in decision-making Shared responsibilities Shared leadership	Effective competition for resources Networking with other organizations Policy influence
Community	Access to resources Open government structure Tolerance for diversity	Coalitions of organizations Pluralistic leadership Social capital

Adapted from Zimmerman, 2000.

other levels. At the individual level, the results of empowerment are psychological, including increased perception of control over one's destiny, a sense of political efficacy, and motivation to act. This type of empowerment occurs when people take action to understand their environment critically and to gain power and control through organizational and community involvement (see this chapter's discussion of conscientization and social movements). At the organizational and community levels, empowerment involves collective problem solving; shared leadership and decision-making; and accessible government, media, and resources (Zimmerman, 2000; Zimmerman et al., 2011; for an example, see Obama, 2022).

Empowerment at the higher ecological levels is a similar concept to **collective efficacy**, which Bandura (1997) defined as "a group's shared belief in its conjoint capabilities to organize and execute the courses of action required to produce given levels of attainments." Collective efficacy may be applied to the levels of family, organization, community, and nation. For example, perceived organizational efficacy could be employees' beliefs that their organization can accomplish its goals. Change in collective efficacy comes through the same mechanisms as change in personal or self-efficacy at the individual level (see Chapter 3). The most effective way to enhance a community's collective efficacy is through success at accomplishing a particular goal. A community could experience enhanced efficacy by mounting a successful campaign of lobbying the city council to pass a clean indoor air act. Models of how other communities accomplished similar goals could also enhance efficacy, as might community leaders persuading the community members to take action (Commers et al., 2007).

Paulo Freire's work (Freire, 1973a, 1973b) on **conscientization** has formed the basis for empowerment models (Martinson et al., 2022; Wallerstein et al., 2015). In conscientization, facilitators lead individuals in small groups to consider their own realities and constraints. Rather than providing individuals with information through traditional, passive teaching, they are made the subjects of their own learning. The process of listening-dialogue-action-reflection moves group members to an understanding of the social forces underlying a problem and an understanding of their responsibility to act.

Critical consciousness, or conscientization, links individual-level and community-level empowerment and is a key method for strengths-based community organization. Using the context of developing literacy for adults in his home country, Brazil, Freire described the method by which critical consciousness emerges (see Freire, 1998). Educaters began the process by being with the people in a local community, discovering the words and phrases they used to describe daily life, and observing the way they lived. Educaters then selected generative words and integrated them to form codes that represented the life of the people. Program participants discussed these codes, which might be pictures, songs, or words, in cultural circles or in learning groups. They framed the discussion in terms of the participants' lives and the root causes of the conditions of their lives. This reflection on root causes gave rise to a political and social understanding that was accompanied by action to transform this reality. The final step of conscientization was the understanding that oppressive reality is a process that can be overcome. This understanding results in praxis, defined as "action based on critical reflection" (Freire, 1973b).

The cycle of listening-dialogue-action-reflection is reflected in community-based participatory research (CBPR) and participatory action research (PAR) approaches widely applied in current health promotion research and practice. Community members participate in different stages of intervention planning, research, development, and implementation, including participation in program advisory committees, data collection, intervention design, participant recruitment, and stages of program adoption and implementation (Hall et al., 2021; McFarlane et al., 2024). Community engagement is a key point in solving planning questions through applying Core Processes (see Chapter 2).

Both CBPR and PAR approaches utilize diverse methods alongside focus groups, interviews, and community events, including photovoice and digital storytelling. For example, Akande et al. (2021) explored the perspectives of an Inuit population in the arctic territories of Canada on the barriers and enablers of healthy diets and physical activity participation through one-on-one semi-structured photo-elicitation interviews. Photo-elicitation was used to initiate conversation on the research topics, and through participants' lived experiences and views, uncover the barriers and enablers of healthy dietary choices and physical-activity participation. This approach was believed to be particularly relevant because of the cultural differences between researchers and the Inuit research participants.

Digital storytelling is a workshop-based, collaborative method in which participants, guided by trained facilitators, create digital stories to articulate their personal experiences and interpretations of health and wellness and is one of the engaging methods increasingly used in health research (Lambert, 2010). Fiddian-Green et al. (2019) describe digital storytelling as a distinct narrative intervention, they illustrate key elements that inform the methodology, and they present a conceptual model to examine how digital storytelling may contribute to increased socioemotional well-being and bolster positive health outcome measures. Their proposed model is informed by elements of narrative theory, Freirian conscientization, multimodality, and social cognitive theory and can serve as a guide for public health practitioners and researchers interested in assessing the potential benefits of digital storytelling as an applied health intervention. Moreover, creative methods like photovoice and storytelling have proven particularly useful in amplifying people's experiences, perspectives, and voices in online research processes, such as those conducted during the COVID-19 pandemic (Valdez & Gubrium, 2020).

Environment-Related Theories by Ecological Levels

With a foundation in systems thinking and theories of power and empowerment, in the following sections we explore environmental theories as organized by social-ecological levels: interpersonal-level theories, organizational-level theories, community-level theories, and societal-level theories.

Interpersonal-Level Theories

Social relationships are the foundation for human existence. Social connection benefits health and longevity (Holt-Lunstad, 2023). Interpersonal-level theories are key to understanding and intervening on social connections and relationships. Social connections at the interpersonal level typically include family members, friends, peers, neighbors, associates, and service providers. Social network theory, social support theory, and social identity theory represent three examples of theories that explain phenomena at the interpersonal level.

Social Network Theory

A social network is an analytic framework for understanding relationships among members of social systems. Networks are classified as personal, based on the ties an individual has with other persons, or whole, based on the relationships among a defined group of people. Personal networks are particularly useful for the study of social support. The whole-network approach shows the network in which the personal network is embedded as a larger system, with a view of cliques of individuals and those persons who span the boundaries across networks. Networks can be horizontal (peers) or vertical (hierarchical) and can provide a way to understand types of social capital and power relationships in organizations (Valente, 2015).

Social networks consist of nodes (individuals, groups, or organizations) that are joined by ties (the relationships among nodes). Community can be understood as networks of networks in which the nodes of the larger network comprise smaller-scale networks. Networks can be defined by their content—whether they are primarily friendship, kinship, sexual, communication, or task oriented. The network also has a structure, including the number of members, the degree of members' similarity to each other, the way they are connected, and their links to other networks (Valente & Pitts, 2017). An individual can play several roles in a network: a group member, a linking agent, or an isolate with few ties to other network members. Linking agents are especially important because, as members of multiple networks, they bring information across network boundaries. Research during the COVID-19 pandemic illustrated how social network characteristics and health outcomes influence each other. Steijvers et al. (2024) found that networks changed in structure and size during the pandemic. The same research group also found that strengthening social networks can mobilize social support for pandemic preparedness behaviors, such as encouraging vaccination.

Social networks provide the means to understand mechanisms for behavior change. Most behavior change models acknowledge that people progress through a motivational, volitional, and maintenance stage (Keller et al., 2020) and that social networks play a pivotal role in each of these stages (Valente, 2015). Also, the more challenging the behavior change, the more people rely on their social networks. Berkman et al. (2000) argue that networks enable behavior change through four key pathways: (1) the provision of social support, (2) the exertion of social influence, (3) fostering social engagement and attachment, and (4) facilitating access to resources and material goods. Additionally, social network techniques can also be used for sustaining behavior change. Because social networks remain in the community once the program is over, the change process continues and is reinforced.

Although social network interventions have been criticized for their lack of generalizability and potential for upscaling, social media and computational tools that leverage computing power to process, analyze, and interpret large data sets, model social systems, and balance social connections to individuals' needs, provide opportunities for informing different types of social network interventions, such as identifying individuals who can act as champions for change, the use of peer-to-peer interaction to create message diffusion (going viral, snowball effects), or providing suggestions to alter the network itself by adding or deleting nodes, adding or deleting links, or rewiring existing links (Valente, 2012; Valente & Pitts, 2017). For example, Shelton et al. (2019) reviewed the use of social network analysis in the development, dissemination, implementation, and sustainability of health behavior interventions for adults. One-third of selected articles explicitly used social network analysis techniques to inform some aspect of interventions, mostly to inform intervention development.

Social Support Theory

The personal social network provides the structure for a variety of social functions, including social influence, control, undermining, comparison, companionship, and support. We focus here on social support—the help provided through social relationships and interactions (Holt-Lunstad & Uchino, 2015). The four main types of social support are emotional (provision of empathy, love, trust, and caring), instrumental (provision of tangible aid and services), informational (provision of advice, suggestions, and information), and appraisal (provision of feedback useful for self-reevaluation and affirmation). Social support is a positive social interaction. However, negative interactions and modeling for unhealthy or deviant behaviors also occur in relationships. Health educators will need a comprehensive view of relevant social networks, including both support and undermining, with regard to the development of interventions and design of health outcomes studies (Holt-Lunstad, 2023).

The extent and nature of social relationships has been linked to health status and physiological processes related to disease outcomes (Holt-Lunstad, 2022a, 2022b; Kelly et al., 2017; Leigh-Hunt et al., 2017; Sendra et al., 2020). The mechanisms underlying these findings have been hypothesized to include modeling and reinforcement of positive health-related behaviors, buffering the effects of stress on health, and providing access to resources to cope with stress. Social-structural conditions such as culture, socioeconomic factors, politics, and social change shape social networks. Social networks in turn provide opportunities for social support, norms and social control, social involvement, person-to-person contagion, and access to resources and material goods (Berkman et al., 2000).

Interventions can be directed toward different types of social networks and the specific types of social support they provide. Small, dense, geographically close, intense networks provide emotional and appraisal support. These networks typically do not have access to the larger society or to information outside the network's domain. On the other hand, large, diffuse, and less intense networks provide more informational support and social outreach (McLeroy et al., 2001). Different types of social support are important at different times in the experience of stressors. For example, with the loss of a job, emotional support that the individual is still loved and remains intact is most important at first. Later, the individual needs informational support regarding other job opportunities or possible career changes. Tangible support, such as loans, transportation, or child care, may also help people when they are job hunting.

Holt-Lunstad and Uchino (2015) identified four types of interventions to increase social support: enhancing existing social network linkages, developing new social network linkages, enhancing networks through indigenous natural helpers and community health workers, and enhancing networks at the community level through participatory problem solving.

The enhancement of existing network linkages can be accomplished by training network members in skills for providing support and by training members of the target group to mobilize and maintain their networks. For example, family members or significant others may be trained to provide support to individuals who are in programs to stop. At the government and society level, legislation can be enacted to support social networks. Examples of such legislation are family leave acts, policies to promote volunteerism, and funding for child and elder care. We describe methods for policy change later in this chapter.

New social network linkages can be developed through mentor programs, buddy systems, and self-help groups. Buddies have been used in diverse settings, for example, in smoking cessation programs, for mothers of very preterm infants, and in worksite programs. Groups such as Alcoholics Anonymous provide access to new social networks designed to provide emotional, instrumental, and informational support for behavioral and life change. Interventions can encourage such networks to reach out to incorporate new members and new information from persons who hold membership in other networks.

Indigenous or natural helpers have been employed to enhance networks, particularly around health issues. Natural helpers are community members to whom other persons turn for advice, emotional support, and tangible aid. Often they agree to become a link between the community and the formal service-delivery system. They may include persons who encounter many people in their role, such as hairstylists, shopkeepers, and clergy. They may also be community volunteers and people with similar problems. Scott et al. (2018) provide a comprehensive review of lay or community health worker interventions. Key features that contribute to positive outcomes in community health worker programs include integration within the community, supportive supervision, ongoing education, and sufficient logistical support and resources.

Finally, social support can be enhanced at the community level through participatory problem-solving processes. For example, McEvoy et al. (2018) describe the systematic process of developing a theory-based tailored peer support intervention to encourage a Mediterranean diet in people high at risk for cardiovascular diseases: the target group preferred a group-based mode of peer support delivery, either alone or in combination with face-to-face mentoring or telephone support. Both meeting face-to-face and meeting as a group were seen as helpful, for different reasons, e.g., trust versus learning from others' experiences.

Interventions may also combine the above types of social support interventions. Shushtari et al. (2023) did a systematic review and meta-analysis to evaluate the effectiveness of social support interventions in improving therapy adherence among people living with HIV. They identified 17 RCTs, representing 4,110 participants in eight countries, and showed a positive effect in increasing adherence to antiretroviral therapy; effect sizes were larger for interventions of longer duration. Support from all sources, except family support alone, had a positive effect on adherence behavior, but only for interventions with multiple sources of support.

Social Identity Theory

Social identity theory (Tajfel & Turner, 1986) provides a theoretical framework that the health promotor can draw upon to develop health interventions that change people's behavior (Haslam et al., 2018; Reynolds et al., 2020). Tarrant et al. (2020) present a new social identity model—called the social identity model of behavior change—and accompanying guidance to support this process.

Tarrant et al. (2020) explain that social identity interventions are based on the relationships between group memberships, social identity, and health (see also Haslam et al., 2018). Social identity is defined as a person's knowledge that they belong to certain social groups and that these groups have some cognitive, emotional, and valued significance (Tajfel & Turner, 1986). People can view themselves as "I" or as "we"; in that last case they identify with a social group. Their perceptions of themselves will then shift, including their norms, values, beliefs, and, in turn, their behaviors. For example, Folk et al. (2016) examined predictors of criminal reoffending and community adjustment among former prisoners and assessed their identification with the criminal community as well as with the wider community. They found that the more the self was overlapping with the criminal community, the higher the reoffending rate one year later, demonstrating the importance of social identification to behavior change.

It may be clear that social identity interventions are group interventions at the interpersonal level, as they aim to change how people respond to the expectations from their relevant groups. It may also be clear that social identity processes are unavoidable and, moreover, can be very supportive for the individual, among others by promoting healthy behaviors. An essential *parameter* of planned group interventions' effectiveness is social identification: Applying "key social identity-building processes that are critical to the design and delivery of group-based interventions" (Tarrant et al., 2020).

How can we promote social identification? Haslam et al. (2018) describe six hypotheses that can make group-based interventions a powerful resource for behavior change:

When people define themselves in terms of shared social identity,

1. ... that identity will focus their energies and imbue them with a sense of meaning, purpose, and worth—**meaning**;
2. ... they will be more likely to perceive themselves in terms of shared social identity, to perceive themselves as similar and connected, and positively oriented toward each other—**connection**;

3. ... they will expect to give each other support, actually give each other support, and construe the support they receive more positively—**support**;
4. ... they will (strive to) enact the norms and values associated with that identity—**norm enactment**;
5. ... they will be more likely to influence each other—**influence**;
6. ... they will, as a group, develop a sense of collective efficacy, agency, and power—**agency**.

Based on these six hypotheses, Tarrant et al. (2020) argue that the planning for this type of group intervention first needs to involve a thorough understanding of the problem and the population that is involved. Then, the group environment needs to encourage the members to see themselves as a collective entity: an "us" rather than a collection of "I"s. Various practical applications can support the promotion of shared social identity, for example mapping similarities between group members, using inclusive language, promoting cooperation, and shared decision-making. Finally, the intervention focus is on helping the group members to realize that the behavior change is "for us" instead of "done to us"—and supporting them to enact this change using evidence-based techniques.

In addition, three key leadership processes are highlighted: (1) **identity reflection** on the things that matter to the group; (2) **identity representation** to help clarify the group's values and goals, aligning the group's social identity with the intervention's objectives; and (3) **identity realization**, taking steps to make the group matter and maximizing its potential to become a resource for promoting change.

An evaluation of this kind of social identity intervention should measure the primary outcomes (e.g., behavior, health), but also the group processes by which these outcomes were achieved. Social identification is the key hypothesized mechanism for these types of interventions and should be measured, preferably at various time points, not only for the evaluation but also for an ongoing measure of the program's success in promoting social identification. Other process measures can also be taken (e.g., social support), depending on the intervention and research focus. In conclusion, "Intervention groups can become a positive resource for behavior change when facilitators engage in social identity management in ways that help group members to develop a sense of shared social identity" (Tarrant et al., 2020).

Organization-Level Theories

An organization can be defined as an organized body of people that can be activated to accomplish goals via coordinated action. Organizations take inputs from the environment, such as human effort, raw materials, information, or financial and social capital, and transform them to produce goods, services, and value for customers, shareholders, and other key partners in the environment. Organizations can be small or large; be for-profit or not-for-profit, governmental or nongovernmental, and publicly held or privately held. All organizations, however, attempt to manage their complex environments to obtain needed resources and to release valued outputs into the environment. The environment, which includes economic, competitive, technological, political, physical, demographic, cultural, and social forces, is constantly changing, and organizations must change in response to maintain their effectiveness and to survive.

Health promotion practitioners sometimes work in organizations with the opportunity to serve as internal change agents. They also work as external change agents with community groups seeking to make changes in organizations. Organization-level theories describe, explain, and predict the complex interaction between organizations and their environments, including the individual level. These theories have potential to explain and ground investigations focused on the role of policies, institutions, funding fluctuations, contract design, procurement processes, and workforce dynamics (Birken, Bunger, et al., 2017). These theories can also be used to enable organizations' adoption, implementation, and sustaining of health promotion interventions. Understanding key aspects of organizations and organizational change is critical to the health promoter's ability to change environmental conditions for individual and community health promotion. Below, we briefly describe a few organization theories of the many that exist to stimulate changes in policy, culture, and other organizational conditions.

Transaction Cost Economics

Transaction cost economics (TCE) examines relationships among organizations, focusing on the interactions between organizational structures, transactions, and their effectiveness (e.g., minimizing costs and delivering high-quality services to clients) (Leeman et al., 2019). Organizations engage in transactions with other organizations to procure goods and services, incurring costs related to activities such as negotiating contracts, monitoring compliance, and implementing financial incentives or penalties. The characteristics of these transactions often inform the choice of governance structures to optimize costs and effectiveness (Shelanski & Klein, 1995).

Governance structures for managing transactions exist on a continuum, ranging from no formal structure to informal agreements, formal contracts, and full integration of goods and services production within an organization's operations. TCE is particularly relevant for guiding decisions made by health plans, integrated delivery systems, nonprofits, and other intermediaries about whether to invest in building practice-level capacity to implement an intervention or to undertake implementation themselves (Leeman & Mark, 2006).

An example of TCE application in healthcare is Zinn et al.'s (2003) study on the factors influencing skilled nursing facilities' decisions about whether to contract with rehabilitation therapists or employ them as staff members. Another example is the study by Khanakwa and Mbonigaba (2022), which explored transaction costs associated with providing HIV and AIDS services in Uganda. Their findings did not support TCE, likely due to the reliance on informal institutions rather than principal-agent sanctions. These results suggest that the level of transaction costs is associated with features of institutional arrangements.

Institutional Theory

Institutional theory explains how environmental pressures drive organizations to adopt similar structures and practices, a phenomenon referred to as "isomorphism" (i.e., the tendency of organizations to resemble other, similar organizations when facing comparable environmental conditions; Dimaggio & Powell, 1983; Leeman et al., 2019). A notable application of institutional theory is D'Aunno et al.'s (1991) study of hybrid clinics offering both mental health and drug abuse treatment. The researchers used institutional theory to analyze the environmental pressures from the mental health and drug abuse sectors and examined how these pressures influenced service delivery in hybrid clinics.

Another example is the systematic review by Kerins et al. (2020), which synthesized evidence on barriers and facilitators to implementing menu labeling interventions from the food service industry's perspective. The most frequently cited barriers were categorized as Consumer Needs & Resources (e.g., lack of customer demand or interest in menu labeling, risk of overwhelming or confusing customers) and Compatibility with Organizational Processes (e.g., lack of standardized recipes, limited space on menus). Facilitators were primarily linked to the constructs of Relative Advantage (e.g., improved business image or reputation) and Consumer Needs & Resources (e.g., customer demand for nutrition information). These findings align with key propositions of institutional theory, which suggest organizations adopt innovations in response to coercion or significant pressure to comply with rules, mandates, or regulations.

Contingency Theory

Contingency theory asserts that the most effective way to structure a task depends on the characteristics of both the task itself and its surrounding environment (Leeman et al., 2019, 2022). Tasks may involve designing, producing, and distributing a good or service. According to the theory, coordination structures for tasks exist along a continuum from programmed structures, which rely on standardized protocols, rules, hierarchical authority, and centralized decision-making, to unprogrammed structures, which involve new professional roles, teams, and communication systems that enable coordination and collaborative, real-time decision-making (Schoonhoven, 1981).

The task environment includes factors both internal and external to the organization. In contexts of high environmental uncertainty, contingency theory suggests that interventions should be less prescriptive and allow for flexible, on-the-spot decision-making during implementation and delivery. An application of this theory is highlighted in Leeman et al.'s (2019) discussion of Schoonhoven's research, which examined how uncertainty about patient inflow influenced operating room coordination to enhance patient outcomes.

Organizational Change Theory

Organizational change theory predicts who initiates and carries out organizational change, how, and under what conditions. As suggested above, managers design a structure and culture to match the environment, choose technology to convert inputs to outputs, and develop strategies to guide the organization to create value. This planned organizational change can be incremental, using methods such as quality improvement and flexible workgroups, or revolutionary, involving methods such as restructuring, reengineering, and innovation (Batras et al., 2016; Boonstra, 2004; Jones et al., 2004).

Lewin (1947) described the change process as having three phases: unfreezing, moving, and refreezing. Unfreezing reduces the forces that maintain the organization's current behavior, often by showing that the behaviors or conditions that organizational members desire are different from those they currently exhibit. During the moving phase, changes in organizational structures and processes lead to new behaviors, values, and attitudes. In refreezing, the organization puts in place norms, policies, and structures that support the new state of equilibrium (Cummings & Worley, 2018). As a caveat, it should be noted that although planned change is described as a rationally controlled and orderly process, in practice it can be messy and unpredictable.

Within the organizational change literature, **Stage Theory** (Butterfoss et al., 2008) suggests that organizations move through a series of stages as they change and that strategies to promote change must be matched to the stage: agenda setting, matching, redefining and restructuring, and clarifying and routinizing. In order: (1) Sensing unsatisfied demands on the system, noting a problem, and bringing it to the surface, (2) Searching for possible responses, seeking solutions to the problem, (3) Evaluating alternatives, judging potential solutions, (4) Deciding to adopt a course of action, selecting one of a number of alternative responses, (5) Initiating action within the system, which requires policy changes and resources necessary for implementation, (6) Implementing the change, which includes putting the innovation into practice and usually requires some organization members to change their work behaviors and relationships, and (7) Institutionalizing the change by including the change in strategic plans, job descriptions, and budgets so that it is a routine part of organizational operations.

The key agents involved in change have been found to differ from stage to stage. Top managers with political skills are important in the early stages, when a problem is recognized and made public, alternative solutions are discussed, and a choice is made and initiated within the organization. Top managers are also important at the institutionalization stage because they have the power to incorporate the changes into organizational structure and routines. Midlevel managers are active during the adoption and early implementation stages, when roles such as obtaining and diffusing information, adapting information and the intervention, mediating between strategy and day-to-day implementation activities, and selling intervention implementation are critical (Birken et al., 2012, 2015). The frontline staff who need to make changes in their day-to-day practices are the focus of the implementation process. Examples of frontline staff are teachers involved in curriculum innovation or food service workers involved in an innovation in preparing cafeteria food.

Flaspohler et al. (2008) examined the capacity staff and organizations needed to adopt and implement prevention programs. These elements are also important to consider in general organizational consultation and technical assistance. The Interactive Systems Framework describes support and delivery systems that are needed to increase general and innovation-specific capacity to carry out prevention efforts (Leeman et al., 2014; Wandersman et al., 2008, 2012). Wandersman et al. (2012) also proposed an evidence-based system for innovation support (EBSIS) to increase the effectiveness and efficiency of support activities within an organization that is intended to build capacity for implementation (Kreuter et al., 2012). EBSIS includes four components for innovation-specific and general capacity building: tools, training, technical assistance, and quality assurance/quality improvement (Ray et al., 2012). Frameworks such as the Consolidated Framework for Implementation Research (Damschroder et al., 2022), the Theoretical Domains Framework (Birken, Powell, et al., 2017), and the Exploration, Preparation, Implementation Sustainment (EPIS) Framework (Moullin & Aarons, 2022) similarly propose conditions for intervention implementation. These frameworks generally suggest that conditions for implementation relate to characteristics of individuals within the implementing organization, features of the intervention to be implemented, features of the organization's inner and outer environments, and the process required for implementation (see Chapter 9).

Institutionalization focuses on the integration of the innovation into organization functions and routines so that it survives beyond the presence of the original program funding, adopters, or program champions (Manning et al., 2014). Institutionalization of an intervention requires mechanisms for becoming embedded in the organization's routines, for example, in the continuing allocation of resources (funding, personnel, materials, facilities, and time), and in the development of objectives, job descriptions, plans, and budgets. In other cases, interventions may be institutionalized outside an organization's boundaries, or the goals of the intervention may be subsumed in other programs. For example, program components may be taken over by community organizations, once the demonstration program is over, as in the historic cases of the Stanford Heart Disease Prevention Program (Jackson et al., 1994) and the Minnesota Heart Health Program (Bracht et al., 1994). Finally, the program continuation goal may be sustainability—to continue the program's effects whether or not the program itself continues intact (Shigayeva & Coker, 2015). For example, in the World Health Organization's historic efforts to eradicate smallpox, the initial program of mass vaccination was followed by surveillance and aggressive follow-up of suspected cases (Fenner et al., 1988).

Stakeholder Theory

We describe stakeholder theory in this section on organizational-level theories; however, stakeholders can be key agents at the community and societal levels as well. Change processes at all levels bring together stakeholders who may differ from each other in their social, political, and ethical paradigms; engagement goals and interests; and types and amounts of power (Brown et al., 2003). Such diversity is critical to the understanding of an issue from multiple perspectives and to the creation of new meanings and intervention opportunities. Stakeholders who cross levels and networks can be particularly important change agents, as they have the potential to produce change in multiple system sectors (Foster-Fishman et al., 2007).

Health promoters, their organizations, and the communities with which they work are frequently external stakeholders of organizations, that is, they exist outside a focal organization but have a direct interest in what the organization does. Stakeholder theory has examined how managers can strategically approach relationships with multiple external stakeholders, but research has also studied how stakeholders can influence organizations, through conducting a stakeholder analysis (Kok et al., 2015). Stakeholder analysis identifies stakeholders and their interests and prioritizes them based on their characteristics and location in social networks outside the organization. The salience of stakeholder participation depends on three attributes: their **power** (ability to impose their will by authority), **legitimacy** (perception that their actions are appropriate), and **urgency** (requirement of immediate attention).

Change-focused stakeholder groups, such as community groups seeking to change organizational policies related to collective conditions, seek to maximize their power, legitimacy, and urgency (Kok et al., 2015). They may forge alliances with other stakeholders, and they may use either community development or social action, a more radical approach to change (see Community-Level Theories section). Community development efforts use persuasion, constructive dialogue, and cooperation. In social action, when mass participation is possible, tactics include boycotts, buycotts (buying from preferred companies), letters or e-mails, petitions, marches, and rallies. When there is less dependence on participatory action, blocking of gates, sabotage, Internet activism, lawsuits, shareholder activism, and negative publicity may be useful tactics.

Besides their use of change agents, Presseau et al. (2022) argue for seeking input from stakeholders during the planning process of health promotion programs, similar to embedding members of the public in all stages of the development process. An example of stakeholder engagement in program design is provided by Saleme et al. (2021), who applied Intervention Mapping with incorporation of stakeholder and user input to design a digital game intervention to support social-emotional skills development and promote prosocial behavior in children aged 8–11 years old. Their key stakeholders included teachers and education experts. They describe how behavioral theory and stakeholder input can be incorporated into a final game design. The final digital game prototype was co-designed with continuous input and insights provided by expert stakeholders and feedback from children. Stakeholder theory provides further foundation for Intervention Mapping's focus on involving stakeholders and community partners throughout the planning, implementation, and evaluation process.

Community-Level Theories

Communities are organized around shared needs and challenges across various domains, including social justice, economic development, health and well-being, education, safety, and environmental sustainability. Communities may be based on geography; on gender, ethnic, or cultural identity; or on an issue, such as the environment, animal rights, food security, or public health. A shared reality or identity is key to the definition of a community. Collaboration and advocacy often play a central role in addressing the shared concerns (Minkler & Wakimoto, 2022b; Obama, 2022). In this section, we first review Community Coalition Theory, which could also be considered an interorganization network theory. Then we discuss theories of social capital and community capacity. Although social capital can be considered an emergent property of social networks, we have included it as a community-level construct because it is so closely intertwined with development of community capacity, which should be a goal of every community change effort. The remainder of this section focuses on social norms, conscientization, and community organization.

Community Coalition Theory

Organizations form partnerships to manage their environments. These interactions may be informal and transient or highly structured with shared decision-making and leadership. Community coalitions are one such form of organization at the community level that include a structured arrangement for organizations to work together to achieve a common goal, usually preventing or ameliorating a community problem (Butterfoss & Kegler, 2022).

Thus, coalitions are an important method for facilitating community empowerment, particularly through four processes: enhancing experience and competence, improving group structure and capacity, removing social and environmental barriers, and increasing environmental support and resources (de Leeuw et al., 2021; Lawlor et al., 2022).

Over the past two decades, community coalitions, funded by governments and foundations, have become a key approach to community problem solving. This has led to some concern that community coalitions have been co-opted by human service organizations and funders, to the detriment of disenfranchised communities (Chavis, 2001). Butterfoss and Kegler (2009) proposed the Community Coalition Action Theory that draws on a large body of empirical research and has been described through a set of "practice-proven propositions" (see Butterfoss & Kegler, 2022, Tables 18.1 and 18.2, pp. 309–313). Coalitions develop through three specific stages: formation, maintenance, and institutionalization. Coalitions recycle through these stages with the recruitment of members, renewal of plans, and addition of new issues. Each stage requires a different set of skills and resources and thus different strategies for training and technical assistance by staff and consultants.

The formation stage is most successful when a convener or lead agency with linkages to the community provides technical assistance, material support, credibility, and valuable contacts. The coalition must also include a deeply committed core group that expands to include community gatekeepers and a broad constituency of participants. The coalition should identify strong staff and member leaders who then develop structures, such as formalized rules, roles, and procedures. During this stage, open and frequent communication, shared and formalized decision-making processes, conflict management, benefits of participation that outweigh the costs, and positive relationships among members will provide a high level of member engagement, pooling of resources, and effective assessment and planning (see Butterfoss & Kegler, 2022, pp. 309–315).

The key tasks of the maintenance stage are sustaining member involvement; pooling member and external resources; and engaging in assessment, planning, and action to achieve coalition goals. There is a synergy in these tasks to promote successful implementation of strategies and community change outcomes. Coalitions are more likely to create community change when they direct interventions at multiple levels (see Butterfoss & Kegler, 2022, pp. 315–318).

At the institutionalization stage, successful coalitions show an impact on health and social outcomes, as well as increases in capacity that they can apply to other issues. Sustainability planning should start early, be carefully managed and governed, and remain an ongoing effort throughout the coalition's lifespan. Key conditions for success include securing diverse funding sources and building credibility with both the constituency and policymakers (see Butterfoss & Kegler, 2022, pp. 318–319).

As Butterfoss and Kegler (2022) highlight, achieving the stage of institutionalization represents a sustainable outcome in its own right. Progress in addressing one community issue can enhance the capacity of local organizations to leverage the skills, partnerships, and resources developed through this process. This increased capacity enables organizations to tackle additional challenges that align with the community's needs and priorities, fostering long-term resilience and adaptability.

Collective Impact Model

More recently, the Collective Impact Model has been introduced to the field of community health promotion (Flood et al., 2015). Originally developed in the business domain, the Collective Impact Model is a framework for addressing complex social problems by bringing together diverse organizations from various sectors to work collaboratively toward a common goal. It relies on five key conditions across phases of action initiation, action organizing, and sustaining action and impact: a common agenda, shared measurement, mutually reinforcing activities, continuous communication, and a backbone support organization. The model states that effective collective impact requires a shared vision and common understanding of the problem among all participants, along with a coordinated but differentiated approach to solutions in which alignment and accountability is ensured by regular and consistent data collection. Open communication should foster trust, shared goals, and motivation, while a dedicated backbone organization with specialized staff is essential to manage the initiative and coordinate the efforts of all involved parties (see also Table 1 and 2 in Flood et al., 2015). Applying the model to a community health initiative could mean that local clinics provide medical services, schools offer health education, and businesses fund well-being programs. A dedicated backbone organization would then ensure these efforts are coordinated and aligned with the common vision.

Social Capital and Community Capacity Theories

Social capital emphasizes the value of relationships and community ties in enabling collective action and improving societal outcomes. It is considered a critical resource for fostering civic engagement, economic development, and overall community well-being. Social capital has been defined variously, for example, as "the ability of actors to secure benefits by virtue of membership in social networks or other social structures" (Portes, 1998), as "the processes and conditions among people and organizations that lead to accomplishing a goal of mutual social benefit" (Green & Kreuter, 2005), and as "features of social organization such as networks, norms, and social trust that facilitate coordination and cooperation for mutual benefit" (Putnam, 2011). The first definition is from the individual perspective and is similar to social support. The latter definitions are from the perspective of the whole network—the collective.

High social capital is manifested in high levels of four interrelated constructs: trust, cooperation, civic engagement, and reciprocity (Jin & Lee, 2013).

Three types of social capital have been described: bonding, bridging, and linking (Claridge, 2018). Bonding social capital refers to trust and cooperation between network members with a shared social identity (see Reynolds et al., 2020). Bridging social capital occurs between people who are not alike in a sociodemographic or social identity sense and yet have relations of respect and mutuality. Linking social capital, a subset of bridging social capital, comprises norms of respect and trusting relationships between people who are interacting across explicit differences in power.

At the collective level, social capital is thought to influence health outcomes by regulating social behavior through informal social control and enabling groups to engage in collective action, known as collective efficacy. While social capital can promote health, it also has the potential to pose risks, such as through the exclusion of outsiders. Kawachi and Berkman (2015) reported that social capital, operationalized as interpersonal trust, norms of reciprocity, and per capita membership in voluntary associations aggregated to the state level, is directly and negatively associated with health outcomes. This seems to be true for social capital at both the individual and collective level (Murayama et al., 2012). Although some evidence calls into question the role of social capital in the promotion of health in a cross-national examination (Kennelly et al., 2003), many researchers agree that it has some role, with the three different types (bridging, bonding, linking) of social capital functioning both as a buffer against negative health effects of low socioeconomic environments and as a driver of health more so for people with a lower as opposed to higher socioeconomic status (Uphoff et al., 2013). Negative associations between social capital and health have also been observed. For instance, disadvantaged groups lacking access to bridging social capital may fare better in environments with weaker social divides than in communities where they face social exclusion. Research in rural communities, however, suggests that social capital functions more effectively as a collective rather than an individual resource. Bridging social ties within economically disadvantaged minority communities play a critical role in overcoming the social and economic isolation caused by segregation (Wilson et al., 2015).

Community capacity is closely related to and inclusive of social capital. It has been defined as "a set of dynamic community traits, resources, and associational patterns that can be brought to bear for community building and community health improvement" (Wendel et al., 2009). Dimensions of community capacity include skills and resources, the nature of social relations, structures and mechanisms for community dialogue, leadership, civic participation, the value system, and learning culture. Central to community capacity are the community's ability to engender leadership and participation, analyze its own thinking processes and change efforts, mobilize resources, experience a sense of connection among people, participate in meaningful rituals, maintain an awareness of previous change efforts and current conditions, and employ power to create change (Flaspohler et al., 2008).

From the perspective of social networks, we emphasize the importance of linking persons to community organizations, such as places of worship, social clubs, schools, political groups, and work settings, in which individuals can voluntarily associate with others to address issues of community concern. It is also important for residents to have loose ties outside their primary networks to bring in new information and resources, and interorganizational meetings and coalitions can foster such ties. For example, statewide meetings of church associations, nonprofit health agency volunteers, political conventions, and joint neighborhood association meetings allow the opportunity for residents to connect with others with similar concerns and interests, to learn about their activities, and to team up to work together. Villalonga-Olives et al. (2018) report on a systematic review on social capital interventions in public health. The majority of these interventions focused on individual-level change (e.g. encouraging social participation), as opposed to community-level change. The majority of interventions sought to directly strengthen social capital to influence health outcomes. There is a clear lack of studies that incorporate a multilevel perspective, and there is a lack of consideration of specific groups that might selectively benefit from social capital interventions. For example, Hussen et al. (2018) employed a community-based participatory research process to develop a novel intervention designed to enhance social capital and engagement in HIV care among young Black gay/bisexual and other men who have sex with men. They define social capital as the net worth of an individual's resource-containing, reciprocal, and trustworthy social network connections, which is an important resilience resource that has been shown to positively impact a range of different health outcomes, including HIV care engagement.

Social Norms Theory

Social norms, expectations of behavior by members of a social group, are a property of a community. They are the social rules that specify what is appropriate or inappropriate in a particular situation (Gross & Vostroknutov, 2022). Unlike codified laws, social norms are informal, unwritten rules of conduct that are shaped and understood through social interaction and mutual negotiation (Chung & Rimal, 2016). Social norms can be explicated at the individual level (i.e., perceived norms) or at the societal level (i.e., collective norms). Perceived norms refer to individuals' perceptions about others' behaviors and attitudes, whereas collective norms refer to commonly accepted rules or standards that define which behaviors are encouraged or discouraged for members of a group (Lapinski & Rimal, 2005; Rimal & Lapinski, 2015). Norms are transmitted to individuals through the process of socialization that occurs primarily in childhood through the family and then continues through institutions, such as churches, voluntary associations, sport clubs, and schools (Chung & Rimal, 2016). To achieve effective normative change, several lessons can be learned from research and practice and are related to how social norms differ from other socially constructed concepts (e.g., attitude), the dual role of social norms in behavioral and societal change showing both direct and indirect impact and having harmful and supportive influence, and the importance of changing social norms from "the inside" (Cislaghi & Heise, 2018).

Different methods have been used to shift social norms, including **mass media portrayals of role models, entertainment-education, behavioral journalism,** and **mobilizing social networks.** In various formats, including soap operas, popular music, films, and comic books, popular characters have modeled norms about health behaviors. Entertainment-education has been applied in popular television shows and television series, in particular to communicate accurate health information. A classic successful example of entertainment-education is the children's program Sesame Street. An example of a long-running program is the Soul City program in South Africa, which started directly after the change of government and the transition to democracy in 1994 with the purpose of inducing social change (Sood et al., 2017). Entertainment-education is using many formats including local street theatre, music, games, and social media, next to traditional channels as radio and television. The most common health topic across programs is sexual and reproductive health, followed at some distance by topics related to diet and nutrition, physical activity, cancer prevention, mental health, and cardiovascular health (Sood et al., 2017). In a meta-analysis of 10 experimental and quasi-experimental studies into the effectiveness of narrated mass media programs in promoting safer sexual practices among youth, Orozco-Olvera et al. (2019) found that entertainment-education narratives had small but significant effects for three sexual behaviors (number of sexual partners, unprotected sex, STI testing and management). Indeed, given their ability to reach large audiences, entertainment-education programs have significant potential to serve as cost-effective communication tools, particularly when compared to resource-intensive or face-to-face interventions (Orozco-Olvera et al., 2019; Sood et al., 2017).

Behavioral journalism uses mass media role-model stories of community members and advice from experts to change norms and increase adoption of behaviors (McAlister, 2017; van Empelen, Kok, Schaalma, et al., 2003; van Empelen, Kok, van Kesteren, et al., 2003). In behavioral journalism, the health educator interviews potential models for descriptions of reasons for their behavior change, skills used, and ways in which the change has been reinforced. The media materials then use those models who are perceived as attractive and similar to members of the priority population and model the right kinds of behaviors. Formats used for behavioral journalism include reality television programs, broadcast and print news media, printed newsletters for special audiences, documentary film and video, digital and mobile communication, and social media. Behavioral journalism is intended for use in concert with community organization and actions to prompt and reinforce the imitation of role models and to facilitate and enable behavior change. Behavioral journalism has also been combined with entertainment-education by using a community network of volunteers who cue people to watch the television documentary stories (Serra-Martinez et al., 2018). These methods increase the visibility of behaviors of opinion leaders and early adopters, increasing the speed of adoption of the behaviors within the population (McAlister, 2017).

Mobilizing social networks is another method used to influence social norms. For example, in a natural-helper model intervention Kelly (2004) and Jones et al. (2008) trained respected and popular patrons of gay bars to adopt protective sexual practices and persuade acquaintances to follow their examples. The researchers considered training 15% of the priority population as opinion leaders to be a critical mass to establish new norms among the bar patrons (Kelly, 2004). This intervention led not only to a change in individual behavior but also to increased norms supportive of protective behavior.

In addition to in-person methods, non-governmental but also non-profit and profit organizations increasingly utilize social media platforms to mobilize resources and advocate for collective action to achieve their goals. Notable is the example of healthcare providers who rapidly organized during the COVID-19 pandemic to address the shortage of personal protective equipment (PPE). They used social media to raise awareness and, within days, with the help of volunteering software engineers launched a website to facilitate the donation, request, and distribution of PPE. This combination of awareness-raising through social media and actionable solutions via the website enabled unprecedented resource mobilization, ultimately protecting both patients and healthcare providers (He et al., 2020).

Community Organization and Community Building

In the opening chapter of the 4th edition of their book *Community Organizing and Community Building for Health and Social Equity*, editors Minkler and Wakimoto (2022b) articulate the relevance and need for people to organize themselves to successfully confront the health, safety and social inequity challenges people face in nowadays world: "In this time of reimagining our world while confronting extraordinary challenges, including historic imbalances in privilege and power, renewed attacks on women's reproductive health, and immigrant and LGTBTQ rights, the importance of community organizing and community building has seldom been clearer" (p. 9). Added to these challenges at the time of writing of this text (July 2025) can be the Russian invasion in Ukraine, the Israel-Palestina conflict, the political interferences in national election campaigns and policy-making by foreign political or economic powers with oligarchic characteristics both on the American and European continent, and the continuous devastating natural and living consequences of climate change. Building further on the call from Pastor et al. (2011, 2018) and Minkler and

Wakimoto (2022a) compile extensive evidence demonstrating how social action through community organizing and community building serves as a catalyst for mobilizing collective power to address the socioeconomic and health inequities that face communities and societies at large.

Minkler and colleagues define **community organizing** as "a process by which communities identify their assets and concerns, prioritize and select issues, and intentionally build power and develop and implement action strategies for change" (Minkler et al., 2019). Reflected in this definition are concepts such as empowerment, social action and Freire's conscientization techniques (see the section on Empowerment theories), but—as Minkler and Wakimoto argue—these do not fully grasp the complexity of successfully organizing communities to remove the social, economic and educational barriers to health and social equity which are reflected in incidents of discrimination, violence, crime, and in figures related to educational attainment, health care access, and life expectancy.

Community building is conceptualized as a process that happens in the community. Rather than bringing external people to the community, community building processes focus on identifying and developing individual and community capacities as well as leveraging community assets already in place, including social capital and the built environment, to help effect change. Minkler et al. (2022) reference Blackwell and Colmenar (2000, p. 162), who define community building through eight principles. These principles emphasize a holistic rather than fragmented approach to strengthening communities, focusing on enhancing problem-solving capacity, fostering strong relationships with resource institutions, and ensuring community participation in policy development and implementation. They also call for explicit attention to minority and disadvantaged groups, the creation of broader regional networks that connect communities, and the integration of monitoring and evaluation systems to measure and sustain progress.

Rothman (2008) developed three models of community organization: locality development, social planning, and social action. Locality development raises consciousness about the underlying causes of problems and identifies strategies for action. It is heavily process oriented, with an emphasis on consensus, cooperation, and development of a sense of community. This model is most akin to the community development tradition in health promotion. Social planning uses information derived from empirical research. It is heavily task oriented, with an emphasis on expert assistance to solve problems. Social action is based on coercive change and seeks to redress imbalances of power. It relies on conflict methods of change, such as demonstrations and boycotts, and the change agent is both an activist and a partisan (Minkler et al., 2022).

For example, Ingabire et al. (2016) studied active community participation in malaria control as the key to achieving malaria pre-elimination in Rwanda. They describe the development, implementation, and evaluation of a community-based malaria elimination project in Ruhuha sector,

Bugesera district, Eastern province of Rwanda. A community-oriented approach was chosen in which self-organization among trained community members was a key element combined with regular training and support visits from local health authorities to ensure effectiveness and continuation. The establishment of community malaria action teams in combination with an environmental intervention by local rice farmers using biological substances for mosquito larval control innovative larval source control intervention contributed to reduction in mosquito density and nuisance bites, increased knowledge and skills for malaria control, as well as program ownership.

Social Movements

The study of social movements overlaps considerably with community organization. It offers insights for understanding the processes of change at the community level, in particular when feelings of collective autonomy are at stake. Social movements have been defined as "collectivities acting with some degree of organization and continuity outside of institutional or organizational channels for the purpose of challenging or defending extant authority, whether it is institutionally or culturally based, in the group, organization, society, culture or world order of which they are a part" (Snow et al., 2004).

Rivera-Rodriguez et al. (2025) developed the Movement Mobilization Model of Collective Autonomy to describe the process of what happens when disadvantaged group members try to gain power in an attempt to protect their collective autonomy. And, as these social movements gain traction, how advantaged groups in turn organize counter-movements to protect social hierarchy and their privileged position within it when they feel that their privileged position and collective autonomy are threatened. The model illustrates the different ways in which real-world power structures shape the way individuals experience and navigate social movements and counter-movements as they unfold in real time. Evidence of disadvantaged group-led social movements and subsequent advantaged group-led counter movements is widely present and visible. Examples include the backlash against the #MeToo movement, which sought to address sexual misconduct and violence against women, accompanied by reduced support for feminist movements among men who perceived a threat to their social status. Similarly, there is widespread religious and politically conservative opposition to comprehensive sexuality education programs in schools and broader sexual health and rights movements. In the United States, pro-life counter-movements have emerged in response to the progress achieved by the abortion rights movement over recent decades. Additionally, the Black Lives Matter protests have faced counter-responses from some White Americans who viewed these movements as restricting their racial group's autonomy (for supporting references, see Rivera-Rodriguez et al., 2025).

Health Advocacy

Advocacy is a primary method used in community organizing and for change at the higher policy level. This method addresses many of the processes that social movement theorists have discussed. Some view advocacy as directed primarily to legislative policy, using the strategies of voting, electioneering, direct lobbying, and grassroots lobbying (Galer-Unti et al., 2004). Others, however, view advocacy as a key component of community organization, with goals other than legislation and consisting of coalition building, leadership development, and extensive public participation. An example is forcing New York City to include lead treatment services and its school system to address the hazards of peeling paint in kindergarten classrooms (Klitzman et al., 2008).

It is important that health promoters choose tactics and activities that fit the type of community organizing they are using, the issue, and the community. Groups must decide the ways in which they intend to accomplish goals, and those activities will likely change over time in response to reactions to actions taken and to shifting external forces. Altman et al. (1994) listed the following approaches to advocacy: coalition building, community development, coordination, education, networking, public awareness, and policy or legislative change. Cohen and Marshall (2017) argue the public health sector is uniquely positioned to take a leading advocacy role in driving and coordinating multi-sectoral efforts to address the social determinants of health inequities. The authors reviewed the extent to which the public health advocacy literature addresses the goal of reducing health and social inequities, but concluded that the empirical literature does not reflect that this is occurring widely. They identified multiple barriers to engaging in advocacy for health equity, including a preoccupation with individual responsibilities for healthy lifestyles and behaviors, a lack of organizational and skillful capacity, and limited evaluation research despite the many theoretical models, frameworks, and professional practice standards supporting health advocacy (Cohen & Marshall, 2017).

According to Blenner et al. (2017), incorporating public health advocacy into public health training, practice, and research serves as a long-term investment for the public's health. These authors developed an advocacy training program that embeds students in community-based organizations for 9 months, providing students with experiential education through the application of advocacy skills and with opportunities to expand and broaden their advocacy efforts. The program directly addresses barriers to engage in advocacy, raising awareness, teaching skills to engage effectively in advocacy, and providing a forum to address perceived ethical dilemmas: "We teach students how to be advocates: true agents of change" (Blenner et al., 2017).

Media Advocacy

Media advocacy seeks to influence the selection and presentation of topics by the media in order to set and achieve a public health agenda

(Dorfman et al., 2022; Dorfman & Krasnow, 2014). Media advocacy is based on three steps: setting the agenda (framing for access), shaping the debate (framing for content), and advancing the policy. This is preceded by being clear about the overall strategy, which can be developed by addressing five key questions (Dorfman et al., 2022): What is the problem or issue? What solution or policy is being proposed? Who holds the power to implement the necessary change? Who needs to be mobilized to exert the required pressure? What specific action will advocates take to reach and persuade the target audience?

The next step is to ensure the media selects and highlights the story (framing for access), which requires developing a comprehensive media strategy. This involves determining the optimal timing for media attention—such as during budget negotiations or just before a critical parliamentary vote—and identifying the most effective channels to reach the target audience. To make these decisions, it is crucial to closely monitor the media landscape, identifying reporters to engage with and understanding which aspects of the message they are likely to cover and which they might overlook. Finally, media advocates must decide on the best approach, whether it involves creating news, leveraging breaking news, writing op-eds, posting blogs, submitting letters, requesting editorials, utilizing social media, or purchasing advertisements (Dorfman et al., 2022).

Developing a message strategy (framing for content) includes what you will say (the message), whom you will say it to (the target or audience), and who says it (the messenger). The message strategy involves shifting the view of health from the individual to the social level and dealing with the complexity of health and social problems so that a public health perspective defines the debate. Designing a message that receives media coverage is challenging at times, for example when it opposes a larger societal frame that can contradict a public health or government-supported perspective. For instance, in Ghana, religious opposition—primarily conveyed through traditional media channels such as radio and television—led to the withdrawal of national comprehensive sexuality education (CSE) guidelines for primary and junior high schools in 2019. This resulted in a shift toward abstinence-only education, which, despite its demonstrated ineffectiveness, has become the dominant narrative. Consequently, the reintroduction of CSE has emerged as a critical focus of public health research and advocacy (Achigibah et al., 2024).

Dorfman et al. (2022) provide the example of violence prevention. The prevailing narrative suggests that acts of violence are inevitable, unpredictable, and therefore unavoidable. Framing for content involves reshaping this story to emphasize that violence is predictable and preventable—if not at the individual level, then certainly at the population level.

The final step in successful media advocacy is then to frame the content so that it reaches the key decision makers whom the advocacy group is trying to influence (advancing the policy). Messages that grab the reporter's attention typically have elements that deviate from the regular information flow, for example because the message is controversial or ironic, describes a breakthrough, provides a new perspective, or touches on community values or assets relevant to the medium's regular audience. To enable easy coverage by the reporter, it is important to provide them with story elements that can be directly used such as visuals and concise media bites (Dorfman et al., 2022).

In the current digital era, the use of social media for advocacy is a logical path to follow. Yet, the number of empirical studies on their use in advocacy is surprisingly low given the potential reach of social media, as seen in some of the examples of social media use in community organization earlier described in this section. Jackson and colleagues conducted a scoping review of academic literature published between 2011 and 2020 and found a mere 22 studies that discussed the public health community's use of social media for public policy advocacy to a considerable extent (Jackson et al., 2021). The authors hypothesized that barriers to engaging in traditional and social media such as lack of training and resources, perceived credibility issues, and reputational repercussions might limit research and scholarship into this topic.

Societal-Level Theories

For the societal level, we examine theories that relate to public policy and its development. Because public policy is usually set by governments, change in policies will often focus on influencing government action at the local, state, or national levels (Ruiter et al., 2020).

Theories of Public Policy

Public policy is "a guide to action to change what would otherwise occur, a decision about amounts and allocations of resources, made at any level of government" (Milio, 1981). Health policy is directly related to public health and health services. Other public policies directed to issues such as economics, housing, or public safety also have much potential to influence health. Milio (1986) viewed economic policy as acting directly on people's biophysical and socioeconomic environments and indirectly through various areas for public policy, such as environmental safety, energy, income maintenance, and health and human services delivery. This framework shows policy as a collective condition of health behavior and health. *Health in All Policies* is a strategy of the European Union that reflects this close linkage of policy to health (Kickbusch, 2003).

Public policy sets options for organizations and for individuals, both directly and indirectly through organizations. According to Milio (1981), policy components should make "the creation and maintenance of healthful environments and personal habits the easiest—the "cheapest" and most numerous—choices for selections by governmental units and corporations, producers and consumers, among all the options available to them." Policy instruments include direct spending, such as grants and contracts; the production of goods and services; regulation and monitoring; and fiscal incentives, such as subsidies, taxation, and tax deductions.

Policy formation is a cyclical process occurring within a system open to the environment (Buse et al., 2023; Freudenberg & Tsui, 2014). In a rational or economic decision-making model, a policy maker would select the most efficient alternative to maximize the most valuable output. However, policy formation is much more complex than that, with many stakeholders and interest groups with varying power and diverse ideologies, insufficient information about policy problems and solutions, and unique contexts for specific issues. Theorists have endeavored to isolate key constructs and their relationships in this process to create hypotheses that can be tested (Jones, 2003). We will discuss several of these theories in the context of a model developed by Longest (2006).

Longest (2006) has identified three intertwined phases of the policy process: policy formulation, policy implementation, and policy modification. Policy formulation includes setting the policy agenda and the development of legislation. Policy implementation includes activities associated with rule making that guide operationalization and implementation of a policy. Policy modification is feedback from individuals, organizations, and interest groups on policy formulation and policy implementation. Health advocates and activated communities have opportunities to influence the policy process at each phase.

The policy process involves the movement from "policy primeval soup" (Kingdon, 2003) to the development of legislation. Cobb and Elder (1983) represented the traditional perspective of the policy process in the so-called Agenda-Building Theory. They suggested that the policy process follows clearly distinguishable steps from problem definition, through alternative specification, to resource allocation and implementation. However, Breton and de Leeuw (2011) concluded in their review: "Although this conceptual framework seems to have served a purpose, it has since become the subject of devastating criticism, predominantly focusing on the fact that the stages heuristic fails to address the dynamics of multiple, interacting, iterative and incremental cycles of action at many different levels of mutual and reciprocal action at the same time." Breton and de Leeuw cited Sabatier (Sabatier, 2007), who defined four parameters to assess appropriate theoretical frameworks of the policy process:

1. Each must do a reasonably good job of meeting the criteria of a scientific theory; that is, its concepts and propositions must be relatively clear and internally consistent, it must identify clear causal drivers, it must give rise to falsifiable hypotheses, and it must be fairly broad in scope (i.e., apply to most of the policy process in a variety of political systems).
2. Each must be the subject of a fair amount of recent conceptual development or empirical testing. A number of currently active policy scholars must view it as a viable way of understanding the policy process.

3. Each must be a positive theory seeking to explain much of the policy process. The theoretical framework may also contain some explicitly normative elements, but these are not required.
4. Each must address the broad sets of factors that political scientists looking at different aspects of public policy making have traditionally deemed important: conflicting values and interests, information flows, institutional arrangements, and variation in the socioeconomic environment (p. 8).

de Leeuw, Clavier, et al. (2014) view health promotion from a policy point of view, often different from a more social psychological perspective. They state that the establishment of policy is key to the implementation of actions for health. Their key arguments are that "(a) policy is not an intervention, but drives intervention development and implementation; (b) understanding policy processes and their pertinent theories is pivotal for the potential to influence policy change; (c) those theories and associated empirical work need to recognize the wicked, multilevel, and incremental nature of elements in the process; and therefore (d) the public health, health promotion, and education research toolbox should more explicitly embrace health political science insights" (de Leeuw, Clavier, et al., 2014). Moreover, de Leeuw (2017) states that health is created outside the healthcare sector. The healthcare sector aims to cure or mediate disease and is ill equipped to deal with the "causes of the causes" of health and disease (i.e., the social, economic, and political determinants that create opportunities for people to make healthy choices). Following up on that line of thinking, Greer et al. (2017) argue that if public health is the discipline that diagnoses and seeks to address social ills, then understanding the political causes and solutions to health problems should be an integral component of the field.

As a practical case example, Drennan et al. (2018) examined contemporary health and social care policies in England to assess how well they addressed health promotion for older adults with early frailty. Their focus was on evaluating whether these policies supported independence and prevented progression toward more severe frailty. The study found that older adults were not consistently identified as a distinct policy priority. This omission could be interpreted positively as an absence of age discrimination or negatively as a lack of attention to the specific needs of certain groups of older individuals. The authors concluded that this lack of policy focus on those in the early stages of frailty creates challenges for publicly funded or supported services. These services may struggle to legitimize health promotion plans for older adults with early frailty in the face of competing priorities, due to the absence of a clear policy rationale (Drennan et al., 2018).

As another practical case example, Mevissen et al. (2018) focused on experiences of sexual prejudice that could threaten the quality of life and psychological well-being of sexual minority youth. They provide a comprehensive overview of how they developed a theory- and evidence-based sexual prejudice reduction program suitable for the Dutch high school context, guided by Intervention Mapping. The aim of this sexual prejudice reduction program is primarily to reduce negative behavior toward lesbian, gay, and bisexual (LGB) individuals, mobilize social support, and strengthen the coping skills of LGB teenagers. However, the description of the program development and testing process can also serve as input for policy makers to develop standards and guidelines on how to systematically design and describe health promotion programs.

Multiple Streams Theory

Kingdon (2003) has investigated how issues reach systemic or governmental agenda status, inserting an element of chance that explains the fluidity and rapid change of the policy-making process. He views this process in terms of three *streams*: politics, problems, and policies (Kingdon, 2003; Zahariadis, 2007). The political stream includes changes in administration, party platforms, elections, and national mood regarding government. The problem stream includes issues within the various policy sectors, such as global warming, the national debt, health care costs, teenage pregnancy, specific diseases, and poor housing infrastructure. Science-based information is used to indicate the seriousness and causes of a problem and to provide evaluative information regarding current policies and programs. Policy solutions, such as pollution controls, universal health insurance, school-based clinics, or cooperative housing, "float around in or near government, searching for problems to which to become attached or political events that increase their likelihood of adoption" (Kingdon, 2003). In the policy stream, science offers ideas for solutions, legitimizes them, and provides information about technical feasibility. Events and ideas in these streams move along independently until there is a change in one stream, such as a change in government, emergence of a large problem, or advocacy of new policies. At this point a window between the streams opens up so that a problem may enter the political stream or a policy may become linked to a problem. The role of the policy advocate is to create, monitor, and capitalize on these opportunities (de Leeuw et al., 2013).

Policy advocates or entrepreneurs promote their proposals and the associated problems and facilitate coupling between the streams, linking problems, policies, and political opportunities together when the windows are open. Characteristics of effective policy advocates are recognized authority; visibility; strong political, communication, and negotiation skills; ability to engage in strategic planning; creativity; relative independence in resources and structure; and persistence (Kingdon, 2003).

In policy advocacy, as in many other arenas, timing is everything, and opportunity knocks for those advocates who are prepared. Much of the success in placing issues on the systemic and institutional agendas and in achieving policy enactment comes from an understanding of when to act and how to frame the issue. Kingdon's notion of policy windows

(Kingdon, 2003) provides a framework for timing. Kingdon said that policy is placed on the agenda when the windows between the three streams—politics (including elections, party platforms, and national mood regarding government), problems (all the issues within different policy sectors, including health, housing, and economic sectors), and policy solutions (such as school-based clinics and universal health insurance)—are open so that the policy can be put forward. For example, newly elected officials may focus on certain problems, for which prepared advocates who have networked with the right gatekeepers can present their solutions. Community advocacy groups can work with each of the streams. For instance, they can support candidates for elected office or influence party platforms, build community demand to address particular problems, and develop and promote well-researched and persuasive policy proposals.

Hoeijmakers et al. (2007) pointed to the importance of organizations in the policy development process. By building on Multiple Streams Theory and the network perspective on policy-making, they argued that influential organizations that have specific national policy interests and fluid resources and that are embedded within communication and resource-exchange networks are the main agents in the national policy process. These organizations are typically corporate entities, such as trade associations, professional societies, labor unions, corporations, public interest groups, government bureaus, and congressional committees. The policy process begins when one or more of these organizations recognizes a condition as a problem or an issue and alerts other organizations to it. The interested organizations then generate options, often as solutions in search of issues. The alternative options are then narrowed to get the policy option onto the governmental agenda for consideration. Each step is a product of negotiation and advocacy.

Powerful corporate entities representing industries such as health insurance, pharmaceuticals, processed foods, and tobacco take positions opposed or aligned with those of health promoters. Developing and maintaining strong entities on behalf of public health—such as public health professional associations, associations representing public health officials, and citizens' groups—and carefully creating alliances where appropriate with corporate groups are strategies necessary to represent health promotion in the policy development process (de Leeuw, 2017).

After policy is enacted into law, it must be operationalized; and advocates, especially strong interest groups, seek to influence this process through lobbying and other forms of influence. Especially important are long-standing working relationships between those implementing policy and the leaders of affected organizations and interest groups. These relationships are marked by the exchange of information and expertise. For complex policies that may affect a number of interest groups, advisory committees and task forces may be set up to help develop the proposed rules. Gaining a seat on these bodies allows for direct input to the process (Kingdon, 2003; Longest, 2006). According to Longest (2006), the success of the operational implementation of the policy rests on the fit between the implementing organizations and policy objectives and on the amount of resources (e.g., authority, fiscal, personnel, information and expertise, and technology) that the organization has. A key consideration is the competence of agency managers related to strategy, leadership, collaboration, and conceptual and technical knowledge and skills. Implementation problems are certain to arise, and management must be able to address these challenges.

The policy-making process is cyclical, and most health policies are the result of modifying previous policies. Policy modification occurs when key partners incorporate feedback from policy implementation and consequences into the policy formulation and policy implementation phases. Rules and practices may be changed or the law may be amended, typically in an incremental fashion. Feedback comes from the groups affected by the policies, especially key interest groups, and from those who formulate and take charge of implementation. Pressure to change can be external, from individuals, organizations, and interest groups, and internal, through oversight by the legislative, executive, and judicial branches. Evaluations of policy implementation and outcomes of policy are often crucial to decisions regarding modification (de Leeuw, Clavier, et al., 2014; Kingdon, 2003).

de Leeuw et al. (2016) suggest a new conceptual gaze at theorizing the policy process. They postulate that alternating between practical, empirical, and theoretical perspectives would create a more powerful conceptual toolbox to capture the dynamic interactions between actors in the different (policy, problem, and politics) streams. de Leeuw et al. (2016) address the criticisms directed at the stages heuristic and suggest that a more appropriate metaphor for policy processes is juggling. While these processes may seem chaotic, they require precise discipline, coordination, and sharp acuity from policy scholars and practitioners to effectively keep all the elements in motion.

Advocacy Coalition Framework

The Advocacy Coalition Framework (Breton et al., 2013; Weible & Sabatier, 2007) focuses on the system of policy-making. The primary focus is the policy subsystem, the set of agents who follow and seek to influence public policy in a given area across a time frame of a decade or more. Agents can be elected and appointed agency officials at all levels of government, interest group leaders, researchers, and important journalists who cover the issue. The agents engage in coordinated activity through advocacy coalitions. Advocacy coalitions are based on deep and unchangeable shared basic values, causal assumptions, and problem perspectives in the particular policy arena, along with more changeable secondary beliefs about how to implement the policy core. A small number of coalitions within a particular policy subsystem compete, promoting conflicting strategies, and policy brokers within the subsystem attempt to find a reasonable compromise to reduce this conflict so that policy can be enacted.

The Advocacy Coalition Framework provides guidance for carrying out policy advocacy. The framework rejects the notion that there are coalitions of convenience formed by agents motivated by short-term self-interest. Instead, core beliefs or ideologies create a stable lineup of allies and opponents. Advocacy coalitions will negotiate on the secondary beliefs, including decisions on administrative rules, budgets, interpretation of statutes, and information about the problem, before shifting on the fundamental policy core. Because of this, the core attributes of a governmental program are unlikely to change if the coalition that instituted that program remains in power. Policy can change through a perturbation from outside the policy subsystem, policy-oriented learning, internal subsystem events that highlight failures in the current subsystem practices, and negotiated agreements between coalitions. In comparison to Kingdon's Multiple Streams Theory, the Advocacy Coalition Framework sees the policy solution stream as much more integrated with the political stream because of the foundation of core normative and policy beliefs.

Khayatzadeh-Mahani et al. (2017), using the Advocacy Coalition Framework, examined why a proposed shisha smoking ban in Iran in 2011, despite reaching the political agenda, failed to achieve significant progress. The health sector led efforts to frame shisha smoking as a public health risk and advocated for a federal ban on its use in public spaces. However, opposition groups countered these efforts effectively. The policy stasis was attributed to (1) disagreements over evidence and conflicting core beliefs between pro- and anti-ban groups; (2) the pro-ban group's failure to mobilize sufficient public support; and (3) institutional constraints, including autocratic governance limiting policy change. The study highlights the role of actors' belief systems and issue framing in policy outcomes and underscores the need for robust public awareness campaigns to shift cultural attitudes toward shisha smoking in Iran.

Summary

This chapter aims to examine and describe theories that inform efforts to change environmental conditions in order to promote healthy behavior. These theories primarily focus on initiating change at the group or collective level. Examples include applying organizational change theory to implement new workplace procedures, using community organization theories to improve access to local health services, and drawing on public policy theories to prioritize health promotion in legislative processes. Following an introduction on systems thinking and power-related theories, the chapter provides an overview of theories at the interpersonal, organizational, community, and societal levels that offer guidance for planning effective change methods to influence conditions external to the individual that facilitate health and health behavior. While the chapter provides a broad overview of relevant environmental theories, understanding specific environmental phenomena may require engagement with additional theories beyond those included here. Further examples of theory application at the environmental level can be found in Kok et al. (2015), Ruiter et al. (2020), and Salmon et al. (2020).

Discussion Questions and Learning Activities

1. Discuss why collective conditions are considered important influences to promote health and health behavior.
2. Describe three examples of collective conditions that may influence health outcomes through individual behavior.
3. Describe three examples of collective conditions that may influence health directly.
4. Explain why agents at environmental levels are considered an important focus for health promotion programs. Give examples of agents for different types of collective conditions.
5. Discuss how systems theory can be helpful for health promotion planners to consider for placing a planned intervention in the context of broader social systems.
6. Explain why the role of power in society is an important consideration in planning health promotion programs.
7. Describe how organization theories could be used to change organizational conditions to promote health behavior and improve health outcomes.
8. Use one of the policy theories to analyze a health issue of current interest, for example health care reform, HIV prevention, or sexuality education.

References

Achigibah, A. D., Amdjadfar, M., Krugu, J. K., Ruiter, R. A. C., & Mevissen, F. E. F. (2024). The end point of it is abstinence: A qualitative analysis of underlying factors influencing Christian leaders' adoption and implementation of sex and sexuality education in Bolgatanga, Ghana. *Culture, Health & Sexuality, 26*, 1301–1315.

Aiyer, S. M., Zimmerman, M. A., Morrel-Samuels, S., & Reischl, T. M. (2015). From broken windows to busy streets: A community empowerment perspective. *Health Education & Behavior, 42*, 137–147.

Akande, V. O., Fawehinmi, T. O., Ruiter, R. A. C., & Kremers, S. P. J. (2021). Healthy dietary choices and physical activity participation in the canadian arctic: Understanding nunavut inuit perspectives on the barriers and enablers. *International Journal of Environmental Research and Public Health, 18*, 1–13.

Altman, D. T., Balcazar, F. E., Fawcett, S. B., Seekins, T. M., & Young, J. Q. (1994). Public health advocacy: Creating community change to improve health. In M. Minkler (Ed.), *Community organizing and community building for health* (2nd ed.). Rutgers University Press.

Bandura, A. (1997). *Self-efficacy: The exercise of control.* WH Freeman & Co.

Bartelink, N., van Assema, P., Jansen, M., Savelberg, H., & Kremers, S. (2023). Health promotion intervention research in complex adaptive systems: The Contextual Action-Oriented Research Approach (CARA). In D. Jourdan & L. Potvin (Eds.), *Global handbook of health promotion research.* Springer International Publishing.

Bartelink, N., van Dongen, B., Kremers, S., Renders, C., van Vlokhoven, B., Koperen, V., & van Assema, P. (2022). Supporting schools during the implementation of the health-promoting school approach: The roles of a healthy school advisor. *Frontiers in Public Health, 10,* 960873.

Batras, D., Duff, C., & Smith, B. J. (2016). Organizational change theory: Implications for health promotion practice. *Health Promotion International, 31,* 231–241.

Berkman, L. F., Glass, T., Brissette, I., & Seeman, T. E. (2000). From social integration to health: Durkheim in the new millennium☆. *Social Science & Medicine, 51,* 843–857.

Birken, S. A., Bunger, A. C., Powell, B. J., Turner, K., Clary, A. S., Klaman, S. L., Yu, Y., Whitaker, D. J., Self, S. R., Rostad, W. L., Chatham, J. R. S., Kirk, M. A., Shea, C. M., Haines, E., & Weiner, B. J. (2017). Organizational theory for dissemination and implementation research. *Implementation Science, 12,* 62.

Birken, S. A., Dimartino, L. D., Kirk, M. A., Lee, S.-Y. D., McClelland, M., & Albert, N. M. (2015). Elaborating on theory with middle managers' experience implementing healthcare innovations in practice. *Implementation Science, 11,* 2.

Birken, S. A., Lee, S.-Y. D., & Weiner, B. J. (2012). Uncovering middle managers' role in healthcare innovation implementation. *Implementation Science, 7,* 28.

Birken, S. A., Powell, B. J., Presseau, J., Kirk, M. A., Lorencatto, F., Gould, N. J., Shea, C. M., Weiner, B. J., Francis, J. J., Yu, Y., Haines, E., & Damschroder, L. J. (2017). Combined use of the Consolidated Framework for Implementation Research (CFIR) and the Theoretical Domains Framework (TDF): A systematic review. *Implementation Science, 12,* 2.

Blackwell, A. G., & Colmenar, R. (2000). Community-building: From local wisdom to public policy. *Public Health Reports, 115,* 161–166.

Blenner, S. R., Lang, C. M., & Prelip, M. L. (2017). Shifting the culture around public health advocacy: Training future public health professionals to be effective agents of change. *Health Promotion Practice, 18,* 785–788.

Boonstra, J. J. (2004). *Dynamics of organizational change and learning.* John Wiley & Sons.

Bracht, N., Finnegan, J. R., Jr., Rissel, C., Weisbrod, R., Gleason, J., Corbett, J., & Veblen-Mortenson, S. (1994). Community ownership and program continuation following a health demonstration project. *Health Education Research, 9,* 243–255.

Breton, E., & de Leeuw, E. (2011). Theories of the policy process in health promotion research: A review. *Health Promotion International, 26,* 82–90.

Breton, E., Richard, L., Gagnon, F., Jacques, M., & Bergeron, P. (2013). Coalition advocacy action and research for policy development. In C. Clavier & E. de Leeuw (Eds.), *Health promotion and the policy process.* Oxford University Press.

Brown, L. D., Bammer, G., Batliwala, S., & Kunreuther, F. (2003). Framing practice-research engagement for democratizing knowledge. *Action Research, 1,* 81–102.

Buse, K., Mays, N., Colombini, M., Fraser, A., Khan, M., & Walls, H. (2023). *Making health policy*. Open University Press.

Butterfoss, F. D., & Kegler, M. C. (2009). Community coalition action theory. In R. J. Diclemente, L. Crosby, & M. C. Kegler (Eds.), *Emerging theories in health promotion practice and research* (2nd ed.). Jossey-Bass.

Butterfoss, F. D., & Kegler, M. C. (2022). Community coalition action theory: Designing and evaluating community collaboratives. In M. Minkler & P. Wakimoto (Eds.), *Community organizing and community building for health and social equity* (4th ed.). Rutgers University Press.

Butterfoss, F. D., Kegler, M. C., & Francisco, V. T. (2008). Mobilizing organizations for health promotion: Theories of organizational change. In K. Glanz, B. K. Rimer, & K. Viswanath (Eds.), *Health behavior: Theory, research, and practice* (4th ed.). Jossey-Bass.

Chavis, D. M. (2001). The paradoxes and promise of community coalitions. *American Journal of Community Psychology, 29*, 309–320.

Chung, A. C. A., & Rimal, R. N. (2016). Social norms: A review. *Review of Communication Research, 4*, 01–28.

Cislaghi, B., & Heise, L. (2018). Theory and practice of social norms interventions: Eight common pitfalls. *Globalization and Health, 14*, 83.

Claridge, T. (2018). Functions of social capital–bonding, bridging, linking. *Social Capital Research, 20*, 1–7.

Cobb, R. W., & Elder, C. D. (1983). *Participation in American politics*. John Hopkins University Press.

Cohen, B. E., & Marshall, S. G. (2017). Does public health advocacy seek to redress health inequities? A scoping review. *Health & Social Care in the Community, 25*, 309–328.

Commers, M. J., Gottlieb, N., & Kok, G. (2007). How to change environmental conditions for health. *Health Promotion International, 22*, 80–87.

Cranley, L. A., Keefe, J. M., Taylor, D., Thompson, G., Beacom, A. M., Squires, J. E., Estabrooks, C. A., Dearing, J. W., Norton, P. G., & Berta, W. B. (2019). Understanding professional advice networks in long-term care: An outside-inside view of best practice pathways for diffusion. *Implementation Science, 14*, 10.

Cummings, T. G., & Worley, C. G. (2018). *Organization development and change*. Cengage Learning.

D'Aunno, T., Sutton, R. I., & Price, R. H. (1991). Isomorphism and external support in conflicting institutional environments: A study of drug abuse treatment units. *Academy of Management Journal, 34*, 636–661.

Damschroder, L. J., Reardon, C. M., Opra Widerquist, M. A., & Lowery, J. (2022). Conceptualizing outcomes for use with the Consolidated Framework for Implementation Research (CFIR): The CFIR outcomes addendum. *Implementation Science, 17*(1), 7.

de Leeuw, E. (2017). Engagement of sectors other than health in integrated health governance, policy, and action. *Annual Review of Public Health, 38*, 329–349.

de Leeuw, E., Clavier, C., & Breton, E. (2014). Health policy – Why research it and how: Health political science. *Health Research Policy and Systems, 12*, 55.

de Leeuw, E., Harris, P., Kim, J., & Yashadhana, A. (2021). A health political science for health promotion. *Global Health Promotion, 28*, 17–25.

de Leeuw, E., Hoeijmakers, M., & Peters, D. T. J. M. (2016). Juggling multiple networks in multiple streams. *European Policy Analysis, 2,* 196–217.

de Leeuw, E., Keizer, M., & Hoeijmakers, M. (2013). Health policy networks: Connecting the disconnected. In C. Clavier & E. de Leeuw (Eds.), *Health promotion and the policy process.* Oxford University Press.

de Leeuw, E., Tsouros, A. D., Dyakova, M., & Green, G. (Eds.). (2014). *Healthy cities, promoting health and equity—Evidence for local policy and practice 'a0.* Copenhagen, Denmark: WHO Regional Office for Europe.

Dimaggio, P. J., & Powell, W. W. (1983). The Iron Cage revisited: Institutional isomorphism and collective rationality in organizational fields. *American Sociological Review, 48,* 147–160.

Dooris, M. (2009). Holistic and sustainable health improvement: The contribution of the settings-based approach to health promotion. *Perspectives in Public Health, 129,* 29–36.

Dooris, M. (2013). Expert voices for change: Bridging the silos—Towards healthy and sustainable settings for the 21st century. *Health & Place, 20,* 39–50.

Dorfman, L., Gonzales, P., & Cuestas, S. M. (2022). Media advocay: A potent strategy for engaging communities in the fight for equitable public policy. In M. Minkler & P. Wakimoto (Eds.), *Community organizing and community building for health and social equity* (4th ed.). Rutgers University Press.

Dorfman, L., & Krasnow, I. D. (2014). Public health and media advocacy. *Annual Review of Public Health, 35,* 293–306.

Dori, D., Sillitto, H., Griego, R. M., McKinney, D., Arnold, E. P., Godfrey, P., Martin, J., Jackson, S., & Krob, D. (2019). System definition, system worldviews, and systemness characteristics. *IEEE Systems Journal, 14,* 1538–1548.

Drennan, V., Walters, K., Avgerinou, C., Gardner, B., Goodman, C., Frost, R., Kharicha, K., Iliffe, S., & Manthorpe, J. (2018). Moving upstream in health promoting policies for older people with early frailty in England? A policy analysis. *Journal of Health Services Research & Policy, 23,* 168–175.

Fenner, F., Henderson, D. A., Arita, I., Jezek, Z., & Ladnyi, I. D. (1988). Lessons and benefits. *Smallpox and Its Eradication,* 1363–1365.

Fiddian-Green, A., Kim, S., Gubrium, A. C., Larkey, L. K., & Peterson, J. C. (2019). Restor(y)ing health: A conceptual model of the effects of digital storytelling. *Health Promotion Practice, 20,* 502–512.

Flaspohler, P., Duffy, J., Wandersman, A., Stillman, L. M., & Maras, M. A. (2008). Unpacking prevention capacity: An intersection of research-to-practice models and community-centered models. *American Journal of Community Psychology, 41,* 182–196.

Flood, J., Minkler, M., Hennessey Lavery, S., Estrada, J., & Falbe, J. (2015). The collective impact model and its potential for health promotion: Overview and case study of a healthy retail initiative in San Francisco. *Health Education & Behavior, 42,* 654–668.

Folk, J. B., Mashek, D., Tangney, J., Stuewig, J., & Moore, K. E. (2016). Connectedness to the criminal community and the community at large predicts 1-year post-release outcomes among felony offenders. *European Journal of Social Psychology, 46,* 341–355.

Foster-Fishman, P. G., Nowell, B., & Yang, H. (2007). Putting the system back into systems change: A framework for understanding and changing organizational and community systems. *American Journal of Community Psychology, 39*, 197–215.

Freire, P. (1973a). *Education of critical consciousness.* Continuum International.

Freire, P. (1973b). *Pedagogy of the oppressed.* Continuum International.

Freire, P. (1998). Reprint: Cultural action for freedom. *Harvard Educational Review, 68*, 476–522.

Freudenberg, N., & Tsui, E. (2014). Evidence, power, and policy change in community-based participatory research. *American Journal of Public Health, 104*, 11–14.

Friel, S., Townsend, B., Fisher, M., Harris, P., Freeman, T., & Baum, F. (2021). Power and the people's health. *Social Science & Medicine, 282*, 114173.

Galer-Unti, R. A., Tappe, M. K., & Lachenmayr, S. (2004). Advocacy 101: Getting started in health education advocacy. *Health Promotion Practice, 5*, 280–288.

Garland, B. H., Majumder, M., Wiemann, C. M., Sanchez-Fournier, B., Babla, J., & Hergenroeder, A. C. (2024). Development of a multi-level/multi-modal intervention for health care transition preparation. *Health Care Transitions, 2*, 100063.

Glenn, B. A., Nonzee, N. J., Herrmann, A. K., Crespi, C. M., Haroutunian, G. G., Sundin, P., Chang, L. C., Singhal, R., Taylor, V. M., & Bastani, R. (2022). Impact of a multi-Level, multi-component, system intervention on HPV vaccination in a federally qualified health center. *Cancer Epidemiology, Biomarkers & Prevention, 31*, 1952–1958.

Grabowski, D., Aagaard-Hansen, J., Rod, M. H., & Jensen, B. B. (2023). Complexity theory in health promotion research: Four essential principles based on Niklas Luhmann's Systems Theory. *Societies, 13*, 253.

Green, L. W., & Kreuter, M. W. (2005). *Health promotion planning: An educational and ecological approach.* McGraw Hill Professional.

Greer, S. L., Bekker, M., de Leeuw, E., Wismar, M., Helderman, J. K., Ribeiro, S., & Stuckler, D. (2017). Policy, politics and public health. *The European Journal of Public Health, 27*, 40–43.

Gross, J., & Vostroknutov, A. (2022). Why do people follow social norms? *Current Opinion in Psychology, 44*, 1–6.

Hall, J., Gaved, M., & Sargent, J. (2021). Participatory research approaches in times of Covid-19: A narrative literature review. *International Journal of Qualitative Methods, 20*, 1–13.

Haslam, C., Jetten, J., Cruwys, T., Dingle, G., & Haslam, S. A. (2018). *The new psychology of health: Unlocking the social cure.* Routledge.

Hawe, P. (2015a). Lessons from complex interventions to improve health. *Annual Review of Public Health, 36*, 307–323.

Hawe, P. (2015b). Minimal, negligible and negligent interventions. *Social Science & Medicine, 138*, 265–268.

Hawe, P., Shiell, A., & Riley, T. (2009). Theorising interventions as events in systems. *American Journal of Community Psychology, 43*, 267–276.

He, S., Ojo, A., Beckman, A. L., Gondi, S., Gondi, S., Betz, M., Faust, J. S., Choo, E., Kass, D., & Raja, A. S. (2020). The story of #GetMePPE and GetUsPPE.org to mobilize health care response to COVID-19: Rapidly deploying digital tools for better health care. *Journal of Medical Internet Research, 22*, e20469.

Hoeijmakers, M., de Leeuw, E., Kenis, P., & de Vries, N. K. (2007). Local health policy development processes in the Netherlands: An expanded toolbox for health promotion. *Health Promotion International, 22,* 112–121.

Holt-Lunstad, J. (2022a). Erratum: Social connection as a public health issue: The evidence and a systemic framework for prioritizing the "Social" in social determinants of health. *Annual Review of Public Health, 1.*

Holt-Lunstad, J. (2022b). Social connection as a public health issue: The evidence and a systemic framework for prioritizing the "Social" in social determinants of health. *Annual Review of Public Health, 43,* 193–213.

Holt-Lunstad, J. (2023). National health guidelines for social connection: What Is the evidence in support and what might the guidelines say? *Policy Insights from the Behavioral and Brain Sciences, 10,* 41–50.

Holt-Lunstad, J., & Uchino, B. N. (2015). *Social support and health behavior.* Jossey-Bass.

Hussen, S. A., Jones, M., Moore, S., Hood, J., Smith, J. C., Camacho-Gonzalez, A., Del Rio, C., & Harper, G. W. (2018). Brothers building brothers by breaking barriers: Development of a resilience-building social capital intervention for young black gay and bisexual men living with HIV. *AIDS Care, 30,* 51–58.

Ingabire, C. M., Hakizimana, E., Kateera, F., Rulisa, A., van den Borne, B., Nieuwold, I., Muvunyi, C., Koenraadt, C. J. M., van Vugt, M., Mutesa, L., & Alaii, J. (2016). Using an intervention mapping approach for planning, implementing and assessing a community-led project towards malaria elimination in the Eastern Province of Rwanda. *Malaria Journal, 15,* 594.

Jackson, C., Fortmann, S. P., Flora, J. A., Melton, R. J., Snider, J. P., & Littlefield, D. (1994). The capacity-building approach to intervention maintenance implemented by the Stanford Five-City Project. *Health Education Research, 9,* 385–396.

Jackson, M., Brennan, L., & Parker, L. (2021). The public health community's use of social media for policy advocacy: A scoping review and suggestions to advance the field. *Public Health, 198,* 146–155.

Jin, B., & Lee, S. (2013). Enhancing community capacity: Roles of perceived bonding and bridging social capital and public relations in community building. *Public Relations Review, 39,* 290–292.

Jones, B. D. (2003). Bounded rationality and political science: Lessons from public administration and public policy. *Journal of Public Administration Research and Theory, 13,* 395–412.

Jones, K., Baggott, R., & Allsop, J. (2004). Influencing the national policy process: The role of health consumer groups. *Health Expectations, 7,* 18–28.

Jones, K. T., Gray, P., Whiteside, Y. O., Wang, T., Bost, D., Dunbar, E., Foust, E., & Johnson, W. D. (2008). Evaluation of an HIV prevention intervention adapted for Black men who have sex with men. *American Journal of Public Health, 98,* 1043–1050.

Kawachi, I., & Berkman, L. (2015). Social cohesion, social capital, and health. In L. F. Berkman, I. Kawachi, & M. M. Glymour (Eds.), *Social epidemiology.* Oxford University Press.

Keller, L., Gollwitzer, P. M., & Sheeran, P. (2020). Changing behavior using the model of action phases. In M. S. Hagger, L. D. Cameron, K. Hamilton, N. Hankonen, & T. Lintunen (Eds.), *The handbook of behavior change.* Cambridge University Press.

Kelly, J. A. (2004). Popular opinion leaders and HIV prevention peer education: Resolving discrepant findings, and implications for the development of effective community programmes. *AIDS Care, 16*, 139–150.

Kelly, M. E., Duff, H., Kelly, S., McHugh Power, J. E., Brennan, S., Lawlor, B. A., & Loughrey, D. G. (2017). The impact of social activities, social networks, social support and social relationships on the cognitive functioning of healthy older adults: A systematic review. *Systematic Reviews, 6*, 259.

Kennelly, B., O'Shea, E., & Garvey, E. (2003). Social capital, life expectancy and mortality: A cross-national examination. *Social Science & Medicine, 56*, 2367–2377.

Kerins, C., McHugh, S., McSharry, J., Reardon, C. M., Hayes, C., Perry, I. J., Geaney, F., Seery, S., & Kelly, C. (2020). Barriers and facilitators to implementation of menu labelling interventions from a food service industry perspective: A mixed methods systematic review. *International Journal of Behavioral Nutrition and Physical Activity, 17*, 48.

Keshavarz Mohammadi, N., Rezaei, Z., Burggraf, L., & Pype, P. (2024). Exploring settings as social complex adaptive systems in setting-based health research: A scoping review. *Health Promotion International, 39*, daae001.

Khanakwa, S., & Mbonigaba, J. (2022). Institutional arrangements for providing HIV and AIDS services in Uganda: A transaction cost economics analysis. *Health Services Insights, 15*, 11786329221096046.

Khayatzadeh-Mahani, A., Breton, E., Ruckert, A., & Labonte, R. (2017). Banning shisha smoking in public places in Iran: An advocacy coalition framework perspective on policy process and change. *Health Policy and Planning, 32*, 835–846.

Kickbusch, I. (2003). Policy innovations for health. In I. Kickbusch (Ed.), *Policy innovations for health*. Springer.

Kingdon, J. W. (2003). *Agenda, alternatives, and public policies*. Longman.

Klitzman, S., Kass, D., & Freudenberg, N. (2008). Coalition building to prevent childhood lead poisoning: A case study from New York City. In M. Minkler (Ed.), *Community organizing and community building for health* (2nd ed.). Rutgers University Press.

Kok, G., Gottlieb, N. H., Panne, R., & Smerecnik, C. (2012). Methods for environmental change; an exploratory study. *BMC Public Health, 12*, 1037.

Kok, G., Gurabardhi, Z., Gottlieb, N. H., & Zijlstra, F. R. H. (2015). Influencing organizations to promote health: Applying stakeholder theory. *Health Education and Behavior, 42*, 123–132.

Kok, G., Zijlstra, F. R. H., & Ruiter, R. A. C. (2014). Changing environmental conditions impacting health—A focus on organizations. In R. J. Burke & A. M. Richardsen (Eds.), *Corporate wellness programs*. Edward Elgar Publishing.

Kreuter, M. E., Casey, C. M., & Bernhardt, J. M. (2012). Enhancing dissemination through marketing and distribution systems: A vision for public health. In R. C. Brownson, G. A. Colditz, & E. K. Proctor (Eds.), *Dissemination and implementation research in health: Translating science to practice*. Oxford University Press.

Lambe, F., Ran, Y., Jürisoo, M., Holmlid, S., Muhoza, C., Johnson, O., & Osborne, M. (2020). Embracing complexity: A transdisciplinary conceptual framework for understanding behavior change in the context of development-focused interventions. *World Development, 126*, 104703.

Lambert, J. 2010. *Digital storytelling: Capturing lives, creating communities*, Digital Diner.

Lapinski, M. K., & Rimal, R. N. (2005). An explication of social norms. *Communication Theory, 15*, 127–147.

Lawlor, J. A., Metta, K. R., & Neal, Z. (2022). What is a coalition? A systematic review of coalitions in community psychology. *Journal of Community & Applied Social Psychology, 32*, 3–18.

Leeman, J., Baquero, B., Bender, M., Choy-Brown, M., Ko, L. K., Nilsen, P., Wangen, M., & Birken, S. A. (2019). Advancing the use of organization theory in implementation science. *Preventive Medicine, 129S*, 105832.

Leeman, J., & Mark, B. (2006). The chronic care model versus disease management programs: A transaction cost analysis approach. *Health Care Management Review, 31*, 18–25.

Leeman, J., Teal, R., Jernigan, J., Reed, J. H., Farris, R., & Ammerman, A. (2014). What evidence and support do state-level public health practitioners need to address obesity prevention. *American Journal of Health Promotion, 28*, 189–196.

Leeman, J., Wangen, M., Kegler, M., Lee, M., O'Leary, M. C., Ko, L. K., Fernández, M. E., & Birken, S. A. (2022). Applying theory to explain the influence of factors external to an organization on the implementation of an evidence-based intervention. *Frontiers in Health Services, 2*, 889786.

Leigh-Hunt, N., Bagguley, D., Bash, K., Turner, V., Turnbull, S., Valtorta, N., & Caan, W. (2017). An overview of systematic reviews on the public health consequences of social isolation and loneliness. *Public Health, 152*, 157–171.

Lewin, K. (1947). Quasi-stationary social equilibria and the problem of social change. In T. M. Newcomb & E. L. Hartley (Eds.), *Readings on social psychology*. Holt, Rinehart & Winston.

Longest, B. B., Jr. (2006). *Health policymaking in the United States*. Health Administration Press.

Luna Pinzon, A., Stronks, K., Dijkstra, C., Renders, C., Altenburg, T., Den Hertog, K., Kremers, S. P. J., Chinapaw, M. J. M., Verhoeff, A. P., & Waterlander, W. (2022). The ENCOMPASS framework: A practical guide for the evaluation of public health programmes in complex adaptive systems. *International Journal of Behavioral Nutrition and Physical Activity, 19*, 33.

Manning, M. A., Bollig-Fischer, A., Bobovski, L. B., Lichtenberg, P., Chapman, R., & Albrecht, T. L. (2014). Modeling the sustainability of community health networks: Novel approaches for analyzing collaborative organization partnerships across time. *Translational Behavioral Medicine, 4*, 46–59.

Marenus, M. W., Marzec, M., & Chen, W. (2023). A Scoping review of workplace culture of health measures. *American Journal of Health Promotion, 37*, 854–873.

Marteau, T. M., Fletcher, P. C., Hollands, G. J., & Munafò, M. R. (2020). Changing behavior by changing environments. In M. S. Hagger, L. D. Cameron, K. Hamilton, N. Hankonen, & T. E. Lintunen (Eds.), *The handbook of behavior change*. Cambridge University Press.

Martinson, M., Su, C., & Minkler, M. (2022). Contrasting organizing approaches: The "Alinsky Tradition" and Freirian organizing approaches. In M. Minkler & P. Wakimoto (Eds.), *Community organizing and community building for health and social equity* (4th ed.). Rutgers University Press.

McAlister, A. (2017). Behavioral journalism in health and risk messaging. In M. Powers (Ed.), *Oxford research encyclopedia of communication*. Oxford University Press.

McEvoy, C. T., Moore, S. E., Appleton, K. M., Cupples, M. E., Erwin, C., Kee, F., Prior, L., Young, I. S., McKinley, M. C., & Woodside, J. V. (2018). Development of a peer support intervention to encourage dietary behaviour change towards a Mediterranean diet in adults at high cardiovascular risk. *BMC Public Health, 18*, 1194.

McFarlane, S. J., Occa, A., Peng, W., Awonuga, O. & Morgan, S. E. 2024. Community-based participatory research (CBPR) to enhance participation of racial ethnic minorities in clinical trials: A 10-Year systematic review. Health Communication. 2022 Aug;37(9):1075–1092. 10.1080/10410236.2021.1943978.

McLeroy, K. R., Gottlieb, N. H., & Heaney, C. A. (2001). Social health in the workplace. In M. P. O'Donnel (Ed.), *Health promotion in the workplace*. Delmar.

Mevissen, F. E. F., van Empelen, P., Watzeels, A., van Duin, G., Meijer, S., van Lieshout, S., & Kok, G. (2018). Development of Long Live Love +, a school-based online sexual health programme for young adults. An intervention mapping approach. *Sex Education, 18*, 47–73.

Milio, N. (1981). *Promoting health through public policy*. F. A. Davis Company.

Milio, N. (1986). Multisectoral policy and health promotion: Where to begin. *Health Promotion, 1*, 129–132.

Minkler, M., Rebanal, R. D., Pearce, R., & Acosta, M. (2019). Growing equity and health equity in perilous times: Lessons from community organizers. *Health Education & Behavior, 46*, 9S–18S.

Minkler, M., & Wakimoto, P. (2022a). *Community organizing and community building for health and social equity*. Rutgers University Press.

Minkler, M., & Wakimoto, P. (2022b). Introduction to community organizing and community building in a new era. In M. Minkler & P. Wakimoto (Eds.), *Community organizing and community building for health and social equity* (4th ed.). Rutgers University Press.

Minkler, M., Wallerstein, N., & Hyde, C. A. (2022). Improving health through community organizing and community building: Perspectives from health education and social work. In M. Minkler & P. Wakimoto (Eds.), *Community organizing and community building for health and social equity* (4th ed.). Rutgers University Press.

Mkhitaryan, S. (2023). *Towards useful complexity in health behavior interventions. Maastricht University*.

Mkhitaryan, S., Giabbanelli, P. J., de Vries, N. K., & Crutzen, R. (2020). Dealing with complexity: How to use a hybrid approach to incorporate complexity in health behavior interventions. *Intelligence-Based Medicine*, 3–4.

Moullin, J. C., & Aarons, G. A. (2022). *Exploration, preparation, implementation, sustainment (EPIS) framework. Implementation science*. Routledge.

Murayama, H., Fujiwara, Y., & Kawachi, I. (2012). Social capital and health: A review of prospective multilevel studies. *Journal of Epidemiology, 22*, 179–187.

Obama, B. (2022). Why organize? Problems and promise in the Inner City. In M. Minkler & P. Wakimoto (Eds.), *Community organizing and community building for health and social equity* (4th ed.). Rutgers University Press.

Orozco-Olvera, V., Shen, F., & Cluver, L. (2019). The effectiveness of using entertainment education narratives to promote safer sexual behaviors of youth: A meta-analysis, 1985-2017. *PLoS One, 14*, e0209969.

Orum, A. M. (1988). Political sociology. In N. J. Smelser (Ed.), *Handbook of sociology*. Sage.

Pastor, M., Benner, C., & Matsuoka, M. (2011). *This could be the start of something big: How social movements for regional equity are reshaping metropolitan America*. Cornell University Press.

Pastor, M., Terriquez, V., & Lin, M. (2018). How community organizing promotes health equity, and how health equity affects organizing. *Health Affairs, 37*, 358–363.

Poland, B., Krupa, G., & McCall, D. (2009). Settings for health promotion: An analytic framework to guide intervention design and implementation. *Health Promotion Practice, 10*, 505–516.

Popay, J., Whitehead, M., Ponsford, R., Egan, M., & Mead, R. (2021). Power, control, communities and health inequalities I: Theories, concepts and analytical frameworks. *Health Promotion International, 36*, 1253–1263.

Portes, A. (1998). Social capital: Its origins and applications in modern sociology. *Annual Review of Sociology, 24*, 1–24.

Presseau, J., Byrne-Davis, L. M. T., Hotham, S., Lorencatto, F., Potthoff, S., Atkinson, L., ... Byrne, M. (2022). Enhancing the translation of health behaviour change research into practice: A selective conceptual review of the synergy between implementation science and health psychology. *Health Psychology Review, 16*, 22–49.

Putnam, R. D. (2011). Bowling alone: America's declining social capital. In R. T. Legates & F. Stout (Eds.), *The city reader* (5th ed.). Routledge.

Ray, M. L., Wilson, M. M., Wandersman, A., Meyers, D. C., & Katz, J. (2012). Using a training-of-trainers approach and proactive technical assistance to bring evidence based programs to scale: An operationalization of the interactive systems framework's support system. *American Journal of Community Psychology, 50*, 415–427.

Reynolds, K. J., Branscombe, N. R., Subašić, E., & Willis, L. (2020). Changing behavior using social identity processes. In M. S. Hagger, L. D. Cameron, K. Hamilton, N. Hankonen, & T. Lintunen (Eds.), *The handbook of behavior change*. Cambridge University Press.

Rimal, R. N., & Lapinski, M. K. (2015). A re-explication of social norms, ten years later. *Communication Theory, 25*, 393–409.

Rivera-Rodriguez, A., Mercado, E., Tropp, L. R., & Dasgupta, N. (2025). When social hierarchy, power, and collective autonomy motivate social movement and counter-movement mobilization among disadvantaged and advantaged groups. *Personality and Social Psychology Review, 30*, 3–28.

Rothman, J. (2008). Multi modes of community intervention. In J. Rothman, J. L. Erlich, & J. Tropman (Eds.), *Strategies of community intervention* (7th ed.). Eddie Bowers.

Ruiter, R. A. C., Crutzen, R., de Leeuw, E., & Kok, G. (2020). Changing behavior using theories at the interpersonal, organizational, community, and societal levels. In M. S. Hagger, L. D. Cameron, K. Hamilton, N. Hankonen, & T. Lintunen (Eds.), *The handbook of behavior change*. Cambridge University Press.

Sabatier, P. A. (2007). The need for better theories. In P. A. Sabatier (Ed.), *Theories of the policy proces* (2nd ed.). Westview Press.

Saleme, P., Dietrich, T., Pang, B., & Parkinson, J. (2021). Design of a digital game intervention to promote socio-emotional skills and prosocial behavior in children. *Multimodal Technologies and Interaction, 5*, 58.

Sallis, J. F. (2018). Needs and challenges related to multilevel interventions: Physical activity examples. *Health Education & Behavior, 45*, 661–667.

Salmon, J., Hesketh, K. D., Arundell, L., Downing, K. L., & Biddle, S. J. H. (2020). Changing behavior using ecological models. In M. S. Hagger, L. D. Cameron, K. Hamilton, N. Hankonen, & T. Lintunen (Eds.), *The handbook of behavior change*. Cambridge University Press.

Schoonhoven, C. B. (1981). Problems with contingency theory: Testing assumptions hidden within the language of contingency theory. *Administrative Science Quarterly, 26*(3), 349–377.

Scott, K., Beckham, S. W., Gross, M., Pariyo, G., Rao, K. D., Cometto, G., & Perry, H. B. (2018). What do we know about community-based health worker programs? A systematic review of existing reviews on community health workers. *Human Resources for Health, 16*, 39.

Sendra, A., Farré, J., & Vaagan, R. W. (2020). Seeking, sharing and co-creating: A systematic review of the relation between social support theory, social media use and chronic diseases. *Social Theory & Health, 18*, 317–339.

Serra-Martinez, Y., Colon-Lopez, V., Velez, C., Valencia-Torres, I. M., Acevedo-Montanez, A., & Fernandez, M. E. (2018). Using Intervention Mapping to design a health education program to increase colorectal cancer screening in Puerto Rico. *Annals of Behavioral Medicine, 52*, 324.

Shelanski, H. A., & Klein, P. G. (1995). Empirical research in transaction cost economics: A review and assessment. *The Journal of Law, Economics, and Organization, 11*, 335–361.

Shelton, R. C., Lee, M., Brotzman, L. E., Crookes, D. M., Jandorf, L., Erwin, D., & Gage-Bouchard, E. A. (2019). Use of social network analysis in the development, dissemination, implementation, and sustainability of health behavior interventions for adults: A systematic review *Social Science &. Medicine, 220*, 81–101.

Shigayeva, A., & Coker, R. J. (2015). Communicable disease control programmes and health systems: An analytical approach to sustainability. *Health policy and planning, 30*, 368–385.

Shushtari, Z. J., Salimi, Y., Sajjadi, H., & Paykani, T. (2023). Effect of social support interventions on adherence to antiretroviral therapy among people living with HIV: A systematic review and meta-analysis. *AIDS and Behavior, 27*, 1619–1635.

Skaggs, A. W., Loehfelm, T. W., Fananapazir, G., Dall'era, M., & Corwin, M. T. (2021). Utilization and yield of CT urography: Are the American Urological Association guidelines for imaging of patients with asymptomatic microscopic hematuria being followed? *AJR American Journal of Roentgenology, 216*, 106–110.

Snow, D. A., Soule, S. A., & Kriesi, H. (2004). Mapping the terrain. In D. A. Snow, S. A. Soule, & H. Kriesi (Eds.), *Blackwell companion to social movements*. Oxford, England: Blackwell.

Sood, S., Riley, A. H., & Alarcon, K. C. (2017). *Entertainment-education and health and risk messaging*. Oxford University Press.

Steijvers, L. C., van Bilsen, C. J., Wagner, S., Stutterheim, S. E., Crutzen, R., Ruiter, R. A., Hoebe, C. J., & Dukers-Muijrers, N. H. (2024). Social networks and COVID-19 vaccination intention in Dutch middle-aged and older adults in 2020: Insights into individual, interpersonal, community, and societal determinants—The SaNAE study. *Vaccine, 20*, 100562.

Tajfel, H., & Turner, J. C. (1986). The social identity theory of intergroup behavior. In S. Worchel & W. G. Austin (Eds.), *Psychology of intergroup relations*. Nelson Hall.

Tarrant, M., Haslam, C., Carter, M., Calitri, R., & Haslam, S. A. (2020). Social identity interventions. In M. S. Hagger, L. D. Cameron, K. Hamilton, N. Hankonen, & T. Lintunen (Eds.), *The handbook of behavior change*. Cambridge University Press.

Turner, J. C. (2005). Explaining the nature of power: A three-process theory. *European Journal of Social Psychology, 35*, 1–22.

Uphoff, E. P., Pickett, K. E., Cabieses, B., Small, N., & Wright, J. (2013). A systematic review of the relationships between social capital and socioeconomic inequalities in health: A contribution to understanding the psychosocial pathway of health inequalities. *International Journal for Equity in Health, 12*, 54.

Valdez, E. S., & Gubrium, A. (2020). Shifting to virtual CBPR protocols in the time of corona virus/COVID-19. *International Journal of Qualitative Methods, 19*, 160940692097731.

Valente, T. W. (2012). Network interventions. *Science, 337*, 49–53.

Valente, T. W. (2015). Social networks and health behavior. In K. Glanz, B. K. Rimer, & K. Viswanath (Eds.), *Health behavior: Theory, research, and practice* (5th ed.). Jossey-Bass.

Valente, T. W., & Pitts, S. R. (2017). An appraisal of social network theory and analysis as applied to public health: Challenges and opportunities. *Annual Review of Public Health, 38*, 103–118.

van der Put, A. C., Mandemakers, J. J., de Wit, J. B., & van der Lippe, T. (2023). Worksite health promotion and work performance: Both awareness and use matter. *Journal of Occupational and Environmental Medicine, 65*, 949–957.

van Empelen, P., Kok, G., Schaalma, H. P., & Bartholomew, L. K. (2003). An AIDS risk reduction program for Dutch drug users: An intervention mapping approach to planning. *Health Promotion Practice, 4*, 402–412.

van Empelen, P., Kok, G., van Kesteren, N. M., van den Borne, B., Bos, A. E., & Schaalma, H. P. (2003). Effective methods to change sex-risk among drug users: A review of psychosocial interventions. *Social Science & Medicine, 57*, 1953–1608.

Vennegoor, G., van Assema, P., Molleman, G. R. M., van Empelen, P., Dieleman, J., & Jansen, M. W. J. (2023a). Conditions for implementation of whole school health promotion in the Netherlands. *European Journal of Public Health, 33*.

Vennegoor, G., van Assema, P., Molleman, G. R., van Empelen, P., Dieleman, J., & Jansen, M. W. (2023b). Fidelity, adaptation and integration of whole-school health promotion within Dutch schools: A cross-sectional survey study. *Health Promotion International, 38*, daad173.

Villalonga-Olives, E., Wind, T. R., & Kawachi, I. (2018). Social capital interventions in public health: A systematic review. *Social Science & Medicine, 212*, 203–218.

Wallerstein, N., Minkler, M., Carter-Edwards, L., Avila, M., & Sánchez, V. (2015). Improving health through community engagement, community organization, and community building. In K. Glanz, B. K. Rimer, & K. Viswanath (Eds.), *Health behavior: Theory, research, and practice* (5th ed.). Jossey-Bass.

Wandersman, A., Chien, V. H., & Katz, J. (2012). Toward an evidence-based system for innovation support for implementing innovations with quality: Tools, training, technical assistance, and quality assurance/quality improvement. *American Journal of Community Psychology, 50*, 445–459.

Wandersman, A., Duffy, J., Flaspohler, P., Noonan, R., Lubell, K., Stillman, L., & Saul, J. (2008). Bridging the gap between prevention research and practice: The interactive systems framework for dissemination and implementation. *American Journal of Community Psychology, 41*, 171–181.

Weber, M. (1974). *The theory of social and economic organization.* Oxford University Press.

Weible, C. M., & Sabatier, P. A. (2007). A guide to the advocacy coalition framework. In F. Fischer, G. J. Miller, & M. S. Sidney (Eds.), *Handbook of public policy analysis: Theory, politics, and methods.* CRC Press.

Wendel, M. L., Burdine, J. N., McLeroy, K. R., Alaniz, A., Norton, B., & Felix, M. R. J. (2009). Community capacity: Theory and application. In R. J. Diclemente, R. A. Crosby, & M. C. Kegler (Eds.), *Emerging theories in health promotion practice and research.* Jossey-Bass.

Wilson, R. L., Wilson, G. G., & Usher, K. (2015). Rural mental health ecology: A framework for engaging with mental health social capital in rural communities. *EcoHealth, 12*, 412–420.

World Health Organization, Canadian Public Health Association, & Health Canada (1986). *Ottawa charter for health promotion* (Vol. 1). *Health Promotion.*

Zahariadis, N. (2007). The multiple streams framework: Structure, limitations, prospects. In P. Sabatier (Ed.), *Theories of the policy process* (2nd ed.). Boulder, CO: Westview Press.

Zimmerman, M. A. (2000). Empowerment theory: Psychological, organizational, and community levels of analysis. In J. Rappaport & E. Seidman (Eds.), *Handbook of community psychology empowerment theory: Psychological, organizational, and community levels of analysis.* Kluwer Academic/Plenum.

Zimmerman, M. A., Stewart, S. E., Morrel-Samuels, S., Franzen, S., & Reischl, T. M. (2011). Youth empowerment solutions for peaceful communities: Combining theory and practice in a community-level violence prevention curriculum. *Health Promotion Practice, 12*, 425–439.

Zinn, J. S., Mor, V., Intrator, O., Feng, Z., Angelelli, J., & Davis, J. A. (2003). The impact of the prospective payment system for skilled nursing facilities on therapy service provision: A transaction cost approach. *Health Services Research, 38*, 1467–1486.

PART TWO

INTERVENTION MAPPING STEPS

CHAPTER 5

INTERVENTION MAPPING STEP 1

Needs and Assets Assessment

INTERVENTION MAPPING STEP 1 TASKS

1. Establish a planning group
2. Conduct a needs and assets assessment
3. Describe the context for the intervention, including the community, population, and setting
4. State intervention goals

Overview

Health promotion intervention planning begins with embracing a *culture of learning.* This includes intentional learning about the targeted health problem and its behavioral and environmental causes; the community and subgroups affected—including the settings and context that shape the problem; and the opportunity for improving health and quality of life (QOL). A *culture of learning* also includes learning about oneself as a health promotion practitioner and embracing *reflexivity* about how to engage in health promotion research and intervention in meaningful ways that bring mutual benefits for all people affected by the health issue.

In this chapter, we describe Step 1 of the Intervention Mapping (IM) framework. This step guides the health promotion planner in conducting *a needs and assets assessment* (NAA) to thoroughly understand a given health problem and to identify community assets that can be leveraged to address it. Foundational to conducting an NAA, and to the IM framework more broadly, is the promotion of community partnerships. Active participation among community partners, including those directly affected by the health issue, is critical to informing, guiding, and leading health intervention planning. We explore the NAA process as organized by the following sections: *Conducting a NAA as part of the intervention planning process; Exploring planning resources for conducting an NAA;* and an in-depth review of *Step 1 tasks.*

Conducting a Needs and Assets Assessment as Part of the Intervention Planning Process

Conducting a NAA is an important if not essential first step for planning health promotion interventions. While definitions vary, an NAA generally encompasses a collaborative and systematic process for determining the nature and extent of health needs in a population/ community; the factors contributing to those needs; and the human, organizational, and community assets available to respond to such needs (Smith et al., 2006). NAAs should be conducted in partnership with communities, as we explore below. While communities are often *geographically defined* (e.g., a neighborhood, city, or county), an NAA can also focus on a specific *community of shared interest*, such as a school (Clarke et al., 2019), workplace (Roemer et al., 2019), clinic setting (Linn et al., 2021), faith-based organization (Berkley-Patton et al., 2018), or *a community of shared experience or identity*, such as Latino immigrant farmworkers (Linville et al., 2020), persons experiencing intellectual and developmental disorders (Bakker et al., 2012), or the transgender community (Salkas et al., 2018).

Reasons for Conducting a Needs and Assets Assessment

An NAA gathers information that clearly describes the needs and assets of a *geographically defined* community or *community of shared interest or experience*. It is usually conducted before taking action and can help planners understand the current situation, informing the development of goals for change. While multiple reasons exist for conducting an NAA—from identifying and prioritizing needs among various health issues as part of a traditional community health assessment (NACCHO, n.d.) to measuring how a public health system is fulfilling its core function to assure access to essential services (Public Health Accreditation Board, 2013). Central to the purpose of an NAA is understanding the discrepancy between what is and what should be in a group or situation as well as the current resources and assets available to address a need (Gilmore & Campbell, 2005). Health inequities, defined as differences in health that are avoidable, unnecessary, unfair, and unjust (Dover & Belon, 2019), represent an important frame to guide the NAA process by helping planners identify and understand health discrepancies and the reasons for these within a defined community.

In describing health needs and inequities, there is a growing shift from a *deficit lens* that emphasizes the individual or at-risk group, toward an *opportunity lens* that focuses on the system that created the inequity, as well as the opportunity for improvement. The Robert Wood Johnson-funded *Health Opportunity and Equity (HOPE) Initiative*, for example, reframed a focus on *health disparities* into a positive frame of *health opportunity* by benchmarking health indicators in relation to the highest performing groups, which may include states or specific racial/ethnic and socioeconomic subgroups within states (Wong Croal et al., 2018). A *health equity and opportunity lens* can guide the NAA by focusing planners on inequitable health conditions and resources and point to opportunities within a given system for improving the situation.

Application and Models of Needs and Assets Assessments

The assessment of health needs represents a core function of public health (Centers for Disease Control and Prevention, n.d.; Public Health Accreditation Board, 2013) that has garnered increased interest in recent years. In the United States, community health needs assessments (CHNA) and community health assessments (CHA) are now required for both federally funded hospitals as part of the Affordable Care Act (IRS, 2019) and for health department accreditation (Public Health Accreditation Board, 2013). Paralleling this focus on NAA is a growing menu of health assessment and planning models. In the field of health promotion, NAA has been a key facet of individual-level and multilevel health promotion intervention planning and behavior change models, such as the *PRECEDE-PROCEED Model* (Green & Kreuter, 1999; Fielding, 2022), *MATCH* (Simons-Morton et al., 1995), *Behavior Change Wheel* (Michie, 2014), and *IM*. At the community level, practice-based health planning models that help guide the NAA process include the *CHANGE Tool* (CDC, n.d.), the *Community Health Assessment Toolkit* (ACHI AHA Improvement, 2017), and *Mobilizing for Action through Planning and Partnerships (MAPP)* (NACCHO, n.d.), among others (for a review of community health planning models, see Pennel et al. (Pennel et al., 2017).

An Intervention Mapping Approach to Needs and Assets Assessment

Traditional CHA often cast a wide net in exploring a range of health problems. For example, planning frameworks such as MAPP aim to provide a comprehensive assessment to identify the top four or five health problems of a community (NACCHO, n.d.). Once these health needs are identified, planners need to delve deeper into understanding the behavioral and environmental influences on the health need or issue (e.g., a health condition such as Type 2 diabetes, a health risk behavior such as smoking, or an environmental condition such as lack of access to health services), as well as the groups most affected by the health issue. IM can complement traditional needs assessments by providing a comprehensive understanding of a selected health issue. Step 1 of IM guides health promotion planners in conducting an NAA via:

- An epidemiologic, behavioral, and social-environmental analysis of factors that influence the health and QOL of a community and at-risk population;

- An assessment of determinants of health behavior for a given health problem—including modifiable determinants such as health beliefs, as well as biologic and demographic factors that may serve to identify priority populations; and
- An exploration of the intervention context, including the environmental factors that influence the problem, the settings where priority populations can be reached, and the strengths and assets of a given community that can be activated to address health needs.

Upon completion of Step 1, planners should present a full description of the health-related problem, QOL issue, health behavior(s), and/or environmental condition(s) influencing the problem in as much detail and complexity as practical within the resources and aims of the project.

Partnering with the Community to Conduct a Needs and Assets Assessment

In Chapter 1, we introduced the importance of partnering with the community in designing, implementing, and evaluating health promotion interventions. Given the growing recognition that the causes of well-being lie in the social determinants of health (Centers for Disease Control and Prevention, 2024e), we need health promotion approaches that embrace community participation as well as an intersectoral approach that can address the social forces that shape health. Beyond the need to bring together diverse sectors to tackle difficult social issues, fields such as *systems science, implementation science,* and *improvement science* underscore the importance of indigenous knowledge and the idea that there are people within systems who know their own people and context (e.g., school, organization, or community) and bring valuable perspectives for planning (Fernandez et al., 2019; Hawe, 2015; Langley et al., 2009; May et al., 2016). In Step 1, health promotion planners explore ways to foster (1) participation and partnership with the community via the establishment of a planning group, as well as (2) methods aimed at generating insights from community members about needs and assets that can be harnessed to achieve project goals.

Exploring Planning Resources for Conducting a Needs and Assets Assessment

> We shape our tools and afterward our tools shape us.
>
> —Marshall McLuhan

The increased interest in NAA has been accompanied by a rich and growing field of health assessment practice, including guiding principles, processes, methods, and planning tools. We encourage health promotion

Table 5.1 Intervention Mapping Step 1—Needs and Assets Assessment (NAA)

Summary of Planning Resources Presented in Chapter 5
Task 1: Establish and work with a planning group ✓ Principles of Collaboration[a] ✓ Linkage System Concept[a] ✓ Stakeholder Mapping[b] ✓ Group Formation Stages[a] ✓ Group Facilitation Processes[b]
Task 2: Conduct an NAA ✓ IM Core Processes[b] ✓ NAA Data Collection Methods[b] ✓ Social-Ecological Perspective[a] ✓ Logic Model of the Problem[c] ✓ Environmental Asset Assessment Framework[c]
Task 3: Describe the context for the intervention, including the community, population, and setting ✓ At-A-Glance Population and Context Table[c] *See Planning Resources for Task 2*
Task 4: State intervention goals ✓ Importance and Changeability Prioritization Framework[c] ✓ SMART Goal Framework[c]

[a] Guiding principles and concepts
[b] Processes and methods
[c] Planning tools.

planners to actively grow their NAA toolbox by exploring planning resources within the IM framework, as well as other NAA resources, including the Centers for Disease Control (CDC) Community Needs Assessment (Center for Global Health, 2013); Community Health Assessment Toolkit (Centers for Disease Control and Prevention, n.d.); Community Toolbox (Center for Community Health and Development (CCHD) Kansas University, n.d.); and MAPP (NACCHO, n.d.) among others.

As introduced in Chapter 2, a key planning resource for Step 1 and all subsequent IM steps are the *IM Core Processes (posing questions, brainstorming, reviewing empirical literature, reviewing theories for additional constructs, assessing and addressing needs for new data, and developing a working list of answers)*. In addition to the Core Processes, we explore in this chapter other planning resources (*guiding principles and concepts, processes and methods, and planning tools*) that are helpful in guiding an NAA and that are specific to the four primary tasks of IM Step 1. Table 5.1 provides a summary of planning resources for Step 1, with further description provided below.

Step 1 Tasks

The four primary tasks for conducting an IM NAA in Step 1 are presented in Box 5.1 and described below.

BOX 5.1. INTERVENTION MAPPING STEP 1 TASKS

1. Establish a planning group
2. Conduct an needs and assets assessment
3. Describe the context for the intervention, including the community, population, and setting
4. State intervention goals

Task 1: Establish a Planning Group

Task 1 of Step 1 consists of establishing a planning group to develop and complete the health NAA, and then to develop and plan implementation and evaluation of the health intervention as part of Steps 2 through 6. Toward this end, health promotion planners should consider both the composition of the planning group as well as the approaches and structures that will be used to enhance group management and processes for engaging project partners. The establishment of a planning group can take many forms, including *community advisory boards* in community-based participatory research (CBPR) (Newman et al., 2011; Turner et al., 2019), *community advisory councils* in healthcare settings (Oldfield et al., 2019), *core change teams* in the field of quality improvement (Silver et al., 2016), and *core planning teams* in community health improvement planning (NACCHO, n.d.), among other forms.

The establishment of a multidisciplinary planning group builds from a simple premise: *that greater participation and partnership with community partners, including those most affected by a given health issue, results in better health promotion interventions and greater benefits for individual and community health.* Participation by community partners, including potential beneficiaries and those who bring perspectives to inform the intervention, helps ensure that a health promotion intervention addresses issues important to a given community, that the intervention is culturally relevant and tailored to specific settings, and that project outcomes and evaluation findings are locally relevant, reflecting community insights and knowledge (Hawe, 2015; Wallerstein et al., 2018).

Importantly, health interventions that actively embrace participation and partnership with community members can build *capacity* for health promotion and other community improvement efforts—for both researchers and community partners—beyond the specific focus of the health intervention. This intentional capacity-building is at the heart of community-engaged research orientations that include CBPR (Wallerstein et al., 2018) and *participatory learning and action* (IIED, 2004), as well as community health planning frameworks such as the *Parallel Track Model* (Vatcharavongvan et al., 2013), which expands the benefits of a health intervention via a parallel track of capacity-building for all involved, regardless whether a given intervention was successful.

Meaningful participation in health promotion planning, implementation, and evaluation can take many forms. Seminal work on citizen participation by Arnstein (Arnstein, 1969) highlights the various degrees of community participation, from *manipulation* at the bottom rung of the ladder to *citizen control* at the top. Acknowledging that there may be various degrees of participation, planners should avoid *token participation* and strive, instead, to create meaningful opportunities for *equitable participation* throughout the planning process. Within the health promotion planning field, participation may be explained as a continuum where, at one end, the health planning group works *with* community members and implementers to understand the problem and its solution; and at the other end, the community members *are* the planners, building from participatory planning models and representing higher levels of participation (Wallerstein et al., 2018).

Guiding Principles for Collaboration

In fostering meaningful participation in health promotion planning, Box 5.2 presents a set of guiding principles for community collaboration identified by leading community-based health promotion professionals (e.g., Belansky et al. (2011); Cargo & Mercer (2008); Green et al. (2022); Minkler (2005); Turner et al. (2019); Wallerstein et al. (2018)). We encourage planners to explore approaches for incorporating these principles into their praxis, which may include forming *organizational structures* that include co-leadership with community partners; incorporating collaboration principles within *work group agreements* (Center for Community Health and Development (CCHD) Kansas University, n.d.), and creating *pause and reflect* spaces throughout the project as part of a *learning agenda* aimed at generating insights about the project process (USAID, n.d.). In applying principles of community collaboration, we embrace the call from community-based researchers for an intentional co-learning and co-creation approach among project partners as well as flexibility, adaptability, and critical reflection for partner engagement across different contexts (Wallerstein et al., 2018).

BOX 5.2. GUIDING PRINCIPLES FOR COMMUNITY COLLABORATION

- Acknowledge personal and institutional histories of planners and priority groups.
- Recognize the community (in its various conceptualizations- see below) as a unit of identity and promote community involvement from the beginning of the project.

- Achieve a balance between knowledge generation and benefits for community partners and priority populations, with an emphasis on mutual benefit of all partners.
- Use an ecological perspective in planning that recognizes and attends to the multilevel and complex determinants of health.
- Incorporate systems development planning principles, using a cyclical and iterative process.
- Facilitate collaborative, equitable influence on the direction and activities of the project through all or most phases.
- Make sure that the project results in learning, capacity-building, and sustainability.
- Show respect for the expertise, values, perspectives, contributions, and confidentiality of everyone in the community.
- Allot time and resources to group function.
- Compensate community participants.
- Disseminate results to all partners and involve them in the dissemination process.
- Address issues of race/ethnicity, racism, social class, LGBTQ discrimination, and other forms of oppression by embracing cultural humility and seeking the voice, guidance, and participation of groups who have been marginalized.

Establishing Effective Project Planning Groups

In considering who should be involved in a health intervention planning group, a growing body of research, theory, and practice underscores the importance of engaging diverse perspectives, individuals, and groups in the development of health interventions (Preskill & Jones, 2009; Rudolph et al., 2013; Turner et al., 2019; Wallerstein et al., 2018). While *stakeholder* has been a common term used to describe anyone who has an interest in the project and can influence its success or failure, given the negative historical roots of this term, we use alternate terms such as community or project partners. Having community partners work together can bring a variety of perspectives and knowledge, nurture feelings of project ownership, and increase the cultural relevance of a given intervention. Below, we describe the *linkage system* concept and *stakeholder (partner) mapping*—helpful approaches for identifying partners for a planning group to lead the NAA and overall intervention planning. First, in Box 5.3 we share an example of the establishment of a planning group with *¡Activate Ya!*, a tobacco-use prevention and physical activity promotion project in Uruguay.

BOX 5.3. ESTABLISHING THE PLANNING GROUP—¡ACTIVATE YA!

Uruguay is a global leader in the fight against tobacco use, which includes accomplishments with the regulation of the sales and marketing of tobacco products, policies governing public use of tobacco, and reduction in tobacco use and related adverse health outcomes (Abascal et al., 2012; Alonso et al., 2018). In supporting Uruguay's tobacco prevention efforts, the *¡Activate Ya!* project aimed to enhance school-based health promotion efforts to reduce youth tobacco use while enhancing physical activity, a key chronic disease prevention behavior that has also been linked to reduced tobacco use (Vatcharavongvan et al., 2013).

Toward this end, a partnership was established between leaders at CIET, a nongovernmental organization based in Uruguay aimed at decreasing chronic disease, and researchers at the UTHealth School of Public Health in Austin, Texas. The primary aim of this partnership was the development and evaluation of *¡Activate Ya!*, a school-based program funded by the US National Institutes of Health. A secondary aim was capacity-building among all project partners for adolescent health research and health promotion practice, following planning models such as the Parallel Track Model that place equal emphasis on co-learning and capacity-building in addition to an initiative's targeted health goal (Vatcharavongvan et al., 2013).

The *¡Activate Ya!* team began their efforts by establishing a planning group composed of individuals and groups related to the *community of interest*: secondary schools located on the outskirts of Montevideo. Members selected for this group included tobacco epidemiologists, adolescent health promotion researchers and practitioners, healthcare providers dedicated to the prevention of tobacco use, and importantly, secondary school teachers and leaders—a key group for the initiative (Springer et al., 2020). In addition to the core planning team, efforts were made to include the voices of school district planners and secondary school students. This planning group—which included both implementers/ program adopters (school staff) and representatives of the target population (students)—follows the linkage system concept (see description, below). Subsequently (Tasks 2–4), the *¡Activate Ya!* planning group led the NAA with the aim of co-learning about youth engagement in tobacco use and physical activity.

A Linkage System The *linkage system* concept provides direction in identifying potential community partners for a planning group. Originally developed by Orlandi and colleagues in describing work groups (Orlandi et al., 1990), a *linkage system* aims to link three primary groups in guiding planning: *a resource group* (developers—which may include content experts and funders), *an intermediate-user group* (potential adopters and implementers), and *an end-user group* (priority population or their advocates). While health intervention planning groups often include experts, they also need the voice of potential adopters (those who make the decision to implement a health intervention in a given setting) and implementers who understand a given intervention setting (e.g., a school, workplace, or faith-based community). The establishment of a linkage system aims to ensure that, once a health intervention is developed, it can be adopted, fully implemented, maintained, and have positive benefits for the priority population. As project planning is an iterative process, and each planning step requires different expertise, project leaders should continually reassess the group's composition.

Stakeholder (Partner) Mapping As a complement to the linkage system concept, stakeholder mapping is a helpful method for identifying partners for a project. Stakeholder mapping has been applied in a variety of fields, including citizen science initiatives (Skarlatidou et al., 2019), management and human resources (Greening & Turban, 2000), and policy development (Falbe et al., 2018). The purpose of stakeholder mapping may vary—from ensuring that needs of different groups are addressed (Cargo & Mercer, 2008)—to better understanding influential groups for a policy initiative (Green et al., 2022). The basic approach can range from a small group process to a larger workshop in which participants come together to brainstorm about a given issue or initiative.

Table 5.2 presents questions to guide the identification of community partners for conducting an NAA based on work by Cargo and Mercer

Table 5.2 Questions to Guide Recruitment of Community Partners for NAA

Planning Group Need	Questions to Consider
Expertise in the health problem or its causes	Who has content knowledge relative to the health problem or its causes? What disciplines can be most helpful in describing problems from an ecological perspective? Who knows about similar problems? Who is well respected for knowledge of this health problem or ones like it? Who has worked on a similar needs assessment or program?
Diverse perspectives and community participation	Who has needs and perspectives related to the problem? When programs are developed related to needs and problems, who are the potential clients, participants, or beneficiaries? Who already works with potential beneficiaries? Who can help the planning group clarify values related to the needs assessment and intervention development? Who can help the planning group balance science, social relevance, and cultural relevance? Who are the potential critics of the program or initiative?
Responsibility and authority	Who will manage the NAA and program development? Who is the funder? Who can become a partner in the assessment and program development? Who can bring resources to the endeavor?
Influence	Who has served as a resource to community members for this problem or related ones? What policy makers have worked on this type of problem? Who are opinion leaders who might have an interest in this type of problem? Who can help the planning team access expertise and other resources of the community? Who can garner support and buy-in for the project?
Commitment to the issue	Who will want to help the NAA team develop and disseminate its conclusions? Who might advocate for the assessment and intervention development? Who has been working on the problem from a practice perspective? Who has been working on the problem from a research perspective? Who could bring creative energy to the project?

(Cargo & Mercer, 2008) and Preskill and Jones (Preskill & Jones, 2009). These questions can help to inform a linkage system framework and stakeholder mapping for planning group composition.

Structuring and Facilitating Effective Project Planning Groups

Once a planning group is established, it must be managed over time to facilitate the successful completion of each step in the IM process. Health promotion planners will need certain skills, including those used in interpersonal communication and group facilitation. Group process skills are briefly covered here, but the successful health promotion planner should pursue further training. We encourage planners to explore additional resources such as the *Community Tool Box* (Center for Community Health and Development (CCHD) Kansas University, n.d.) and *Facilitating Intentional Group Learning* (Preskill et al., 2017).

Once the planning group is established, initial activities may include defining members' responsibilities, choosing an organizational structure, deciding how to make decisions, agreeing to tasks, and proposing a timeline (CCHD.b, n.d.; Newman et al., 2011). In some cases, groups will function as a whole; for other tasks, members may break into smaller working and advisory groups. Common best practices of high-performing groups include:

- Effective two-way communication *among* group members, rather than strictly to and from group members and the leader.
- Distribution of leadership and responsibility for group function among *all* members, including the generation of goals and agendas.
- Setting goals that reflect both individual and group needs.
- Fostering group cohesion through structure and facilitation techniques that incorporate team building, inclusionary decision-making/problem-solving, and support for members (CCHD.b, n.d.; Johnson & Johnson, 2012).

Stages of Group Formation To effectively facilitate group processes, it is helpful for facilitators to understand the general stages of group formation. Tuckman's (Tuckman, 1965) seminal small group development model identifies four primary stages: (1) *forming* (orientation of purpose, tasks, and each other; need for guidance), (2) *storming* (members gain trust and begin voicing opinions, with the emergence of disagreements and conflict), (3) *norming* (establishment of group norms and movement toward common goals), and (4) *performing* (clarity of vision and purpose and achievement of common goals).

By gauging the stage of a group at various points in the planning process, facilitators can better understand group behavior and be more intentional about selecting activities to enhance group process. In the forming stage, for example, *team-building activities* can help foster group cohesion and build trust (Ingalls, 2018). In the storming and norming stages, establishing *community agreements* (values and expectations for how the team will work together) (CCHD.d, n.d.) can help enhance reflexivity and collaboration. In the performing stage, *recognition of group accomplishments*—both small and large—can provide positive reinforcement, among other benefits (CCHD.c, n.d.). We encourage planners to continually grow their skills and toolbox for enhancing group processes.

Group Facilitation Because group work is at the heart of intervention planning, all groups require group facilitation skills among team members. While team members will bring diverse expertise, group facilitation is an essential skill that all health promotion planners should develop. Three core group facilitation domains have been identified in the literature (Bradford, 1976; Johnson & Johnson, 2012; Toseland & Rivas, 2008): *communication, task functions*, and *maintenance and team-building functions*, highlighted in Table 5.3.

Communication is foundational for a good group process. This includes listening to others' ideas with a willingness to review and make transparent one's own assumptions about the health problem and its solutions, as well as providing a space for intentional reflection. As Avery and colleagues (Avery et al., 2001) share in their book, *Teamwork Is an Individual Skill*, we may be dealt "bad teams," yet our individual behaviors can help any team become more functional. These behaviors begin with strong communication processes as outlined in Table 5.3, which range from using first-person language in *owning a statement* to being able to acknowledge lack of *congruence* in the group's verbal and nonverbal communication, to actively *requesting information* about how communication is delivered (*feedback*) (Johnson & Johnson, 2012; Bradford, 1976; Toseland & Rivas, 2008). In fostering positive communication within the group, facilitators should consider their own behaviors—including how they "share the stick" (i.e., allow everyone in the group to be heard) in encouraging other group members to participate (IIED, 2004).

Task Functions, Group Maintenance, and Team Building Every planning group has two necessary types of activities: those related to the work at hand *(task functions)* and those related to group process *(group maintenance and team-building functions)* (Bradford, 1976).

Task functions are whatever actions must be accomplished to do the group's work. Effective facilitators employ a range of techniques to help groups complete their tasks, including *developing the agenda*; *initiating* discussion about a given topic; *coordinating* (joining two ideas within a group discussion), *partializing* ideas (pointing out differences between ideas), and *summarizing* and *synthesizing*, among other functions.

Good facilitation also requires effective **group maintenance and team-building skills**, which often occur simultaneously with task functions but may also require dedicated time, effort, and skills (Bradford, 1976).

Table 5.3 Group Facilitation Processes

Process	Description
	Communication
Owning a statement	Using first-person singular pronouns (I or me)
Completeness and specificity	Clearly stating all necessary information, including the context or frame of reference, intention or goal, and assumptions
Congruence	Making verbal and nonverbal communication congruent
Redundancy	Using more than one channel of communication (written, oral, or graphic) to clarify meaning
Requesting feedback	Asking for information about how a communication is being understood
Frame of reference	Making the communication appropriate to the receiver's frame of reference
Feelings	Describing feelings by name
Describing behavior	Describing behavior of another person without evaluating or interpreting
	Task functions
Developing the agenda	Enabling the group to list activities, set priorities, and budget time
Initiating	Beginning a discussion that includes both substantive offerings (such as the background of an issue) and methodological offerings (such as the suggestion to begin by brainstorming)
Information seeking	Eliciting pertinent information by asking for information, keeping issues from closing prematurely, encouraging members to speak, and accepting both people and ideas
Opinion giving	Allowing opinions to be freely given and valued by the group as coming from the members' experience
Elaboration	Asking for elaboration on a partially stated idea
Coordination	Joining together ideas from two or more members (ideas that might seem disparate at first)
Partializing	Pointing out the fine differences between two ideas that might seem the same at first glance
Evaluating	Evaluating ideas but not people
Structuring	Deciding and facilitating the ways in which a group can work, such as by using subgroups
Energizing	Moving a group through a "stuck" point by restructuring the work or process. For example, introducing a process such as brainstorming, using humor, expressing feelings, or giving or getting feedback
Summarizing	Summing up the points, progress, and needs of the group orally in the meeting and in meeting notes, summaries, and action items after the meeting
Synthesizing	Making meaning of various ideas expressed in the group
	Maintenance and team-building functions
Gatekeeping	Making opportunities for participation by the less talkative members of the group
Encouraging	Encouraging members to participate in the group
Harmonizing	Seeking common goals or common ground in a conflict
Consensus seeking	Modifying group decisions and plans until group members are relatively comfortable and supportive
Giving feedback	Sharing with the whole group a direct, specific, immediate description of impact of group or individual communication
Standard setting	Setting and revisiting group norms regarding efficiency, fairness, power, and communication
Processing	Setting aside the final minutes of a meeting for reviewing how the work progressed and how it can be improved

Investing in group maintenance and team-building aims to enhance the relationships among group members, including feelings of inclusivity, group norms, predictability of procedures, and issues of participation and trust. Examples of facilitation processes for group maintenance and team building include *gatekeeping*, in which the facilitator encourages participation from less talkative group members, *harmonizing*, in which facilitators seek common goals or mitigate conflict and *consensus seeking*, among others (Table 5.3). In our own work with the Travis County CATCH project (Springer et al., 2013), we found that creating community agreements (*standard setting*) as well as incorporating ice-breakers and reflection during our team meetings (*energizing, encouraging*, and *processing*) helped foster cohesion and group process.

Other important considerations for working in participatory groups are the facilitation of power/equity, and inclusive decision-making (Johnson & Johnson, 2012). Effective participatory groups are more likely to base power and influence on ability and information rather than position in the group. They build tactics into their practice that equalize influence (i.e., the loudest member having a disproportionate impact on group function) by setting group norms and using facilitation processes.

The *group facilitation processes* outlined in Table 5.3, coupled with the IM Core Processes, can help to optimize group decision-making and planning at each step, while providing a starting point for a productive group. Below we provide examples of participatory methods for generating ideas and reaching group consensus.

Processes for Idea Generation Central to facilitating project work groups and health promotion intervention planning is engaging project partners in the generation of ideas. In the IM framework, idea generation is guided by the *Core Processes* that include *brainstorming* within the planning group as well as *primary data collection* from community partner groups. In generating good ideas, we embrace the scientist Linus Pauling's famous saying that, "The best way to a good idea is to have a lot of ideas." Indeed, idea generation is a key phase for sparking innovation via planning frameworks such as Design Thinking's "ideation" phase (Hasso Plattner Institute of Design, 2010), which explores multiple ideas before acting on one of them. And yet a common challenge that planning groups face is the tendency to jump on one idea, need, or solution without fully exploring a range of possibilities.

Below we describe selected methods for facilitating idea generation while maintaining active community participation in the NAA process and other planning steps. We encourage health promotion planners to explore additional resources for participatory learning, such as *Facilitating Intentional Group Learning* (Preskill et al., 2017), *Liberating Structures* (Lipmanowicz & McCandless, 2014), and others (Center for Community Health and Development (CCHD) Kansas University, n.d.; IIED, 2004).

- ***Brainstorming or Free Association*** encourages group members to generate ideas in response to a question (Preskill & Jones, 2009). A common approach called "off-the-wall thinking" encourages participants to respond to an anchoring question on sticky notes and place them on a wall or use electronic technologies for display. With ideas written in participants' own words, the group then conducts "affinity grouping" to link similar ideas. Then groups may engage in a prioritization process such as *dotmocracy* in which participants place sticky dots next to their favorite ideas.

- ***Nominal Group Technique*** is also enacted in response to a posed question, with ideas generated independently by each member and then shared collectively (Moon, 1999). This prevents group members from taking turns which can interfere with idea generation (production blocking). Stimulus questions might include, for example, "In this neighborhood, what health threats concern you the most?" Following individual brainstorming, members give answers one at a time, round-robin style. The facilitator records the answers, using a board or large pad. After the list of answers is clarified, group members make preliminary rankings, which they record and discuss. Group members then vote a second time, yielding a final prioritization. A more formal approach to this process—concept mapping—uses multidimensional scaling and cluster analysis to develop a visual display of themes or categories (Thompson & Burke, 2020).
- ***Small and Large Group Participatory Inquiry Methods,*** such as Gallery Walks and World Café, are participatory inquiry approaches widely used in community health planning that generally consist of several steps. First, the large group is divided into smaller groups and then presented different open-ended questions, assigning each group one question to explore in depth. Next, each small group posts their ideas for the question and invites participants from all groups to circulate and add additional thoughts. Finally, a plenary discussion takes place about the ideas generated for each station. Project partners with the Austin/Travis County Community Health Improvement initiative engaged in a gallery walk-type activity as part of their CHA which provided input on their primary health needs, priority populations, and proposed solutions (Austin/Travis County Community Health Assessment, 2017).
- ***Data Walks*** are an increasingly popular method for generating ideas and providing further context from the perspective of project partners (Preskill et al., 2017). The method consists of posting data (e.g., bar charts, pie charts) on different walls or providing them directly to small group tables and having participants review findings and respond to questions. The 2019 *Youth-led Community Health Learning Initiative* engaged high school students from Central Texas in a data walk to explore health indicators to provide further context for health disparities and to prioritize health issues (Springer et al., 2022).

Processes for Consensus Building Consensus is the process of choice for most decisions made by a health promotion planning team. Most decisions require group members to understand and weigh evidence regarding a certain course of action and to evaluate the group's options based on that evidence. Voting and majority rule are not usually effective because they do not encourage full discussion or incorporate minority opinions in the decision-making. To reach consensus, group members need to listen attentively in order to understand differences of opinion among the members; help each interested person clearly, fully, and persuasively present a position; critically consider all positions presented; encourage members' willingness to change their minds when they have been logically persuaded of the merit of someone else's argument; tolerate and even encourage intellectual conflict/avoid premature closure of arguments; and focus on the goal of reaching the best possible decision (Johnson & Johnson, 2012). Well-functioning groups make the best decisions possible by embracing conflict in ways that build upon and extend the consensus-building process.

Task 2: Conduct a Needs and Assets Assessment

Once the planning group is established, **Task 2 of IM Step 1 consists of conducting the NAA.** While we separate below the description of a needs assessment from an assets assessment, both are commonly conducted concurrently to increase efficiency.

Conducting a Needs Assessment

Before conducting the needs assessment, an important first step is to identify an NAA framework(s). In IM, we use a modified PRECEDE model based on the original work by Green and Kreuter (Green & Kreuter, 1991, 1999, 2005) (Figure 5.1). The modified PRECEDE model, known as *the logic model of the problem* within IM, is a population-based epidemiologic planning framework that is ecological in perspective. This model is a helpful framework to identify and analyze health and QOL problems, including their behaviors and environmental determinants.

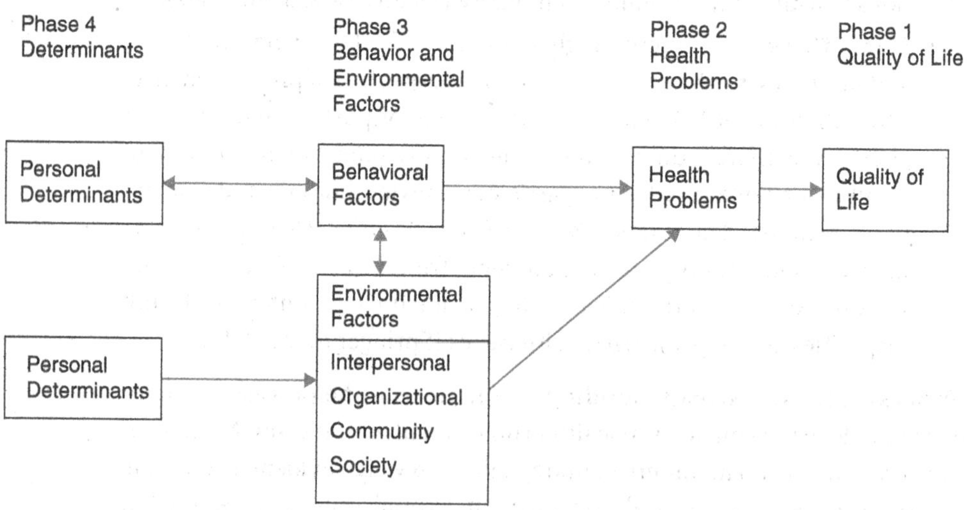

Figure 5.1 Logic Model of the Problem

Planners conduct the needs assessment by using the IM Core Processes introduced in Chapter 2. Within each phase of the *logic model of the problem*, the planning group will: pose questions; brainstorm what the planning group already knows in relation to the posed question; search the literature for empirical evidence and evaluate the strength of the evidence; access and use theory when appropriate, such as when questions concern determinants; conduct new research; and develop a final summary of answers to the posed questions. Below, we elaborate on the application of the logic model of the problem for guiding the health needs assessment.

Guiding Health Needs Assessment Using a Logic Model of the Problem

The overarching aim of the IM *logic model of the problem* is to provide a framework for comprehensively assessing factors that influence the health problem at both the individual and environmental levels. While the IM logic model of the problem builds from the PRECEDE model, an important distinction is that IM separates the *assessment of the causes* of the health problem as part of the *logic model of the problem* (Step 1) from the *identification of factors associated with* the positive health outcome or solution, which are explored in Step 2 via the *logic model of change*. For example, predisposing, enabling, and reinforcing factors of the positive health behavior or health outcome—key factors within the PRECEDE model—are incorporated as environmental factors or personal determinants of the IM *logic model of change* in Step 2. The IM *logic model of the problem* is similar to other *conceptual health risk models* that aim to identify and understand the influence of environmental, social, and psychological risk factors on disease outcomes (Linder & Sexton, 2011).

The *logic model of the problem* (Figure 5.1) is helpful in guiding the assessment process, which often begins with social and epidemiologic descriptions of adverse QOL issues and health problems. When completed, the model can be read from left to right as a logic or causal model of the health problem and adverse QOL conditions. For example, in addressing premature mortality and morbidity from cardiovascular disease, the planning group would explore the impact of this health issue on QOL-related issues, such as loss of productive years of life. Next, the planners would support the description of the health problem and QOL issues with data and would begin finding evidence of behavioral and environmental causes- with environmental causes explored across social-ecological levels (interpersonal, organizational, community, and societal). Lastly, planners would explore personal determinants of behavior of the at-risk population and individuals who can influence environmental conditions (i.e., environmental agents). Personal determinants reside at the individual level and include factors such as knowledge, attitudes, beliefs, values, perceptions, and skills that influence behavior (see Chapter 3).

"Entering" the Logic Model of the Problem A key consideration in completing the needs assessment is where to begin, or "enter," the logic model. On the far-right side, with assessing the QOL in the community? Toward the center, with health problems or risks? Or with behavioral or environmental causes? Although the PRECEDE logic model is often developed from right to left, specifying where the planning group is entering the model is helpful to further "anchor" the process. For example, in our work with the Travis County CATCH Middle School project (Springer et al., 2013), we entered the model in the "health phase" because our overall aim was reducing childhood obesity and promoting healthy weight. We then moved to the right to ask what adverse QOL issues are impacted by childhood obesity, and then to the left to ask what behavioral and environmental factors influence childhood obesity. Key behaviors that influence childhood obesity include physical inactivity and unhealthy eating (Springer et al., 2013) with growing evidence of other behaviors such as lack of sleep (Morrissey et al., 2020). Because obesity is influenced by multiple behaviors, had we entered the behavioral phase with a focus solely on physical inactivity, our causal model for understanding childhood obesity would be incomplete and underspecified given the key role of other behaviors listed here.

Alternatively, planners may be specifically focused on reducing physical inactivity in a given population. Planners would then enter the logic model of the problem in the behavioral phase, and then move to the right of the model by asking what adverse health issues may arise from physical inactivity, such as diabetes and hypertension, among others (Institute of Medicine, 2005; Save the Children US, USAID, US Agency for International Development 2020). Planners would then list not just obesity, but all adverse health conditions arising from physical inactivity. Specifying where the planning group is entering the logic model of the problem is helpful in leading planners to comprehensively explore phases of the model in relation to the targeted issue.

It is perfectly legitimate to begin in the middle of the logic model of the problem with a behavioral or environmental risk so long as there is strong epidemiologic evidence for the causal relation between the risk factor and one or more health problems. No matter where one begins the needs assessment, one will need to cover all phases of the model, including the relation of the behavioral or environmental factor to health and QOL.

Describing the Priority Population and Community of Interest

The NAA process is instrumental in helping the planning group further define the partner community, the population at risk, and other environmental agents (e.g., parents or teachers) for the focus of health improvement efforts. This process is iterative; it may begin with the identification of a geographically defined partner community, then further define the priority populations within a given community. We introduce here the importance of describing the partner community and priority populations to prepare planners for this important step.

In describing the partner community, it is helpful to first understand the different definitions of "community." Three common definitions we introduced above include: (1) a *geographically defined community,* (2) a *community of shared interest-* such as a school, workplace, or faith-based group, and (3) a *community of shared experience,* such as groups who share a common history, health problem, or trauma (Goodman et al., 2014; Wallerstein et al., 2018). Health promotion planners often begin with a geographically defined community—or a community of interest or shared experience within a geographically defined community—and then conduct an NAA in partnership with the community to identify priority health needs and at-risk groups. Alternatively, planners may begin by identifying a health issue (e.g., tobacco use), conduct an epidemiologic assessment of the problem to identify higher-risk groups, and then identify where to reach those populations via a geographically defined community or community of interest. Regardless of the approach, the NAA aims to help the planning group further define both the community and the population(s) at risk for the topic of interest.

While the health and QOL analysis—as guided by the *logic model of the problem* framework—is always focused on the at-risk population, the NAA aims to identify other priority populations for intervention planning within both the behavioral and environmental phases of the model. For example, while children represent a key at-risk population for infectious diseases preventable by immunizations and would thus represent a key priority group within the behavioral phase, *parents* have the ability to make decisions and take actions for their children's health. As such, parents would also represent a key priority population for an immunization intervention within the behavioral phase of the model.

The NAA also identifies other priority populations for the focus of an intervention that includes *environmental agents* within the environmental phase of the logic model of the problem; these individuals have the ability to influence the environment and/or influence the at-risk population directly. In the case of immunizations, key environmental agents may include the school nurse at the interpersonal level, the board of education at the organizational level, and state legislators to set policy at the societal level. Upon completion of the NAA, both the community and priority populations—including the at-risk populations and initial identification of potential environmental agents—should be well described.

Describing Health Problems and Quality of Life

Most health promotion planners begin a needs assessment with some understanding of both the selected health risk (e.g., smoking) or problem (e.g., cardiovascular disease), along with the population groups that have it. They use concepts from epidemiology to further define the nature of the health problem and affected populations, with guiding questions that include:

- What is the problem?
- Who has it?
- What are the incidence, prevalence, and distribution of the problem?
- What are the demographic characteristics of the population at risk?
- Is there a defined geographic community or community of shared interest? What are its characteristics, including its resources and strengths?
- What segments of the population experience an excess burden from the health problem?
- Where can the at-risk groups be reached?

Guided by the *health* and *QOL* phases of the logic model of the problem (*phases 1 and 2* in Figure 5.1), the planner needs to understand how the health problem is exhibited in the population, and what it means to those who have it. In the process of conducting the needs assessment, the planning group will constantly seek to deepen its understanding of the impact of the problem dimensions of health problems include (but are not limited to): disability, discomfort, fertility, fitness, morbidity, mortality, and physiological risks (Fielding, 2022; Green & Kreuter, 2005). Dimensions of QOL include, but are not limited to, effects of illness on both *individual-level* QOL indicators, such as absenteeism from work, school performance, activities of daily living, stigma, isolation and alienation, discrimination, happiness, and self-esteem, as well as *societal-level* QOL indicators, such as healthcare cost and health-related productivity loss.

To better understand and describe the *health problem*, the planning group will use both quantitative and qualitative methods and sources to assess the prevalence of the problem across subgroups as well as personal interviews to explore *QOL effects*. The first step is to describe demographically who has the health problem and for whom it represents an excess burden.

Rates and Risk *Rate* and *risk* measures and related statistics are helpful for describing the health problem. While we provide a brief description here, we refer the reader to epidemiology texts to explore these concepts further (Centers for Disease Control and Prevention, n.d.; Friis & Sellers, 2013; L G, 2009). The extent of the health problem is usually described as a rate, the number of events (people experiencing a problem) over a period of time per population of 1,000 or 100,000. A rate can be incidence, the number of new cases over a specified time period, or prevalence, the number of existing cases at a single point. Usually, both types of rates are needed to fully understand a problem (Centers for Disease Control and Prevention, n.d.; Friis & Sellers, 2013; L G, 2009).

Rates can be compared across group characteristics and geographic areas to answer questions such as: Is this an important problem in a specific community? Is it more or less prevalent in this community than in others?

Is it more prevalent here than in communities that are demographically similar? Rates may need to be adjusted by demographic variables, such as age and gender, and are often reported as age-specific and weighted to match the age distribution in the population of interest (L G, 2009).

Risk ratios can also provide insights into the association between a risk factor (e.g., smoking) and a health outcome (e.g., lung cancer). *Relative risk compares the "*. . . risk of a health event (disease, injury, risk factor, or death) among one group with the same risk in another group" (Centers for Disease Control and Prevention, n.d.). Another frequently used measure of association is the *odds ratio*, a measure of how strongly an event (e.g., lung cancer) is associated with exposure (e.g., tobacco use) (Centers for Disease Control and Prevention, n.d.; Tenny & Hoffman, 2020). The odds ratio is based on the likelihood of the event occurring in an exposed group versus a non-exposed group (Tenny & Hoffman, 2020).

In recent years, the *disproportionality ratio* has gained popularity given its ability to clearly communicate the excess burden of a given issue for a specific group. Disproportionality refers to "the under representation or over-representation of a racial or ethnic group compared to its percentage in the total population" (Girvan et al., 2019; Huggins-Hoyt et al., 2019). Commonly used within the education and social service fields to describe racial/ethnic social and health inequities (Girvan et al., 2019; Huggins-Hoyt et al., 2019), disproportionality ratios have been included in community health dashboards for organizations such as the Community Advancement Network based in Austin, Texas as a way to identify, monitor and set goals to reduce racial/ethnic health and social disparities (Community Advancement Network, n.d.).

Describing Possible Behavioral and Environmental Causes of Health Problems

In exploring possible causes of the health problem or QOL issue, *phase 3* of the logic model of the problem framework (Figure 5.1) guides planners to identify both behavioral and environmental risk factors that influence the health problem. In doing so, health promotion planners aim to answer several key questions: "What are the risk behaviors that influence the health problem? What are the environmental factors that directly influence the health problem or indirectly influence the health problem by influencing the risk behavior?" In identifying behavioral and environmental risk factors, health promotion planners will engage their planning group with the IM *Core Processes*, which include reviewing the empirical literature as well as collecting primary data to explore environmental factors that shape behaviors and health outcomes both directly and indirectly.

Describing Behavior of the At-Risk Group Some behaviors may be causally related to the health problem. For example, a large body of evidence shows that smoking is associated with cardiovascular disease and a variety of cancers. Furthermore, as the number of cigarettes smoked increases, the association increases. Such a dose-response relationship provides a higher level of evidence.

Describing Environmental Risk The *environment*—in all its forms (e.g., social, physical, information, and policy) and levels (interpersonal, organizational, community, and societal)—plays a key role in influencing health and related behavior (Sallis & Owen, 2015). For this reason, in addition to describing health risk behaviors for a given health condition or outcome, planners will also identify *environmental* risk factors as part of the NAA process. In assessing environmental influences within the logic model of the problem, it is important to first recognize that environmental factors can influence health *directly* through disease-causing exposures (e.g., air pollution on physical health) or *indirectly* by influencing health-related behavior (e.g., limited access to supermarkets and low fruit and vegetable consumption).

An ecological framework as conceptualized by ecological levels (interpersonal, organizational, community, and societal) (Figure 5.1) and settings provides helpful guidance for comprehensively understanding environmental influences on a given disease condition or health-related behavior. For example, health promotion research on youth e-cigarette prevention helps to illustrate the influence of different ecological levels on behavior. At *the interpersonal level,* peer and family member e-cigarette use has been found to increase teen use (Wang et al., 2018). At *the organizational level,* school-level context and social norms influence the behavior (Shorten & Smith, 2017; Springer et al., 2018). At the *community level,* marketing of e-cigarettes close to schools has been associated with student e-cigarette use (Giovenco et al., 2016). Lastly, at *the societal level,* youth living in a state with state-level e-cigarette retail licensing policies use e-cigarettes at higher rates compared to those living in states without such policies (Azagba et al., 2020).

In addition to the direct effects of the environment influencing individual-level outcomes, each ecological level can also influence any lower level. For example, at the organizational level, healthcare providers might lack incentives for preventive care. This *organizational* characteristic could influence providers to omit discussing prevention in their *interpersonal* interactions with patients. Individuals with control over social or physical conditions in a given setting are referred to as *environmental agents.* As we shall discuss in Chapter 6 and Step 2, environmental agents may differ from program implementers and are often themselves the focus of change in a health promotion intervention.

Describing Determinants of Behavioral and Environmental Risks

Once the behavioral and environmental risk factors are identified, *phase 4* of the logic model of the problem (Figure 5.1) guides the health promotion planner to explore factors that cause—or in some way modify—the behavior or the environmental risk. Here, the planner asks: *Why do members of the at-risk group engage in behaviors that increase their risk of a health problem? Why do agents in the environment create or maintain unhealthy environmental conditions?* We refer to these factors as personal "determinants," which are intrapersonal factors that reside within the individual (people at risk or the environmental agent) and include, for example, knowledge, attitudes, beliefs, values, perceptions, and skills that influence behavior (see Chapter 3). We use the term determinants as our focus is on changeable factors that can lead to improved outcomes (see Crutzen et al. (2017)). While biologic and demographic factors are important to consider within the needs assessment process, these factors are not often easily modifiable. Instead, in this phase we are interested in those factors that *can be changed* or *modified* by interventions that influence the ways people think and behave.

In identifying determinants of behavior for the at-risk population and environmental agents, we underscore here again the wisdom of Kurt Lewin's adage that nothing is as useful as a good theory. As an example, in exploring *why* some people choose to follow COVID-19 guidelines (e.g., mask-wearing, social distancing, hand washing) during the COVID-19 pandemic and others do not, we could apply the IM Core Processes. These processes may include: brainstorming within our planning group to identify initial reasons, searching the empirical evidence to confirm evidence for determinants, searching theory to confirm our initial list and identify additional determinants, and collecting additional primary data with the priority population. Initial psychosocial factors found to be associated with *not* following guidelines (stated in the negative as we are in the logic model of the problem) based on a nationally representative sample of US adults include lower self-efficacy for not following guidelines, lower perceptions of social endorsement of the guidelines, negative attitudes related to guidelines, and weaker intentions to follow guidelines (Bogg & Milad, 2020) key theoretical constructs found in theories that include Social Cognitive Theory and Theory of Reasoned Action. We encourage readers to further explore behavior-oriented theories that focus on understanding (and changing) behavior of the at-risk group or environmental agents (Chapter 3) as well as environmental theories that focus on understanding (and changing) environmental conditions to enhance health outcomes (Chapter 4).

Upon evaluating the empirical evidence for a given determinant, planners may find that much of the empirical evidence for a given determinant is cross-sectional (i.e., collected at a single time point, precluding inferences of causality), or that the evidence does not relate specifically to the relevant health topic, or that the evidence is not based on the population of interest. As such, planners must weigh the strength of the evidence to judge whether a case for causation can be argued. Where the empirical literature is sparse, health promotion planners are encouraged to collect primary data (one of IM's Core Processes in which planning groups collect new data via surveys, focus groups, or other methods) to confirm determinants identified via the empirical literature and theory as well as explore additional potential determinants of a given behavior. Box 5.4 provides an example of exploring personal determinants via focus groups from the *¡Activate Ya!* study of physical activity in an adolescent population.

BOX 5.4. EXPLORING PERSONAL DETERMINANTS—*¡ACTIVATE YA!*

As part of the needs assessment of the *¡Activate Ya!* Study, a school-based health promotion intervention with secondary school students in Uruguay (Springer et al., 2020), the planning team conducted focus groups with young people to explore potential personal determinants, including perceived barriers, of youth physical activity (PA) engagement. The opportunity to learn directly from young people resulted in rich insights and findings about personal determinants, including *perceived lack of accessibility and availability* of PA opportunities, *competing interests and preferences* for some youth (such as video games), *perceptions of low safety* for girls to engage in PA in their neighborhoods, and *verguenza,* a factor cited by girls that refers to being embarrassed to exercise in public and in front of boys (Parobii et al., 2018). Qualitative research methods such as focus groups can provide deeper insights into the determinants of a given risk behavior and why an environmental agent (or agents, such as a board of education) may maintain or fail to address an adverse environmental condition.

Acquiring Needs Assessment Data

Needs assessments often require multiple data sources to address questions posed for each phase of the logic model of the problem. To comprehensively understand a given health issue and the multiple phases within the model, planners need both qualitative and quantitative data. This may include *archival data* such as organizational records, demographic data, census data, disease registries, medical records, and public-use databases; *noninteractive primary data collection* such as written, Internet-based, or mailed surveys; and *interactive primary data collection* such as focus groups, key informant interviews, and community forums. In selecting the approach, planners should consider the data available from other sources; cost, time, and other constraints; degree of interaction desired with respondents; and which project partners should be involved.

Combining Qualitative and Quantitative Data

In this section, we describe a mixed-methods approach for combining qualitative and quantitative data, followed by a brief overview of common methods for conducting an NAA. We also refer the reader to other helpful resources that present needs assessment methods in greater detail (NACCHO, n.d.; Center for Community Health and Development (CCHD) Kansas University, n.d.)

In Box 5.5 we provide a summary of needs assessment methods used in the *¡Activate Ya!* school-based tobacco prevention and PA promotion program. We encourage planners to also explore other recent needs assessments guided by IM that span a variety of topic areas, including self-management of osteoarthritis (Hurley et al., 2016), youth mental health (Brooke et al., 2020), and medication information transfer for long-term care patients (Kerstenetzky et al., 2018) among many others.

BOX 5.5. CONDUCTING THE NEEDS ASSESSMENT—*¡ACTIVATE YA!*

In conducting the needs assessment as part of the *¡Activate Ya!* school-based tobacco prevention and PA promotion program in Uruguay, the logic model of the problem provided key phases of inquiry to guide the assessment. Planners entered the model in the behavioral phase with a specific focus on youth tobacco use (smoking) and physical inactivity, exploring the adverse health and QOL issues that result from youth tobacco use and inactivity (Phases 1 and 2 of the logic model of the problem), gaining deeper understanding of the context and environmental factors that shape youth tobacco use and inactivity (Phase 3), and exploring the personal determinants of why youth in Uruguay engage in tobacco use and inactivity (Phase 4). While it is common to target one specific health risk behavior, the *¡Activate Ya!* team conducted a concurrent needs assessment to assess both tobacco use and inactivity/PA, given the study's focus on understanding how increased PA may serve as a protective behavior against tobacco use.

As a first step, the team conducted a *review* of empirical literature, policy, and epidemiologic data on tobacco use and PA in Uruguay as well as a review of psychosocial-related determinants of youth tobacco use and PA engagement. They then collected primary data through *focus groups* with Uruguayan secondary school students (to better understand the context of PA and tobacco and the psychosocial determinants of these behaviors); *personal interviews* with teachers, school principals, and district leaders (to explore the barriers and facilitating factors within the school and afterschool context); and *participant observation* of the school context (Parobii et al., 2018; Peterson et al., 2019; Springer et al., 2020). Lastly, multiple *meetings were held with the planning team* to analyze, review, and provide context to the findings.

The needs assessment produced rich insights and findings regarding key personal determinants (see Box 5.4) and environmental factors that shape tobacco use and leisure-time PA, such as the importance of *peer influence* as a key environmental factor that contributed to tobacco use, including the social context of tobacco use via *previas*—the "pre-party" in which youth often consume tobacco (Peterson et al., 2019); the *lack of opportunities for PA* outside of Physical Education (PE) class, which included limited time during the school day for free-play opportunities, limited active learning in classes, lack of extracurricular activities available via schools, and economic barriers to community resources such as gyms (Parobii et al., 2018; Peterson et al., 2019; Springer et al., 2020).

A mixed-methods approach intentionally combines qualitative and quantitative research methods with the aim of more fully understanding a given health issue (Shorten & Smith, 2017). It allows for greater triangulation, corroboration, and confirmation of data in ways that increase the validity of findings (Creswell & Plano, 2018), synergistic integration of data that provides a deeper and more nuanced understanding of the topic, and a deeper understanding of context (Creswell & Plano, 2018).

The characteristics of mixed-methods research designs (Creswell & Plano, 2018; Halcomb & Hickman, 2015; Shorten & Smith, 2017) provide helpful guidance for designing a mixed methods needs assessment approach. Two basic types of designs include *concurrent designs* and *sequential designs*. Under a *concurrent design* (aka *convergent parallel design*), qualitative and quantitative data are collected at the same time but analyzed independently. A concurrent *nested design* (aka *embedded design*) consists of embedding qualitative methods within a predominantly quantitative approach, or vice-versa, with aims that include confirming, cross-validating, or corroborating findings within a single study (Halcomb & Hickman, 2015). Advantages of concurrent designs include shorter data collection timeframes, as qualitative and quantitative data are collected at the same time. Disadvantages include the inability of either data collection approach to inform the other (Halcomb & Hickman, 2015).

While concurrent designs allow for a more complete understanding of a given topic (Creswell & Plano, 2018), sequential designs have the advantage of allowing one type of data collection (e.g., personal interviews) to inform another type (e.g., a survey), with one disadvantage being the longer time frame required to collect the data (Halcomb & Hickman, 2015; Shorten & Smith, 2017). The two basic sequential designs are *sequential exploratory designs* and *sequential explanatory designs*. A *sequential exploratory design* (qualitative to quantitative methods) allows quantitative methods to build from qualitative findings (Creswell & Plano, 2018; Halcomb & Hickman, 2015; Shorten & Smith, 2017). Under a *sequential explanatory* design (quantitative to qualitative methods), qualitative data are collected to explain quantitative data (Creswell & Plano, 2018; Halcomb & Hickman, 2015). In our work with the *Youth-led Community Health Learning Initiative*, youth from Central Texas engaged in data walks (a participatory inquiry method described above) and photovoice (a technique that combines digital photography and youth-generated narratives). This approach provided further context for the quantitative health indicator findings for the partner community in relation to a comparison community and the state of Texas (Springer et al., 2022).

Finding and Using Archival Data

Archival or secondary data are data that have been collected for a purpose other than the needs assessment. Many governmental, health, social service, and education agencies collect data describing health problems and demographics that can be useful to the needs assessor; these can include census-type data, in which the goal is to describe every event or person—for example, birth and death records—or they can be survey-type data, in which an attempt is made to capture a representative sample of the population of interest. Archival sources can be local, regional, national, or international and can be obtained directly from the agency responsible for collection and analysis, with many datasets now made publicly available online. For example, local health departments collect census and other data such as birth and death records. National agencies such as the CDC in the

United States collect a variety of data on disease incidence and prevalence as well as survey data regarding disease risk. In addition to health-specific data, there are an increasing number of data portals that provide access to a range of social determinant-related data (e.g., CDC-SDOH).

Collecting Primary Data

In this section, we provide a general description of various primary data collection methods that can be helpful for conducting the NAA.

Planning Group One of the first places to look for information is from the planning itself. Multidisciplinary planning groups that include perspectives from the resource group, potential intervention implementers, and priority populations bring valuable insights about all aspects of the endeavor See the section above on *Structuring and Facilitating Effective Project Planning Groups* for an example of participatory inquiry methods that can be used to elicit input from group members.

Surveys While hard-copy and telephone surveys continue to be a standard method for conducting surveys, Internet-based surveys, including email-based, smartphone-based, and now ecological momentary assessment surveys, have rapidly gained popularity (Runyan et al., 2013). Surveys use structured forms or interview protocols that employ a variety of scales and response modes. As with all data collection activities, questions on surveys should be carefully linked to the purpose of the study. Key issues to consider include the validity and reliability of items and scales, appropriate sampling, and the ability to achieve high response rates (Dillman et al., 2008). In conducting needs assessment surveys for community-based planning, health departments in the United States have been implementing Rapid Needs Assessments such as Community Assessment for Public Health Emergency Response (CASPER), which provides household-level information.

Interviews Interviews can be highly structured (much like a survey), or moderately unstructured, using a general guide outlining the set of issues to be addressed. Interviews based on elicitation rather than a rigid protocol of questions have the advantage of allowing the respondent opportunities for free expression, with attitudes more likely to be revealed; this method (unstructured) requires skilled interviewers and qualitative data analysts. As with surveys, it is important to determine the purpose of the interview and to select the sample carefully. *Mall intercept* interviews, in which potential respondents are approached in public places, are frequently used for structured interviews with convenience samples. Innovative methods for capturing community voices (such as video) can further enhance and inform the community needs assessment process (Cain et al., 2017).

Ethnographic Methods Ethnographic methods are particularly useful in describing marginalized settings and hard-to-reach populations, such as commercial sex workers, drug users, people engaging in HIV-risk behaviors, or individuals who are experiencing homelessness (Cain et al., 2017). Methods such as participant observation, in-depth interviews, focus groups, and analysis of written texts focus on the description of a culture through the experiences and perspectives of individuals in their own language and on their own terms. Rapid-assessment techniques, drawing significantly from anthropological and sociological methods, have been applied in the planning and evaluation of a variety of international programs in such areas as nutrition and primary healthcare, reproductive health, AIDS, epilepsy, hunger, water and sanitation, emergency relief, and community engagement for childhood obesity prevention (Burton et al., 2019; Cifuentes et al., 2006; Scrimshaw & Hurtado, 1992).

Appreciative Inquiry (AI) Building on the science of positive psychology, this approach focuses on identifying and activating the strengths within an organization or community (Cooperrider & Fry, 2020), one that seeks the root causes for success instead of failure (Ludema et al., 2003). The method focuses on asking questions that "... elevate a system's cooperative capacity to apprehend strengths and positive potentials, unite around greater meanings and shared goals, and activate the kind of generative designs that serve to open those systems to better and more valued possibilities" (Cooperrider & Fry, 2020). The main inquiry involves (1) asking a main question with a series of tightly focused sub-questions or probes regarding the group's positive *high-point* experiences or accomplishments, and then (2) eliciting scenarios regarding what the entity would be like if the high-points occurred more routinely. AI has been widely applied in healthcare, academic, and social-sector settings, with recent public health examples that include understanding teaching strategies developed by PE teachers to re-engage students (Gray et al., 2019) and enhancing person-centered dementia care in hospitals (Scerri et al., 2019).

Focus Groups Focus groups are a commonly used qualitative method in which a moderator leads a group in discussion, often guided by a 5–10 question interview guide. Focus groups represent a rich and helpful method for exploring the health needs, strengths, and opportunities for health promotion intervention among other factors for the NAA and intervention development process (Gilmore & Campbell, 2005; Krueger & Casey, 2009; Santa Maria et al., 2014). The goal of a focus group is to stimulate discussion among 6–12 fairly homogenous people to ascertain opinions and attitudes related to the topic of interest. Key steps in planning and conducting focus groups include the development of a focus group guide; recruitment of participants, conducting the focus groups, including introductions, facilitation, and recording; transcription of focus groups; and analysis of textual data (Krueger & Casey, 2009). The number of groups that should be conducted is based on factors such as ensuring that different segments of the community are represented and determining whether saturation has been reached (i.e., no new themes are being generated). While in-person focus groups continue to be a common approach, virtual groups have grown in popularity (Dangerfield II et al., 2021; Thrul et al., 2017).

In the *¡Activate Ya!* study (Springer et al., 2020), focus groups were conducted with Uruguayan secondary school students to co-learn about the personal determinants (knowledge, attitudes, practices) of tobacco use and PA, as well as the environmental influences and context of these behaviors. Focus groups were stratified by grade level, gender, and socioeconomic status to provide rich comparisons to further understand engagement in these behaviors (Parobii et al., 2018; Peterson et al., 2019).

Delphi Technique This survey method uses an iterative process to build consensus in a group, which is often comprised of experts or people with knowledge of a given domain. The method begins with a first round of mailed or online surveys that solicits responses to a limited number of questions; the second round is informed by first-round analysis and asks clarifying questions; a third round often involves ranking of preferences, with the eventual aim of generating a consensus on a given topic. This method has been used in various facets of intervention planning, including needs assessment, policy determination, and resource allocation, with examples that include prioritization of health issues for intervention (Gilmore & Campbell, 2005; Hsu & Sandford, 2019; Keeney et al., 2011).

Geographic Methods Geographic information systems (GIS) are a commonly used tool to geocode, map, and analyze health data in relation to place. Recent advances in technology have expanded its use to a more general audience through online GIS platforms (Highfield et al., 2011). Online systems allow users with and without specialized skill sets to access public health data (e.g., incidence and mortality) and statistics through online maps, both of which are critical for supporting data-driven community needs assessment. In addition, public participation GIS (PPGIS) focuses on the inclusion of the community in the collection, analysis, and use of spatial data (Gwede et al., 2010). For example, Friedman et al. (2014) used PPGIS to show practitioners and other community partners the density of Federally Qualified Health Centers (FQHCs) in relation to four types of cancer to facilitate the assessment of where to locate new FQHCs (Friedman et al., 2014). In combining traditional GIS data with images, audio, and text, *story maps* provide a rich platform to tell a more comprehensive story about health and are particularly useful for mixed-methods community assessments and for conveying information to a lay audience (ESRI, n.d.).

Synthesizing Needs Assessment Data to Create the Logic Model of Problem

While the planning group often begins with an initial logic model based on the group's input and use of brainstorming, following the needs assessment the group will analyze data to develop a comprehensive understanding of the problem, the priority population(s), and the context. As

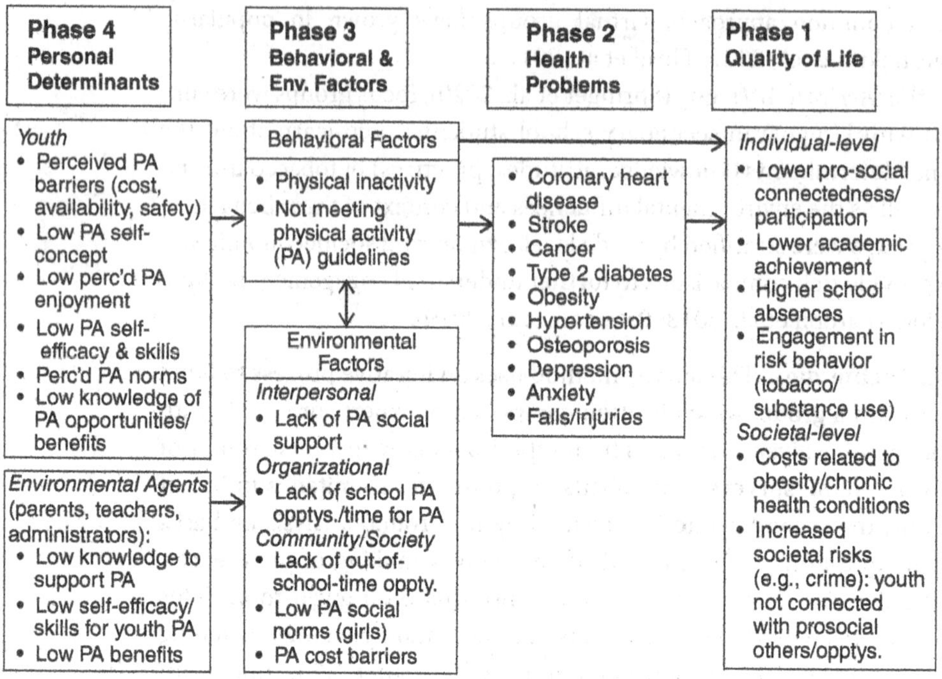

Figure 5.2 Abbreviated Logic Model of the Problem—Youth Physical Inactivity, *iActivate Ya!*

described above, *the logic model of the problem* provides a helpful framework for both *guiding* as well as *synthesizing key findings* from the needs assessment to describe potential influences on the target health problem and health and QOL impacts of the health problem. Figure 5.2 presents an abbreviated model of the problem with a specific focus on physical inactivity in Uruguayan students as part of the ¡Activate Ya! study (Springer et al., 2020).

Balancing the Needs Assessment with an Assets Assessment

In addition to conducting an assessment of the health problem, **Task 2 of Step 1 also consists of conducting an assessment of the partner community's assets,** broadly defined as any resource that can be used to improve the QOL of individuals or communities (Center for Community Health and Development (CCHD) Kansas University, n.d.; Springer & Evans, 2016). Spearheaded in part by seminal work on asset mapping in the field of community organizing during the 1990s (McKnight & Kretzmann, 1996), assets assessment reframes community assessment *from* a deficit approach to one that values, builds from, and harnesses local resources, capacities, and strengths for community health and development. This shift from a deficit to a strength-based approach has been embraced within the field of health promotion, with examples that include work on *community capacity* (Goodman et al., 1998), *social capital* (Kawachi et al., 1997), and *developmental assets* for adolescent health (Scales & Leffert, 1999). Incorporating assets assessment into health promotion planning offers multiple benefits, including the opportunity to:

- *Activate existing individual and community strengths* by moving from a deficit orientation in which communities are viewed as clients in need of services to an empowerment approach in which solutions and capacities that exist within individuals and communities can be further activated via the assessment and planning process (McKnight & Kretzmann, 1996; Springer & Evans, 2016).
- *Increase effectiveness of the proposed intervention on health outcomes* by harnessing individual and environmental assets while providing insights about the factors associated with positive health, building from positive deviance (Wishik & Vynckt, 1976) and resilience perspectives (Rutter, 1987).
- *Enhance implementation and sustainability of the health promotion intervention* by exploring how to "interweave" the intervention within the environments and settings of the priority population so that the intervention "sticks" and does not attenuate over time (Hawe et al., 2009; Saunders et al., 2013; Springer & Evans, 2016; Springer et al., 2017).

Conducting an Assets Assessment

In identifying assets that can be harnessed for health intervention planning, planners should identify a conceptual framework that can guide the assessment. In the field of community development, Kretzmann and McNight's Asset-Based Community Development framework categorizes assets according to *individuals* (e.g., skills and capacities), *associations* (e.g., voluntary organizations), *institutions, physical assets* (e.g., land and infrastructure), and *connections* (Kretzmann & McKnight, 1996). Building from this work, Green and Haines (Green & Haines, 2016) propose seven types of capital that can guide assets assessment: *human, social, physical, financial, environmental, political,* and *cultural.* In the field of adolescent health, the Search Institute defines assets in terms of internal assets (e.g., personal assets such as skills) and external assets (e.g., community assets such as opportunities) that help prevent youth risk behaviors and foster resilience (Scales & Leffert, 1999). Below, we share a basic conceptual framework for guiding assets assessment for health promotion planning.

Environmental Asset Assessment Framework Informed by ecological models of health behavior (Sallis & Owen, 2015) and systems theory (Hawe, 2015; Hawe et al., 2009; May et al., 2016), the *Environmental Asset Assessment Framework* (Springer & Evans, 2016) builds from the premise that our health and health behavior are shaped by settings and the multiple environments within settings (policy, information, social, and physical). Designing interventions in relation to context, therefore, holds promise for enhancing the environmental conditions that influence health, in addition to increasing cultural relevance, sustainability, and overall impact of interventions. This framework guides health planners to ***first identify settings*** where the target populations can be reached (e.g., school, worksite, faith-based institution, neighborhood), and then to ***explore assets of various environments*** within those settings. Figure 5.3 presents a *settings and environments* framework for identifying environmental assets for intervention planning, with illustrations from the CTAN BOOST—an initiative aimed at promoting child PA, healthy eating, and social-emotional wellness in out-of-school time (OST) settings (Springer & Evans, 2016).

In conducting an assets assessment, our work with the *Youth-led Community Health Learning Initiative* began with key informant interviews with community leaders and participatory mapping with our youth co-investigators to first ***define the geographic community*** and explore ***potential settings*** for reaching the priority population (Springer et al., 2022). Key findings from this NAA included the importance of schools and the school district as a center of community and *promising setting* for health promotion; the defining of our *geographic community* based on school district boundaries for this unincorporated area; the importance of the partner community as a *setting* to spend time with family; and *the need* for youth and families to travel to the neighboring community for leisure-time activities, healthcare, and groceries due to lack of opportunities in the partner community (Springer et al., 2022). In Task 3 below, the planning group will build from the assets assessment to describe the geographic community, priority populations, and potential intervention settings.

Once the geographic community and settings are defined, the second step of the Environmental Asset Assessment Framework consists of ***exploring the specific environmental assets*** within those settings that can be leveraged for the intervention, including assets within *the policy,*

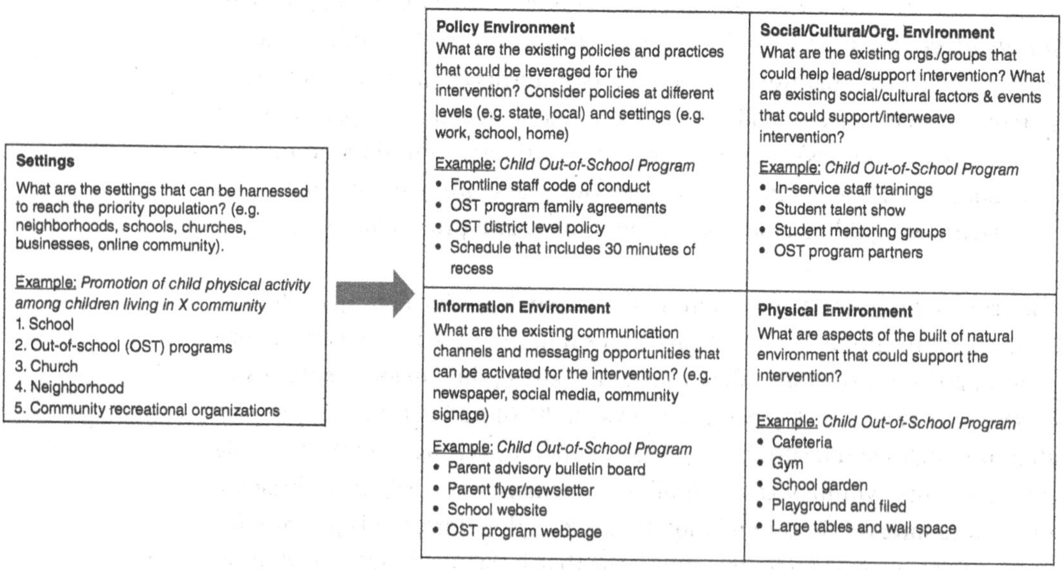

Figure 5.3 Environmental Asset Assessment Framework with Examples from the CTAN BOOST Project (Springer & Evans, 2016)

information, social, and physical environments. Examples of environmental assets include:

- *Policies and practices* within the policy environment of an organization, community, state, or nation that can be leveraged, such as state legislation mandating support for breastfeeding within the workplace (N.A, n.d.).
- *Communication channels* within the information environment, such as the use of electric bills to promote PA messaging in Sao Paulo, Brazil (Matsudo et al., 2002).
- *Existing groups* and *organizations* within the social environment, such as cultural organizations to lead community wellness efforts of Filipino-Americans in California (Dirige et al., 2013).
- *Physical spaces, design of those spaces, and other physical assets* within the physical environment, such as the redesign of the cafeteria serving line to promote healthier food options for children (Frerichs et al., 2015).

By mapping assets via a settings and environments framework, the planning group can incorporate existing assets to support the intervention (Sallis et al., 2006; Springer & Evans, 2016; Springer et al., 2017). For example, assessing environmental assets can help to inform: the *environmental outcomes* for the intervention (e.g., enhancing a current policy with language specific to the intervention); the *potential environmental agents* (e.g., partnering with existing organizations to lead the intervention); and the *practical applications* for delivering the intervention (e.g., harnessing existing communication channels). Figure 5.3 provides a template for an initial *environmental asset map* to identify settings where the priority population can be reached, and to list assets within those settings. Below, we describe each type of environment and share examples of tools that can be used to assess assets within these environments.

Assessing *Policy* Environmental Assets In addition to exploring state and national policies that can support a given health topic at the societal level (often referred to as "Big P"), we encourage planners to explore "little p" policy assets within lower ecological levels (community, organization, interpersonal) that can provide a platform for "interweaving" the health intervention, such as an *employee handbook* within a workplace that could incorporate policies to discourage soda drinking in front of students; *campus improvement plans* to incorporate organizational practices such as a Fresh Fruit Friday or before-school open gym policy within the school setting; or even *parent-child agreements* such as setting TV-watching limits within the household (Springer & Evans, 2016; Springer et al., 2010, 2017). Several instruments have been developed to examine policies and practices in different sectors, such as the *School Health Policies and Practices Study*, a national survey in the United States of school health policies and practices at the state, district, school, and classroom levels (Centers for Disease Control and Prevention, 2016).

Assessing *Social-Environmental* Assets The social environment broadly refers to social and cultural organizations within a defined setting, such as a geographic community (e.g, Houston), neighborhood organizations, parent-teacher associations, and other community groups, as well as the more specific factors social and organizational assets that influence health and health behavior (e.g., work schedules) (Springer & Evans, 2016). Goodman and colleagues' seminal work on *community capacity* identifies multiple dimensions of the social environment posited to enhance health promotion interventions, including citizen participation, leadership, skills, social and interorganizational networks, social capital, and community history, values, and power (Goodman et al., 1998). Tools for assessing social-environmental assets include the *Asset Mapping User Guide,* which includes which includes multiple examples of community assets and methods for mapping assets (Doner et al., n.d.).

Assessing *Information* Environmental Assets The information environment can take on many forms, including written, symbolic, verbal, and nonverbal messaging, with communication channels that span local television and radio stations, community newspapers, organizational newsletters, and social media. Key informant interviews, household surveys, and participatory inquiry workshops can help identify relevant communication channels for a new intervention. Assessing communication channels represents a growing area of health research and practice (Hillyer et al., 2017; Tam et al., 2018; Tucker et al., 2016).

Assessing *Physical* Environmental Assets The physical environment, defined broadly as features of the built and natural environments, has received increased attention in recent years for its effects on health (Glanz et al., 2016) including physical health (Anderson et al., 2017; Cerin et al., 2017), mental health (Francis et al., 2012; Younan et al., 2016), and social health (Child et al., 2015). Environmental audits of *worksites (Centers for Disease Control and Prevention,* 2024d; *Freak-Poli et al.,* 2020*)* and *schools (Saluja et al.,* 2018*),* for example, provide measures for assessing features of these settings that influence health behaviors, such as dietary behaviors, PA, tobacco, and breastfeeding.

Task 3: Describe the Context for the Intervention, Including the Community, Population, and Setting

A growing body of evidence highlights the influence of the context that surrounds us on our health and health-related behaviors, including where we live, study, work, pray, and play (Centers for Disease Control and Prevention, 2024c). In addition to evidence that shows the influence of geographic residence on health behavior, health-related outcomes, and life expectancy (Andersen et al., 2018; Chetty et al., 2016; Decker et al., 2018; Ludwig et al., 2011), a growing body of research also finds that our health and behaviors can be shaped by the specific organizational settings within geographically defined communities, including evidence of effects of schools (Springer et al., 2015, 2018), workplace (Proper & van Oostrom, 2019; van de Ven et al., 2020), and faith-based institutions (Hays & Aranda, 2016; Robertson-James et al., 2018). Planners are in a unique position to co-learn about and harness the environmental context, including place, settings, and the environments within place and settings, in designing interventions for individual-level and population-level health promotion.

In Task 3 of Step 1, the health planning group describes the context for the intervention, including the community, population, and setting. Building on the NAA (Task 2), in Task 3, the planning group aims to further clarify and describe the priority populations for the intervention, which includes specification of the at-risk group along with the potential environmental agents, and a description of the context for the intervention. In describing the at-risk group(s), the planning group builds from the descriptive epidemiology of the health problem by specifying the subgroups with higher risk for a *given health behavior*, *exposure to an adverse environmental condition*, or *adverse health or QOL condition*, which may include considerations of age, gender, sex, race/ethnicity, socioeconomic status, and geographic location. The planning group also specifies the environmental agents who should be considered for the intervention, including those who may directly influence the at-risk group (e.g., healthcare providers, teachers, parents), and those who have influence over an environmental condition, such as a city council or other decision-making entity.

In addition to describing the priority populations, Task 3 of Step 1 involves the synthesis of findings from the NAA to describe the overall environmental context of the intervention, which includes specifying the geographic community and the potential settings to reach the priority populations and deliver the intervention. In exploring this broader context, the group should also consider the *forces of change* that affect the context, which include current trends and events such as legislation, the economy, technology, and even pandemics. The MAPP *Forces of Change Assessment* provides helpful guidance in this process (NACCHO, n.d.). Table 5.4 presents an example *At-A-Glance Description of Context and Population* table from the ¡Activate Ya! study in Uruguay (Springer et al., 2020). Data for this table can be gleaned from the NAA methods described above.

Task 4: State Intervention Goals

The final task for IM Step 1 is to state intervention goals by prioritizing the QOL, health, behavioral, and environmental factors identified in the NAA that will become the key targets of the intervention. In setting priorities, we embrace the wisdom of the American philosopher, psychologist, and education reformer John Dewey who once said: "A problem well stated is a problem half solved." Upon completion of the NAA, the planning team should have a comprehensive understanding of the health problem(s) and priority populations to develop *well-stated intervention goals* to address the health problem, which are essential to guide the overall intervention and evaluation of the intervention.

Table 5.4 Initial *At-A-Glance* Description of Context and Population—*¡Activate Ya! Youth Tobacco Prevention and Physical Activity Promotion Program*

Population and Context	Findings from Needs and Assets Assessment (Task 2)
Priority populations	
At-Risk Population(s) *(Consider age, gender, SES, race/ethnicity, other characteristics)*	Secondary school students (ages 11–15 years) in low to mid-income semi-urban communities in Uruguay
Potential Environmental Agents *(Consider those who may directly influence the at-risk population as well as those who have influence over an environmental condition)*	1. Classroom teachers and PE teachers 2. Principals and School District Leaders 3. Parents/Guardians 4. CIET (chronic disease prevention nongovernmental organization based in Uruguay)
Context	
Geographically Defined Community	Semi-urban area of Montevideo, Uruguay *(*community name not included for protection of human subjects)*
Settings *(Consider the settings where you can reach the population and that may also serve to deliver the intervention)*	1. Public and private secondary schools 2. Out-of-school settings (sports fields and public parks)
Forces of Change *(Trends and events that affect context, along with the threats and opportunities posed by these forces of change)*	**Threats** 1. Tobacco industry push-back on recent legislation 2. Limited school schedule for additional activities 3. Teacher protests *(a threat and opportunity)* **Opportunities** 1. Recent tobacco regulation and PE mandates 2. One laptop per child policy (Plan Ceibal) 3. *Espacio Adolescente*: a "free space" within the school schedule for healthy adolescent development activities.

Adapted from Springer et al. (2020).

Importance and Changeability Framework for Prioritizing Goals

Once the planning group has completed the NAA and clearly defined the health issue of interest, the behavioral and environmental causes of the issue, the population groups most at risk, and the overall intervention context, the planning group begins to think about what factors should be prioritized and explicitly targeted by the intervention, which represents a key focus of Step 2. In making this bridge to Step 2, we state the initial intervention goals, which may become further refined as we proceed with the subsequent IM steps, recognizing the iterative nature of the planning process.

A useful framework for prioritizing the behavioral and environmental factors and developing goals for a given intervention is the application of an *importance and changeability* prioritization framework, originally developed by Green and Kreuter (Green & Kreuter, 1991, 1999, 2005). Under this framework, behaviors and environmental conditions that are both more important (i.e., are causally related to a health issue based on existing evidence) and more changeable (i.e., the level of ease or difficulty in changing a factor based on evidence and expert input) will be a high priority for the focus of the intervention. Factors that are more important and less changeable may be a priority for innovative interventions for which evaluation is key. Factors that are less important but more changeable may be deemed as lower priorities except to demonstrate initial change. Factors that are both less important and less changeable should not be prioritized. This analysis should be carefully conducted so that factors that are important but hard to change are not neglected.

SMART Framework for Stating Intervention Goals

Within the IM framework, we define intervention goals as changes in QOL, health, behavioral, or environmental factors identified via the needs assessment. Looking back at the modified PRECEDE *logic model of the problem*, planners target how much change can be expected in indicators over a specified time frame. These goals also become the main targets for the evaluation of the intervention. The ultimate intervention goals are usually related to health or QOL—with common health indicators that include morbidity, mortality, incidence, prevalence, disability, and physiological risk factors; however, planners should also include behavioral and environmental goals as well, given their key roles in influencing health and QOL. Of note, if the time period is too long to assess intervention effects on QOL and health within the intervention time frame (e.g., an intervention aimed at preventing HIV or cancer), then planners may decide to define goals specifically in terms of behavior or environment, provided these behaviors or environmental conditions have a strong link to health outcomes.

A useful framework for guiding the development of intervention goals is the *SMART Goals* framework, which is an acronym for *Specific* (goals should be as specific as possible, including specification of targeted outcomes and populations), *Measurable* (goals should ideally include an indicator or measure to assess whether goals have been attained), *Achievable* (goals should be feasible, both overall and within the timeframe), *Relevant* (goals should align with evidence of their importance, values and long-term objectives), *and Time-bound* (goals should be based on a realistic timeframe for accomplishment). In writing intervention goals, it is also common to include a comparison group, depending on the evaluation design. Health promotion planners may consider consulting authority recommendations for a given health or behavior, which can provide the foundation for a given goal, such as recommendations for fruit and vegetable consumption. Planners may also consider state, national, or global health goals for a given health issue, such as targeted goals for breastfeeding.

In Box 5.6, we provide example intervention goals for the *¡Activate Ya! program*. These include a statement (with a strong verb) of what will change in a specified population and where, by how much, and by what period of time. The amount of expected change and the time frame should be empirically justifiable, which may include conducting a review of the literature to identify evidence of the amount and time needed to achieve change for a given outcome as well as consulting with experts.

BOX 5.6. STATING INTERVENTION GOALS—*¡ACTIVATE YA!*

Building from the NAA process, the *¡Activate Ya!* team set intervention goals as a final task of Step 1. While the *¡Activate Ya!* program had a dual focus of tobacco prevention and PA promotion among Uruguayan secondary school students, we provide below example goals for the PA focus of the intervention. A health goal is also included as an example, yet measuring intervention effects on health was beyond the scope and funding resources of the *¡Activate Ya!* study.

- Health Goal: Upon completion of two years of implementation of the *¡Activate Ya!* program based in X geographic place in Uruguay (de-identified), increase the percentage of healthy weight secondary school students as assessed by BMI-for-age-and-sex percentiles by 5% in intervention schools compared to comparison schools.
- Behavioral Goal: At the end of two years of implementation of the *¡Activate Ya!* program based in X schools and X geographic place of Uruguay (de-identified), increase the percentage of secondary students meeting PA recommendations of 60 minutes of daily PA by 10% compared to same-age students attending comparison schools.
- Environmental Goal: At the end of two years of implementation of the *¡Activate Ya!* program based in X geographic place of Uruguay, increase the number and frequency of PA opportunities provided throughout the day (targets: one or more daily classroom activity breaks/active learning lessons; and one or more days of after school programming with active games) in intervention schools compared with comparison schools.

In summary, specifying intervention goals as part of Task 4 of Step 1 is a key facet of intervention planning that will guide the overall development of the intervention. Once the intervention goals are defined, they will serve as the foundation for guiding the development of the expected behavioral and environmental outcomes and objectives as part of Step 2. In addition, the intervention goals will inform the major outcome evaluation questions in Step 6, which pertain to whether the intervention accomplished its goals.

FOR OUR CHILDREN EXAMPLE: STEP 1

We use the ***For Our Children*** or, in Spanish, ***Por Nuestros Hijos* (PNH)** program as an example throughout the book to illustrate the development of an intervention guided by IM (Rodriguez et al., 2018a, 2018b, 2019, 2020; McGlone et al., 2017). PNH is a theory-based program designed to educate Hispanic/Latino parents about the human papillomavirus (HPV) and motivate them to vaccinate their adolescent children (11–17 years) (Rodriguez et al., 2018a). This program was developed by the Center for Health Promotion and Prevention Research at the University of

Texas Health Science Center School of Public Health with funding from the Cancer Prevention and Research Institute of Texas (CPRIT). We present this example step by step at the end of each IM step (Chapters 5 through 10) starting in this chapter with Step 1.

Task 1. Establish a Planning Group

The PNH intervention is a multi-component program that targets both providers and parents of age-eligible children with the goal of increasing HPV vaccination among Hispanic/Latino/a/e (heretofore referred to as "Hispanic") children ages 11–17. In developing the PNH program, the planning group used the IM core processes throughout each planning step. In establishing the planning group (Task 1), the team drew on longstanding relationships with *community and healthcare partners* to participate as part of the core team that would be involved in decisions about the intervention (the *planning group*). The *planning group* consisted of a multidisciplinary team including health promotion researchers, epidemiologists, behavioral scientists, community leaders, healthcare providers, a representative from a community health worker organization, clinic partners (including an outreach coordinator), and lay health workers who were also parents of age-eligible children. Each member of the group was selected to guide program development and implementation given their unique perspective and experience in areas including HPV vaccination, health promotion planning and implementation, community engagement, and healthcare delivery in community primary care clinics. Since the components of the intervention were developed consecutively (i.e., the parent component was developed first, and the provider component followed), the planning group for each component varied somewhat. When developing the parent component, the group included parent participants, and when developing the provider component, the group included clinicians. The larger planning group for each component met periodically, with a smaller design group—primarily made up of health educators—meeting weekly during the intensive design phase.

Task 2. Conduct a Needs and Assets Assessment

In conducting the *NAA* (Task 2), the planning group began by developing a logic model of the problem. The IM *logic model of the problem* (also called the *risk* model), helped the initial sorting of ideas that emerged as the planning group identified potential factors hindering HPV vaccination and how lack of HPV vaccination can lead to health problems (HPV-related cancer) and QOL issues (see Figure 5.4). Because the project was funded to improve HPV vaccination and behavior, the planning group was clear that they would be entering the logic model of the problem at the behavioral phase. They initially discussed whether they would be focusing only on people who were unvaccinated (vaccine uptake) or also include those who had not completed vaccination (two- or three-shot series depending on the age of the child). The planning group chose to focus on parents of unvaccinated children first, since at least one vaccine could offer substantial protection, thus deciding to focus on vaccine uptake.

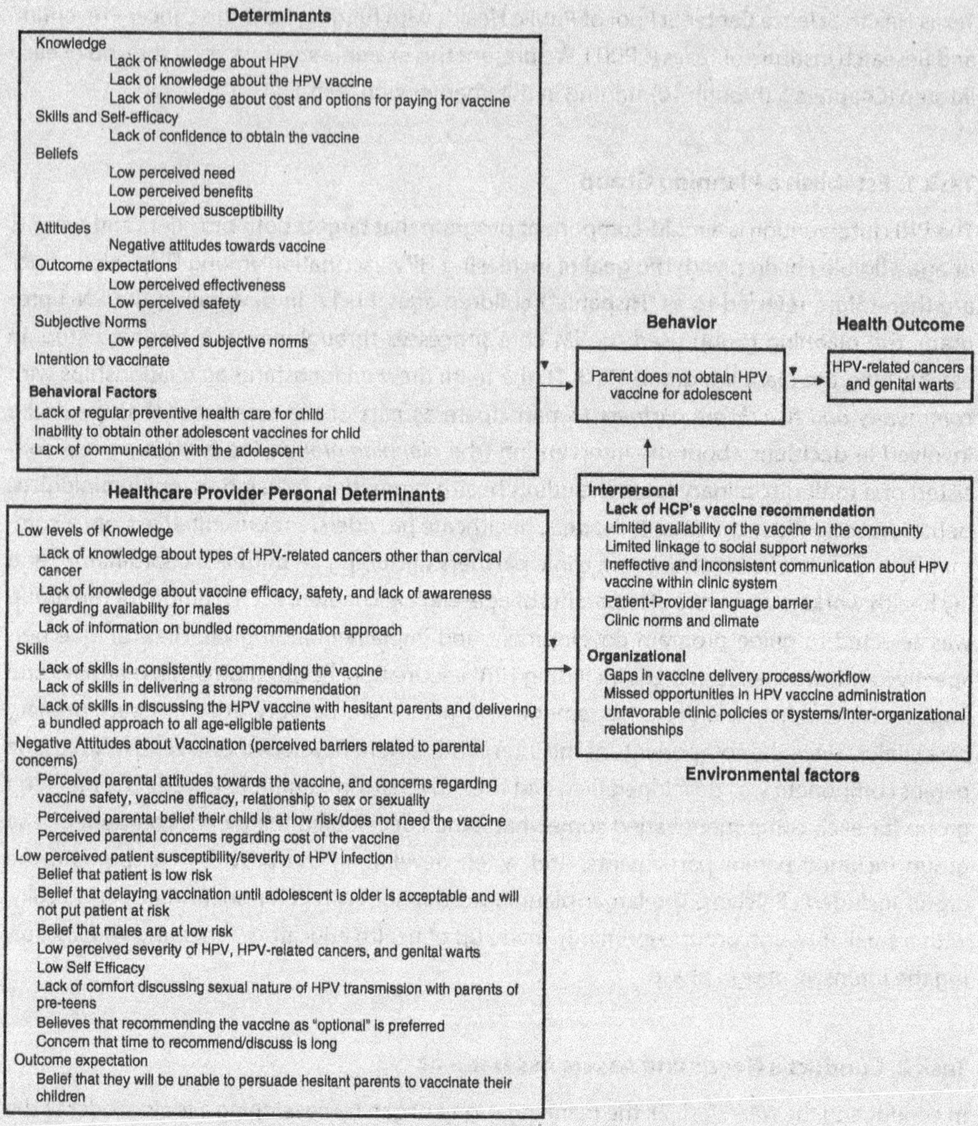

Figure 5.4 Por Nuestros Hijos/For Our Children Logic Model of the Problem

For an intervention that seeks to influence the health of children/adolescents, parents are usually considered an environmental agent at the interpersonal level influencing behavior. However, in this case, since the behavior (agreeing to vaccinate their children) is *controlled* by the parent, and children and adolescents less than 18 years of age cannot obtain the vaccine independently, the planning group decided to focus the intervention (and develop the logic model of the problem) from the perspective of parent behavior. Thus, they defined the risk behavior of interest as *Hispanic parents do not obtain the HPV vaccine for their children.*

Moving to the right of the logic model of the problem, the planning group then described the *health problems* associated with not getting vaccinated (HPV infection) and the QOL implications of HPV infection and associated conditions caused by HPV infection. Using the IM *core processes*, the planning group began brainstorming answers to questions about what environmental factors influence HPV vaccination of Hispanic adolescents. For example, an important factor negatively influencing parents' decision to vaccinate was that they rarely received a strong recommendation from the child's doctor. Moving to the left in the model, the planning group then asked and brainstormed answers to questions about *personal determinants* for why parents/adolescents do not engage in HPV vaccination uptake and the personal determinants related to why providers were not making appropriate HPV vaccination recommendations. Brainstormed answers to these questions were discussed and used to fill out the key sections (boxes) of the preliminary logic model of the problem.

Overview of Needs Assessment Methods

Following the brainstorming sessions, the planning group reviewed the literature and available data sources related to vaccination and held focus groups and in-depth interviews with parents from the priority population. Questions included: What is the prevalence of HPV vaccination among Hispanic adolescents in the area of focus? What behavioral and environmental factors and personal determinants are associated with Hispanic parents not obtaining the HPV vaccine for their adolescent children? And what behavioral, environmental, and personal determinants are associated with healthcare providers not strongly recommending the HPV vaccine to the parents of their adolescent patients?

The planning group conducted seven focus groups and seven in-depth interviews with parents. They also conducted three in-depth interviews per clinic (seven clinics total) which included interviews with physicians, nurses and/or medical assistants, and front desk staff/ appointment schedulers. The purpose of the qualitative inquiry was to explore parents' and providers' knowledge, attitudes, and beliefs about HPV, the HPV vaccine, and HPV-related cancers. Other objectives of the interviews were to understand patient flow at each clinic, current vaccine recommendation practices, barriers to making a strong recommendation, factors influencing providers' comfort with talking to parents about HPV (e.g.,11–12 versus older adolescents), and other implementation issues.

The planning group also explored and documented organizational and human resource assets as part of the social/organizational environment of the partner clinics that could be leveraged for the program or its delivery. They evaluated clinic processes for administering HPV vaccination, including any available resources the clinic could leverage to deliver the vaccine. They generated health delivery process maps unique to each clinic to illustrate key individuals, activities, and resources in the clinical process. They also documented each step of the appointment process from patient check-in to check-out, the different types of staff involved, and the roles and responsibilities for each step of the process. The group assessed whether the clinic provided health education through a lay health worker or provided outreach services as well as the resources required to carry out outreach activities.

The asset mapping included considerations of potential intervention delivery. The planning group assessed, for example, if there was anyone within the clinic who could function as a clinic/immunization champion whose role would be to encourage program adoption and implementation and support HPV vaccine delivery at the clinic. Recruitment of clinic/immunization champions is an effective implementation strategy to promote the uptake of HPV vaccination (Bonawitz et al., 2020). To assess the physical environmental assets, the planning group explored the physical layout of the clinic and, in particular, space and opportunities within the process of patient flow, where education by a lay health worker may occur. They also worked with the clinics to determine the best way to obtain information from the electronic medical record (EMR) to obtain data needed for the evaluation of the program. This generally included establishing a relationship with the individual responsible for managing the clinic's EMR system. The planning group identified two immunization champions to support the implementation of the intervention: a clinic coordinator (who could be involved in the delivery of the intervention materials) and a C-suite leader (who could influence provider behavior).

Describing Health Problems, Quality of Life, and the Population at Risk

The *priority population* for PNH comprised Hispanic parents of children aged 11–17 in Texas whose children had not initiated their HPV vaccine series. Using the modified PRECEDE model to guide the needs assessment, the planning group used secondary data sources, empirical literature reviews, and community input to describe *health problems* and *QOL issues* related to the lack of HPV vaccination among adolescents.

The planning group described the impact of HPV infections on health. HPV can cause six different types of cancers: cervical, vaginal, vulvar, penile, anal, and oropharyngeal. HPV infection is responsible for 90% of all cervical cancers and 60% of all penile cancers (Centers for Disease Control and Prevention, 2025). Hispanic men and women were disproportionately affected by HPV-associated cancer compared to their non-Hispanic counterparts, particularly in Texas. Between 2014 and 2018, the incidence of cervical cancer among Hispanic women in the United States was 9.3 per 100,000 compared to 6.7 per 100,000 among their non-Hispanic White counterparts (National Cancer Institute, 2021; National Cancer Institute, n.d.). In Texas, the incidence among Hispanic women was 10.5 per 100,000 compared to 7.6 per 100,000 among non-Hispanic White women (Texas Cancer Registry, 2020). Additionally, Hispanic women had disproportionately higher incidence rates than women of other races and ethnicities and the second-highest cervical cancer mortality rate behind Black women (Shoemaker & White, 2016). Disparities also existed between Hispanic and non-Hispanic White men in Texas. For example, between 2013 and 2017, HPV-related penile cancer incidence rates were higher among Hispanic men compared to non-Hispanic White men in Texas (1.4 versus 0.7 per 100,000) (Texas Cancer Registry, 2020; Viens et al., 2016).

As it relates to QOL, the planning group documented the potential impact of cervical cancer and its treatment including negative short- and long-term effects on an individual's economic, social, and psychological well-being, including lowered ability to find or maintain employment (Cohen et al., 2017); high financial distress due to hospitalization, ER visits, and treatments (Cohen et al., 2017; Marion et al., 2022; Shankaran et al., 2018); physical limitations as a result of the disease (Bjelic-Radisic et al., 2012; Le Borgne et al., 2013; Wenzel et al., 2005) and/or treatments (Frumovitz et al., 2005); and mental health issues related to prolonged treatment (Janda et al., 2010; Park et al., 2007).

Finally, recognizing the health problems and QOL issues related to the lack of HPV vaccination, a systematic review of reviews informed the planning group's understanding of HPV vaccination as well as the modifiable factors at multiple levels that could be intervened upon to increase HPV vaccination initiation and coverage (Rodriguez et al., 2020). This review also highlighted important clinical factors associated with the successful implementation of patient- and provider-level interventions.

Describing the Risk Behavior of the Priority Population

As noted above, parents' decision not to initiate HPV vaccination for their children was the *primary risk behavior* targeted by the program. HPV vaccination has been shown to prevent HPV infections (Centers for Disease Control and Prevention, 2024a); however, vaccination rates remain low. According to the 2015–2019 National Immunization Survey–Teen, only 53.7% of Hispanic adolescents in the United States are fully vaccinated against HPV (Centers for Disease Control and Prevention, 2020). Texas ranked 31 of 50 in HPV vaccination rates (Centers for Disease Control and Prevention, 2024b), with only 45.4% of Hispanic adolescents being fully vaccinated (Elam-Evans et al. 2020; Pingali et al., 2021). The CDC Advisory Committee for Immunization Practices recommends that healthcare providers administer the HPV vaccine series to adolescent males and females at ages 11–12 concurrent with other recommended vaccines and complete the series prior to age 13. Despite the national recommendations, the HPV vaccine is undervalued as a strategy, resulting in low uptake and missed opportunities to prevent HPV-related cancers (President's Cancer Panel, 2018). The HPV vaccine has the potential to reduce the number of cancers linked to HPV by preventing over 90% of malignancies when administered before exposure (Markowitz et al., 2013).

Describing Determinants Affecting Parental Acceptance of HPV Vaccine

Moving again to the left of the logic model of the problem (Figure 5.4), the planning group then explored the *determinants* of parents' lack of acceptance of HPV vaccination by asking, "Why don't parents vaccinate their adolescents?" Overall, Hispanic mothers in the United States are more accepting of vaccination than their White non-Hispanic counterparts (Galbraith et al., 2016); however, in addition to access issues, HPV vaccination for this group can be negatively impacted by parental beliefs and concerns. The literature review indicated that Hispanic parents delayed HPV vaccination due to concerns that the vaccine would promote sexual initiation among their daughters (Fernandez et al., 2014; Madhivanan et al., 2016; Rodriguez et al., 2018). Parental perception that their child was not at risk (Galbraith et al., 2016; Morales-Campos et al., 2021) and that the vaccine was not necessary because the child was too young or not sexually active (Galbraith et al., 2016; Warner et al., 2015) has been cited as causes for delaying HPV vaccination in this population. Concerns about vaccine safety and effectiveness (Morales-Campos et al., 2021; Rodriguez et al., 2018; Vollrath et al., 2018) were also negatively associated with initiation. Lastly, lack of knowledge regarding HPV, the HPV vaccine, and HPV-related diseases was found to be associated with parental hesitation to vaccinate their child (Colón-López et al., 2017; Madhivanan et al., 2016). On the other hand, parents who were aware (Kepka et al., 2012) of the vaccine and were given a vaccine recommendation (Kim & LeClaire, 2019; Loke et al., 2017; Ryan et al., 2018; Vollrath et al., 2018) by the provider, were aware that medical plans and coupons covered vaccine expenses, believed that the vaccine was covered by insurance (Kepka et al., 2012; Reiter et al., 2009), and believed that the vaccine prevents disease, particularly genital warts (Vanderpool et al., 2011), were more likely to accept the HPV vaccine.

Findings from focus groups with parents aligned with the literature in that Hispanic parents reported low levels of knowledge about HPV, HPV-related cancers, and the HPV vaccine. Concerns about vaccine safety and side effects were also confirmed. Regarding susceptibility, parents of girls perceived that their daughters were too young to get vaccinated and therefore not at risk; however, parents of boys believed that their sons were soon to be sexually active and that vaccinating them could prevent HPV transmission. Lastly, parents believed that parents like them needed more information on how to initiate a conversation about HPV and the HPV vaccine with their child's healthcare provider.

Describing Environmental Factors Affecting Parental Acceptance of HPV Vaccine

The decision to get one's child vaccinated has been associated with parents' interaction with healthcare services, including regular visits to a healthcare provider and previous receipt of other vaccines, such as meningitis and Measles, Mumps, Rubella (MMR) vaccines (Newman et al., 2018). At the *interpersonal level*, providers play an important role in HPV vaccine uptake; specifically, their recommendation for the vaccine is the most important driver of parental decisions to vaccinate their child/adolescent (Morales-Campos et al., 2021; Newman et al., 2018; Vamos et al., 2021). Parents are more likely to refuse or delay vaccination when they do not receive a high-quality and strong recommendation from a healthcare provider (Gilkey et al., 2016).

Organizational factors are also crucial in HPV vaccination uptake, particularly the role of clinic staff in the decision-making process. Nurses and medical assistants are often the first health professionals to meet with patients. Clinic-level factors that are important to consider include the types of information presented to parents by medical assistants and nurses, formal and informal patterns of communication about the vaccine among the clinical and non-clinical staff (Selove et al., 2017), and clinic norms and climate for HPV vaccination (Selove et al., 2017). Given that the strength of the recommendation varies widely across physicians and other clinic staff (Shay et al., 2018), the planning group realized that it was important to understand the practice culture and the multi-layered context under which HPV vaccines are recommended. The planning group conducted process mapping and interviews with providers and clinic staff to better understand the organizational factors that could be influencing HPV vaccinations, particularly provider recommendation.

Describing Determinants of Environmental Factors

Providing a strong recommendation from a provider in a presumptive manner is one of the most important predictors of parents obtaining the HPV vaccine for their child. Unfortunately, healthcare providers often fail to do so during adolescent clinic visits (Dempsey et al., 2018; Gilkey et al., 2016; Savas et al., 2021). Many providers delay recommending the HPV vaccine, only offering it to older adolescents (Allison et al., 2013) and use a risk-based approach to recommending the vaccine resulting in many missed clinical opportunities to vaccinate. The literature review and interviews helped the planning group to better understand factors negatively influencing provider recommendation of HPV vaccination. Factors influencing lack of strong recommendations for the HPV vaccine include low levels of provider knowledge of HPV and the HPV vaccine, negative attitudes about the safety and efficacy of vaccines, apprehension with discussing the HPV vaccine risks and benefits with parents, discomfort discussing sexuality and sexually transmitted infections with parents or adolescents (Valentino & Poronsky, 2016; Zimet et al., 2013), perceptions about parental concerns, perceptions about parental attitudes toward the HPV vaccine, and questions about the need to vaccinate their child (Quinn et al., 2012; Valentino & Poronsky, 2016). Providers report numerous challenges associated with providing care to children of vaccine-hesitant parents (Diekema, 2013). Providers are likely to view vaccine hesitancy as an inconvenient (Hughes et al., 2011) and time-consuming (McRee et al., 2014) problem, discouraging them from routinely recommending the HPV vaccine (Kempe et al., 2011; McRee et al., 2014). Providers are also less likely to recommend the vaccine to uninsured and underinsured patients as they are concerned about the cost to parents, cost to the clinic, and inadequate insurance coverage and reimbursement (Quinn et al., 2012).

Task 3. Describe the Context for the Intervention, Including the Community, Population, and Setting

While the ultimate beneficiary of the program would be adolescents, the primary target identified through the planning process was parents. Since parent and provider interaction is significantly associated with vaccine initiation, providers were another intervention target, and community clinics were an important *setting* for health promotion and education. The PNH program was designed as a large multilevel intervention that draws on previous work to address factors influencing HPV vaccination at both parent and provider levels (Rodriguez et al., 2018). The initial setting was community health centers within the Greater Houston metropolitan area (*the initial geographic community*) with the intent of making it available throughout Texas. It was designed to be used in community clinics including those within the Harris Health System (the county safety net system) as well as FQHCs and private and community clinics.

Task 4. State Intervention Goals

The planning group was ultimately interested in decreasing the incidence of HPV-related cancers and genital warts. However, the evaluation time frame was not long enough to assess the intervention's effect on these health outcomes. Instead, the planning group chose to focus on vaccine initiation (behavioral) and provider recommendation (environmental) as the primary intervention goals. Previous interventions within clinical settings that aimed to increase vaccination coverage demonstrated differences ranging between 8% and 47% with a median of 15% in vaccination coverage between intervention and comparison groups (Shefer et al., 1999). Studies documenting the annual change in provider recommendation rates ranged between 3% and 11% with an average of 6% annually (Caldwell et al., 2021; Cataldi et al., 2021; Osazuwa-Peters et al., 2015; Shefer et al., 1999; Stokley et al., 2014). Based on the needs assessment conducted, the planning group determined that the *primary intervention goals* should include the following:

- Behavioral Goal: After two years of implementation of the PNH intervention, the percentage of Houston metropolitan area Hispanic adolescents in the intervention group who have initiated the HPV vaccine series will be 15% higher than Hispanic adolescents in the nonintervention group (or those who received standard care).
- Environmental Goal: After two years of implementation of the PNH intervention, the percentage of Houston metropolitan area healthcare providers in the intervention group who have recommended the HPV vaccine for their age-eligible patients will be 10% higher than healthcare providers in the nonintervention group.

Summary

Chapter 5 describes Step 1 of the IM framework, which involves four key tasks: (1) Establish a planning group; (2) Conduct an NAA; (3) Describe the context for the intervention, including the community, population, and setting; and (4) State intervention goals. A key focus of Step 1 involves engaging in deep learning about the health problem prior to proposing solutions, including learning about the multiple influences of the health problem, the priority populations most affected, and the context of the problem. In leading the NAA, Step 1 begins with engaging project partners and establishing a participatory planning group; we provide in this chapter a detailed description of the processes useful in facilitating such a planning group to carry out the NAA.

Guided by a modified PRECEDE model (Fielding, 2022; Green & Kreuter, 2005), or "*logic model of the problem*" conceptual framework, the planning group conducts a needs assessment with a population-based epidemiologic perspective to describe the health problem—such as morbidity and mortality, disease risk, and burden of disease—in at-risk groups. The assessment includes an analysis of causation of health problems at multiple levels as well as consideration of multiple determinants of health-related behavior and environment. While the health and QOL analysis always focuses on the population at risk of the health problem, Step 1 also explores the role of environmental agents who directly influence the health problem (e.g., at an interpersonal level) or have influence over environmental conditions that influence the problem (e.g., at organizational, community or societal levels), building from a multilevel perspective.

In conducting the assessment, Step 1 promotes a mixed-methods approach that builds from the *IM core processes* and incorporates qualitative and quantitative modes of inquiry. Specifically, we describe several data collection methods that can inform the NAA, including surveys, interviews, ethnographic methods, and focus groups, among other methods. We also describe a basic framework for conducting an assets assessment to identify assets rooted in various environments *(policy, information, social/cultural /organizational, and physical)* that can be harnessed for intervention planning. The final task of Step 1 involves prioritizing health outcomes and behavior and environmental factors identified in the needs assessment using *an importance and changeability framework,* and then stating intervention goals as guided by the *SMART goal framework.* The statement of intervention goals provides a link to Step 2 in IM, which begins with specifying behavioral and environmental outcomes for the proposed intervention.

Discussion Questions and Learning Activities

1. Discuss why an NAA is so critical to planning a health promotion program.
2. Explain why it is important for health promotion program planners to balance a needs assessment with an assessment of community assets and needs. Give examples of types of environmental assets.
3. Describe how you would establish a planning group and who you would include to develop a health promotion intervention of your choice. Briefly describe a process for how you would use the planning group to help conduct the NAA.
4. Describe the population at risk for the problem you selected in terms of demographic variables. Provide a rationale for why this population was chosen. Briefly describe the setting for a proposed health promotion intervention.
5. Indicate the phase of needs assessment at which you are entering the *logic model of the problem* (e.g., QOL, health, behavior, or environment). First, describe the factor with which you are beginning your model and then describe each of the other factors and their relation to each other.
6. Describe two indicators of QOL of the selected population. Describe two methods you would use to determine whether these indicators are important to this population. Explain why you selected these methods.

7. Describe health problem(s) that could affect the QOL for the population. Select at least one of these problems to be addressed by a health promotion program and explain the epidemiologic basis for giving the selected problem(s) priority. Describe the health problem and the incidence/prevalence of the problem in this population. Is it higher compared to other populations? Is there a greater burden of disease? If you cannot find data for your chosen population, construct estimates based on comparable populations.
8. Describe behaviors and environmental conditions that are likely causal factors for the health problem selected above. Document and provide references to support the possibility of a causal relationship.
9. From the list generated in Question 8, select the most important behaviors(s) and environmental condition(s) for programmatic focus based on a rating process where you determine the importance (in terms of relation to the health problem) and the changeability of each factor. Present a rationale and evidence.
10. State program goals that would serve as an indicator for the program achieving measurable improvements in health outcomes, QOL outcomes, or behavioral and environmental impact. Consider the time period and use the research literature to justify the amount of change you expect to occur.
11. Specify determinants of the risk behavior and environmental conditions using selected behavioral or social science theories and available empirical evidence.
12. Diagram *a logic model of the problem* that illustrates the causal pathways for how different factors influence increased risk for health problems that have an impact on QOL for a specified population.

References

Abascal, W., Elba, E., Goja, B., Gonzalez Mora, A., Sica, A., Triunfo, P., & Harris, J. E. (2012). Tobacco control campaign in Uruguay: A population-based trend analysis. *The Lancet, 380*(9853), 1575–1582.

ACHI AHA Improvement. (2017). Community health assessment toolkit. https://assesstoolkit.org/. Accessed July 6, 2020.

Allison, M. A., Dunne, E. F., Markowitz, L. E., O'Leary, S. T., Crane, L. A., Hurley, L. P., et al. (2013). HPV vaccination of boys in primary care practices. *Academic Pediatrics, 13*(5), 466–474.

Alonso, R., Pineros, M., Laversanne, M., Musetti, C., Garau, M., Barrios, E., et al. (2018). Lung cancer incidence trends in Uruguay 1990-2014: An age-period cohort analysis. *Cancer Epidemiology, 55*, 17–22.

Andersen, S., Blot, W., Shu Xo Sonderman, J., Steinwandel, M., Hargreaves, M., & Zheng, W. (2018). Associations between neighborhood environment, health behaviors, and mortality. *American Journal of Preventive Medicine, 54*(1), 87–95.

Anderson, H., Christiansen, L., Klinker, C., Ersboll, A., Troelsen, J., Kerr, J., et al. (2017). Increases in use and activity due to urban renewal: Effect of a natural experiment. *American Journal of Preventive Medicine, 53,* e81.

Arnstein, S. R. (1969). A ladder of citizen participation. *Journal of the American Planning Association, 35*(4), 216–224.

Austin/Travis County Community Health Assessment. (2017). Community health assessment: Austin/Travis county: Austin public health and community partners. https://austintexas.gov/sites/default/files/files/Health/CHA-CHIP/ATC_CHA_Dec2017_Report_Final.pdf. Accessed July 3, 2020.

Avery, C., Walker, M., & O'Toole, E. (2001). *Teamwork is an individual skill: Getting your work done when sharing responsibility.* Berrett-Koehler Publishers.

Azagba, S., Shan, L., & Latham, K. (2020). E-cigarette retail licensing policy and e-cigarette use among adolescents. *Journal of Adolescent Health, 66*(1), 123–125.

Bakker, M., Van Dijk, A., & Wicherts, J. M. (2012). The rules of the game called psychological science. *Perspectives on Psychological Science, 7,* 543–554.

Belansky, E., Cutforth, N., Chavez, R., Waters, E., & Bartlett-Horch, K. (2011). An adapted version of intervention mapping (AIM) is a tool for conducting community-based participatory research. *Health Promotion Practice, 12*(3), 440–455.

Berkley-Patton, J., Bowe Thompson, C., Bradley-Ewing, A., Marcie, B., Booker, A., Catley, D., et al. (2018). Identifying health conditions, priorities, and relevant multilevel health promotion intervention strategies in African American churches: A faith community health needs assessment. *Evaluation and Program Planning, 67,* 19–28.

Bjelic-Radisic, V., Jensen, P. T., Vlasic, K. K., Waldenstrom, A.-C., Singer, S., Chie, W., et al. (2012). Quality of life characteristics in patients with cervical cancer. *European Journal of Cancer, 48*(16), 3009–3018.

Bogg, T., & Milad, E. (2020). Slowing the spread of COVID-19: Demographic, personality, and social cognition predictors of guideline adherence in a representative U.S. sample. *Society for Health Psychology, 39*(12), 1026–1036.

Bonawitz, K., Wetmore, M., Heisler, M., Dalton, V. K., Damschroder, L. J., Forman, J., et al. (2020). Champions in context: Which attributes matter for change efforts in healthcare? *Implementation Science, 15*(1), 1–10.

Bradford, L. (1976). *Making meetings work: A guide for leaders and group members.* San Diego, CA: University Associates.

Brooke, L., Lin, A., Ntoumanis, N., & Gucciardi, D. (2020). The development of a sport-based life skills program for young people with first episode psychosis: An intervention mapping approach. *Mental Health and Physical Activity, 19,* 100330.

Burton, W., Twiddy, M., Sahota, P., Brown, J., & Bryant, M. (2019). Participant engagement with a UK community-based preschool childhood obesity prevention programme: A focused ethnography study. *BMC Public Health, 19,* 1–14.

Cain, C., Orionzi, D., O'Brien, M., & Trahan, L. (2017). The power of community voices for enhancing community health needs assessments. *Health Promotion Practice, 18*(3), 437–443. Ngo, A. D., McCurdy, S. A., Ross, M. W., Markham, C., Ratliff, E. A., Pham, H. T. B. (2007). The lives of female sex workers in Vietnam: Findings from a qualitative study. *Culture, Health & Sexuality,* 9(6), 555–570.

Caldwell, A. C., Madden, C. A., Thompson, D. M., Garbe, M. C., Roberts, J. R., Jacobson, R. M., et al. (2021). The impact of provider recommendation on human papillomavirus vaccine and other adolescent vaccines. *Human Vaccines & Immunotherapeutics*, *17*(4), 1059–1067.

Cargo, M., & Mercer, S. (2008). The value and challenges of participatory research: Strengthening its practice. *Annual Review of Public Health*, *29*, 325–350.

Cataldi, J. R., O'Leary, S. T., Markowitz, L. E., Allison, M. A., Crane, L. A., Hurley, L. P., et al. (2021). Changes in strength of recommendation and perceived barriers to human papillomavirus vaccination: Longitudinal analysis of primary care physicians, 2008-2018. *The Journal of Pediatrics*, *234*(149–57), e3.

CCHD.b. (n.d.). Developing an organizational structure for the initiative. Community tool box. https://ctb.ku.edu/en/table-of-contents/structure/organizational-structure/overview/main. Accessed July 3, 2020.

CCHD.c. (n.d.). Rewarding accomplishments. Community toolbox. https://ctb.ku.edu/en/table-of-contents/maintain/reward-accomplishments. Accessed July 27, 2020.

CCHD.d. (n.d.). Promoting coordination, cooperative agreements, and collaborative agreements among agencies. Community toolbox. https://ctb.ku.edu/en/table-of-contents/implement/improving-services/coordination-cooperation-collaboration/main. Accessed July 27, 2020.

CDC. (n.d.). Community health assessment and group evaluation (CHANGE) tool. https://www.cdc.gov/public-health-gateway/php/public-health-strategy/public-health-strategies-for-community-health-assessment-models-frameworks-tools.html. Accessed July 3, 2020.

Center for Community Health and Development (CCHD) Kansas University. (n.d.). Community assessment. Community toolbox. https://ctb.ku.edu/en/table-of-contents/assessment. Accessed July 3, 2020.

Centers for Disease Control and Prevention. (2016). School health policies and practices study. https://archive.cdc.gov/www_cdc.gov/healthyyouth/data/shpps/index.htm. Accessed July 3, 2020.

Centers for Disease Control and Prevention. (2020). Supplementary tables for Estimated Vaccination coverage with selected vaccines and doses among adolescents aged 13–17 years—national immunization survey–teen (NIS-Teen), United States, 2019. https://www.cdc.gov/teenvaxview/publications/nis-teen-coverage-estimates-tables-2019.html Accessed January 15, 2020.

Centers for Disease Control and Prevention. (2024a). HPV vaccination. https://www.cdc.gov/hpv/vaccines/index.html. Accessed July 20, 2025.

Centers for Disease Control and Prevention. (2024b). TeenVAXView: Vaccination coverage among adolescents (13–17 years). https://www.cdc.gov/teenvaxview/interactive/index.html. Accessed July 29, 2025.

Centers for Disease Control and Prevention. (2024c). About Healthy Places. https://www.cdc.gov/healthy-places/php/about/index.html. Accessed July 20, 2025.

Centers for Disease Control and Prevention. (2024d). Community Planning for Health Assessment: CHA & CHIP. https://www.cdc.gov/public-health-gateway/php/public-health-strategy/public-health-strategies-for-community-health-assessment-health-improvement-planning.html. Accessed July 20, 2025.

Centers for Disease Control and Prevention. (2024e). Social determinants of health: Know what affects health. https://www.cdc.gov/socialdeterminants/index.htm. Accessed July 20, 2025.

Centers for Disease Control and Prevention. (2025). Cancers linked with HPV each year. https://www.cdc.gov/cancer/hpv/cases.html. Accessed July 20, 2025.

Centers for Disease Control and Prevention. (n.d.). Lesson 3- measures of risk: Section 5- measures of association. https://archive.cdc.gov/www_cdc.gov/csels/dsepd/ss1978/lesson3/section5.html. Accessed September 13, 2022.

Centers for Disease Control and Prevention CDC. (n.d.). 10 essential public health services.

Center for Global Health (U.S.). (2013). Field Epidemiology Training Program. 2013. Community needs assessment : facilitator/mentor guide. Centers for Disease Control and Prevention. https://stacks.cdc.gov/view/cdc/24069. Accessed November 20, 2025.

Cerin, E., Nathan, A., van Cauwenberg, J., Barnett, D., & Barnett, A. (2017). The neighbourhood physical environment and active travel in older adults: A systematic review and meta-analysis. *International Journal of Behavioral Nutrition and Physical Activity, 14*(15).

Chetty, R., Stepner, M., & Abraham, S. (2016). The association between income and life expectancy in the United States: 2001–2014. *Journal of the American Medical Association, 315*(16), 1750–1766.

Child, S., Schoffmann, D., Kaczynski, A., Forthofer, M., Wilcox, S., & Baruth, M. (2015). Neighborhood attributes associated with the social environment. *American Journal of Health Promotion, 30*(8), 634–637.

Cifuentes, E., Alamo, U., Kendall, T., Brunkard, J., & Scrimshaw, S. (2006). Rapid assessment procedures in environmental sanitation research: A case study from the northern border of Mexico. *Canadian Journal of Public Health, 97*(1), 24–28.

Clarke, A., Beenstock, J., Lukacs, J., Turner, L., & Limmer, M. (2019). Major risk factors for sexual minority young people's mental and physical health: Findings from a county-wide school-based health needs assessment. *Journal of Public Health, 41*(3), e274–e282.

Cohen, J., Harper, A., Nichols, E. M., Rao, G. G., Mohindra, P., & Roque, D. M. (2017). Barriers to timely completion of radiation therapy in patients with cervical cancer in an urban tertiary care center. *Cureus, 9*(9).

Colón-López, V., Fernández-Espada, N., Vélez, C., Gonzalez, V. J., Diaz-Toro, E. C., Calo, W. A., et al. (2017). Communication about sex and HPV among Puerto Rican mothers and daughters. *Ethnicity & Health, 22*(4), 348–360.

Community Advancement Network. (n.d.). Community advancement network. canatx.org. Accessed July 3, 2020.

Cooperrider, D., & Fry, R. (2020). Appreciative inquiry in a pandemic: An improbable pairing. *The Journal of Applied Behavioral Science, 56*(3), 266–271.

Creswell, J., & Plano, C. V. (2018). *Designing and conducting mixed methods research* (3rd ed.). Los Angeles, CA: SAGE Publications.

Crutzen, R., Peters, G.-J. Y., & Noijen, J. (2017). Using confidence interval-based estimation of relevance to select social-cognitive determinants for behavior change interventions. *Frontiers in Public Health, 5*, 165.

Dangerfield, D., II, Wylie, C., & Anderson, J. (2021). Conducting virtual, synchronous focus groups among black sexual minority men: Qualitative study. *JMIR Public Health and Surveillance, 7*(2), e22980.

Decker, M., Isquick, S., Tilley, L., Zhi, Q., Gutman, A., Luong, W., . . . Neighborhoods matter. (2018). A systematic review of neighborhood characteristics and adolescent reproductive health outcomes. *Health & Place, 54*, 178–190.

Dempsey, A. F., Pyrznawoski, J., Lockhart, S., Barnard, J., Campagna, E. J., Garrett, K., et al. (2018). Effect of a healthcare professional communication training intervention on adolescent human papillomavirus vaccination: A cluster randomized clinical trial. *JAMA Pediatrics, 172*(5), e180016–e.

Diekema, D. S. (2013). Provider dismissal of vaccine-hesitant families: Misguided policy that fails to benefit children. *Human Vaccines & Immunotherapeutics, 9*(12), 2661–2662.

Dillman, D., Smyth, J., & Christian, L. (2008). *Internet, mail and mixed-mode surveys: The tailored design method* (3rd ed.). Hoboken, NJ: John Wiley & Sons.

Dirige, O., Carlson, J., Alcaraz, J., Moy, K., Rock, C., Oades, R., et al. (2013). Siglang Buhay: Nutrition and physical activity promotion in Filipino-Americans through community organizations. *Journal of Public Health Management and Practice, 19*(2), 162–168.

Doner A, Rosing H, Hopes K, and Dwywe-Voss R. (n.d.) Asset mapping user guide: Overview. Community Catalyst Initiative. https://drive.google.com/file/d/1zfYfVWDhIrJD90s9bUU8mGmXYyod2Xa4/view. Accessed August 19, 2025.

Dover, D., & Belon, A. (2019). The health equity measurement framework: A comprehensive model to measure social inequities in health. *International Journal for Equity in Health, 18*(36), 1–12.

Elam-Evans, L. D., Yankey, D., Singleton, J. A., et al. (2020). National, regional, state, and selected local area vaccination coverage among adolescents aged 13–17 years—United States, 2019. *Morbidity and Mortality Weekly Report, 69*, 1109–1116. doi:10.15585/mmwr.mm6933a1

ESRI. (n.d.). Story maps. http://storymaps.arcgis.com/en/. Accessed July 23, 2020.

Falbe, F., Minkler, M., Dean, R., & Cordeiero, J. (2018). Power mapping: A useful tool for understanding the policy environment and its application to a local soda tax initiative. In N. Wallerstein, B. Duran, J. G. Oetzel, & M. Minkler (Eds.), *Community-based participatory research for health: Advancing Social and Health Equity* (pp. 405–410). Wiley.

Fernandez, M., Melvin, C., Leeman, J., Ribisl, K., Allen, J., Kegler, M., et al. (2014). The cancer prevention and control research network: An interactive systems approach to advancing cancer control implementation research and practice. *Cancer Epidemiology, Biomarkers & Prevention, 23*(11), 2512–2521.

Fernandez, M. E., Ten Hoor, G. A., Van Lieshout, S., Rodriguez, S. A., Beidas, R. S., Parcel, G., et al. (2019). Implementation mapping: Using intervention mapping to develop implementation strategies. *Frontiers in Public Health, 7*, 158.

Fielding, J. E. (2022). *Health program planning, implementation, and evaluation: Creating behavioral, environmental, and policy change.* JHU Press.

Francis, J., Wood, L., Knuiman, M., & Giles-Corti, B. (2012). Quality or quantity? Exploring the relationship between public open space attributes and mental health in Perth, Western Australia. *Social Science & Medicine, 74*(10), 1570–1577.

Freak-Poli, R., Brand, M., Boelsen-Robinson, T., Huse, O., de Courten, M., & Peeters, A. (2020). Development and piloting of a checklist for healthy eating and physical activity in the workplace (CEPAW). *Health Promotion International, 36*(1), 8–19.

Frerichs, L., Brittin, J., Sorensen, D., Trowbridge, M. J., Yaroch, A. L., Siahpush, M., et al. (2015). Influence of school architecture and design on healthy eating: A review of the evidence. *American Journal of Public Health, 105*(4), e46–e57.

Friedman, D. B., Brandt, H. M., Freedman, D. A., Adams, S. A., Young, V. M., & Ureda, J. R. (2014). Innovative and community-driven communication practices of the south Carolina cancer prevention and control research network. *Preventing Chronic Disease, 11*, e127.

Friis, R., & Sellers, T. (2013). *Epidemiology for public health practice.* Burlington, MA: Jones & Bartlett Publishing.

Frumovitz, M., Sun, C. C., Schover, L. R., Munsell, M. F., Jhingran, A., Wharton, J. T., et al. (2005). Quality of life and sexual functioning in cervical cancer survivors. *Journal of Clinical Oncology, 23*(30), 7428–7436.

Galbraith, K. V., Lechuga, J., Jenerette, C. M., Moore, L. A. D., Palmer, M. H., & Hamilton, J. B. (2016). Parental acceptance and uptake of the HPV vaccine among African-Americans and Latinos in the United States: A literature review. *Social Science & Medicine, 159*, 116–126.

Gilkey, M. B., Calo, W. A., Moss, J. L., Shah, P. D., Marciniak, M. W., & Brewer, N. T. (2016). Provider communication and HPV vaccination: The impact of recommendation quality. *Vaccine, 34*(9), 1187–1192.

Gilmore, G., & Campbell, M. (2005). *Needs and capacity assessment strategies for health education and health promotion* (3rd ed.). Sudbury, MA: Jones and Bartlett.

Giovenco, D. P., Casseus, M., Duncan, D. T., Coups, E. J., Lewis, M. J., & Delnevo, C. D. (2016). Association between electronic cigarette marketing near schools and e-cigarette use among youth. *Journal of Adolescent Health, 59*(6), 627–634.

Girvan, E. J., McIntosh, K., & Smolkowski, K. (2019). Tail, tusk, and trunk: What different metrics reveal about racial disproportionality in school discipline. *Educational Psychologist, 54*(1), 40–59.

Glanz, K., Handy, S. L., Henderson, K. E., Slater, S. J., Davis, E. L., & Powell, L. M. (2016). Built environment assessment: Multidisciplinary perspectives. *SSM—Population Health, 2*, 24–31.

Goodman, R. M., Speers, M. A., McLeroy, K., Fawcett, S., Kegler, M., Parker, E., et al. (1998). Identifying and defining the dimensions of community capacity to provide a basis for measurement. *Health Education & Behavior, 25*(3), 258–278.

Goodman, R. A., Bunnell, R., & Posner, S. F. (2014). What is "community health"? Examining the meaning of an evolving field in public health. *Preventive Medicine, 67*, S58–S61.

Gray, S., Treacy, J., & Hall, E. T. (2019). Re-engaging disengaged pupils in physical education: An appreciative inquiry perspective. *Sport, Education and Society, 24*(3), 241–255.

Green, G. P., & Haines, A. L. (2016). *Asset Building & Community Development* (4th ed.). Los Angeles, CA: Sage Publications.

Green, L., & Kreuter, M. (1991). *Health promotion planning: An educational and environmental approach* (2rd ed.). Mountain View, CA: Mayfield.

Green, L., & Kreuter, M. (1999). *Health program planning: An educational and ecological approach* (3rd ed.). Mountain View, CA: Mayfield.

Green, L., & Kreuter, M. (2005). *Health program planning: An educational and ecological approach* (4th ed.). New York, NY: McGraw-Hill.

Green, L., Gielen, A., Peterson, D., Kreuter, M., & Ottoson, J. (2022). *Health program planning, implementation, and evaluation.* Baltimore, MD: Johns Hopkins University Press.

Greening, D. W., & Turban, D. B. (2000). Corporate social performance as a competitive advantage in attracting a quality workforce. *Business & Society, 39*(3), 254–280.

Gwede, C. K., Menard, J. M., Martinez-Tyson, D., Lee, J.-H., Vadaparampil, S. T., Padhya, T. A., et al. (2010). Strategies for assessing community challenges and strengths for cancer disparities participatory research and outreach. *Health Promotion Practice, 11*(6), 876–887.

Halcomb, E., & Hickman, L. (2015). *Mixed methods research. Nursing Standard: Promoting excellence in nursing care.* University of Wollongong.

Hasso Plattner Institute of Design (2010). *An introduction to design thinking process guide.* Institute of Design at Stanford.

Hawe, P. (2015). Lessons from complex interventions to improve health. *Annual Review of Public Health, 36*(1), 307–323.

Hawe, P., Shiell, A., & Riley, T. (2009). Theorising interventions as events in systems. *American Journal of Community Psychology, 43*(3–4), 267–276.

Hays, K., & Aranda, M. P. (2016). Faith-based mental health interventions with African Americans: A review. *Research on Social Work Practice, 26*(7), 777–789.

Highfield, L., Arthasarnprasit, J., Ottenweller, C. A., & Dasprez, A. (2011). Interactive web-based mapping: Bridging technology and data for health. *International Journal of Health Geographics, 10*(1), 69.

Hillyer, G. C., Schmitt, K. M., Lizardo, M., Reyes, A., Bazan, M., Alvarez, M. C., et al. (2017). Electronic communication channel use and health information source preferences among Latinos in northern Manhattan. *Journal of Community Health, 42*(2), 349–357.

Hsu, C.-C., & Sandford, B. A. (2019). The Delphi technique: Making sense of consensus. *Practical Assessment, Research and Evaluation, 12,* 10. doi:10.7275/pdz9-th90

Huggins-Hoyt, K. Y., Briggs, H. E., Mowbray, O., & Allen, J. L. (2019). Privatization, racial disproportionality and disparity in child welfare: Outcomes for foster children of color. *Children and Youth Services Review, 99,* 125–131.

Hughes, C. C., Jones, A. L., Feemster, K. A., & Fiks, A. G. (2011). HPV vaccine decision making in pediatric primary care: A semi-structured interview study. *BMC Pediatrics, 11*(1), 1–9.

Hurley, D. A., Murphy, L. C., Hayes, D., Hall, A. M., Toomey, E., McDonough, S. M., et al. (2016). Using intervention mapping to develop a theory-driven, group-based complex intervention to support self-management of osteoarthritis and low back pain (SOLAS). *Implementation Science, 11*(1), 56.

IIED. (2004). Participatory learning and action: Critical reflections, future directions. https://pubs.iied.org/pdfs/9440IIED.pdf. Accessed July 3, 2020.

Ingalls, J. S. (2018). Improvisational theater games: Performatory team-building activities. *Journal of Physical Education, Recreation & Dance, 89*(1), 40–45.

Institute of Medicine (2005). *Preventing childhood obesity: Heath in the balance.* Washington, DC: National Academies Press. https://doi.org/10.17226/11015

IRS. (2019). Requirements for 501(c)(3) hospitals under the affordable care act—section 501(r). https://www.irs.gov/charities-non-profits/charitableorganizations/requirements-for-501c3-hospitals-under-the-affordable-care-act-section-501r. Accessed July 3, 2020.

Janda, M., Gebski, V., Brand, A., Hogg, R., Jobling, T. W., Land, R., et al. (2010). Quality of life after total laparoscopic hysterectomy versus total abdominal hysterectomy for stage I endometrial cancer (LACE): A randomised trial. *The Lancet Oncology, 11*(8), 772–780.

Johnson, D. W., & Johnson, F. P. (2012). *Joining together: Group theory and group skills* (11th ed.). Upper Saddle River, NJ: Pearson.

Kawachi, I., Kennedy, B. P., Lochner, K., & Prothrow-Stith, D. (1997). Social capital, income inequality, and mortality. *American Journal of Public Health, 87*(9), 1491–1498.

Keeney, S., Hasson, F., & McKenna, H. (2011). *The Delphi technique in nursing and health research.* Oxford, UK: Wiley Online Library.

Kempe, A., Daley, M. F., McCauley, M. M., Crane, L. A., Suh, C. A., Kennedy, A. M., et al. (2011). Prevalence of parental concerns about childhood vaccines: The experience of primary care physicians. *American Journal of Preventive Medicine, 40*(5), 548–555.

Kepka, D., Berkowitz, Z., Yabroff, K. R., Roland, K., & Saraiya, M. (2012). Human papillomavirus vaccine practices in the USA: Do primary care providers use sexual history and cervical cancer screening results to make HPV vaccine recommendations? *Sexually Transmitted Infections, 88*(6), 433–435.

Kerstenetzky, L., Birschbach, M. J., Beach, K. F., Hager, D. R., & Kennelty, K. A. (2018). Improving medication information transfer between hospitals, skilled-nursing facilities, and long-term-care pharmacies for hospital discharge transitions of care: A targeted needs assessment using the intervention mapping framework. *Research in Social and Administrative Pharmacy, 14*(2), 138–145.

Kim, K., & LeClaire, A.-R. (2019). A systematic review of factors influencing human papillomavirus vaccination among immigrant parents in the United States. *Health Care for Women International, 40*(6), 696–718.

Kretzmann, J., & McKnight, J. P. (1996). Assets-based community development. *National Civic Review, 85*(4), 23–29.

Krueger, R., & Casey, M. (2009). *Focus groups: A practical guide for applied research* (4th ed.). Thousand Oaks, CA: Sage.

L G (2009). *Epidemiology*. Philadelphia, PA: Saunders.

Langley, G. J., Moen, R. D., Nolan, K. M., Nolan, T. W., Norman, C. L., & Provost, L. P. (2009). *The improvement guide: A practical approach to enhancing organizational performance.* John Wiley & Sons.

Le Borgne, G., Mercier, M., Woronoff, A.-S., Guizard, A.-V., Abeilard, E., Caravati-Jouvenceaux, A., et al. (2013). Quality of life in long-term cervical cancer survivors: A population-based study. *Gynecologic Oncology, 129*(1), 222–228.

Linder, S. H., & Sexton, K. (2011). Conceptual models for cumulative risk assessment. *American Journal of Public Health, 101*(S1), S74–S81.

Linn, M., Huber, J., Olgun, G., & Larson, K. (2021). Determining social needs for pediatric patients in a Sioux falls pediatric clinic. *South Dakota Medicine, 74*(6), 250–254.

Linville, D., McClure, H., Martinez, C., & Mena Morales, C. (2020). Latinx immigrant farmworker community health promotion: A needs assessment. *Health Promotion Practice, 21*(3), 372–382.

Lipmanowicz, H., & McCandless, K. (2014). *The surprising power of liberating structures: Simple rules to unleash a culture of innovation.* Seattle, WA: Liberating Structures Press.

Loke, A. Y., Kwan, M. L., Wong, Y.-T., & Wong, A. K. Y. (2017). The uptake of human papillomavirus vaccination and its associated factors among adolescents: A systematic review. *Journal of Primary Care & Community Health, 8*(4), 349–362.

Ludema, J., Whitney, D., Mohr, B., & Griffin, T. (2003). *The appreciative inquiry summit: A practitioner's guide for leading large-group change.* San Francisco, CA: Berrett-Koehler.

Ludwig, J., Sanbonmatsu, L., Gennetian, L., Adam, E., Duncan, G. J., Katz, L. F., et al. (2011). Neighborhoods, obesity, and diabetes—a randomized social experiment. *New England Journal of Medicine, 365*(16), 1509–1519.

Madhivanan, P., Pierre-Victor, D., Mukherjee, S., Bhoite, P., Powell, B., Jean-Baptiste, N., et al. (2016). Human papillomavirus vaccination and sexual disinhibition in females: A systematic review. *American Journal of Preventive Medicine, 51*(3), 373–383.

Marion, S., Aviki, E., & Chino, F. (2022). Financial toxicity of surgical treatment for gynecological cancer: A growing malignancy. *Gynecologic Oncology, 166*(2), 197–199.

Markowitz, L. E., Hariri, S., Lin, C., Dunne, E. F., Steinau, M., McQuillan, G., et al. (2013). Reduction in human papillomavirus (HPV) prevalence among young women following HPV vaccine introduction in the United States, national health and nutrition examination surveys, 2003–2010. *Journal of Infectious Diseases, 208*(3), 385–393.

Matsudo, V., Matsudo, S., Andrade, D., Araujo, T., Andrade, E., de Oliveira, L. C., et al. (2002). Promotion of physical activity in a developing country: The Agita São Paulo experience. *Public Health Nutrition, 5*(1a), 253–261.

May, C. R., Johnson, M., & Finch, T. (2016). Implementation, context and complexity. *Implementation Science, 11*(1), 141.

McGlone, M. S., Stephens, K. K., Rodriguez, S. A., & Fernandez, M. E. (2017). Persuasive texts for prompting action: Agency assignment in HPV vaccination reminders. *Vaccine, 35*(34), 4295–4297.

McKnight, J. L., & Kretzmann, J. P. (1996). *Mapping community capacity.* Evanston, IL.

McRee, A.-L., Gilkey, M. B., & Dempsey, A. F. (2014). HPV vaccine hesitancy: Findings from a statewide survey of health care providers. *Journal of Pediatric Health Care, 28*(6), 541–549.

Michie, S. (2014). Implementation science: Understanding behaviour change and maintenance. *BMC Health Services Research, 14*(Suppl 2), O9.

Minkler, M. (2005). Community-based research partnerships: Challenges and opportunities. *Journal of Urban Health, 82*(2), ii3–ii12.

Moon, R. (1999). Finding diamonds in the trenches with the nominal group process. *Family Practice Management, 6*(5), 49–50.

Morales-Campos, D. Y., Snipes, S., Villarreal, E. K., Crocker, L., Guerrero, A., & Fernandez, M. (2021). Cervical cancer, human papillomavirus (HPV), and HPV vaccination: Exploring gendered perspectives, knowledge, attitudes, and cultural taboos among Mexican American adults. *Ethnicity & Health, 26*(2), 206–224.

Morrissey, B., Taveras, E., Allender, S., & Strugnell, C. (2020). Sleep and obesity among children: A systematic review of multiple sleep dimensions. *Pediatric Obesity, 15*(4), e12619.

NACCHO. (n.d.). Mobilizing action through planning and partnerships (MAPP). https://www.naccho.org/programs/public-health-infrastructure/performance-improvement/community-health-assessment/mapp. Accessed July 3, 2020.

National Cancer Institute (2021). *Seer cancer statistics review, 1975-2018—table 1.25 and SEER*explorer.* Bethesda, MD: National Cancer Institute. [based on November 2020 SEER data submission, posted to the SEER website, April 1]. Available from: https://seer.cancer.gov/csr/1975_2018/

National Cancer Institute. (n.d.). All cancer sites combined, recent trends in SEER age-adjusted incidence rates, 2000-2019: National cancer institute—surveillance, epidemiology, and end results program. https://seer.cancer.gov/explorer/. Accessed January 15, 2024.

Newman, S. D., Andrews, J. O., Magwood, G. S., Jenkins, C., Cox, M. J., & Williamson, D. C. (2011). Community advisory boards in community-based participatory research: A synthesis of best processes. *Preventing Chronic Disease, 8*(3), A70–A.

Newman, P. A., Logie, C. H., Lacombe-Duncan, A., Baiden, P., Tepjan, S., Rubincam, C., et al. (2018). Parents' uptake of human papillomavirus vaccines for their children: A systematic review and meta-analysis of observational studies. *BMJ Open, 8*(4), e019206.

Oldfield, B. J., Harrison, M. A., Genao, I., Greene, A. T., Pappas, M. E., Glover, J. G., et al. (2019). Patient, family, and community advisory councils in health care and research: A systematic review. *Journal of General Internal Medicine, 34*(7), 1292–1303.

Orlandi, M., Landers, C., Weston, R., & Haley, N. (1990). Diffusion of health pro motion innovations. In K. Glanz, F. M. Lewis, & B. K. Rimer (Eds.), *Health behavior and education: Theory, research, and practice* (1st ed., pp. 288–313). San Francisco, CA: Jossey-Bass.

Osazuwa-Peters, N., López, J., Rice, S., Tutlam, N., Tokarz, S., & Varvares, M. A. (2015). No change in physician discussions with patients about the human papillomavirus vaccine between 2007 and 2013. *Journal of Cancer Policy, 5*, 18–22.

Park, S. Y., Bae, D. S., Nam, J. H., Park, C. T., Cho, C. H., Lee, J. M., et al. (2007). Quality of life and sexual problems in disease-free survivors of cervical cancer compared with the general population. *Cancer: Interdisciplinary International Journal of the American Cancer Society, 110*(12), 2716–2725.

Parobii, I., Springer, A., Harrell, M., Martinez, G. L., Traversa, F., Alers, N., et al. (2018). Exploring physical activity engagement in secondary school students in Montevideo, Uruguay: A qualitative study. *International Journal of Child and Adolescent Health, 11*(1), 47–56.

Pennel, C. L., Burdine, J. N., Prochaska, J. D., & McLeroy, K. R. (2017). Common and critical components among community health assessment and community health improvement planning models. *Journal of Public Health Management and Practice, 23*, S14–S21.

Peterson, E., Harrell, M., Springer, A., Medina, J., Martinez, L., Perry, C., et al. (2019). Uruguayan secondary school students speak up about tobacco: Results from focus group discussions in and around Montevideo. *Global Health Promotion, 26*(2), 15–24.

Pingali, C., Yankey, D., Elam-Evans, L. D., Markowitz, L. E., Williams, C. L., Fredua, B., et al. (2021). National, regional, state, and selected local area vaccination coverage among adolescents aged 13–17 years—United States, 2020. *Morbidity and Mortality Weekly Report, 70*(35), 1183.

President's Cancer Panel (2018). *HPV vaccination for cancer prevention: Progress, opportunities, and a renewed call to action.* Bethesda, MD: National Cancer Institute.

Preskill, H., & Jones, N. (2009). *A practical guide for engaging stakeholders in developing evaluation questions.* Princeton, NJ: Robert Wood Johnson Foundation.

Preskill, H., Gutierrez, E., & Mack, K. (2017). Facilitating intentional group learning: A practical guide to 21 learning activities. http://www.fsg.org/tools-and-resources/facilitatingintentional-group-learning. Accessed July 3, 2020.

Proper, K., & van Oostrom, S. (2019). The effectiveness of workplace health promotion interventions on physical and mental health outcomes—a systematic review of reviews. *Scandinavian Journal of Work, Environment & Health, 45*(6), 546–559.

(Public Health Accreditation Board). (2013). PHAB standards: An overview. https://www.phaboard.org/wp-content/uploads/2018/11/Overview.pdf. Accessed July 3, 2020.

Quinn, G. P., Murphy, D., Malo, T. L., Christie, J., & Vadaparampil, S. T. (2012). A national survey about human papillomavirus vaccination: What we didn't ask, but physicians wanted us to know. *Journal of Pediatric and Adolescent Gynecology, 25*(4), 254–258.

Reiter, P. L., Brewer, N. T., Gottlieb, S. L., McRee, A.-L., & Smith, J. S. (2009). Parents' health beliefs and HPV vaccination of their adolescent daughters. *Social Science & Medicine, 69*(3), 475–480.

Robertson-James, C., Sawyer, L., Mertus, S., Robertson, D., Congleton, S., Watkins, S., et al. (2018). The role of health policies in faith-based institutions in promoting health and changing food practices: The philadelphia ujima experience. *Project MUSE, 12*(4), 419–429.

Rodriguez, S. A., Roncancio, A. M., Savas, L. S., Lopez, D. M., Vernon, S. W., & Fernandez, M. E. (2018a). Using intervention mapping to develop and adapt two educational interventions for parents to increase HPV vaccination among Hispanic adolescents. *Frontiers in Public Health, 6*, 164.

Rodriguez, S. A., Savas, L. S., Baumler, E., Nyitray, A. G., Mullen, P. D., Vernon, S. W., et al. (2018b). Parental predictors of HPV vaccine initiation among low-income Hispanic females aged 11–17 years. *Vaccine, 36*(33), 5084–5090.

Rodriguez, S. A., Savas, L. S., Loomba, P., Vernon, S. W., & Fernandez, M. E. (2019). Low-income Hispanic parent recall of daughters' HPV vaccination status: Correlates of accurate reporting of daughters' HPV-vaccine naïve status compared with electronic health records. *Vaccine, 37*(23), 2998–3001.

Rodriguez, S. A., Mullen, P. D., Lopez, D. M., Savas, L. S., & Fernandez, M. E. (2020). Factors associated with adolescent HPV vaccination in the US: A systematic review of reviews and multilevel framework to inform intervention development. *Preventive Medicine, 131*, 105968.

Roemer, E. C., Kent, K. B., Mummert, A., McCleary, K., Palmer, J. B., Lang, J. E., et al. (2019). Validity and reliability of the updated CDC worksite health scoreCard. *Journal of Occupational and Environmental Medicine, 61*(9), 767–777.

Rudolph, L., Caplan, J., Mitchell, C., Ben-Moshe, K., & Dillon, L. (2013). Health in all policies: Improving health through intersectoral collaboration. https://nam.edu/wp-content/uploads/2015/06/BPH-HiAP.pdf. Accessed July 3, 2020.

Runyan, J., Steenbergh, T., Bainbridge, C., Daugherty, D., Oke, L., & Fry, B. (2013). A smartphone ecological momentary assessment/intervention "app" for collecting real-time data and promoting self-awareness. *PLoS One, 8*(8), e71325.

Rutter, M. (1987). *Psychosocial resilience and protective mechanisms.* London, UK: American Orthopsychiatric Association.

Ryan, C., Duvall, K. L., Weyant, E. C., Johnson, K. R., & Wood, D. (2018). Human papillomavirus vaccine uptake, knowledge, and acceptance for youth: A systematic review of Appalachia. *Journal of Community Health, 43*(3), 616–624.

Salkas, S., Conniff, J., & Budge, S. L. (2018). Provider quality and barriers to care for transgender people: An analysis of data from the Wisconsin transgender community health assessment. *International Journal of Transgenderism, 19*(1), 59–63.

Sallis, J., & Owen, N. (2015). Ecological models of health behavior. In K. Glanz, B. K. Rimer, & K. Viswanath (Eds.), *Health behavior: Theory, research, and practice* (pp. 43–64). 11: Jossey-Bass.

Sallis, J. F., Cervero, R. B., Ascher, W., Henderson, K. A., Kraft, M. K., & Kerr, J. (2006). An ecological approach to creating active living communities. *Annual Review of Public Health, 27*, 297–322.

Saluja, K., Rawal, T., Bassi, S., Bhaumik, S., Singh, A., Park, M. H., et al. (2018). School environment assessment tools to address behavioural risk factors of non-communicable diseases: A scoping review. *Preventive Medicine Reports, 10*, 1–8.

Santa Maria, D., Swartz, M. C., Markham, C., Chandra, J., McCurdy, S., & Basen-Engquist, K. (2014). Exploring parental factors related to weight management in survivors of childhood central nervous system tumors. *Journal of Pediatric Oncology Nursing, 31*(2), 84–94.

Saunders, R. P., Evans, A. E., Kenison, K., Workman, L., Dowda, M., & Chu, Y. H. (2013). Conceptualizing, implementing, and monitoring a structural health promotion intervention in an organizational setting. *Health Promotion Practice, 14*(3), 343–353.

Savas, L. S., Farias, A. J., Healy, C. M., Shegog, R., Fernandez, M. E., Frost, E. L., et al. (2021). Wording matters when pediatricians recommend HPV vaccination. *Journal of Applied Research on Children: Informing Policy for Children at Risk, 12*(2), 5.

Save the Children US, USAID, US Agency for International Development. (2020). Planning pause & reflect sessions. https://resourcecentre.savethechildren.net/document/planning-pause-reflect-sessions-practical-guidance-for-your-project. Accessed: July 3, 2020.

Scales, P., & Leffert, N. (1999). *Developmental assets: A synthesis of the scientific research on adolescent development.* Search Institute.

Scerri, A., Innes, A., & Scerri, C. (2019). Using appreciative inquiry to implement person-centred dementia care in hospital wards. *Dementia, 18*(1), 190–209.

Scrimshaw, S., & Hurtado, E. (1992). *Rapid assessment procedures: Qualitative methodology for planning and evaluation of health related programmes.* Boston, MA: International Nutrition Foundation for Developing Countries.

Selove, R., Foster, M., Mack, R., Sanderson, M., & Hull, P. C. (2017). Using an implementation research framework to identify potential facilitators and barriers of an intervention to increase HPV vaccine uptake. *Journal of Public Health Management and Practice: JPHMP, 23*(3), e1.

Shankaran, V., Leahy, T., Steelquist, J., Watabayashi, K., Linden, H., Ramsey, S., et al. (2018). Pilot feasibility study of an oncology financial navigation program. *Journal of Oncology Practice, 14*(2), e122–e129.

Shay, L. A., Baldwin, A. S., Betts, A. C., Marks, E. G., Higashi, R. T., Street, R. L., et al. (2018). Parent-provider communication of HPV vaccine hesitancy. *Pediatrics, 141*(6).

Shefer, A., Briss, P., Rodewald, L., Bernier, R., Strikas, R., Yusuf, H., et al. (1999). Improving immunization coverage rates: An evidence-based review of the literature. *Epidemiologic Reviews, 21*(1), 96–142.

Shoemaker, M. L., & White, M. C. (2016). Breast and cervical cancer screening among Hispanic subgroups in the USA: Estimates from the National Health Interview Survey 2008, 2010, and 2013. *Cancer Causes & Control, 27*(3), 453–457.

Shorten, A., & Smith, J. (2017). Mixed methods research: Expanding the evidence base. *Evidence-Based Nursing, 20*(3), 74–75.

Silver, S., Harel, Z., McQuillan, R., Weizman, A., Thomas, A., Chertow, G., et al. (2016). How to begin a quality improvement project. *Clinical Journal of the American Society of Nephrology, 11*(5), 893–900.

Simons-Morton, B., Greene, W., & Gottlieb, N. (1995). *Introduction to health education and health promotion*. Prospect Heights, IL: Waveland Press.

Skarlatidou, A., Suskevics, M., Gobel, C., Pruse, B., Tauginiene, L., Mascarenhas, A., et al. (2019). *The value of stakeholder mapping to enhance co-creation in citizen science initiatives*. Citizen Science: Theory and Practice.

Smith, B. J., Tang, K. C., & Nutbeam, D. (2006). WHO health promotion glossary: New terms. *Health Promotion International, 21*(4), 340–345.

Springer, A. E., & Evans, A. E. (2016). Assessing environmental assets for health promotion program planning: A practical framework for health promotion practitioners. *Health Promotion Perspective, 6*(3), 111–118.

Springer, A. E., Kelder, S. H., Barroso, C. S., Drenner, K. L., Shegog, R., Ranjit, N., et al. (2010). Parental influences on television watching among children living on the Texas–Mexico border. *Preventive Medicine, 51*(2), 112–117.

Springer, A. E., Kelder, S. H., Byrd-Williams, C. E., Pasch, K. E., Ranjit, N., Delk, J. E., et al. (2013). Promoting energy-balance behaviors among ethnically diverse adolescents: Overview and baseline findings of the central Texas CATCH middle school project. *Health Education & Behavior, 40*(5), 559–570.

Springer, A. E., Li, L., Ranjit, N., Delk, J., Mehta, K., & Kelder, S. H. (2015). School-level economic disadvantage and obesity in middle school children in central Texas, USA: A cross-sectional study. *International Journal of Behavioral Nutrition and Physical Activity, 12*(1), S8.

Springer, A., Evans, A., Ortuno, J., Salvo, D., & Arevalo, M. (2017). Health by design: Interweaving health promotion into environments and settings. *Frontiers in Public Health, 5*, 1–10.

Springer, A. E., Davis, C., Van Dusen, D., Grayless, M., Case, K. R., Craft, M., et al. (2018). School socioeconomic disparities in e-cigarette susceptibility and use among central Texas middle school students. *Preventive Medicine Reports, 11*, 105–108.

Springer, A. E., Harrell, M. B., Martínez Gomensoro, L., Traversa Fresco, M., Rogers, S., Florines, M., et al. (2020). ¡Activate Ya! Co-learning about school-based tobacco prevention and physical activity promotion in secondary school students in Uruguay. *Global Health Promotion, 27*(2), 63–73.

Springer, A. E., Marshall, A. N., Randolph, R., Wilkinson, A. V., Rosenbluth, B., Cortez, A., et al. (2022). Exploring models for youth engagement in community health planning: The youth-led community health learning initiative. *Project MUSE, 16*(2), 155–168.

Stokley, S., Jeyarajah, J., Yankey, D., Cano, M., Gee, J., Roark, J., et al. (2014). Human papillomavirus vaccination coverage among adolescents, 2007–2013, and postlicensure vaccine safety monitoring, 2006–2014—United States. *Morbidity and Mortality Weekly Report, 63*(29), 620.

Tam, G., Huang, Z., & Chan, E. Y. Y. (2018). Household preparedness and preferred communication channels in public health emergencies: A cross-sectional survey of residents in an Asian developed urban city. *International Journal of Environmental Research & Public Health, 15*(8), 1598.

Tenny, S., Hoffman, M. (2020). Odds ratio. StatPearls. https://www.ncbi.nlm.nih.gov/books/NBK431098/. Accessed February 18, 2021.

Texas Cancer Registry (2020). *HPV-associated cancers in Texas, 2013-2017*. Austin, TX: Texas Department of State Health Services. [Available from: https://www.dshs.texas.gov/sites/default/files/tcr/data/modifiable/HPV-Associated-Cancers-in-Texas.pdf].

Thompson, J. R., & Burke, J. G. (2020). Increasing community participation in public health research: Applications for concept mapping methodology. *Project MUSE, 14*(2), 243–250.

Thrul, J., Belohlavek, A., Hambrick, D. A., Kaur, M., & Ramo, D. E. (2017). Conducting online focus groups on Facebook to inform health behavior change interventions: Two case studies and lessons learned. *Internet Interventions, 9*, 106–111.

Toseland, R., & Rivas, R. (2008). *An introduction to group work practice* (6th ed.). Boston, MA: Allyn & Bacon.

Tucker, J. A., Cheong, J., & Chandler, S. D. (2016). Selecting communication channels for substance misuse prevention with at-risk African-American emerging adults living in the southern United States. *Journal of Child & Adolescent Substance Abuse, 25*(6), 539–545.

Tuckman, B. W. (1965). Developmental sequence in small groups. *Psychological Bulletin, 63*(6), 384–399.

Turner, B., Valerio, M., Rochat, A., Winkler, P., Rodriguez, N., Avant, K., et al. (2019). *Underserved populations: Advancing health, engaging, and developing (UP AHEAD) research handbook*. Society for Public Health Education.

Valentino, K., & Poronsky, C. B. (2016). Human papillomavirus infection and vaccination. *Journal of Pediatric Nursing, 31*(2), e155–e166.

Vamos, C. A., Vázquez-Otero, C., Kline, N., Lockhart, E. A., Wells, K. J., Proctor, S., et al. (2021). Multi-level determinants to HPV vaccination among Hispanic farmworker families in Florida. *Ethnicity & Health, 26*(3), 319–336.

Vanderpool, R. C., Casey, B. R., & Crosby, R. A. (2011). HPV-related risk perceptions and HPV vaccine uptake among a sample of young rural women. *Journal of Community Health, 36*(6), 903–909.

Vatcharavongvan, P., Hepworth, J., & Marley, J. (2013). The application of the parallel track model in community health promotion: A literature review. *Health & Social Care in the Community, 21*(4), 352–363.

van de Ven, D., Robroek, S. J. W., & Burdorf, A. (2020). Are workplace health promotion programmes effective for all socioeconomic groups? A systematic review. *Occupational and Environmental Medicine, 77*(9), 589–596.

Viens, L. J., Henley, S. J., Watson, M., Markowitz, L. E., Thomas, C. C., Thompson, T., et al. (2016). Human papillomavirus-associated cancers—United States, 2008–2012. *Morbidity and Mortality Weekly Report, 65*(26), 661–666.

Vollrath, K., Thul, S., & Holcombe, J. (2018). Meaningful methods for increasing human papillomavirus vaccination rates: An integrative literature review. *Journal of Pediatric Health Care, 32*(2), 119–132.

Wallerstein, N., Duran, B., Oetzel, J., & Minkler, M. (2018). *Community-based participatory research for health: Advancing social and health equity* (3rd ed.). San Francisco, CA: Jossey-Bass.

Wang, J.-W., Cao, S.-S., & Hu, R.-Y. (2018). Smoking by family members and friends and electronic-cigarette use in adolescence: A systematic review and meta-analysis. *Tobacco Induced Diseases, 16*(February), 1–11.

Warner, E. L., Lai, D., Carbajal-Salisbury, S., Garza, L., Bodson, J., Mooney, K., et al. (2015). Latino parents' perceptions of the HPV vaccine for sons and daughters. *Journal of Community Health, 40*(3), 387–394.

Wenzel, L., DeAlba, I., Habbal, R., Kluhsman, B. C., Fairclough, D., Krebs, L. U., et al. (2005). Quality of life in long-term cervical cancer survivors. *Gynecologic Oncology, 97*(2), 310–317.

Wishik, S. M., & Vynckt, S. (1976). The use of nutritional 'positive deviants' to identify approaches for modification of dietary practices. *American Journal of Public Health, 66*(1), 38–42.

Wong Croal, N., Smedley, B., Andrulis, D., Woolf, S., Siddiqui, N., Wilson, K., et al. (2018). *Advancing health opportunity and equity across the United States: A state-by-state comparison*. National Collaborative for Health Equity Texas Health Institute Virginia Commonwealth University Center on Society and Health.

Younan, D., Tuvblad, C., Li, L., Wu, J., Lurmann, F., Franklin, M., et al. (2016). Environmental determinants of aggression in adolescents: Role of urban neighborhood greenspace. *Journal of the American Academy of Child and Adolescent Psychiatry, 55*(7), 591–601.

Zimet, G. D., Rosberger, Z., Fisher, W. A., Perez, S., & Stupiansky, N. W. (2013). Beliefs, behaviors and HPV vaccine: Correcting the myths and the misinformation. *Preventive Medicine, 57*(5), 414–418.

CHAPTER 6

INTERVENTION MAPPING STEP 2

Intervention Outcomes and Objectives

INTERVENTION MAPPING STEP 2 TASKS

1. State desired behavioral and environmental outcomes
2. Specify performance objectives for behavioral and environmental outcomes
3. Select determinants for behavioral and environmental outcomes
4. Construct matrices of change objectives

Overview

In Step 1, the needs assessment helps planners develop a *risk model* or *logic model of the problem*, that defines the causes of a health problem and related quality-of-life (QOL) issues for a specific population. The assets assessment identifies potential settings, environments, and resources that may be leveraged within a health promotion intervention. In Step 2, building from these needs and assets assessments (NAAs), the planner shifts focus to a *health-promoting model* or *logic model of change*.

In Step 2, the planner first specifies the desired outcomes in terms of individual health-promoting behaviors and environmental conditions that are needed to enhance health and QOL. Once the desired change is specified, the planners write *performance objectives* for each behavioral and environmental outcome; these performance objectives describe exactly what the priority populations (i.e., at-risk population members and environmental agents at different levels) need to do to accomplish improvements in behavioral and environmental outcomes. The planners then develop *matrices of change objectives*—these are created by intersecting performance objectives and personal determinants (the factors such as behavioral capability, attitudes, beliefs, and self efficacy that influence behavior). These matrices contain specific objectives that describe the desired change in the determinant needed to accomplish the performance objective. These change objectives represent the immediate targets for a health promotion intervention at the individual level as well as at different environmental levels to promote, protect, and improve health.

This chapter guides the reader in using the Core Processes (see Chapter 2), along with information from the NAA, to create sound theory- and evidence-informed matrices. These matrices provide detailed "blueprints" to guide the development of a multilevel intervention in subsequent IM steps (explained further in Chapters 7 and 8).

Partnering with the Community

Partnering with community members and other interested parties—including policy makers, potential implementers, and potential intervention beneficiaries—throughout the planning process is critical for developing health promotion interventions that are feasible, engaging, and sustainable in "real world" settings (Harden et al., 2018). In Step 2, combining community insight with Step 1 NAA findings allows planners to identify important and changeable behavioral and environmental outcomes.

Community engagement is critical for identifying relevant settings (e.g., homes, schools, clinics, or worksites) within environmental levels that provide widespread access to the at-risk population; engagement of these settings will lead to an increased likelihood that an intervention will be implemented with fidelity. For example, in developing a large-scale, community-based intervention to decrease COVID-19 testing disparities in southeast Texas, the multidisciplinary planning group included behavioral scientists, epidemiologists, biostatisticians, public health department officials, community-based healthcare and social service providers, and an extensive community advisory group. This helped ensure that the perspectives of community members and other interested parties were appropriately incorporated into the planning and implementation process.

Interweaving Health Promotion Within and Across Ecological Levels and Settings

Interweaving, defined as weaving or blending together, is a common practice for health promotion planners when designing health promotion interventions in relation to people's ecological context (Springer et al., 2017). Step 2 continues this use of an ecological framework to plan health promotion interventions. Most health issues are caused by a web of factors that occur across multiple "ecological" or environmental levels (interpersonal, organizational, community, or societal). Some environmental conditions influence behaviors, either directly or indirectly. For example, marketing and state-level retail licensing policies effect e-cigarette use among adolescents, impacting health *indirectly* (Azagba et al., 2020; Giovenco et al., 2016). Other conditions, such as air quality, impact health *directly* by exacerbating asthma or other respiratory conditions (Beelen et al., 2014; Shah et al., 2013; Song et al., 2019).

Complex multi-causal health problems, such as smoking or poor asthma management, require complex interventions, with interacting intervention components that address multiple behaviors among the at-risk population or among environmental agents at different levels (Craig et al., 2008; Mkhitaryan et al., 2020; Petticrew, 2011). These are often *multilevel* interventions, designed to address both individual-level factors (such as attitudes toward smoking cessation or asthma self-management) as well as the physical or social environment (such as the healthcare systems that individuals access) (Paskett et al., 2016). For the greatest impact, complex or multilevel interventions should occur across ecological levels simultaneously or in close succession. Strategically intervening across ecological levels has the potential to produce stronger, synergistic effects than working at only one level (Mathieu & Taylor, 2007; Paskett et al., 2016; Sallis et al., 2006; Stange et al., 2012). These "levels" of intervention are represented in Step 2's *matrices of change objectives*. They delineate what needs to change across ecological levels (individual, interpersonal, organizational, community, and/or societal) to improve health.

Findings from the Step 1 assets assessment help planners identify existing settings within an ecological level (e.g., schools, worksites, or hospitals, are all at the organizational level) and specific assets within those settings (e.g., policy, information, social/cultural/organizational, and physical assets) that may be leveraged within a health promotion intervention. For example, existing assets that might be leveraged for a school-based intervention include a parent/teacher organization within the school's social/organizational environment, and morning announcements for students within the school's information environment (Springer et al., 2017). Interweaving health promotion within and across multiple ecological levels and settings is critical for achieving health and health behavior change (Paskett et al., 2016; Sallis et al., 2006; Springer et al., 2017).

The Logic Model of Change

Starting in Step 2, the planners begin to develop a *logic model of change* to illustrate *how* the health promotion intervention is intended to produce change to promote, protect, and improve health. This is in contrast to the logic model of the *problem* that was completed in Step 1, which is designed to more fully understand the problem and its contributing factors as part of the NAA. This logic model of change is expanded in Steps 3, 4, and 5, respectively, with the addition of theoretical change methods, intervention components, and implementation strategies, to fully illustrate pathways of intervention effect and specify areas for evaluation (Step 6). The logic model of change (see Figure 6.1) is developed from right to left, starting with the intervention goals for health and QOL to be achieved by the health promotion intervention. Moving to the left, planners then state the behavioral and environmental changes necessary to achieve health and QOL outcomes.

Moving further to the left in the logic model, the planners specify the performance objectives needed to achieve the behavioral and environmental outcomes. *Performance objectives* are statements of what a program

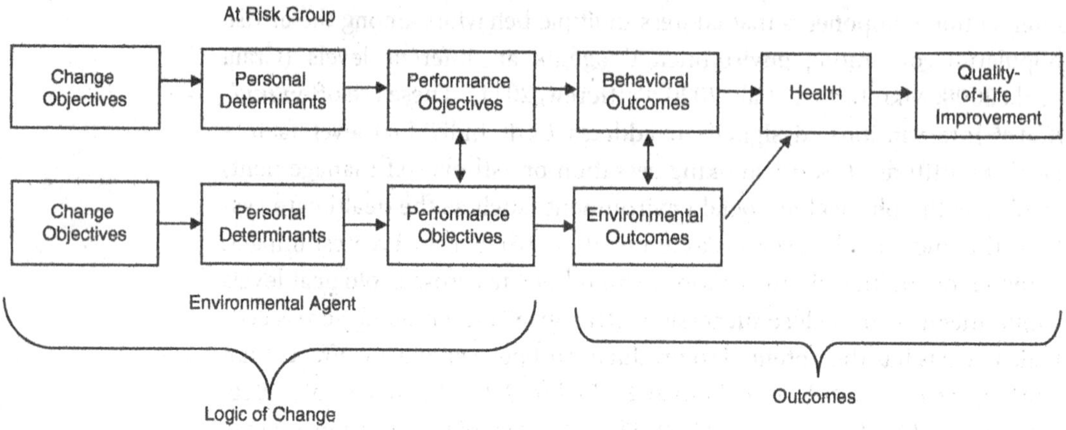

Figure 6.1 Logic Model of Change

participant will do, or how an individual will modify the environment. Planners then identify the personal determinants (for example, attitudes, or self-efficacy), that influence the behavior of an individual or environmental agent's behavior and cross these with the performance objectives to create "change objectives."

Change objectives provide the "blueprint" for a health promotion intervention as they specify exactly what needs to change in the determinants of the specified behavioral or environmental outcomes to bring about improvements in health and QOL. The planning group will build upon these matrices in Steps 3 and 4 to bring their multilevel intervention to life.

Step 2 Tasks

The four primary tasks for conducting Step 2 are presented in Box 6.1 and described below.

BOX 6.1. INTERVENTION MAPPING STEP 2 TASKS

1. State desired behavioral and environmental outcomes
2. Specify performance objectives for behavioral and environmental outcomes
3. Select determinants for behavioral and environmental outcomes
4. Construct matrices of change objectives

Task 1: State Desired Behaviors and Environmental Outcomes

The first task in Step 2 of Intervention Mapping (IM) is to state desired program outcomes for health behaviors and environmental conditions to improve health and QOL.

The needs assessment (see Chapter 5) aims to build an explanatory *risk model*, or *logic model of the problem*, that clearly defines the behaviors and environmental conditions associated with a health issue. The logic model of change is, in a sense, the opposite of the logic model of the problem. Rather than listing the problematic (or negative) behavior(s), environments, and determinants of a health problem; instead, it describes the desired changes (or *positive* outcomes) in determinants, behaviors, environmental conditions, health, and QOL outcomes we expect to see as a result of the intervention. To create a *logic model of change*, the planners often "do the flip" by looking at the various elements in the risk model and restating them in a positive way—essentially describing the expected change or goal following a successful health promotion intervention. Thus, starting in Step 2, the planning shifts to focus on *health-promoting* behaviors and environmental conditions. For example, a behavioral cause of lung cancer is smoking but the behavioral outcome for an intervention could be either not starting to smoke or smoking cessation (DHHS, 2012). Likewise, in the logic model of the problem or risk model you might list a negative environmental condition that could stimulate or support smoking, and (in the logic model of change) you would list environmental changes expected as a result of an intervention such as increased price of cigarettes, smoke-free policies, or implementation of a comprehensive state tobacco control program (U.S. Department of Health and Human Services, Centers for Disease Control and Prevention, Office on Smoking and Health, General OotS, 2014; Stevens et al., 2017). Well-defined behavioral and environmental outcomes will lead to better-specified performance objectives in the next task.

Identifying Health-Related Behaviors of the At-Risk Group

One of the difficulties in planning health promotion interventions is confusion over what is meant by the term *behavior*. Health has been defined as a state of complete physical, mental, and social well-being and not merely the absence of disease or infirmity (WHO, 1948). Health promotion interventions seek to impact behaviors that enhance well-being or prevent disease across three broad categories:

- Primary Prevention: Behaviors to promote well-being or prevent a disease from ever occurring; for example, healthy nutrition, physical activity (PA), and vaccinations.
- Secondary Prevention: Screening to identify disease in the earliest stages before the onset of signs and symptoms; the priority population is healthy-appearing individuals with subclinical forms of a disease; for example, mammography, a Papanicolaou (Pap) smear or human papillomavirus (HPV) testing, and regular blood pressure measurement.
- Tertiary Prevention: Managing disease post-diagnosis to slow or stop disease progression; the priority population is symptomatic individuals

or those living with a chronic condition; for example, self-management and treatment adherence behaviors, and rehabilitation (Kisling & Das, 2022).

Below, we describe these three categories and provide examples to provide context for our discussion about stating desired behavioral outcomes.

Primary Prevention Behaviors Primary prevention behaviors include health-promoting and disease-prevention behaviors aimed at enhancing or protecting health and well-being. Examples of health-promoting behaviors include exercising, getting sufficient sleep, and using sunscreen. Other primary prevention behaviors, such as handwashing and wearing a seat belt, protect against a potential risk (Alzyood et al., 2020; Febres et al., 2020; Shakya et al., 2020).

Primary prevention may also focus on reducing risk behaviors, such as altering poor eating habits. For example, heart disease is associated with raised blood pressure (a physiological risk factor), which is strongly influenced by diet (a behavioral risk factor). Moderate reductions in salt intake have been shown to significantly reduce blood pressure, and lower salt consumption is associated with fewer cardiovascular events (Cappuccio et al., 2019). Similarly, the US 2020–2025 dietary guidelines recommend consuming less than 10% of calories from saturated fats to decrease disease risk (USDA, 2020). Primary prevention may also focus on harm reduction, such as wearing condoms during sexual intercourse to reduce the risk of acquiring a sexually transmitted infection (Workowski & Bolan, 2015) or encouraging Ecstasy users to test pills for dose and content to reduce the risk of overdose (Palamar & Barratt, 2019).

Secondary Prevention Behaviors Secondary prevention behaviors, such as screening and early detection, are especially important for diseases in which early signs or symptoms are not apparent. When symptoms are not present or not easily detected by laypeople, screening can identify individuals at high risk for the disease or detect the disease process early so that appropriate medical treatment can be started to prevent more severe illnesses or mortality (USPST, 2014). For example, colorectal cancer (CRC) screening can reduce both the incidence and mortality of CRC through early detection and removal of precancerous lesions (USPST, 2014; American Cancer Society, 2020). Tests for blood pressure and blood cholesterol levels screen for elevated risk for cardiovascular disease (Chobanian et al., 2003; Labarthe, 1998). Screening tests are also used to detect infectious diseases such as sexually transmitted infections (STIs) including HIV (DiNenno et al., 2017; USPST, 2014), genetic diseases such as Tay-Sachs disease (Natowicz & Prence, 1996), cystic fibrosis (Chandrasekharan et al., 2010), and inherited cancer susceptibility (Robson et al., 2015).

Screening and early detection range from self-administered tests to complicated medical procedures, but almost all require some behavior by the person at risk. Generally speaking, interventions are designed to motivate individuals to participate in self-administered screening or to seek out and attend screening procedures by health professionals in accordance with current screening guidelines (USPST, 2014; Serra et al., 2017; Smith et al., 2019). The exact nature of the behavior is specific to the screening method and the purpose of the screening. Some screening involves a one-time or infrequently repeated behavior (i.e., going to a healthcare facility and having blood taken to be examined by a laboratory or healthcare professional); others may require more frequent screening (e.g., blood sugar levels or blood pressure).

Tertiary Prevention Behaviors Tertiary prevention behaviors aim to reduce the effects of a disease once it is established in an individual. Improvement in treatment adherence and self-management behaviors are often the goals of patient education. Individuals who receive healthcare for a diagnosed condition need to be able to follow a healthcare professional's recommended prescription and treatment plans and patient education can help in this regard. Adherence is the extent to which the patient follows through with the recommended action (Bernard Vrijens et al., 2012; Evangelista & Shinnick, 2008); historically, adherence to medical recommendations is often incomplete. For example, people who are prescribed medications to be self-administered typically take only about half their prescribed doses (Nieuwlaat et al., 2014; Zullig et al., 2015). Improving adherence to medical regimens is therefore a critical goal for health promotion interventions, and a specific field of patient education.

Adherence is a subset of self-management. Patients and their families are often required to engage in daily tasks and decision-making that is more complex than simply adhering to a set of instructions. They must manage their condition (e.g., arthritis, asthma, and epilepsy) when they are at home or outside the healthcare facility, independently of the healthcare provider (McGee et al., 2020). Self-management encompasses an array of behaviors to manage symptoms, treatment regimens, disease consequences (physical and psychosocial), and lifestyle factors to reduce the impact of a chronic condition on daily life (Clark & Zimmerman, 2014; Clark et al., 2014; Dineen-Griffin et al., 2019; Harrington & Valerio, 2014; Heijmans et al., 2015; Rust et al., 2015). Self-management is associated with improvements in clinical indicators, health-related QOL, self-efficacy (confidence to self-manage), disease knowledge, and control (Dineen-Griffin et al., 2019).

Improvements in cancer screening, early detection, and treatment will result in an estimated 26 million cancer survivors in 2040. These individuals face a wide range of medical and psychosocial challenges that need to be planned for and appropriately managed, including the threat of cancer recurrence and secondary malignancies, and increased risk for comorbidities, such as obesity, type 2 diabetes, and cardiovascular disease (Shapiro, 2018). Cancer survivorship starts at the time of diagnosis and lasts throughout the lifespan (NCI, 2021). Health-promoting behaviors, for example, PA, may reduce the risk of cancer recurrence and comorbidities

(Campbell et al., 2019), and other behaviors, such as the practice of yoga among cancer patients, have been shown to improve physical and psychological symptoms, QOL, and markers of immunity (Agarwal & Maroko-Afek, 2018).

Stating Behavioral Outcomes

Behavioral outcomes should be stated in terms of the behavior(s) to be engaged in by the priority population as a result of the health promotion intervention. They should be closely related to the behavioral intervention goals that were stated at the end of Step 1. However, unlike the intervention goals, which will be used to evaluate the impact of the intervention (*what* will change, for *whom*, by *how much*, over what *time*), the behavioral outcomes concisely state the behavior an at-risk individual must accomplish to achieve the health and QOL goals. Ideally, behavioral outcomes are identified based on evidence from previous studies of *causal association* between the behavior and improved health outcomes, and evidence that they are *changeable*. If recommended guidelines exist for a specific behavior and population, such as nutrition, PA, or screening (USPST, 2014; USDA, 2020; DHHS, 2018), these guidelines should be used to help state the behavioral outcome to ensure that the dose, intensity, or timing of behavior change that is required to achieve health benefits is accomplished. For example, the US Department of Health and Human Services (DHHS) PA Guidelines for Americans include activity level recommendations for children and adolescents (DHHS, 2018). Based on these guidelines, a behavioral outcome to increase PA among youth could be stated as: "Children and adolescents aged 6–17 years engage in 60 minutes or more of moderate-to-vigorous intensity physical activity a day." The following statements are examples of health-related behavioral outcomes:

- Sexually active individuals in new relationships use condoms correctly and consistently when having sexual intercourse until being tested negative for STIs including HIV.
- Mothers exclusively breastfeed infants for the first six months.
- People living with HIV take antiretroviral medications as prescribed by a healthcare provider.
- Adults consume less than 10% of calories from added sugars.
- Women ages 40–74 years obtain a mammogram every other year (Force UPST, 2024).

Some interventions may address multiple behavioral outcomes to achieve the overall desired health outcome(s). For example, in Your Game, Your Life, a school-based intervention to reduce teen pregnancy, HIV, and STIs, the planners identified five important and changeable behavioral outcomes to promote adolescent sexual health: (1) choose not to have sex, (2) use condoms correctly and consistently if having sex, (3) use long-acting reversible contraception (LARC) or other effective contraceptive methods along with condoms if having sex, (4) go to a clinic for sexual and reproductive health services (HPV vaccination, LARC or other birth control method, HIV/STI testing), and (5) have healthy peer and dating relationships (Markham et al., 2017).

We usually include the behavior of individuals who influence the priority population or at-risk group as part of the environment at the interpersonal level (e.g., a doctor recommending a mammogram). However, for some health issues or behaviors, particularly those in which individuals who are at risk have little to no agency, an environmental agent, such as a parent, may be included within the "behavioral outcome". When the child is too young or does not have the ability to make a behavioral decision, for example, for adolescent HPV vaccination, the at-risk population is early adolescents; however, parental consent is required for adolescents to be vaccinated. Thus, the behavioral outcome may be, "Parents obtain the human papillomavirus (HPV) vaccine for their son or daughter" (Pot et al., 2018; Rodriguez et al., 2018).

Identifying and Stating Environmental Outcomes

In the needs assessment (Chapter 5), we referred to those aspects of the environment that were directly associated with a health problem, or indirectly associated with a health problem through a risk behavior, as *environmental conditions*. However, when stating how the environment needs to change as a result of an intervention, we refer to them as *environmental outcomes*—at the interpersonal, organizational, community, and/or societal ecological levels. Building upon Step 1 findings, the planning group with input from community members and other interested parties identifies specific settings within these ecological levels to maximize reach to the at-risk group (e.g., homes, schools, hospitals, worksites, or community centers) (Harden et al., 2018; Springer et al., 2017). They also identify evidence of *association* between environmental outcomes and improved behavioral or health outcomes, and evidence of *changeability*. Ideally, planners identify evidence of a causal association; however, especially with environmental outcomes, they often rely on observational or correlational data as evidence of association. Planners may also use theory to help identify important potential environmental influences on behavior and health (see Chapter 4).

Addressing multiple environmental outcomes across different ecological levels (e.g., parental communication about contraceptive use at the interpersonal level and provision of contraceptives at the school organizational level) allows planners to create interactions of influence on a specific health behavior or health outcome (Sallis & Owen, 2015).

Interpersonal Level The first place to consider environmental outcomes is in the behavior of individuals in the interpersonal environment of the at-risk group. Humans are embedded in social systems that change as people develop. Families are the primary influence on socialization of children and continue to have an effect on behavior throughout life. As children grow older, peer groups become more important, beginning with playmates and continuing with friends, neighbors, coworkers, and members of organizations with which they affiliate (such as churches, social clubs, and service groups). Certain individuals may hold special influence in accordance with the roles they play, such as teachers, coaches, religious leaders, or healthcare providers. In aggregate, these environmental agents may have a profound impact on the behavior of an individual.

Interpersonal environmental outcomes can also be considered as social constructs such as *social support.* Researchers have extensively studied social support as a protective factor for many health outcomes (Beets et al., 2010; Holt-Lunstad & Uchino, 2015; Kwan & Gordon, 2016; Milgrom et al., 2019; Sedivy et al., 2017). The types of functional support served by social relationships include ***emotional, informational, belonging,*** and ***tangible*** or ***instrumental*** support (Holt-Lunstad & Uchino, 2015). Similarly, social connectedness can influence behavioral and health outcomes. For example, Springer and colleagues found that higher perceived school cohesion was inversely related to peer victimization and bullying among Colombian high school students, even after controlling for individual-level student-school connectedness (Springer et al., 2015). The social environment may also provide modeling and reinforcement for the practice of specific health behaviors (Bandura, 1986, 2006). Thus, the presence or absence of support from important *others* within the individuals' immediate interpersonal environment may have an influence on individual health behavior as well as on health outcomes.

In an intervention developed to sustain exclusive breastfeeding for infants at risk of asthma, the planning group chose to intervene at the interpersonal level, focusing on the newborn's father as an environmental agent to provide breastfeeding support. Although they identified other external agents as important social influences (e.g., grandmothers and friends) they chose to address these through the behavioral outcomes for the mother herself, and through the partner supporting her when she was confronted by opinions against breastfeeding. They worded their environmental outcome as: "Partner supports mother to sustain exclusive breastfeeding for six months" (Mesters et al., 2018).

Me & You: Building Healthy Relationships, a school-based intervention for early adolescents, is an example of how intervention planning provided emotional and instrumental support for children's health behaviors by addressing parents at the interpersonal level (Peskin et al., 2018, 2019). The behavioral outcome for their at-risk population (early adolescents) was: "Students will have healthy peer and dating relationships (i.e., that are free of emotional, physical, and sexual violence)." At the interpersonal level, they developed an associated *environmental outcome* for parents/caregivers to support the children's behavior change, "Parents will communicate with their child about healthy peer and dating relationships."

Organizational Level Elements of organizational environments that influence health behaviors or the actions of environmental agents include norms, policies, practices, and facilities (Sallis & Glanz, 2009; Sallis et al., 2006; Stetler et al., 2008). Policies, for example, can exert strong control over behavior—worksite bans on smoking have been shown to reduce smoking prevalence among workers (Bauer et al., 2005; Helakorpi et al., 2008; Hopkins et al., 2010). Similarly, combinations of preventive healthcare policies and healthcare facility characteristics (such as service hours) can improve access to care for patients. A systematic review conducted in developed countries revealed that initiatives aimed at improving access to after-hours primary care had a notable impact on healthcare utilization. Specifically, enhanced access to after-hours primary care was associated with a significant increase in the utilization of primary care services (Hong et al., 2020).

The Me & You: Building Healthy Relationships planners developed an organizational-level *environmental outcome* for school staff (teachers, school nurses, counselors, social workers, and school leadership) to provide instrumental and emotional support to students and to create a safe school environment: "School staff will recognize dating violence among youth, respond appropriately, and refer students to resources."

Utilizing organizational change theories can aid in understanding the complex interactions within and between organizations and their individuals' contextual factors. In particular, organizational theories can explain how policies, institutions, funding, and workforce dynamics impact implementation. The Organizational Theory for Implementation Science framework developed by (Birken et al., 2023) identifies six domains and associated constructs from organizational change theories that are critical to consider in implementation practices. While developed to understand implementation, because it is focused on organizational functioning it is also useful for understanding environmental influences at the organizational level.

In a study by (Valaitis et al., 2018), organizational-level theory was applied to examine the impact of organizational climate and staff morale on service delivery within a program for homeless persons with serious mental illness. Organizational climate was assessed using measures of teamwork, supervisor support, and staff cohesion, and staff morale was evaluated through measures of job satisfaction and burnout. By examining these organizational factors, the study aimed to understand their influence on service delivery outcomes, such as client engagement and retention in treatment. Analyses identified associations between organizational climate, staff morale, and service delivery outcomes, highlighting the importance of organizational-level factors in shaping the quality of care provided to vulnerable populations.

Community Level The community environment contains conditions that affect the health of populations, either directly or indirectly, through behavior. Examples of these conditions include the availability of work and income, the quality and quantity of housing, access to healthcare, availability of healthy foods and recreational resources, smoking and other health ordinances, law enforcement, judicial practices, and treatment resources for social problems such as child abuse, violence, and drug addiction. Community-based interventions can increase social capital and community capacity to form and maintain problem-solving relationships and implement local policies (Bolton et al., 2017; Springer et al., 2012). Examples of supportive environments that communities have achieved through health promotion projects include increasing PA options and healthful food availability (Coffield et al., 2015; Rollins et al., 2021; Simoes et al., 2017; van den Berg et al., 2019), reducing exposure to second-hand smoke (Alagiyawanna et al., 2017), and reducing alcohol consumption and alcohol-related harm (Porthe et al., 2020). To address complex health issues, such as obesity, community partners may organize around multiple environmental outcomes. For example, The Go! Austin/Vamos! Austin coalition-led obesity initiative (van den Berg et al., 2019) organized community partners into four sectors, each with its own community-level (environmental) outcome:

- Community nutrition sector increases easy access (geographic and financial) to healthy food.
- PA sector increases easy access to safe PA facilities and programs.
- School sector provides children with an environment that promotes healthy eating and PA.
- Early childhood sector provides preschool-aged children with an environment that promotes healthy eating and PA.

Additional examples of health-related community-level outcomes are:

- Community members support laws targeting underage drinking.
- Off-premise alcohol outlets comply with underage drinking laws.
- Tobacco retailers comply with point-of-sale advertising restrictions for tobacco products.
- Corner stores in low-income communities provide healthy food options.

Societal Level The societal level focuses on legislation, enforcement, regulation, and resource allocation as well as policies, programs, and facilities of large political and geographic groups. "Big P – Little P" is one way to distinguish between large and small policy decisions. Big P refers to state, national, or international policy change, including legislative and executive actions. For example, the US Congress and the executive branch revises the Supplemental Nutrition Assistance Program (SNAP) income eligibility limits. Little P policies are typically made at the department or agency level and address organizational practices, priorities, or regulations. For example, a city health department may implement a policy to screen all pregnant women for substance use or prioritize medication-assisted treatment for pregnant women with opioid addiction (Collins, 2019).

Little P policy changes are typically less labor- and time-intensive than Big P policy changes; however, the impact of Big P policy making can be far-reaching, since it affects a larger population. Legislation that influences tobacco use includes minors' access laws, clean air acts, and tobacco excise taxes. These laws, along with lawsuits against tobacco companies by states and individuals, have been pivotal to the success of the tobacco control movement (DHHS, 2020). For example, since passing novel tobacco retailer licensing regulations in 2016, Philadelphia, Pennsylvania, has seen significant decreases in tobacco retailer density and the number of tobacco outlets near schools (Lawman et al., 2020). Other state and federal agencies—including those for health, human services, education, agriculture, transportation, and food and drugs—originate regulations, policies, and programs that affect health status. The following statements are examples of health-related societal-level outcomes:

- State legislators prohibit smoking in all enclosed public places in the state
- The federal government prohibits distribution and sale of flavored e-cigarette products including fruit and mint flavors

Task 2: Specifying Performance Objectives

The second task in IM Step 2 is to subdivide behaviors and environmental outcomes into performance objectives.

Once the program planners have defined the program's behavioral and environmental outcomes, they write *performance objectives* for each outcome. Performance objectives are observable sub-behaviors that an individual (or environmental agent) must perform to achieve an overall behavioral or environmental outcome. Performance objectives enable planners to evolve their description from simply a broadly stated behavioral or environmental outcome to a stated behavioral or environmental outcome accompanied by a detailed description of its components. For example, to achieve the behavioral outcome, "Use condoms correctly and consistently when having sex," a sexually active individual must first: obtain a condom; have the condom readily available; communicate with their partner about condom use ahead of time; use the condom correctly, and maintain condom use for each act of intercourse. Each of the items in this list could be considered a "performance objective." The use of performance objectives is not new, nor is it unique to health promotion. For example, in business management, quality assurance defines a standard of performance to maintain certain levels of service or production (Armstrong, 2015). In the area of training, participants must perform at a criterion level for a program to be successful. Although the term *performance objective* may not be applied exactly the same way in each of these examples, they are all used to further delineate behavioral and environmental program outcomes.

Specifying Performance Objectives for Behaviors

When planners state behavioral outcomes, they are written as broad conceptualizations: "Engage in moderate-to-vigorous intensity physical activity for 60 minutes a day." As planners continue toward intervention development, they use performance objectives to clarify the exact performance or sub-behaviors it would take to achieve the behavioral outcome. To determine the performance objectives, planners ask: "What do the participants in this intervention need to do to perform the behavioral outcome?" For example, reducing daily sodium intake is a health-promoting behavior, but many sub-behaviors or components make up that broader behavior. To perform the behavior, an individual would need to take many actions, including the following: read food labels; select low-sodium foods; limit or substitute salt for spices in recipes, and inquire about sodium content at restaurants. These sub-behaviors, specified by action words, become the *performance objectives.* They refine, focus, and make more specific what the intervention participants and environmental agents should do as a result of the intervention.

Changing health-related behaviors usually requires complex multistep processes. Specifying performance objectives helps program planners to sequence the behavioral learning process when the learner needs to learn one part before another, and to include all necessary supports for the behavior. For example, the following performance objectives were stated for *Puerto Ricans ages 50 and older to adhere to CRC screening guidelines* (behavioral outcome) (adapted from Serra et al., 2017):

PO.1. Make an appointment with the provider

PO.2. Arrange transportation

PO.3. Discuss CRC and CRC screening with the provider

PO.4. Request FIT/FOBT* or obtain referral for colonoscopy

PO.5. Complete FIT/FOBT*

PO.6. Make an appointment for colonoscopy

PO.7. Prepare for colonoscopy per directions

PO.8. Obtain colonoscopy

PO.9. Keep appointment to discuss results with the provider

*FIT, fecal immunochemical test; FOBT, fecal occult blood test

To help new mothers *sustain exclusive breastfeeding for six months for infants at risk of asthma* (behavioral outcome), the planning group identified the following performance objectives for the expectant mother (Mesters et al., 2018):

PO.1. Talk about 6 m-EBF* with care providers (e.g., midwives)

PO.2. Commit before delivery to 6 m-EBF after delivery

PO.3. Start and continue 6 m-EBF after delivery on demand

PO.4. Counteract social criticism toward 6 m-EBF

PO.5. Buy or hire and use a breast pump to express milk

PO.6. Transport, store, and prepare breast milk safely

PO.7. Remind individuals in the environment to not give solid food to infant

PO.8. Give solid food after 6 m-EBF

6 m-EBF, six-month exclusive breastfeeding

Specifying Performance Objectives for Environmental Outcomes

The process for writing performance objectives for environmental outcomes parallels the process for writing performance objectives for health behaviors. The basic question when stating performance objectives for environmental outcomes is: "What does someone (e.g., school district superintendent) or some decision-making body (e.g., a school board) in the environment need to do to accomplish the environmental outcome?" This general question addresses *who* is doing the action to accomplish the objective, because the agent may be different for each of the performance objectives. This is somewhat different from the question asked about performance objectives for the health-related (individual) behavior, because that question assumes a reference to the behavior of the at-risk population. Environmental change, in contrast, usually requires people *outside of* the at-risk population to take action to modify the environmental conditions.

The environmental agent is the individual who has control over, or can influence, a modification in the environmental factor. This agent might be, for example, a family member, healthcare provider, social service provider, clinical manager, policy maker, lawmaker, or resource controller. Different environmental agents may come into play at different environmental levels. At the beginning of the planning process, there may be limited information to identify who are the agents responsible for modifying a specific environmental condition. We suggest starting with whatever information may be available about potential agents, and stating the "who" in terms of general groups of people (e.g., city council members) or appropriate positions of responsibility (e.g., clinic directors)—that is, roles or agents that may be able to accomplish the performance objective. As work on the intervention progresses the planning group will have more information and context to help them determine which individual agent will perform the modification in the environment. This may be ascertained by direct observation, by records review, or through direct dialogue with key informants or planning group members who are familiar with the process at hand.

The Me & You: Building Healthy Relationships intervention provides a good example of various environmental agents at different environmental levels. The performance objectives listed in Table 6.1 were constructed to

Table 6.1 Examples of Environmental Performance Objectives for the Me & You: Building Healthy Relationships Study

Interpersonal Environment
Environmental outcome 1: Parents will communicate with their child about healthy peer and dating relationships.
Parents and caregivers will:
1.1. Create the appropriate times, locations, and activities to talk with their child about healthy peer and dating relationships.
1.2. Use effective communication strategies when talking with their child (e.g., active listening, being nonjudgmental).
1.3. Discuss having healthy peer and dating relationships (e.g., conflict resolution, problem-solving, effective communication).
1.4. Discuss strategies for managing their emotional responses appropriately (e.g., love, anger, anxiety, stress, depression, jealousy) in peer and dating relationships.
1.5. Discuss strategies for getting out of unhealthy peer and dating relationships.
1.6. Establish and discuss rules regarding how their child will spend time in friendship and dating activities (i.e., where, when, with whom) and use media (TV, internet, video games, music).
Organizational Environment
Environmental outcome 2: School staff (teachers, nurses, counselors, social workers, school leadership) will recognize DV among youth, respond appropriately, and refer to resources
School staff will:
2.1. Plan to respond appropriately to youth dating violence incidents
2.2. Use active listening when engaging with youth in discussions about their relationship experiences
2.3. Answer questions and concerns youth may have about relationships
2.4. Provide resources for youth
2.5. Maintain confidentiality standards with youth
2.6. Identify and adhere to reporting laws

Peskin et al. (2018) / with permission of Elsevier.

provide early adolescents with a safe and supportive environment at home (interpersonal level) and at school (organizational level). At the interpersonal level, the focus was on action to be taken by the parents/caregivers. At the organizational level, the focus was on action to be taken by school personnel. The environmental outcomes for parents and teachers were fairly simple. However, the stated performance objectives added specificity that enabled the program planners to more effectively communicate the essential components the intervention should address. Note that each performance objective states who will perform the action.

As part of the Go! Austin/Vamos! Austin coalition-led obesity initiative (van den Berg et al., 2019), representatives from the City of Austin Parks and Recreation Department, Police Activity League, Tenants' Council, Austin Parks Foundation, and Austin Interfaith established the following *community-level* performance objectives to *increase easy access to safe PA facilities and programs* (environmental outcome). They stated: "Members of the Physical Activity Sector will ...

- Improve and activate local parks, playgrounds, and recreation facilities
- Ensure parks, playgrounds, trails, and recreation facilities are safe, well lit, maintained, and accessible.
- Where appropriate, ensure functioning street lamps and park lights that create pleasant light throughout the night.
- Ensure that park adoption team and neighbors support adequate investment and attention to parks from public officials and local leadership."

Performance objectives also provide an opportunity to interweave specific assets (policy, information, social/cultural/organizational, and physical assets) identified in Step 1 into intervention planning. For example, in the Fun Families intervention for elementary school-aged children, planners used an environmental asset frame within the home setting to guide identification of POs that supported the interpersonal environmental outcome, "Parents support their child to reduce television (TV) viewing to less than 2 hours a day," as recommended by the American Academy of Pediatrics (Escobar-Chaves et al., 2010). The performance objectives for parents included:

- Limit TV viewing to less than two hours a day (policy)
- Do not allow TV with meals (policy)
- Post TV viewing schedule in family area (information)
- Turn off TV when nobody is watching (social/cultural)
- Reduce parent's own TV watching (social/cultural)
- Engage in fun, non-media related activities (social/cultural)
- Do not provide TV in the child's bedroom (physical)

Our last example concerns performance objectives across all ecological levels to reduce stigmatization (Table 6.2) (see the section on Stigma

Table 6.2 Performance Objectives to Reduce Stigmatization

Interpersonal Level
PO1. Friends and family express empathy when interacting with people with a stigmatized identity or condition.
PO2. Friends and family provide instrumental and emotional social support.
PO3. Friends and family support person if disclosing.
Organizational Level
PO4. Coworkers express empathy when interacting with people with a stigmatized identity or condition.
PO5. Healthcare providers and managers maintain confidentiality about stigmatized identity or condition.
PO6. Managers develop non-discrimination policies that protect all employees' rights.
Community Level
PO7. Opinion leaders communicate norms for treating every community member with respect.
PO8. Community members express empathy when interacting with people with a stigmatized identity or condition.
PO9. Community members provide social support.
Societal Level
PO10. Elected officials develop and implement anti-discrimination policies that protect individuals' rights.

and Discrimination in Chapters 3 and 7). Note that each performance objective clearly specifies who is the responsible environmental agent, as multiple agents are involved at different levels. Stigma is highly detrimental to the psychological and social well-being, as well as the health, of individuals with a stigmatized condition or identity such as HIV, mental illness, substance use dependence, and gender identity. For example, the stigmatization of people with HIV functions as an environmental factor that impedes HIV prevention, HIV testing, linkage to care, and treatment adherence (Been et al., 2016; Gesesew et al., 2017; Katz et al., 2013; Sweeney & Vanable, 2016; Thapa et al., 2017). Stigmatization can occur at all levels, starting with public stigma at the interpersonal level and then moving to structural or institutional stigma at the organizational, community, and societal level (Bos et al., 2013; Roozen et al., 2020). It can also be internalized and anticipated by people with HIV (Bos et al., 2013; Roozen et al., 2020).

People with a stigmatized identity or condition, however, can also act in ways that reduce stigmatizing behavior by others, or the impact of that behavior on them. Examples include seeking social support (Stutterheim et al., 2011); voluntarily disclosing to others, when prepared to do so (Dima et al., 2014; Lyimo et al., 2014; Stutterheim et al., 2017); and actively coping with stigma by using downward comparison, external attribution, or shift in comparison level (Stutterheim et al., 2012).

Using the Core Processes to Write Performance Objectives

The process for breaking down a health-related behavior or an environmental condition into sub-behaviors is not always obvious. The Core Processes presented in Chapter 2 serve as guides for writing performance objectives, as applied in the steps outlined below.

Formulating a question is the starting point. For a health-related behavior, the question is: *What do the participants of this program need to do to perform the health-related behavior*? For environmental outcomes, the question is: *What does someone in the environment need to do to accomplish the environmental outcome*? The answers to these questions form a logical sequence of smaller steps (this list is the basis for the performance objectives) that are necessary to perform the behavior or achieve the environmental outcome. An initial list can also come from the literature. For example, many countries have guidelines for approaches to treat various illnesses, which can be helpful in constructing illness-management performance objectives. An example of guidelines in the United States can be found at *guidelines.gov*.

Searching the research and practice literature by topic can also be helpful in creating or refining an initial list of performance objectives. Finally, the planning group will review the list of performance objectives and reduce it to a set of objectives essential for performing the behavior or achieving the environmental outcome. This step is important because each performance objective is the basis for further work. Each will be linked with determinants to form change objectives. Nonessential (interesting but not necessary) performance objectives will expand the subsequent planning and potentially diffuse the intervention's focus.

Using Theory as a Basis for Performance Objectives Sometimes theory provides a rationale for performance objectives. For example, *self-management behavior change theory* specifies several processes that could themselves be incorporated into performance objectives for specific behaviors. These include goal setting, making plans or implementation intentions, self-monitoring, comparison to a personal standard, self-evaluation, self-control, and reward (Gollwitzer et al., 2014; Shegog et al., 2013). For example, consider an intervention designed to help a priority population to become more physically active. The performance objectives may incorporate specific advice regarding a particular type of PA, but such a list of specific behaviors might be long and unmanageable. A self-regulatory approach (Plaete et al., 2015) would look quite different from a list of specific dos and don'ts, and it may include the following performance objectives:

- Choose strategies to increase PA level
- Start pursuing PA goals
- Monitor and evaluate PA levels
- Maintain or adapt PA goals to a higher level
- Adapt PA goals and strategies when unable to reach initial goals

Health educators may also find it useful to consider the self-regulatory process when designating health-promoting behaviors for the self-management of chronic disease. Kroese and colleagues (Kroese et al., 2014) applied self-regulatory processes and proactive coping in their implementation of the Beyond Good Intentions intervention for diabetes management. The intervention uses a five-step approach of goal setting, barrier recognition, problem-solving, plan formulation, and self-evaluation to target a behavior critical to diabetes self-management, including health eating, PA, or medical regimens. In another example, the self-regulatory processes of goal setting, self-monitoring, and judging were used to develop the Self-Regulatory Illness Management of Depression model intervention for the self-management of depression (Hagerty et al., 2020). These processes informed the session objectives for the intervention which were critical in attaining self-management of depressive symptoms.

Program planners may also consider using a social determinants of health (SDOH) framework to develop performance objectives. These include factors related to economic stability, healthcare access and quality, neighborhood and built environment, as well as social and community context (ODPHP, 2021). For example, an organizational outcome for a healthcare setting might be, "Clinic staff support patients to adhere to their treatment plan." Using a SDOH lens, related performance objectives may include:

- Metro provides free rides for patients to attend clinic visits (transportation).
- Clinic social worker reviews safety net options to cover clinic costs (economics, insurance).
- Clinic social worker enrolls patient in no- or low-cost medication plan with health insurance or pharmaceutical company (economics, financial barriers).
- Nurse navigator follows up to ensure the patient receives necessary social services (housing, food security).

Using Clinical Guidelines or Counseling Models as a Basis for Performance Objectives In healthcare settings, program planners may use evidence-based clinical guidelines or counseling models to inform the development of performance objectives. For example, the "5As" model of behavior change provides a sequence of evidence-based clinician and office practice behaviors (Assess, Advise, Agree, Assist, Arrange) that can be applied in primary care settings to address a broad range of behaviors and health conditions (Glasgow et al., 2006). Halliday and colleagues (2021) used a modified "5As" model to develop performance objectives for diabetes educators to: *identify and address diabetes distress in adults with Type 1 or Type 2 diabetes (behavior outcome).* Specifically, they wanted diabetes health professionals to:

- ASK about diabetes distress
- ASSESS for diabetes distress using a validated questionnaire
- ADVISE about diabetes distress
- ASSIST with developing an achievable action plan
- ASSIGN to another health professional
- ARRANGE follow-up care

Generating and Validating Performance Objectives

Performance objectives are the building blocks of a health promotion intervention. Thus, *before* investing time and resources into designing the intervention materials, it is important to ensure that program planners are targeting the "right" performance objectives at all levels. Planners will need to collect new data to generate and determine the validity of their performance objectives. What do potential participants in the intervention actually do, or say they do, when performing the behavior? Data may also be collected from service providers, key informants, or potential program implementers; surveys and interviews are good methods for this purpose. Through focus groups or interviews, potential participants can be asked whether the performance objectives fit with their views of how they would go about performing the health-related behaviors. Feedback from individuals who have had both successful and unsuccessful experiences with health behavior or environmental outcomes can be very helpful.

An often overlooked, but in some cases essential, source of information about performance objectives is direct observation of the health behavior or environmental outcomes. For some health problems, there may be a limited amount of information, experience, or documentation of how the related health behavior is performed or how environmental outcomes break down into component parts. Observation of performance in natural, as well as in simulated, settings, can be very helpful. For example, program planners developing a nutrition improvement program for schoolchildren can spend time in the school cafeteria observing how children select, trade, modify, and eat (or do not eat) healthy food.

Performance objectives may also be validated by using quantitative methods to predict health-related behaviors within the priority population. This approach is illustrated by a classic study conducted by van Empelen and Kok (van Empelen & Kok, 2008) to explain condom use among adolescents. In writing their performance objectives, they relied on experts, in addition to theoretical and empirical evidence. From the evidence available, they derived performance objectives that may describe the behavioral outcome (condom use) for the priority population, and then conducted a prospective study among 400 high school students to validate these objectives. Among sexually active students with *steady sex partners*, condom use was mediated by *buying* and *carrying* condoms and by *communicating about condom use* (performance objectives) (van Empelen & Kok, 2008). However, when focusing on condom use with *casual sex partners*, the researchers did not find the predicted sequence of performance objectives; actual condom use with casual sex partners was predicted only by the decision to use condoms, not by buying, carrying, or communicating about condoms. Does this mean that these performance objectives are not important? No! The data showed that adolescents simply do not prepare ahead of casual sexual encounters and that young people are more willing to engage in unsafe sex. Thus, although the researchers were not able to validate the sequence of performance objectives in the case of casual sex, they were able to show that the lack of such performance objectives enhances risk-taking behavior (i.e., not using condoms). This study might suggest the need to consider additional or different performance objectives for casual sex. These findings were further validated by Carvalho and colleagues (Carvalho et al., 2015) who reported similar preparatory behavior for condom use among heterosexual young men.

Planners should engage communities throughout the planning process and the development and validation of performance objectives is a critical point in which the involvement of members of the priority populations as well as the environmental agents is essential. These individuals should be part of the planning group and planners should intentionally involve community members to describe the actions necessary to engage in behaviors and environmental actors can help describe and comment on performance objectives related to making environmental changes.

Task 3: Selecting Personal Determinants

The third task in Step 2 is to select important and changeable determinants of health behaviors and environmental outcomes.

Personal determinants are the internal or intrapersonal factors that motivate and enable individuals to perform specific behaviors. They are helpful in responding to the question, "Why would the at-risk population or environmental agent engage in X protective health behavior or change Y environmental condition?" Personal determinants, sometimes referred to as psychosocial factors, usually include cognitive factors (such as self-efficacy, attitudes, beliefs, and values) and capabilities (such as behavioral capability or skills). A person's perceptions about the environment also represent personal determinants. For example, beliefs or perceptions about social norms (perceived social norms) are a personal determinant that may or may not reflect reality. Personal determinants can be changed or influenced by interventions that involve influencing how people think about or have the capacity to change a behavior or the environment.

Those factors that rest *outside* of the individual, yet influence behavior, are considered environmental conditions and are addressed in IM as environmental outcomes, as discussed in the previous section. These environmental conditions may include such factors as observed social influences (such as norms, social support, and reinforcement) or structural influences (such as access to resources, policies, and organizational climate). The individuals at risk of a health problem are not usually able to control these conditions directly; therefore, change is not likely to be accomplished unless action is taken by agents or groups within the various levels of the environment. As such, personal determinants can be identified as important influences for changing a health behavior in the at-risk population, and personal action to be taken by agents who can exert change in the environment.

Using Core Processes to Select Determinants

Determining an appropriate set of evidence- and theory-informed determinants for the performance objectives—for personal behaviors and the environmental outcomes—requires the use of the Core Processes (see Chapter 2). Briefly, Core Processes involve: (1) asking a question, (2) generating a provisional list of answers, and (3) validating the answers against the empirical evidence in the literature, theory, and new data, in that specific order.

In the needs assessment (see Chapter 5), the planner will have already asked and answered questions about determinants regarding the risk behavior(s) and environmental risk factors, and thus should have a viable starting list of personal determinants to help in two important questions (*Process 1*):

- Why would a person perform a particular risky behavior?
- Why do certain environmental risk factors exist?

In Step 2, planners are posing questions about the determinants of *health-promoting* behavior and environmental outcomes that will support the health behavior or affect health directly.

- Why would people perform the health-promoting behavior or performance objectives?
- Why would a certain environmental agent make an environmental modification?

To answer these planning questions, the planning group, along with input from community members and other interested parties, creates a provisional list of answers (*Process 2*) based on their own knowledge or observations and then conducts a review of the literature to find empirical support for the list of answers (*Process 3*), while incorporating theories and constructs as appropriate. For example, if *self-efficacy* was defined in the literature review as a possible determinant of the behavior, then referencing Social Cognitive Theory (SCT) (Bandura, 1986, 2004)—for which self-efficacy is a central element—would be useful (construct approach). A review of the full SCT may suggest other constructs that might be considered as important determinants of behavior (general theory approach).

Planners should also collect data from the at-risk group and environmental agents directly to identify additional determinants and to understand how determinants manifest in a particular group. Qualitative methods, such as focus groups or interviews, can be helpful in generating new ideas for determinants or in verifying some of the findings from the research literature (Peters, 2014). Quantitative data collection, using questionnaires that measure the determinants and the behavior of interest, can be especially helpful in judging the strength of the association between potential determinants and behavior. As described in Chapter 2, planners may use both types of data collection to identify potential determinants, as well as their relative importance for influencing change.

Rating Importance of Determinants

After identifying a list of potential determinants, the next step is to select those determinants that are most relevant, and those which can be woven into a future intervention (to impact a specific behavior/environmental outcome) with efficacy and efficiency (i.e., cost/benefit).

Determinants that have weak evidence of association with the performance objectives or no logical or theoretical basis for their causal relation to the performance are unlikely to be important foci for an intervention. This is of concern for one primary reason: resources are finite and consideration must be given not only to the *development of content* for the intervention but also to the *deliverability* of the intervention. The latter is especially relevant in case: (1) there are additional costs per participant (e.g., delivering an intervention in a face-to-face setting with a health professional) and (2) the amount of intervention content to which participants can be exposed (i.e., even if the costparticipant is low, this may be a reason for "taking a determinant out of consideration"). Thus, it is important to use a systematic process to select determinants to be targeted in an intervention *before* developing intervention content.

In validating and prioritizing determinants, planners can start by using evidence to rate each in terms of *importance* (i.e., the strength of association between the determinant and the behavior, and whether there is room for improvement in the determinant) and *changeability* (i.e., how likely it is that a health promotion intervention is going to bring about improvement in the determinant). The application of an *importance and changeability framework*, as highlighted in Step 1 (see Chapter 5), is a helpful process for prioritization of behaviors and environmental conditions. Table 6.3 shows an example of information used to assess the importance and changeability of determinants for an intervention that was designed to promote HPV vaccination acceptability among mothers of adolescent girls (Pot et al., 2018; van Keulen et al., 2013).

As much as possible, the basis for rating importance and changeability should be based on evidence from the research literature. Sometimes, the literature will not adequately discuss a proposed determinant, and the planner will need to collect data from the at-risk group and from others in the field. For example, Confidence Interval-Based Estimation of Relevance (CIBER) is an approach based on the visualization of confidence intervals for the means and correlation coefficients for all determinants simultaneously. This visualization facilitates comparison, which

Table 6.3 Judging Importance and Changeability of Determinants of Performance Objectives for HPV Vaccination

Determinants	Importance	Changeability	Evidence for Importance
Knowledge	+	+++	Precondition for informed decision
Risk perception	++	+	$R2 = .23, p < .001$
Attitude	+++	+	$R2 = .62, p < .001$
Beliefs	++	+	$R2 = .47, p < .001$
Outcome expectations	+	+	$R2 = .09, p < .001$
Descriptive norms	+	+	$R2 = .11, p < .001$
Subjective norms	++	+	$R2 = .46, p < .001$
Self-efficacy	+	+	$R2 = .06, p < .001$
Relative effectiveness of HPV vaccination	++	++	$R2 = .36, p < .001$

Note: Importance = the strength of the evidence for the causal relationship between the determinant and the behavior we want to change; changeability = the strength of the evidence that the proposed change can be realized by a program; + means: not very important, not easy to change; ++ means: important, changeable; +++ means: very important, changeable.

is necessary when making selections (see (Crutzen et al., 2017), for how-to guidance).

Assessing evidence for *changeability* for the proposed determinants can be challenging and is typically based on a review of effect sizes and change-over-time reported in previous intervention studies. When looking at determinants, it is important to focus on the magnitude of change rather than simply statistical significance, since findings from large samples are often characterized by extreme statistical significance despite small or even trivial effect sizes. The degree of practical significance is generally determined by the size of the observed effect, not the p-value (Lantz, 2013).

Alternatively, when data are not available, decisions to retain or delete determinants from consideration may be based entirely on a theoretical or conceptual basis. When prioritizing determinants based solely on theoretical/conceptual bases, reviewing experimental work can provide empirical support for deciding on the changeability of a determinant (e.g., the meta-analytic review of the causal effects of manipulations of the Theory of Planned Behavior (TPB) variables on intention and behavior) (Sheeran et al., 2016). Also, the evidence may be strong for one determinant (such as self-efficacy), but the literature may provide little evidence to support the importance of a related factor (such as outcome expectations). However, the theoretical literature suggests that these two constructs are interrelated suggesting that it may be important to address both with methods to promote change (Bandura, 1986, 1997).

Some personal determinants and environmental conditions have a reciprocal relationship. For example, subjective norms are considered personal determinants because they derive from an individual's perception of the norms for behavior and are subject to his or her control. The actual norms for behavior are considered environmental conditions because they are external to the individual and outside her or his control. Both subjective norms and actual norms may influence health behavior; however, the processes for change may be very different. On the one hand, actual norms are very difficult to change and require environmental change methods. Subjective norms, on the other hand, may be influenced by intervention methods that focus on how individuals think about and perceive norms. If subjective norms and actual norms are both considered influences of behavioral outcomes for a health promotion intervention, the program planners can approach change by selecting subjective norms as a determinant of behavior and linking it to specific performance objectives. On the other hand, the planners may decide that it is important and possible to change the actual norms and address them as an environmental outcome for one or more of the environmental levels.

In some situations, the actual norms are supportive of the health behavior but the perception of the norms by the priority population is not consistent with the actual norms. For example, in the United States, young adolescents tend to overestimate the proportion of youth smokers, thinking that many adolescents smoke, when in reality less than 5% of high school students currently smoke (CDC, 2024). The focus of many smoking prevention programs is to correct the perception of what is normative for youth smoking. In other situations, it is difficult to modify an environmental condition; program planners must decide whether to plan for an intervention for an environmental outcome or to prepare the at-risk population to deal with the environmental condition. For example, financial resources may be an important environmental condition and skills in coping with resource limitations may be a personal determinant.

Task 4: Constructing Matrices of Change Objectives

In this final task for Step 2, program planners construct separate *matrices of change objectives* for each level of intervention for which they have written performance objectives (individual, interpersonal, organizational, community, and/or societal). The final number of matrices of change objectives is different for each intervention and is influenced by the problem's complexity, the span of the program across levels, and the population's diversity.

To select intervention levels for which matrices will be needed, program planners ask: "At what levels of intervention (individual, interpersonal, organizational, community, and/or societal) is it necessary to achieve the performance objectives?" For example, in the intervention developed to sustain exclusive breastfeeding for infants at risk of asthma, the planners created matrices for the individual (Table 6.4) and interpersonal (Table 6.5) levels. If they wanted to influence change at the organizational (e.g., worksite or clinic), community, and/or policy levels, they would have developed additional matrices of change for the respective levels.

Differentiating the Intervention Population

Sometimes, because of differences in the various subgroups (different ages, levels of experience, ethnic/racial background), different matrices of change objectives may be needed. To decide whether or not one set of matrices is appropriate for all the subgroups in your priority population, planners consider the question of whether or not to "differentiate" the population of interest. To differentiate a population means to make a distinction between one or more subgroups in your priority population due to substantial differences in either the performance objectives or determinants of health-related behavior or environmental outcomes. The rationale for differentiating subpopulations is based on the premise that populations comprise individuals and groups with different characteristics and needs, all of which must be considered in relation to a health problem, and to a health promotion intervention. The greater these differences, the less likely that a single intervention will fit everyone in the intervention population. If a subgroup has different behaviors or environmental conditions, the program planner must develop separate matrices of change objectives for that

Table 6.4 Partial *Matrix of Change Objectives (Individual Level)* for Women who Exclusively Breastfeed for six months (6 m-EBF)

Behavior: Mothers will exclusively breastfeed (EBF) infant for six months				
	Personal Determinants			
Performance Objectives (Mothers)	**Behavioral Capability**	**Self-Efficacy**	**Attitude**	**Perceived Norms**
PO.1. Talk about 6 m-EBF intention with care providers (e.g., midwives)	BC.1. List questions to ask care provider about 6 m-EBF for children predisposed to allergy or asthma	SE.1. Express confidence in talking with care provider about 6m-EBF	Not applicable	PN1. Recognize that other expectant mothers talk with care provider about pros and cons of 6 m-EBF
PO.2. Commit before delivery to 6 m-EBF after delivery	BC.2.a. Describe health–social advantages of 6 m-EBF BC 2.b. Describe benefits of EBF for mother and child	SE.2. Express confidence in dealing with people not in favor of 6 m-EBF	ATT.2.a. Recognize that giving 6 m-EBF is hard but achievable ATT.2.b. Express positive feelings that 6 m-EBF will benefit mother and child	PN.2.a. Expect that partner will agree and support 6 m-EBF PN. 2.b. Recognize that other expectant mothers commit to 6m-EBF before delivery
PO.3. Start and continue 6 m-EBF after delivery (on demand)	BC.3.a. Describe that an EBF-child has its own feeding schedule BC.3.b. Describe signals that child wants to be fed BC.3.c. Describe what to do with physical complaints of mother or child BC.3.d. Describe what to plan for to EBF at work	SE.3. Express confidence in the ability to start and continue breastfeeding, despite challenges	ATT.3. Recognize that EBF will be enough for a child to grow on	PN.3.a. Expect positive remarks/support about 6 m-EBF by partner PN.3.b. Recognize that other mothers continue 6m-EBF on demand
PO.4. Counteract social criticism toward 6 m-EBF	BC.4.a. List ways to counteract social criticism toward 6m-EBF	SE.4. Express confidence in the ability to recognize and counteract social criticism	Not applicable	PN.4.a. Recognize that other women who BF and postpone solid food go through the same experience
PO.5. Buy or hire and use a breast pump to express breast milk	BC.5.a. Describe where to buy or hire a breast pump BC.5.b. Describe how to use a pump to express breast milk	SE.5. Express confidence that they can express milk with a breast pump	ATT.5. Express positive feelings that using a breast pump will make it easier to EBF	PN.5. State that other mothers use breast pump to maintain EBF
PO.7. Remind other individuals in environment to not give solid food to infant	Not applicable	SE.7. Express confidence in keeping others from giving child solid food	Not applicable	PN.7. Describe expectation that partner will support refraining others to give child solid food

Mesters et al. (2018) / Frontiers Media /CC-BY-4.0.

subgroup and conduct a parallel planning process. If there are substantially different performance objectives or determinants for one subgroup as compared to another you may decide to "differentiate the population" and thus create separate matrices for each subgroup. If subgroups differ only on

Table 6.5 Partial Matrix for Change Objectives (Interpersonal Level) for Partners of Women who Provide Exclusive Breastfeeding for six Months (6 m-EBF)

Interpersonal Outcome: Partners Support Mother to Exclusively Breastfeed for six Months				
	Personal Determinants			
Performance Objectives (Partners)	**Behavioral Capability**	**Self-Efficacy**	**Outcome Expectations**	**Attitude**
PO.1. Support postponement of solid food	BC.1. Describe health and social advantages of 6 m-EBF (and postponement of solid food)	SE.1. Express confidence in dealing with people not in favor of 6 m-EBF and/or postponement of solid food	OE.1. Expect that 6 m-EBF will decrease child's risk for asthma and allergies	ATT.1. Express positive feelings that EBF will be enough for infant to grow on
PO.2. Stand by mother who receives criticism because of 6 m-EBF	BC.2. List ways to counter criticism of 6 m-EBF	SE.2. Express confidence in dealing with people not in favor of 6 m-EBF	Not applicable	ATT.2. Express positive feelings toward importance of 6 m-EBF for mother and child

Mesters et al. (2018) / Frontiers Media /CC-BY-4.0.

a few performance objectives and/or determinants, the planner can use the same matrices but make a note that certain performance objectives or change objectives pertain to a specific subgroup.

Differentiating a population often occurs simultaneously with writing performance objectives, or exploring determinants, because of the question that guides the differentiation process: *Are either performance objectives or determinants substantially different for subgroups?* For example, when planning an early childhood obesity prevention intervention, performance objectives for toddlers, pre-kindergartners, and primary-grade children might be substantially different based on their respective stages of cognitive, physical, and autonomy development (Charlesworth, 2017). This might result in developing a different matrix of change objectives for each age group. Similarly, when planning a smoking cessation intervention based on the stages of change, the performance objectives and determinants for individuals in the Pre-contemplation, Contemplation, Preparation, Action, and Maintenance stages would be substantially different (DiClemente & Prochaska, 1998), resulting in five distinct matrices of change objectives.

The decision of whether or not to differentiate a population should be very carefully considered, because each differentiation into one or more subgroups will expand the details of the planning process and potentially increase the program's complexity and costs. If identified differences in the subpopulations are not great, planners can often accommodate them within the intervention with a few variations to address differences. For example, the performance objectives required to use condoms correctly and consistently (buy or obtain a condom, carry a condom, talk with your partner ahead of time, and use a condom for every sexual act) are similar for male and female adolescents, and slight differences in personal determinants by gender could be accommodated within the same matrix of change objectives, with minor modifications.

Some of the variables that may be important to consider in the differentiation of a population are the ones that were mentioned in the needs assessment. These include age and gender, geographic location, socioeconomic status, education, and cultural group. In addition, using theories and models that describe processes of behavior change, such as stages of change models, or organizational change (DiClemente & Prochaska, 1998; Nidecker et al., 2008) will in many cases enhance a planner's ability to develop change objectives that successfully define what needs to change at the different ecological levels. It is important to note that deciding not to differentiate the population does not mean that the planners cannot still make various versions of targeted materials to reflect different subgroups' preferences for images, language, etc. These decisions will be made in IM Step 4.

Constructing Matrices of Change Objectives

To this point, the planner has made a preliminary decision about the number of matrices for the project, based on population differentiation and levels of environmental change.

The question that leads to the formation of a change objective for personal determinants is: *What needs to change related to X determinant for the intervention participants to do Y performance objective?* For example, Table 6.6 shows a partial matrix from the Me & You: Building Healthy Relationships intervention for middle school students. For students, the first performance objective is, "Identify and evaluate their own behavior within past and current peer and/or dating relationships," which is paired with the determinant of "behavioral capability." The question used to address this cell can be worded this way: *What needs to change related to behavioral capability for the participants to be able to identify and evaluate their own behavior in past and current peer and/or dating relationships?* Answers to this question led to the following change objectives (Table 6.6):

- List actions that constitute unhealthy behaviors (e.g., hitting, choking, substance use, bullying, stalking, verbal threats, unwanted sexual touching, constant texting).
- List actions that constitute healthy behaviors (e.g., support, trust, respecting physical boundaries and sexual limits, active consent).
- Describe how evaluating their own behaviors will be helpful for being in a healthy relationship.
- List actions that constitute own healthy and unhealthy behaviors in past and current peer and/or dating relationships.

In Step 3, the change objectives described in this process will become the targets for program change methods and practical applications to increase knowledge.

Table 6.6 Partial Matrix of Change Objectives for Students in the Me & You Study

Behavioral Outcome: Students will have healthy peer and dating relationships (i.e., that are free of emotional, physical, and sexual violence)					
	Personal Determinants				
Performance Objectives (Students)	**Behavioral Capability**	**Self-Efficacy**	**Adaptive Thinking**	**Subjective Norms**	**Gender Role Expectations**
PO.1. Identify and evaluate their own behaviors within past and current peer and/or dating relationships.	BC.1.a. List actions that constitute unhealthy behaviors (e.g., hitting, choking, substance use, bullying, stalking, verbal threats, unwanted sexual touching, constant texting) BC.1.b. List actions that constitute healthy behaviors (e.g., support, trust, respecting physical boundaries and sexual limits, active consent)	SE.1. Express confidence in ability to identify and evaluate their behaviors within relationships.	AT.1. Describe how thought processes influence past and current behaviors in peer and/or dating relationships.	SN.1. Recognize that peers identify and evaluate their behaviors within relationships	GRE.1. List ways gender role beliefs influence their behavior within past and/or current relationships.
PO.2. Identify and evaluate peers' and/or dating partner's behaviors within past and current peer and/or dating relationships	BC.2.a. List healthy and unhealthy behaviors of peer and/or dating partner of past and current relationships	SE.2. Express confidence in the ability to identify and evaluate peer and/or dating partner behaviors within past and current relationships	AT.2. Recognize how their own thought processes can affect their ability to identify and evaluate peer and dating partner behavior	SN.2. Recognize that peers identify and evaluate peer and/or dating partner behaviors within past and current relationships	GRE.2. List ways gender role beliefs influence peer and/or dating partner behavior within past and current relationships
PO.3. Use effective communication strategies to foster healthy peer and dating relationships (e.g., conflict resolution, problem-solving, and active consent)	BC.3.a. Describe effective communication strategies to foster healthy relationships BC.3.b. Identify appropriate contexts in which to use effective communication strategies	SE.3.a. Express confidence in ability to use effective communication strategies to foster healthy relationships SE.3.b. Express confidence that can recognize appropriate contexts in which to use these strategies	Not applicable	SN.3. Recognize that peers also use effective communication strategies to foster healthy relationships	GRE. 3. State that both males and females have responsibility to use effective communication strategies to foster healthy relationships

PO.4. Manage emotional responses (e.g., love, anger, anxiety, stress, depression, jealousy) to foster healthy peer and dating relationships.	BC.4.a. List types of emotions BC.4.b. Define what is an emotional response BC.4.c. Describe how to manage emotional responses to foster healthy peer and dating relationships BC.4.d. Recognize the signs and situations for when to manage emotional responses	SE.4.a. Express confidence in ability to manage emotional responses SE.4.b. Express confidence to recognize the signs and situations for when to manage emotional responses	AT.4. Recognize that how we think about events affects how we feel about them	SN.4. Recognize that peers also manage emotional responses	GRE.4. State that both males and females have responsibility to manage emotional responses
PO.5. Avoid peers and potential dating partners that engage in unhealthy relationship behaviors	BC.5.a. Identify peers/potential dating partners that engage in unhealthy relationship behaviors BC.5.b. Identify where they come in contact (e.g., school, unsupervised parties, places where peers do drugs) BC.5.c. List strategies (e.g., clear no, alternative actions) to avoid peers/potential dating partners that engage in unhealthy relationship behavior	SE.5. Express confidence in ability to use strategies to avoid peers and potential dating partners that engage in unhealthy relationship behaviors	AT.5. Avoid others who trigger maladaptive thoughts about yourself or situations	SN.5. Recognize that peers avoid other peers and potential dating partners that engage in unhealthy relationship behaviors	Not applicable

Adapted from Peskin et al. (2018) / with permission of Elsevier.

For each behavioral outcome and environmental outcome, the planner enters the performance objectives down the left side of a matrix and the determinants across the top. The next task is to assess each cell of the matrix to judge whether the determinant is likely to influence the accomplishment of the performance objective. It is unlikely that each determinant will be an important influence on every performance objective. Because change objectives are needed for those cells in which the determinant is likely to influence the accomplishment of the performance objective, this task can be a process of review and elimination. One way that the planner accomplishes this task is to look at each cell, decide whether a change in a particular determinant is necessary for the performance objective, put an "X" or "Not applicable" through unimportant cells, and then write change objectives for the cells that remain. The planner then writes change objectives for the personal determinants.

Writing Change Objectives

The examples above show that change objectives are stated with action verbs. Table 6.7 includes words to help with this task (Caffarella, 1985). Change objectives begin with a verb that defines the action, followed by a statement of the expected result of the intervention. The purpose of stating a change objective in this manner is to make as specific as possible what change in the determinant needs to be achieved to accomplish the performance objective. Planners who write change objectives with an action verb and specified change in the determinants have a clear direction to the next steps in the IM process: selecting intervention methods and translating methods into practical applications.

Table 6.7 List of Action Words for Writing Change Objectives: Organized by Levels of Complexity of Learning Tasks

Knowledge	Understand	Applications	Analysis	Synthesis	Evaluation
Define	Describe	Apply	Analyze	Arrange	Appraise
Label	Discuss	Demonstrate	Appraise	Assemble	Assess
List	Explain	Dramatize	Calculate	Collect	Choose
Name	Express	Execute	Categorize	Compose	Compare
Recall	Identify	Illustrate	Compare	Construct	Conclude
Record	Interpret	Implement	Contrast	Create	Critique
Repeat	Locate	Interpret	Debate	Design	Estimate
State	Recognize	Modify	Diagram	Formulate	Evaluate
Tell	Report	Operate	Differentiate	Manage	Judge
	Restate	Practice	Distinguish	Organize	Justify
	Review	Predict	Examine	Plan	Measure
	Summarize	Schedule	Experiment	Prepare	Rate
	Translate	Sketch	Inspect	Propose	Revise
		Use	Inventory	Relate	Score
			Question	Set up	Select
			Relate		Value
			Solve		
			Test		

The program planners for Me & You developed similar matrices of change objectives at the interpersonal level for parents; and at the organizational level for teachers and other school staff who play a role in creating a supportive environment to help students participate in healthy peer and dating relationships (Table 6.8).

Table 6.8 Partial Matrices of Change Objectives for Interpersonal and Organizational Outcomes in the Me & You Study

Interpersonal Outcome: Parents/Caregivers will Communicate with their Child about Healthy Peer and Dating Relationships				
	Personal Determinants			
Performance Objectives (Parents/ Caregivers)	**Behavioral Capability**	**Skills**	**Perceived Benefits**	**Perceived Barriers**
PO.1. Create the appropriate times, locations, and activities to talk with their child about healthy peer and dating relationships (respond)	BC.1.a. State potential times, locations, and activities to talk with their child about healthy relationships K.1.b. Recognize the characteristics of a teachable moment	S.1.a. Demonstrate ability to identify times, locations, and activities to talk about healthy relationships with their child S.1.b. Demonstrate ability to identify and act on teachable moments to discuss healthy relationships with their child	PBen.1.a. State that approaching child about healthy relationships at an appropriate time/ location will ensure that the discussion has a better chance of being received by their child	PBar.1.a. Recognize barriers to finding appropriate times, locations, and activities to discuss healthy relationships with their child PBar.2.b. List ways to overcome barriers
PO.2. Use effective communication strategies when talking with their child (e.g., active listening, being nonjudgmental) (respond)	BC.2.a. List the characteristics of effective and ineffective communication BC.2.b. Describe why it is important that they use effective communication strategies	S.2. Demonstrate ability to use effective communication strategies when talking with their child about healthy relationships	PBen.2.a. Describe how using effective communication strategies when talking with their child will result in better, high-quality discussions and greater connectedness with their child	PBar.2.a. Recognize barriers to using effective communication skills with their child (e.g., discomfort, insecurity, inexperience, competing priorities, lack of knowledge, parenting style) PBar.2.b. List ways to overcome barriers
PO.3. Discuss strategies for having healthy peer and dating relationships (e.g., conflict resolution, problem-solving, effective communication) (respond)	BC.3.a. State characteristics of healthy and unhealthy relationships BC.3.b. List strategies that foster healthy relationships BC.3.c. Anticipate questions their child may have about relationships BC.3.d. State ways to respond to questions to which they do/ do not have an answer	S.3.a. Demonstrate ability to discuss with their child strategies for having healthy relationships S.3.b. Demonstrate ability to effectively respond to child's questions & discuss their concerns about relationships	PBen.3.a. Describe how discussing strategies for having healthy relationships will increase child's ability to make healthy choices with respect to relationships, and handle difficult situations in a positive way (e.g., without looking like a wimp, avoid risky situations)	PBar.3.a. List ways to overcome barriers to discussing healthy relationship strategies with their child (e.g., talk when in the car, speak in the third person, make generalizations, talk early and often)

(continued)

Table 6.8 (*Continued*)

Organizational Outcome: School Staff (Teachers, Nurses, Counselors, Social Workers, School Leadership) will Recognize Dating Violence Among Youth, Respond Appropriately, and Refer to Resources				
	Personal Determinants			
Performance Objectives (School Staff)	**Behavioral Capability**	**Skills**	**Perceived Benefits**	**Perceived Barriers**
PO.1. Plan to respond appropriately to youth dating violence incidents (recognize)	BC.1.a. List the characteristics of healthy/unhealthy dating relationships BC.1.b. List types and prevalence of dating violence (physical, emotional, sexual) BC.1.c. List ways school staff can respond appropriately to DV incidents	S.1. Demonstrate the ability to evaluate youth relationships	PBen.1. a. Explain that identifying DV incidents will help you respond appropriately	Not applicable
PO.2. Use active listening when engaging with youth in discussions about their relationship experiences (respond)	BC.2.a. State characteristics of active listening between youth and school staff (e.g., ask questions, nodding, face the person, open your posture, lean in, maintain eye contact) BC.2.b. State importance of actively and non-judgmentally listening to youth feelings and opinions	S.2.a. Demonstrate ability for effective active listening	PBen.2.a. Describe how effective active listening to youth will reduce likelihood of him/her failing to communicate or miscommunicating important information about current beliefs, values, and behaviors related to healthy relationship	PBar.2.a. Anticipate increased need for time, patience, and self-control than typical staff-youth interaction to actively listen to youth PBar.2.b. Recognize that distractions can make it difficult to actively listen to youth
PO.3. Answer questions and concerns youth may have about relationships (respond)	BC.3.a. List potential questions and concerns youth may have about relationships BC.3.b. State ways to respond to questions and concerns (both those you have answer for and those you do not)	S.3. Demonstrate ability to use effective communication strategies when talking with youth to use these strategies	PBen.3.a. Describe how answering questions and concerns about relationships will promote healthy relationships and reduce youth DV	PBar.3. Anticipate increased need for patience, self-control, time, and self-management of embarrassment when answering questions and concerns about relationships
PO.6. Identify and adhere to reporting laws (refer)	BC.6.a. State the behaviors that require reporting (school, district, state, federal) BC.6.b. List steps to adhering to reporting laws if youth discloses	S.6.a. Demonstrate ability to state behaviors that require reporting S.6.b. Demonstrate ability to list steps to adhere to reporting laws if youth discloses	PBen.6. Describe how adhering to the reporting laws will protect the youth and staff	PBar.6.a. Anticipate barriers to adhering to reporting laws (lack of time, fear, etc.) PBar.6.b. List ways to overcome barriers

Adapted from Peskin et al. (2018) / with permission of Elsevier.

Dealing with Automaticity in the Matrix of Change Objectives As discussed in Chapter 3, automaticity (impulsivity, habits, or prejudice) is not a standard determinant but a characteristic of the behavior and mostly outside of an individual's awareness. Theory predicts that automatic reactions can be overcome by reflective reactions, coping skills, and control motivation. In Step 2, automaticity may best be handled in terms of specific performance objectives which are derived from methods to change habitual, automatic, and impulsive behaviors (see Chapter 7, Table 7.6) in combination with awareness, attitudes, social norms, and (social) coping skills, and (control) self-efficacy. Those performance objectives may, for example, be derived from theories of self-regulation: monitor, compare, plan, implement, and recycle (Clark, 2003; Rothman et al., 2004). Changing a habitual chain by moving the cookie jar from its normal place is a performance objective; being confident and able to implement that coping response are change objectives. Table 6.9 provides a simulated matrix of change objectives to establish a healthy diet.

Table 6.9 Examples of Cells from a Simulated Matrix to Address a Habitual Behavior

Behavior: Establish a Healthy Diet			
Performance Objectives	**Awareness**	**Attitudes**	**Self-Efficacy and Skills**
PO.1. Monitor food intake	A.1. Acknowledge the habitual character of eating high-fat food, especially snacks	ATT.1. Express positive feelings about monitoring food intake	SSE.1.a. Demonstrate ability to monitor food intake. SSE.1.b. Express confidence in ability to correctly monitor one's own food intake
PO.2. Decide if discrepancies exist	Not applicable	Not applicable	SSE.2.a. Demonstrate the ability to evaluate fat content of food intake SSE.2.b. Express confidence in ability to evaluate fat content of food intake
PO.3. Make plan, e.g., change a stimulus that elicits or signals a behavior	A.3. Acknowledge the need to change environmental cues	ATT.3. Recognize the advantages of changing behavior	SSE.3. Express confidence in ability to generate coping strategies to deal with habitual behaviors
PO.4. Take action, e.g., moving the cookie jar from its normal place	Not applicable	Not applicable	SSE.4.a. Demonstrate the ability to recognize automaticity in behavior chains and identify points for cue altering SSE.4.b. Express confidence in ability to recognize automaticity in behavior chains and identify points for cue altering
PO.5. Evaluate (and Recycle to Monitoring)	A.5. Explain the importance of self-evaluation skills	ATT.5. Express positive feelings about evaluating and returning to self-monitoring if necessary	SSE.5.a. Demonstrate ability to evaluate implemented coping strategies and return to self-monitoring if necessary SSE.5.b. Express confidence in ability to evaluate implemented coping strategies and return to self-monitoring if necessary

Identifying Environmental Agents and Program Implementers

A common source of confusion for program planners is the distinction between involving agents in the environment to make environmental changes versus having them implement components of an intervention program. For example, in a school-based program such as Me & You: Building Healthy Relationships, teachers may be both agents to change the environmental conditions and program implementers (Peskin et al., 2018). The organizational component of the intervention included performance and change objectives for providing a safe school environment, and for recognizing and referring students to appropriate resources if they were experiencing difficulties. This was part of the school's environmental change program. They were thus important agents at the organizational level. However, the teachers also implemented a classroom curriculum that enabled students to engage in healthy relationships. A training program helped prepare the teachers to implement the intervention. Program implementation is not part of the planning done in Step 2 but is addressed in Step 5, following a similar set of tasks focused on implementation outcomes rather than health behavior or environmental change outcomes.

Creating a Logic Model of Change

At the end of Step 2, program planners begin to create a *logic model of change* for their health promotion intervention. In contrast to the *logic model of the problem* developed in Step 1, which depicts pathways of problem causation, the *logic model of change* illustrates pathways of program effects. Program planners use information from Step 1 regarding desired health and QOL outcomes and information from the previous tasks in Step 2 (behavior and environmental outcomes, performance objectives, determinants, and change objectives) to begin populating a logic model of change, which is read from left to right. As described in Chapter 2, there is a tool available to help develop a logic model of change: the acyclic behavior change diagram (ABCD) (Metz et al., 2022). Using this tool—which is helpful during the planning process—also provides insight into the rationale of the intervention, and fosters replicability of health promotion interventions (Peters et al., 2012).

In Chapter 5, we learned about the ¡Activate Ya! school-based PA promotion and tobacco prevention intervention developed in partnership with Uruguayan community health leaders and secondary schools. Figure 6.2 presents an abbreviated logic model of change for the PA focus of the ¡Activate Ya! intervention, which builds from the *logic model of the problem* by *flipping that model* to now focus on the positive health-promoting changes that the intervention aims to achieve.

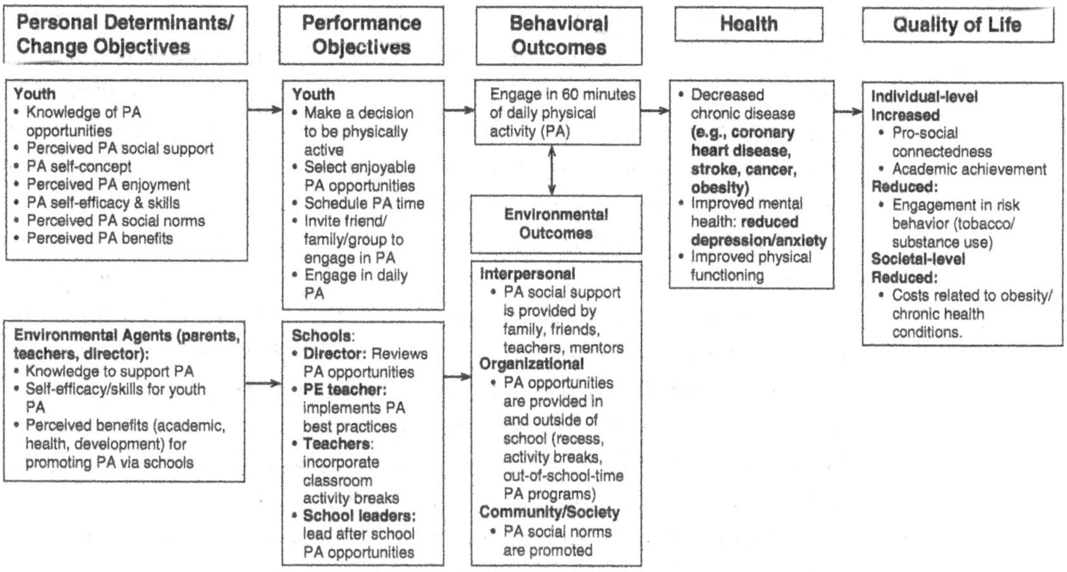

Figure 6.2 Logic Model of Change for ¡Activate Ya! Physical Activity Component

Using Matrices of Change Objectives for Program Evaluation

Each task in Step 2 produces information that is used to guide the program evaluation (see Chapter 10). In the first task, the planners specified the behavioral and environmental outcomes that the program would address. For program evaluation, these outcomes are measured to determine the impact of the program on behavior and environmental conditions (Peskin et al., 2014, 2019).

In Task 2 of IM Step 2, the planners further delineated the behaviors and environmental outcomes by writing performance objectives. These performance objectives help define the critical components and necessary prerequisites for the performance of the behavior and environmental outcomes. Evaluation questions can be asked to determine whether intervention participants achieved the performance objective, which provides valuable information to better understand an intervention's effectiveness. For example, if the behavior was performed, then responses to questions about the performance objectives help the evaluators to know the relative importance of specific sub-steps of the behavior. If the behavior was not performed, then the responses may help explain why the intervention did not have an effect on behavior and may provide important information to guide revisions of the intervention. In some cases, the performance objectives help in defining behavioral or environmental outcomes and can be used to construct evaluation questions to measure the behavior. For example, eating a low-fat diet so that less than 30% of calories are from fat cannot be effectively measured without more specific questions about what and how much was eaten, which can be guided by performance objectives such as "drink low-fat milk instead of whole milk."

In the final task in Step 2, the planners create matrices of change objectives that the intervention will address. These matrices can also be used to guide the development of measures to evaluate the most immediate impact of the intervention. Accomplishment of the change objectives is intended to influence changes in the personal determinants of the performance objectives. For effect evaluation, the evaluator will want to know whether the intervention was successful in influencing changes in the determinants. The change objectives in the matrix cells can be used to help identify existing valid and reliable instruments to measure the determinants. For example, planners can use the change objectives for *self-efficacy* to identify existing measures to assess participants' self-efficacy before and after participating in the intervention. This same principle can be applied to the identification of measures to assess other determinants, such as subjective norms, attitudes, and beliefs.

It is most difficult to evaluate the effectiveness of a health promotion intervention if the planners have not clearly stated the intervention's objectives and outcomes. Step 2 of IM provides the program evaluators with clearly stated behaviors and environmental outcomes, performance objectives, and change objectives that are used as outcome variables in the program evaluation.

FOR OUR CHILDEN EXAMPLE: STEP 2

Task 1: State Desired Behavioral and Environmental Outcomes

Following the NAA for the ***For Our Children*** or, in Spanish, ***Por Nuestros Hijos* (PNH)** project introduced in Chapter 5, the program planners identified the primary health-related behavioral outcome that the program sought to influence. In the case of vaccination among children and adolescents under age 18 years, the decision-maker is the parent. Thus, even though typically the parent would be considered an environmental agent (at the interpersonal level), in this case, the planning group put parental behavior (getting the child vaccinated) as the primary behavioral outcome, which they stated as: *Parents will obtain the HPV vaccine for their adolescent children*. In the environment, receiving a healthcare provider's recommendation was identified as a critical factor (at the interpersonal level) influencing parental decisions to vaccinate their children. Thus, they stated the environmental outcome as: *Healthcare providers will vaccinate all eligible adolescent patients against HPV according to Advisory Committee on Immunization Practices (ACIP) guidelines.*

Task 2: Specify Performance Objectives for Behavioral And Environmental Outcomes

The team considered the question: What do parents need to do to get their child vaccinated against HPV? First, they proceeded to list the various steps (or sub-behaviors) related to the action of vaccinating the child and created a list of performance objectives (Table 6.10). Similarly, to identify performance objectives at the interpersonal level, the team asked the

Table 6.10 Behavioral & Environmental Outcomes for Por Nuestros Hijos Project and Associated Performance Objectives

Behavioral Outcome: Parents will obtain the HPV vaccine for their adolescent children.
Partial Performance Objectives (PO)
PO.1. Parents make an appointment with a healthcare provider.
PO.2. Parents discuss the HPV vaccine with the provider.
PO.2.a. Parents ask the provider any questions or concerns they may have about their son/daughter receiving the HPV vaccine.
PO.3. Parents identify payment mechanisms for the HPV vaccine.
PO.4.a. Parents obtain the first HPV vaccine dose for son/daughter (for people who can vaccinate the same day).
PO.4.b. Parents obtain the first HPV vaccine dose for son/daughter (for people who cannot vaccinate the same day).
PO.5. Parents take their sons/daughters to receive the 2nd dose and 3rd dose (if needed) of the HPV vaccine.
PO.5.a. Parents make follow-up appointment(s).
PO.5.b. Parents and sons/daughters go to appointment(s).
Environmental Outcome (EO): Healthcare Providers will Vaccinate all Eligible Adolescent Patients* Against HPV in Accordance with ACIP Guidelines.
Partial Performance Objectives
PO.1. Check EMR or ask Medical Assistant/Nurse at every encounter to identify if the patient is eligible for HPV vaccination during sick as well as preventive visits.
PO.2. Consistently deliver strong "bundled and unqualified" HPV vaccination recommendation to parents of all eligible adolescent patients* during all patient encounters.
PO.2.a. Deliver bundled HPV vaccination recommendation with Tdap and MCV, if adolescent is ages 11–12.
PO.2.b. Deliver unqualified recommendations for HPV vaccine initiation, if patients ages 13–17 have not initiated HPV vaccination.
PO.3. Identify specific parental concerns if they express vaccine hesitancy and decision to delay vaccination.
PO.4. Communicate tailored message to address specific concerns or hesitancies of parents/ older adolescents.
PO.5. Evaluate provider's (their own) perceived parental concerns vis-à-vis actual parental concerns about HPV vaccine.
PO.6. Identify specific ways to overcome their own provider concerns related to providing HPV vaccine recommendations.
PO.7. Place HPV vaccine order and route order to Medical Assistant/Nurse.
PO.8. Administer (or have other clinic personnel administer) the HPV vaccine.
PO.9. Remind parents to schedule 2nd dose (or a nurse visit), and 3rd dose if needed, before leaving the clinic.
PO.9.a. For adolescents ages 11–14: Two dose schedules at 0 and 6–12 months.
PO.9.b. For adolescents ages 15 years and older: Three dose schedules at 0, 1–2 months, and 6 months.

* Adolescents ages 11–12 and adolescents ages 13–17 who have not initiated HPV vaccination.

question: What do healthcare providers need to do to help get adolescent patients vaccinated against HPV?

Task 3: Select Determinants for Behavioral and Environmental Outcomes

The planning group then discussed determinants associated with parental decisions and actions to vaccinate their children against HPV. They used the Core Processes described in Chapter 2–ask a question, generate a provisional list of answers, validate the answers against the empirical evidence in the literature and theory, and collect new data. The planners worked first to identify determinants of parental behavior and then on determinants of a strong provider recommendation. They brainstormed a preliminary list of factors influencing the health-promoting behavioral and environmental outcomes by asking themselves, "Why would parents [providers] vaccinate their children [adolescent patients] against HPV? Also, why would parents [providers] do these performance objectives (the sub-tasks leading up to vaccination)?" The planning group also reviewed data collected in Step 1 needs assessment, focus groups, and interviews (Chapter 5, Por Nuestros Hijos) to remind themselves about the reasons parents (providers) were not vaccinating their children (adolescent patients). They added relevant determinants to their preliminary list based on this review.

The group then reviewed the literature to find empirical support for the working list of determinants as well as to identify additional relevant determinants. An existing systematic review of reviews that identified modifiable individual, provider, and clinic-level characteristics linked with HPV vaccine uptake and environmental outcomes enriched this validation process. (Rodriguez et al., 2020) Also informed by their literature review, the group modified the preliminary list using theoretical constructs from the SCT, such as behavioral capability (knowledge and skills), self-efficacy, and outcome expectations; the TPB, such as attitudes and normative beliefs; and the Health Belief Model (HBM), such as perceived susceptibility and severity, and perceived benefits and barriers. Constructs from these three theories aligned most closely with the determinants they had compiled. As the final step, the planning group carefully analyzed and refined their list of determinants, walking through a prioritization process to inform the final list of determinants that would be the focus of behavior change in their intervention. This process included assessing the strength of the evidence for the association between each determinant and the behavior, the level of importance of each determinant with respect to changing behavior, and the likelihood that the determinant could be influenced through intervention. Tables 6.11 and 6.12 provide examples of the brainstorming and prioritization process the group worked through to generate the final list of determinants for parents and healthcare providers, respectively.

Task 4: Construct Matrices of Change Objectives

The planners created a matrix for the priority population, that is, parents of adolescent children, and two separate matrices for healthcare providers (medical doctors/physicians/nurse practitioners, and medical assistants/nurses/other clinic staff) at the interpersonal level. In most cases the change objectives for parents of boys vs. girls remained the same; however, the planning group differentiated change objectives where relevant for boys vs. girls. For example, change objectives concerning the benefits of vaccination to adolescent girls included protection from cervical, oropharyngeal, and anal cancers, and genital warts, whereas benefits for adolescent boys included protection from penile, oropharyngeal, and anal cancers, and genital warts. Partial matrices are shown in Tables 6.13 and 6.14. The planners created a logic model of change for the PNH project (Figure 6.3) based on the health and QOL outcomes identified in Step 1 and matrices of change objectives identified in Step 2. Subsequent information from Steps 3, 4, and 5 will be added to the model to complete the logic of change and to guide evaluation planning.

Table 6.11 Partial Work to Generate List of Determinants Affecting Parental Acceptance of HPV Vaccine

1. Original Provisional List	2. Additions from Empirical Literature	3. Theoretical Additions (Some from Empirical Literature)	4. Additions From New Research	5. Final Determinant List
HPV-related barriers • Lack of adequate awareness of HPV, cervical cancer, and associated factors • Lack of awareness of HPV vaccine and the risk and benefits • Low maternal perceived risks of HPV infection/STI **HPV vaccine-related barriers** • Concerns about vaccine cost • Concerns about vaccine safety and side effects • Lack of access to clinics or healthcare provider **Facilitators** • Belief that HPV vaccine is effective • Belief that vaccine is normative and accepted by others • Mother's belief that daughter was at high risk for HPV • Mother's belief that vaccine prevents disease and/or protects against genital warts • Maternal desire to protect daughter against or prevent cervical cancer • Parental desire to protect boys from harm in general	**HPV-related barriers** • Belief that daughter is too young • Moral concerns • Fear that HPV would cause daughters to *mature* faster • Lack of time to see the doctor **HPV vaccine-related barriers** • Lack of HPV vaccine recommendation healthcare provider, especially for boys • Fear that HPV vaccine would cause future infertility. • Perception that vaccine is relatively new • Belief that daughter is not at risk of HPV because she is not sexually active • Lack of perceived benefit or need to vaccinate sons • Belief that HPV vaccine will hasten sons' sexual activity **Facilitators** • Mother's concern for HPV, cervical cancer, STI and genital warts • Maternal personal belief about pap testing and HPV vaccine • Maternal beliefs that the vaccine protects against cancer and protects child's health • Mother's willingness to communicate with daughter about STI, cervical cancer, or sex • Mothers of boys believe that the HPV vaccine can prevent transmission to future female partners • Parents' history of seeking preventive care for themselves and/or their children	• Behavioral capability (SCT) • Attitudes (SCT, TRA/TPB) • Self-efficacy (SCT, TRA/TPB) • Skills (SCT, TRA/TPB) • Perceived risk (HBM) • Perceived benefits (HBM) • Perceived susceptibility/ severity (HBM) • Fear/Threat (HBM) • Perceived barriers (HBM) • Subjective and social norms (TRA/TPB) • Outcome expectations (SCT) • Beliefs about vaccine safety (HBM) • Intention to vaccinate (TRA/TPB) • Health seeking behavior • Parent-child communication • Vaccine access and availability	• Belief that child's personal characteristics would prevent them from acquiring an STI • Belief that obtaining the HPV vaccine could lead to sexual activity and promiscuity • Belief that society would see their daughter as promiscuous if she got the HPV vaccine. • Belief that child's healthcare provider was not easy to talk to or lacked information about vaccine • Lack of long-term study results • Belief about vaccine affordability • More likely to vaccinate their child if vaccine were free • Competing priorities (e.g., compliance with the 3-dose schedule would be hard to keep up with and child would miss too much school)	• Behavioral Capability (SCT) • Attitudes (SCT, TRA/TPB) • Self-Efficacy (SCT, TRA/TPB) • Skills (SCT, TRA/TPB) • Perceived Benefits/Barriers (HBM) • Perceived Susceptibility (HBM) • Normative Beliefs (TRA/TPB) • Outcome Expectations (SCT)

Table 6.12 Partial Work to Generate List of Determinants Affecting Provider Recommendation/Administration of HPV Vaccine

1. Original Provisional List	2. Additions from Empirical Literature	3. Theoretical Additions (Some from Empirical Literature)	4. Additions From New Research	5. Final Determinant List
HPV-related barriers • Lack of awareness about types of HPV-related cancers other than cervical cancer **HPV vaccine-related barriers** • Lack of awareness about vaccine efficacy and safety • Apprehension discussing sex with parents or youth • Belief that the HPV vaccine is associated with risky sexual behaviors • Belief in vaccine misconceptions • Time to recommend/discuss is long **Facilitators** • Parents accept the HPV vaccine as safe • Parents accept the HPV vaccine as effective • Other providers bundle the recommendation • Importance of CDC recommendations • HPV vaccination is recommended by professional organizations • HPV vaccination is supported by professional organizations	**HPV-related barriers** • Lack of awareness about vaccine availability for males • Lack of skills in discussing HPV vaccine with hesitant parents • Lack of skills in discussing sex/sexuality/STIs with parents and adolescents • Lack of skills recommending bundled vaccination • Low perceived severity of HPV-related cancers and genital warts • Perceived parental concerns regarding vaccine safety and vaccine efficacy • Gender bias in recommending vaccine • Lack of skill delivering a strong recommendation • Concerns with cost and insurance reimbursement **Facilitators** • Awareness of HPV-related cancers besides cervical cancer • Expect bundling the recommendation saves time • Addressing hesitancies will lead to increased vaccination • Parents will have positive attitudes about the HPV vaccine • Other providers vaccinate both older and younger girls and boys • Other providers vaccinate their own children	• Behavioral Capability (SCT) • Beliefs (HBM) • Attitudes (SCT, TRA/TPB) • Skills (SCT, TRA/TPB) • Self-efficacy (SCT, TRA/TPB) • Outcome expectations (SCT) • Perceived Social Norms/ Normative beliefs (TRA/TPB) • Perceived severity/seriousness (HBM) • Perceived parental barriers (HBM)	• Lack of information on bundled recommendation approach • Lack of skills delivering a bundled approach to all age-eligible patients • Delaying vaccination until adolescent is older • Belief that they may not be able to change parents' minds • Perceived parental belief their child is at low risk/does not need the vaccine • Belief that patient is at low risk • Identifying and addressing hesitancies will lead to increased vaccination • Recommending HPV with other adolescent vaccines will increase vaccinations	• Behavioral Capability (SCT) • Attitudes (SCT, TRA/TPB) • Self-Efficacy (SCT, TRA/TPB) • Skills (SCT, TRA/TPB) • Perceived Severity (HBM) • Normative Beliefs (TRA/TPB) • Outcome Expectations (SCT)

Table 6.13 Partial Matrix for Behavioral Outcome: Parents Obtain HPV Vaccine for Adolescent Children

	Personal Determinants						
Performance Objectives The parent will:	**Behavioral Capability (BC)**	**Attitude (A)**	**Skills & Self-Efficacy (SSE)**	**Perceived Benefits/ Barriers (Pbe) (Pba)**	**Perceived Susceptibility (PS)**	**Normative Beliefs (NB)**	**Outcome Expectations (OE)**
PO.2. Parents discuss the HPV vaccine with a healthcare provider	BC.2.a. Describe ways to initiate a conversation about the HPV vaccine with their child's physician	A.2.a. Express belief that doctor will take time to discuss concerns about the HPV vaccine	SSE.2.a. Express confidence in and demonstrate the ability to initiate a discussion about HPV and HPV vaccine and ask for provider specifications even if it is not mentioned	Pbe.2.a. Acknowledge that benefits of discussing HPV and HPV vaccine with the doctor outweigh barriers and feelings of discomfort or fear	PS.2.a. Express belief that their son/ daughter could be at risk of HPV infection at some point in their life	NB.2.a. Express belief that other parents like them are discussing the HPV vaccine with their son's/daughter's physician	OE.2.a. Express belief that discussing the HPV vaccine with a healthcare provider will address their concerns
PO.2.a. Parents ask the physician any questions or concerns about their son/daughter receiving the HPV vaccine		A.2.b. Express belief that discussing the HPV vaccine with healthcare provider will address concerns	SSE.2.b. Express confidence in and demonstrate ability to ask questions about the HPV vaccine for son/ daughter				
PO.4.a. Parents obtain the first HPV vaccine dose for son/daughter (for people who can vaccinate the same day)	BC.4a.a. State that they can get the vaccine for their son/daughter during the same appointment	A.4a.a. Express belief that vaccinating their son/ daughter during the same appointment could be beneficial and time/cost-effective	SSE.4a.a. Express confidence in and demonstrate the ability to request the vaccine while at the doctor's office	Pbe.4a.a. Acknowledge that the benefits of getting the HPV vaccine at the same visit outweigh the barriers of getting the vaccine during the same visit	Not applicable	NB.4a.a. Express belief that other parents like them vaccinate their daughter/son against HPV during the same visit	OE.4a.a. Express belief that if they request the HPV vaccine for their child, they will be able to obtain it during the same visit
PO.4.b. Parents obtain the first HPV vaccine dose for son/daughter (for people who cannot vaccinate the same day)	BC.4b.a. Describe where to call or go to obtain the vaccine for their son/daughter BC.4b.b. State that they may need to make an appointment to vaccinate their son/ daughter against HPV	A.4b.a. Express belief that it is important to make an appointment to obtain the vaccine A.4b.b. Express belief that it is their responsibility to obtain the appointment for vaccination	SSE.4b.a. Express confidence in and demonstrate the ability to make the appointment SSE.4b.b. Express confidence in and demonstrate the ability to keep child's appointment	Pbe.4b.a. Acknowledge that the benefits of keeping an appointment outweigh the barriers of getting to the appointment	Not applicable	NB.4b.a. Express belief that other parents like them are making & keeping appointments to vaccinate their son/ daughter against HPV	OE.4b.a. Express belief that if they make an appointment for their son/daughter to obtain the HPV vaccine, they will be able to keep the appointment

Table 6.14 Partial Matrix for Interpersonal Environmental Outcome: Medical Doctors/Physicians/Nurse Practitioners Vaccinate Eligible Patients

Performance Objectives MDs/Physicians/Nurse Practitioners will:	Personal Determinants					
	Behavioral Capability (BC)	**Skills and Self-Efficacy (SSE)**	**Attitudes (A)**	**Outcome Expectations (OE)**	**Perceived Severity (PSEV)**	**Normative Beliefs (NB)**
PO.2. Consistently deliver strong "bundled" and "unqualified" HPV vaccination recommendation to parents of all eligible patients at time of visit PO.2.a. Deliver bundled HPV vaccination recommendation with Tdap and MCV, if adolescent aged 11–12 PO.2.b. Deliver unqualified recommendations for HPV vaccine initiation, if patients 13–17 have not initiated	BC.2.a. Describe CDC recommendation that providers deliver strong "bundled and unqualified" HPV vaccine recommendation for all eligible patients BC.2.b. Describe CDC recommendation to provide a "bundled" recommendation with Tdap and MCV, if adolescent aged 11–12 BC.2.c. Describe that receiving a strong "bundled and unqualified" recommendation for the HPV vaccine is a significant predictor of vaccine uptake BC.2.d. Describe that part of a strong recommendation includes a cancer prevention message	SSE.2.a. Express confidence in and demonstrate ability to deliver a strong "bundled and unqualified" HPV vaccine recommendation to all eligible patients SSE.2.b. Express confidence in and demonstrate ability to deliver a bundled vaccine recommendation with Tdap and MCV, if adolescent aged 11–12 SSE.2.c. Express confidence in and demonstrate ability to deliver unqualified HPV vaccine recommendation for HPV vaccine initiation, if patients 13–17 have not initiated	A.2.a. Express belief that parents are receptive to provider recommendations for HPV vaccine A.2.b. Express belief that parents have positive attitudes toward the HPV vaccine A.2.c. Express belief that parents have a perceived need for the HPV vaccine for their children A.2.d. Express belief that parents have positive attitudes toward preventative care for adolescents	OE.2.a. Express belief that delivering a strong "bundled and unqualified" HPV vaccine recommendation will reduce parental or patient hesitancy and refusal of vaccine OE.2.b. Express belief that delivering a "bundled and unqualified" HPV vaccination recommendation with Tdap and MCV can save time during appointment OE.2.c. Express belief that delivering a "bundled and unqualified" HPV vaccine recommendation with Tdap and MCV will reduce parental or patient hesitancy and refusal of the HPV vaccine OE.2.e. Express belief that delivering a "bundled and unqualified" HPV vaccine recommendation at current appointment will increase vaccination rates in clinic	PSEV.2.a. Describe why delivering a strong "bundled" and "unqualified" HPV vaccine recommendation to all eligible patients is critical to tackle HPV-associated diseases	NB.2.a. Describe why delivering a strong "bundled and unqualified" HPV vaccine recommendation with Tdap and MCV is recommended by the CDC NB.2.b. Describe why delivering a strong "bundled and unqualified" HPV vaccine recommendation supports the clinic's commitment to increasing vaccination rates among all eligible patients. NB.2.c. Describe why delivering a strong "bundled and unqualified" HPV vaccine recommendation is recommended by the CDC and other professional organizations NB.2.d. Express belief that Clinic Leadership wants all physicians to give a strong bundled, unqualified recommendation for HPV vaccine for all eligible patients

PO.3. Identify specific parental concerns if they express vaccine hesitancy and decision to delay vaccination PO.3.a. Identify specific concerns of older adolescent (>=15yrs) if they express vaccine hesitancy	BC.3.a. Describe common parental and adolescent (>=15yrs) concerns about HPV vaccine BC.3.b. Describe common parental/patient-related reasons to delay vaccination for adolescents (i.e., vaccine safety, efficacy, side effects, sexual disinhibition)	SSE.3.a. Express confidence in and demonstrate ability to identify parental and adolescent (>=15yrs) concerns or hesitancy toward HPV vaccine for adolescents		OE.3.a. Express belief that identifying and addressing parental concerns or hesitancy toward HPV vaccine will reduce vaccine refusal OE.3.b. Express belief that addressing parental and adolescent (>=15yrs) concerns will not take much time		NB.3.a. Express belief that other providers are identifying parental concerns about the HPV vaccine and reasons to delay vaccination
PO.4. Communicate tailored message to address specific concerns or hesitancies of parents/ older adolescents (>=15yrs), if present	BC.4.a. Describe recommended responses and talking points to address common parental/ older adolescents hesitancies about the HPV vaccine for adolescents BC.4.b. Describe recommended responses and talking points to address common parental/ older adolescents concerns about the HPV vaccine for adolescents	SSE.4.a. Express confidence in and demonstrate ability to tailor responses to hesitancies of parents/ older adolescents (>=15yrs) about the HPV vaccine SSE.4.b. Express confidence in and demonstrate ability to tailor responses to concerns of parents/ older adolescents (>=15yrs) about the HPV vaccine	A.4.a. Express belief that parents/older adolescents are receptive to tailored messages addressing their hesitancies A.4.b. Express belief that parents/older adolescents are receptive to tailored messages addressing their concerns	OE.4.a. Express belief that providing tailored responses to address common parental /older adolescents hesitancies can reduce hesitancy and refusal for the HPV vaccine OE.4.b. Express belief that providing tailored responses to address common parental /older adolescents concerns can reduce refusal for the HPV vaccine	Not applicable	Not applicable

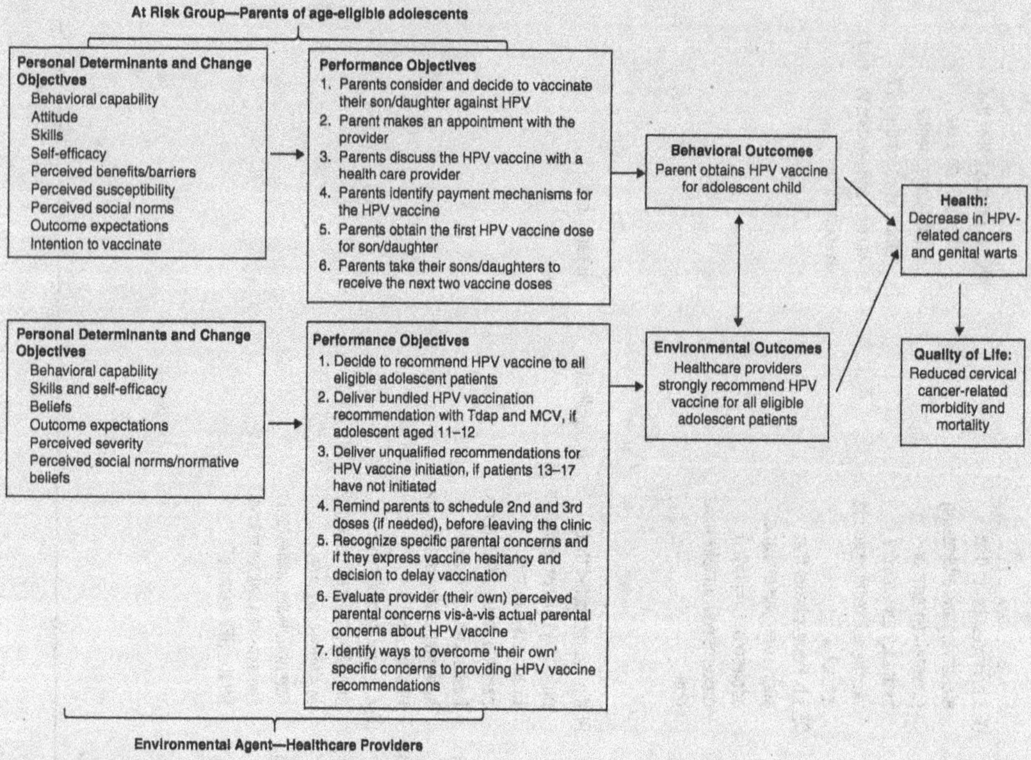

Figure 6.3 Por Nuestros Hijos Logic Model of Change

Summary

In Step 2 of Intervention Mapping, a transition is made from the needs assessment conducted in Step 1 to assessing what should change to prevent a health issue or improve health and quality-of-life outcomes. This transition is a shift from a logic model for causes of a health problem to a logic model for what changes will be addressed by an intervention. The starting points for this assessment are the program goals for health and quality-of-life stated at the end of Step 1. The first task in this step is to state the behavioral and environmental outcomes (BO and EO) that need to be achieved to reach the program goals for improved health and quality-of-life. The second task is to subdivide each behavioral and environmental outcome into performance objectives (PO) that specify exactly what needs to change by whom so that the overall behavioral and environmental outcomes are accomplished.

The third task in Step 2 is to select potential important and changeable determinants for each behavioral and environmental outcome. Determinants are intrapersonal factors derived from behavioral science theory and evidence from empirical studies that suggest a change in the factors may influence a change in the behavior of the at-risk group or of environmental agents capable of changing environmental conditions. The final task is to create a matrix of change objectives for each behavioral and environmental outcome by linking the selected determinants to the performance objectives and forming cells to write change objectives. These change objectives represent what needs to be modified as a result of the intervention to influence performance objectives to achieve the behavioral and environmental outcomes. Thus, the matrix of change objectives describes the most immediate change to be addressed by the intervention and provides the detail for the selection of intervention methods and practical applications for the health promotion program in Step 3. In addition, the matrix of change objectives provides a basis for formulating questions and measurement instruments for the evaluation of the health promotion intervention.

Most program planning will require multiple matrices to address the behavior of the at-risk population as well as describe each level of the environment to be addressed by the intervention. In some cases, it is necessary to break down the population into subpopulations due to important differences in behavior, performance objectives, or determinants and to create separate matrices of change objectives for each group. The final product of Step 2 of the Intervention Mapping process is a set of matrices that specifies the immediate objectives of a health promotion intervention.

Discussion Questions and Learning Activities

1. In Step 2 of IM, the program planners make the transition from a risk model created in Step 1 to a change model that describes what the intervention will change to achieve the health outcome goal. Construct a logic model that illustrates the causal pathways for influencing achievement of the health outcome goal and impact on QOL.
2. Explain why it is important to be very specific when stating behavioral and environmental outcomes.
3. Give examples of the questions planners can use to: (a) state the behavioral and environmental outcomes to be achieved by a health promotion program; (b) subdivide behavioral and environmental outcomes into performance objectives (PO); and (c) write change objectives for the cells of the matrices.
4. For the health problem and population you selected for the needs assessment in Step 1 (Chapter 5), state the behavioral and environmental outcomes to be accomplished by the intervention. What will your intervention try to change? Justify your decisions using evidence from the literature.
5. Priority population differentiation: Whom is this intervention meant to affect? Are there important subgroups? On what variables should the population be grouped? Explain the rationale for differentiation or non-differentiation into subgroup for planning the program.

6. PO: Specify PO for the health behavioral and environmental outcomes for at least one of the priority groups you have differentiated. Briefly describe the process you would use to validate these PO.
7. Specify determinants of health behaviors and environmental outcomes. Specify and justify, using theory and empirical findings, the most important personal determinants for each behavioral outcome and environmental outcome (i.e., those most important to address in your program). Describe any new research you would plan to supplement what you are able to ascertain from the literature.
8. Change Objectives: For each health behavioral and environmental outcome, create matrices to write change objectives and give at least one example in each relevant cell of the matrix.

References

Agarwal, R. P., & Maroko-Afek, A. (2018). Yoga into cancer care: A review of the evidence-based research. *International Journal of Yoga, 11*(1), 3–29.

Alagiyawanna, A., Rajapaksa-Hewageegana, N., & Gunawardena, N. (2017). The impact of multiple interventions to reduce household exposure to second-hand tobacco smoke among women: a cluster randomized controlled trial in Kalutara district, Sri Lanka. *BMC Public Health, 17*(1), 810.

Alzyood, M., Jackson, D., Aveyard, H., & Brooke, J. (2020). COVID-19 reinforces the importance of handwashing. *Journal of Clinical Nursing, 29*(15-16), 2760.

American Cancer Society. (2020). Colorectal Cancer Screening Test. Early Detection, Diagnosis, and Staging: American Cancer Society. https://www.cancer.org/cancer/colon-rectal-cancer/detection-diagnosis-staging.html.

Armstrong, P. (2015). *Bloom's taxonomy*. Nashville: Vanderbilt University Center for Teaching.

Azagba, S., Shan, L., & Latham, K. (2020). E-cigarette retail licensing policy and e-cigarette use among adolescents. *Journal of Adolescent Health, 66*(1), 123–125.

Bandura, A. (1986). *Social foundations of thought and action: A social cognitive theory*. Englewood Cliffs, NJ: Prentice-Hall.

Bandura, A. (1997). *Self—efficacy: The exercise of control 'a0*. New York, NY: W.H. Freeman.

Bandura, A. (2004). Health promotion by social cognitive means. *Health Education & Behavior, 31*(2), 143–164.

Bandura, A. (2006). On integrating social cognitive and social diffusion theories. In A. Singhal & J. Dearing (Eds.), *Communication of innovations: A journey with Ev Rogers* (pp. 111–134). Thousand Oaks, CA: Sage.

Bauer, J. E., Hyland, A., Li, Q., Steger, C., & Cummings, K. M. (2005). A longitudinal assessment of the impact of smoke—free worksite policies on tobacco use. *American Journal of Public Health, 95*(6), 1024–1029.

Beelen, R., Raaschou-Nielsen, O., Stafoggia, M., Andersen, Z. J., Weinmayr, G., Hoffmann, B., et al. (2014). Effects of long-term exposure to air pollution on natural-cause mortality: an analysis of 22 European cohorts within the multi-centre ESCAPE project. *The Lancet, 383*(9919), 785–795.

Been, S. K., va de Vijver, D. A. M. C., Nieuwkerk, P. T., Brito, I., Stutterheim, S. E., Bos, A. R. R., Wolfers, M. E. G., Pogany, K., & Verbon, A. (2016). Risk factors for non-adherence to cART in immigrants with HIV living in the Netherlands: Results from the ROtterdam ADherence (ROAD) project. *Public Library of Science (PLoS One), 11*(10), e0162800.

Beets, M. W., Cardinal, B. J., & Alderman, B. L. (2010). Parental social support and the physical activity—related behaviors of youth: a review. *Health Education & Behavior, 37*(5), 621–644.

Bernard Vrijens, B., Geest, S. D., Hughes, D. A., Przemyslaw, K., Demonceau, J., Ruppar, T., Dobbels, F., Fargher, E., Morrison, V., Lewek, P., Matysjaszcyk, M., Mshelia, C., Clyne, W., Aronson, J. K., & Urquhart, J. (2012). A new taxonomy for describing and defining adherence to medications. *British Journal of Clinical Pharmacology, 73*(5), 691–705.

Birken, S. A., Wagi, C. R., Peluso, A. G., Kegler, M. C., Baloh, J., Adsul, P., et al. (2023). Toward a more comprehensive understanding of organizational influences on implementation: the organization theory for implementation science framework. *Frontiers in Health Services, 3*, 1142598.

Bolton, K. A., Kremer, P., Gibbs, L., Waters, E., Swinburn, B., & de Silva, A. (2017). The outcomes of health-promoting communities: Being active eating well initiative—a community-based obesity prevention intervention in Victoria. *Australia. International Journal of Obesity, 41*, 1080–1090.

Bos, A., Pryor, J., Reeder, G., & Stutterheim, S. (2013). Stigma: Advances in theory and research. *Basic and Applied Social Psychology, 35*(1), 1–9.

Caffarella, R. (1985). *Planning programs for adult learners: A practical guide for educators, trainees, and staff developers 'a0.* San Francisco, CA: Jossey-Bass.

Campbell, K. L., Winters-stone, K. M., Wiskemann, J., May, A. M., Schwartz, A. L., Courneya, K. S., Zucker, D. S., Matthews, C. E., Ligibel, J. A., Gerber, L. H., Morris, G. S., Patel, A. V., Hue, T. F., Perna, F. M., & Schmitz, K. H. (2019). Exercise guidelines for cancer survivors: Consensus statement from international multidisciplinary roundtable. *Medicine and Schience in Sports and Exercise, 51*(11), 2375–2390.

Cappuccio, F. P., Beer, M., & Strazzullo, P. (2019). Population dietary salt reduction and the risk of cardiovascular disease. A scientific statement from the european salt action network. *Nutrition, Metabolism, and Cardiovascular Diseases, 29*, 107–114.

Carvalho, T., Alvarez, M. J., Barz, M., & Schwarzer, R. (2015). Preparatory behavior for condom use among heterosexual young men: A longitudinal mediation model. *Health Education & Behavior, 42*(1), 92–99.

Centers for Disease Control and Prevention (CDC). (2024). *Youth Online- YRBS.* Centers for Disease Control and Prevention. https://youthonline.cdc.gov/

Chandrasekharan, S., Heaney, C., James, T., Conover, C., & Cook-Deegan, R. (2010). Impact of gene patents and licensing practices on access to genetic testing for cystic fibrosis. *Genetics in Medicine, 12*(4), S194.

Charlesworth, R. (2017). *Understanding child development* (10th ed.). Boston, MA: Cengage Learning.

Chobanian, A. V., Bakris, G. L., Black, H. R., Cushman, W. C., Green, L. A., Izzo, J. L., Jr., et al. (2003). Seventh report of the joint national committee on prevention, detection, evaluation, and treatment of high blood pressure. *Hypertension, 42*(6), 1206–1252.

Clark, N. (2003). Management of chronic disease by patients. *Annual Review of Public Health, 24*(1), 289–213.

Clark, N., & Zimmerman, B. (2014). A social cognitive view of self-regulated learning about health. *Health Education & Behavior, 41*(5), 485–491.

Clark, N. M., Gong, M., & Kaciroti, N. (2014). A model of self—regulation for control of chronic disease. *Health Education & Behavior, 41*(5), 499–508.

Coffield, E., Nihiser, A. J., Sherry, B., & Economos, C. D. (2015). Shape up somerville: Change in parent body mass indexes during a child—targeted, community—based environmental change intervention. *American Journal of Public Health, 105*(2), e83–e89.

Collins, S. (2019) Big P, little p—a guide to policy engagement at all levels. Association of Maternal & Child Health Programs.

Craig, P., Dieppe, P., Macintyre, S., Michie, S., Nazareth, I., & Petticrew, M. (2008). Developing and evaluating complex interventions: The new medical research council guidance. *British Medical Journal, 337*, a1655.

Crutzen, R., Peters, G.-J. Y., & Noijen, J. (2017). Using confidence interval-based estimation of relevance to select social-cognitive determinants for behavior change interventions. *Frontiers in Public Health*, 5.165.

DiClemente, C. C., & Prochaska, J. O. (1998). Toward a comprehensive transtheoretical model of change 'a0. In W. Miller & N. Heather (Eds.), *Treating addictive behaviors* (pp. 3–24). New York, NY: Plenum Press.

Dima, A. L., Gibbons, C., Kleppe, M., Byrka, K., De Bruin, M., & Johnston, M. (2014). The opportunities item response theory (IRT) offers to health psychologists methods in health psychology symposium IV. *European Health Psychologist, 16*(6), 249–259.

Dineen-Griffin, S., Garcia-Cardenas, V., WIlliams, K., & Benrimoj, S. I. (2019). Helping patients help themselves: A systematic reivew of self management support strategies in primary health care practice. *PLoS One, 14*(8), e0220116.

DiNenno, E. A., Prejean, J., Irwin, K., Delaney, K. P., Bowles, K., Martin, T., Tailor, A., Dumitru, G., Mullins, M. M., Hutchinson, A. B., & Lansky, A. (2017). Recommendations for HIV screening of gay, bisexual, and other men who have sex with men—United States, 2017. *Morbidity and Mortality Weekly Report (MMWR), 66*(31), 830–832.

Escobar-Chaves, S. L., Markham, C. M., Addy, R. C., Greisinger, A., Murray, N. G., & Brehm, B. (2010). The fun families study: Intervention to reduce children's TV viewing. *Obesity, 18*(1), S99.

Evangelista, L. S., & Shinnick, M. A. (2008). What do we know about adherence and self-care? *The Journal of Cardiovascular Nursing, 23*(3), 250–257.

Febres, J. D., García-Herrero, S., Herrera, S., Gutiérrez, J., López-García, J. R., & Mariscal, M. A. (2020). Influence of seat-belt use on the severity of injury in traffic accidents. *European Transport Research Review, 12*(1), 1–12.

Gesesew, H. A., Gebremedhin, A. T., Demissie, T. D., Kerie, M. W., Sudhakar, M., & Mwanri, L. (2017). Significant association between perceived HIV related stigma and late presentation for HIV/AIDS care in low and middle-income countries: A systematic review and meta-analysis. *Public Library of Science (PLoS One).*, *12*(3), e0173928.

Giovenco, D. P., Casseus, M., Duncan, D. T., Coups, E. J., Lewis, M. J., & Delnevo, C. D. (2016). Association between electronic cigarette marketing near schools and E-cigarette use among youth. *Journal of Adolescent Health, 59*(6), 627–634.

Glasgow, R. E., Klesges, L. M., Dzewaltowski, D. A., Estabrooks, P. A., & Vogt, T. M. (2006). Evaluating the impact of health promotion programs: Using the RE-AIM framework to form summary measures for decision making involving complex issues. *Health Education Research, 21*(5), 688–694.

Gollwitzer, P. M., Martiny-Huenger, T., & Oettingen, G. (2014). Affective consequences of intentional action control. In A. J. Elliot (Ed.), *Advances in motivation scienceà0* (Vol. 1, pp. 49–84). San Diego, CA: Academic Press.

Hagerty, B. M., Bathish, M. A., & Kuchman, E. (2020). Development and testing of a self-regulation model for recurrent depression. *Journal of Health Psychology, 25*(10-11), 1732–1742.

Halliday, J. A., Speight, J., Russell-Green, S., Eric, O., Hagger, V., Morris, A., Sturt, J., & Hendieckx, C. (2021). Developing a novel diabetes distress e-learning program for diabetes educators: An intervention mapping approach. *Translational Behavioral Medicine, 11*, 1264.

Harden, S. M., Smith, M. L., Ory, M. G., Smith-Ray, R. L., Estabrooks, P. A., & Glasgow, R. E. (2018). RE-AIM in clinical, community, and corporate settings: Persceptives, strategies, and recommendations to enhance public health impact. *Frontiers in Public Health, 22*, 6.

Harrington, K. F., & Valerio, M. A. (2014). A conceptual model of verbal exchange health literacy. *Patient Education and Counseling, 94*(3), 403–410.

Heijmans, M., Waverijn, G., Rademakers, J., van der Vaart, R., & Rijken, M. (2015). Functional, communicative and critical health literacy of chronic disease patients and their importance for self—management. *Patient Education and Counseling, 98*(1), 41–48.

Helakorpi, S. A., Martelin, T. P., Torppa, J. O., Patja, K. M., Kiiskinen, U. A., Vartiainen, E. A., & Uutela, A. K. (2008). Did the tobacco control act amendment in 1995 affect daily smoking in Finland? Effects of a restrictive workplace smoking policy. *Journal of Public Health (Oxford, England), 30*(4), 407–414.

Holt-Lunstad, J., & Uchino, B. (2015). Social support and health behavior. In K. Glanz, B. Rimer, & K. Viswanath (Eds.), *Health behavior: Theory, research and practice* (5th ed., pp. 183–204). San Francisco, CA: Jossey-Bass.

Hong, M., Thind, A., Zaric, G. S., & Sarma, S. (2020). The impact of improved access to after-hours primary care on emergency department and primary care utilization: A systematic review. *Health Policy, 124*(8), 812–818.

Hopkins, D. P., Razi, S., Leeks, K. D., Kalra, G. P., Chattopadhyay, S. K., Soler, R. E., Force, T., & on Community Preventive S (2010). Smokefree policies to reduce tobacco use: A systematic review. *American Journal of Preventive Medicine, 38*(2), S275–S289.

Katz, I. T., Ryu, A. E., Onuegbu, A. G., Psaros, C., Weiser, S. D., Bangsberg, D. R., & Tsai, A. C. (2013). Impact of HIV-related stigma on treatment adherence: Systematic review and meta-synthesis. *Journal of the International AIDS Society, 16*, 18640.

Kisling, L. A., & Das, J. M. (2022). *Prevention strategies*. StatPearls: StatPearls Publishing.

Kroese, F. M., Adriaanse, M. A., Vinkers, C. D. W., van de Schoot, R., & de Ridder, D. T. D. (2014). The effectiveness of a proactive coping intervention targeting self-management in diabetes patients. *Psychology & Health, 29*(1), 110–125.

Kwan, M. Y., & Gordon, K. H. (2016). The effects of social support and stress perception on bulimic behaviors and unhealthy food consumption. *Eating Behaviors, 22*, 34–39.

Labarthe, D. R. (1998). *Epidemiology and prevention of cardiovascular diseases: A global challenge*. Gaithersburg, MD: Aspen.

Lantz, B. (2013). The large sample size fallacy. *Scandinavian Journal of Caring Sciences, 27*, 487–492.

Lawman, H. G., Henry, K. A., Scheeres, A., Hillengas, A., Coffman, R., & Strasser, A. A. (2020). Tobacco retail licensing and density 3 years after license regulations in PHiladelphia, Pennsylvania (2012-2019). *American Journal of Public Health, 110*(4), 547–553.

Lyimo, R. A., Stutterheim, S. E., Hospers, H. J., de Glee, T., van der Ven, A., & de Bruin, M. (2014). Stigma, disclosure, coping, and medication adherence among people living with HIV/AIDS in Northern Tanzania. *AIDS Patient Care and STDs, 28*(2), 98–105.

Markham C. M., Peskin, M., Shegog, R., Cuccaro, P., Gabay, E. K., Johnson-Baker, K., Swain-Ogbonna, H. I., Edwards, S., & Tortolero SR. (2017) Reducing sexual risk among racial/ethnic-minority ninth grade students: Using intervention mapping to modify an evidenced-based curriculum. *Journal of Applied Research on Children: Informing Policy for Children at Risk, 8*(1), 2.

Mathieu, J. E., & Taylor, S. R. (2007). A framework for testing meso-mediational relationships in organizational behavior. *Journal of Organizational Behavior: The International Journal of Industrial, Occupational and Organizational Psychology and Behavior, 28*(2), 141–172.

McGee R. E., Shegog R., & Sajatovic M. (2020) Self-management strategies – beyond AEDs. In J. French, P. Engel, & N. Moshe (Eds.), *Section 7 General Treatment Considerations. Epilepsy: A comprehensive textbook.* (3rd ed.). Lippincott Williams & Wilkins *In press*.

Mesters, I., Gijsbers, B., & Bartholomew, L. K. (2018). Promoting sustained breastfeeding of infacts at risk for asthma: Explaining the "active ingredients" of an effective program using intervention mapping. *Frontiers in Public Health, 6*, 87.

Metz, G., Peters, G.-J. Y., & Crutzen, R. (2022). Acyclic behavior change diagrams: A tool to report and analyze interventions. *Health Psychology and Behavioral Medicine, 10*(1), 1216–1228.

Milgrom, J., Hirshler, Y., Reece, J., Holt, C., & Gemmill, A. W. (2019). Social support—a protective factor for depressed pernatal women? *International Journal of Environmental Research and Public Health, 16*, 1426.

Mkhitaryan, S., Giabbanelli, P. J., de Vries, N. K., & Crutzen, R. (2020). Dealing with complexity: How to use a hybrid approach to incorporate complexity in health behavior interventions. *Intelligence-Based Medicine, 3*, 100008.

Natowicz, M. R., & Prence, E. M. (1996). Heterozygote screening for Tay—Sachs disease: Past successes and future challenges. *Current Opinion in Pediatrics, 8*(6), 625–629.

National Cancer Institute (NCI) (2021). *Office of cancer survivorship.* National Cancer Institute.

Nidecker, M., DiClemente, C. C., Bennett, M. E., & Bellack, A. S. (2008). Application of the transtheoretical model of change: Psychometric properties of leading measures in patients with co—occurring drug abuse and severe mental illness. *Addictive Behaviors, 33*(8), 1021–1030.

Nieuwlaat, R., Wilczynski, N., Navarro, T., Hobson, N., Jeffery, R., Keepanasseril, A., Agoritsas, T., Mistry, N., Iorio, A., Jack, S., Sivaramalingam, B., Iserman, E., Mustafa, R. A., Jedraszewski, D., Cotoi, C., & Haynes, R. B. (2014). Interventions for enhancing medication adherence. *The Cochrane Database of Systematic Reviews, 11,* CD000011.

Office of Disease Prevention and Health Promotion (ODPHP) (2021). *Social Determinants of Health.* https://health. gov/healthypeople/priority- areas/ social- determinants-health.

Palamar, J. J., & Barratt, M. J. (2019). Prevalence of reagent test-kit use and perceptions of purity among ecstasy users in an electronic dance music scene in New York City. *Drug and Alcohol Review, 38,* 42–49.

Paskett, E., Thompson, B., Ammerman, A. S., Ortega, A. N., Marsteller, J., & Richardson, D. (2016). Multilevel interventions to address health disparities show promise in improving population health. *Health Affairs, 35*(8), 1429–1434.

Peskin, M. F., Markham, C. M., Gabay, E. K., Shegog, R., Cuccaro, P. M., Temple, J. R., et al. (2018). Using intervention mapping to develop "Me & You: Building Healthy Relationships," a healthy relationship intervention for early middle school students. In D. A. Wolfe & J. R. Temple (Eds.), *Adolescent dating violence* (pp. 467–501). San Diego: Academic Press.

Peskin, M. F., Markham, C. M., Shegog, R., Baumler, E. R., Addy, R. C., Temple, J. R., Hernandez, B., Cuccaro, P. M., Thiel, M. A., Gabay, E. K., & Tortolero-Emery, S. R. (2019). Adolescent dating violence prevention program for early adolescents: The me & you randomized controlled trial, 2014-2015. *AJPH Open-Themed Research, 109*(10), 1419.

Peskin, M. F., Markham, C. M., Shegog, R., Baumler, E. R., Addy, R. C., & Tortolero, S. R. (2014). Effects of the it's your game...keep it real program on dating violence in ethnic-minority middle school youths: A group randomized trial. *American Journal of Public Health, 104*(8), 1471–1477.

Peters, G.-J. Y. (2014). A practical guide to effective behavior change: How to identify what to change in the first place. *The European Health Psychologist, 16,* 142–155.

Peters, G.-J. Y., Abraham, C., & Crutzen, R. (2012). Full disclosure: Doing behavioural science necessitates sharing. *The European Health Psychologist, 14,* 77–84.

Petticrew, M. (2011). When are complex interventions 'complex'? When are simple interventions 'simple'? *European Journal of Public Health, 21*(4), 397–399.

Plaete, J., De Bourdeaudhuij, I., Verloigne, M., Oenema, A., & Crombez, G. (2015). A self-regulation ehealth intervention to increase healthy behavior through general practice: Protocol and systematic development. *JMIR Research Protocols, 4*(4), e4835.

Porthe, V., Garcia-Subirats, I., Ariza, C., Villalbi, J. R., Bartroli, M., Juarez, O., & Diez, E. (2020). Community-based interventions to reduce alcohol consumption and alcohol-related harm in adults. *Journal of Community Health, 46*(3), 565–576.

Pot, M., Ruiter, R. A. C., Paulussen, T. W. G. M., Heuvelink, A., de Melker, H. E., van Vliet, H. J. A., & van Keulen, H. M. (2018). Systematicallly developing a web-based tailored intervention promoting HPV-vaccination acceptability among mothers of invited girls using intervention mapping. *Frontiers in Public Health, 6*, 226.

Robson, M. E., Bradbury, A. R., Arun, B., Domchek, S. M., Ford, J. M., Hampel, H. L., Lipkin, S. M., Syngal, S., Wollins, D. S., & Lindor, N. M. (2015). American society of clinical oncology policy statement update: Genetic and genomic testing for cancer susceptibility. *Journal of Clinical Oncology, 33*(31), 3660.

Rodriguez, S. A., Mullen, P. D., Lopez, D. M., Savas, L. S., & Fernandez, M. E. (2020). Factors associated with adolescent HPV vaccination in the US: A systematic review of reviews and multilevel framework to inform intervention development. *Preventive Medicine, 131*, 105968.

Rodriguez, S. A., Savas, L. S., Baumler, E., Nyitray, A. G., Mullen, P. D., Vernon, S. W., & Fernandez, M. E. (2018). Parental predictors of HPV vaccine initiation among low-income Hispanic females aged 11–17 years. *Vaccine, 36*(33), 5084–5090.

Rollins, L., Carey, T., Proeller, A., Adams, M. A., Hooker, M., Lyn, R., Taylor, O., Holden, K., & Akintobi, T. H. (2021). Community-based participatory approach to increase African Americans' access to healthy foods in Atlanta. *GA. Journal of Community Health, 46*, 41–50.

Roozen, S., Stutterheim, S., Bos, A., Kok, G., & Curfs, L. (2020). Understanding the social stigma of fetal alcohol spectrum disorders: From theory to interventions. *Foundations of Science*. doi:10.1007/s10699-020-09676-y

Rothman, A., Baldwin, A., & Hertel, A. (2004). Self-regulation and behavior change. In R. Baumeister & K. Vohs (Eds.), *Handbook of self-regulation: Research, theory, and applications* (pp. 130–148). New York, NY: Guilford Press.

Rust, C. F., Davis, C., & Moore, M. R. (2015). Medication adherence skills training for african—american breast cancer survivors: The effects on health literacy, medication adherence, and self—efficacy. *Social Work in Health Care, 54*(1), 33–46.

Sallis, J., & Owen, N. (2015). Ecological models of health behavior. In K. Glanz, B. Rimer, & K. Viswanath (Eds.), *Health behavior: Theory, research, and practice* (pp. 43–64). 11: Jossey-Bass.

Sallis, J. F., Cervero, R. B., Ascher, W., Henderson, K. A., Kraft, M. K., & Kerr, J. (2006). An ecological approach to creating active living communities. *Annual Review of Public Health, 27*, 297–322.

Sallis, J. F., & Glanz, K. (2009). Physical activity and food environments: Solutions to the obesity epidemic. *Milbank Quarterly, 87*(1), 123–154.

Sedivy NZ, Podlogar, T., Kerr, D. C., & De Leo D. (2017). Community social support as a protective factor against suicide: A gender-specific ecological study of 75 regions of 23 European countries. *Health & Place, 48*, 40–46.

Serra, Y. A., Colón-López, V., Savas, L. S., Vernon, S. W., Fernández-Espada, N., Vélez, C., et al. (2017). Using intervention mapping to develop health education components to increase colorectal cancer screening in Puerto Rico. *Frontiers in Public Health, 5*, 324.

Shah, A. V. V., Langrish, J. P., Nair, H., McAllister, D. A., Hunter, A. L., Donaldson, K., Newby, D. E., & Mills, N. L. (2013). Global association of air pollution and heart failure: A systematic review and meta-analysis. *The Lancet, 382*, 1039–1048.

Shakya, I., Shults, R. A., Stevens, M. R., Beck, L. F., & Sleet, D. A. (2020). State-level seat belt use in the United States, 2011–2016: Comparison of self-reported with observed use and use by fatally injured occupants. *Journal of Safety Research, 73*, 103–109.

Shapiro, C. L. (2018). Cancer survivorship. *The New England Journal of Medicine, 379*, 2438–2450.

Sheeran, P., Maki, A., Montanaro, E., Avishai-Yitshak, A., Bryan, A., Klein, W., et al. (2016). The impact of changing attitudes, norms, and self-efficacy on health-related intentions and behavior: A meta-analysis. *Health Psychology, 35*(11), 1178–1188.

Shegog, R., Bamps, Y. A., Patel, A., Kakacek, J., Escoffery, C., Johnson, E. K., & Ilozumba, U. O. (2013). Managing epilepsy well: emerging e—tools for epilepsy self—management. *Epilepsy & Behavior, 29*(1), 133–140.

Simoes, E. J., Hallal, P. C., Siqueira, F. V., Schmaltz, C., Menor, D., Malta, D. C., Duarte, H., Hino, A. A., Mielke, G. I., Pratt, M., & Reis, R. S. (2017). Effectiveness of a scaled up physical activity intervention in Brazil: A natural experiment. *Preventive Medicine, 103*, 566–572.

Smith, R. A., Andrews, K. S., Brooks, D., Fedewa, S. A., Manassaram-Baptiste, D., Saslow, D., & Wender, R. C. (2019). Cancer screening in the united states; 2019: A review of current american cancer society guidelines and current issues in cancer screening. *A Cancer Journal for Clinicians, 69*, 184–210.

Song, S., Shon, Z., Kang, Y., Kim, K., Han, S., Kang, M., & Oh, I. (2019). Source apportionment of VOCs and their impact on air quality and health in the megacity of Seoul. *Environmental Pollution, 247*, 763–774.

Springer, A., Evans, A., Ortuno, J., Salvo, D., & Arevalo, M. (2017). Health by design: Interweaving health promotion into environments and settings. *Frontiers in Public Health, 5*, 1–10.

Springer, A. E., Evans, A. E., Ortuño, J., Salvo, D., & Varela Arévalo, M. T. (2017). Health by design: Interweaving health promotion into environments and settings. *Frontiers in Public Health, 5*, 268.

Springer, A. E., Jaramillo, M. C. C., Gomez, Y. O., Case, K., & Wilkinson, A. (2015). School social cohesion, student-school connectedness, and bullying in Colombian adolescents. *Global Health Promotion, 23*(4), 37–48.

Springer, A. E., Kelder, S. H., Ranjit, N., Hochberg-Garrett, H., Crow, S., & Delk, J. (2012). Promoting physical activity and fruit and vegetable consumption through a community—school partnership: The effects of marathon kids'ae on low—income elementary school children in Texas. *Journal of Physical Activity and Health, 9*(5), 739.

Stange, K. C., Breslau, E. S., Dietrich, A. J., & Glasgow, R. E. (2012). State-of-the-art and future directions in multilevel interventions across the cancer control continuum. *Journal of the National Cancer Institute Monographs, 44*, 20–31.

Stetler, C. B., McQueen, L., Demakis, J., & Mittman, B. S. (2008). An organizational framework and strategic implementation for system—level change to enhance research—based practice: QUERI series. *Implementation Science, 3*(1), 1–11.

Stevens, V. L., Diver, W. R., Stoklosa, M., Flanders, W. D., Westmaas, J. L., Jemal, A., Drope, J. M., Gapstur, S. M., & Jacobs, E. J. (2017). *A prospective cohort study of cigarette prices and smoking cessation in older smokers*. American Association for Cancer Research.

Stutterheim, S. E., Bos, A. E., Pryor, J. B., Brands, R., Liebregts, M., & Schaalma, H. P. (2011). Psychological and social correlates of HIV status disclosure: The significance of stigma visibility. *AIDS Education and Prevention, 23*(4), 382–392.

Stutterheim, S. E., Bos, A. E., Shiripinda, I., de Bruin, M., Pryor, J. B., & Schaalma, H. P. (2012). HIV-related stigma in African and Afro-Caribbean communities in the Netherlands: Manifestations, consequences and coping. *Psychology & Health, 27*(4), 395–411.

Stutterheim, S. E., Brands, R., Baas, I., Lechner, L., Kok, G., & Bos, A. E. R. (2017). HIV status disclosure in the workplace: Positive and stigmatizing experiences of health care workers living with HIV. *The Journal of the Association of Nurses in AIDS Care, 28*(6), 923–937.

Sweeney, S. M., & Vanable, P. A. (2016). The association of HIV-related stigma to HIV medication adherence: A systematic review and synthesis of the literature. *AIDS and Behavior, 20*, 29–50.

Thapa, S., Hannes, K., Cargo, M., Buve, A., Aro, A. R., & Mathei, C. (2017). Building a conceptual framework to study the effect of HIV stigma-reduction intervention strategies on HIV test uptake: A scoping review. *The Journal of the Association of Nurses in AIDS Care, 28*(4), 545–560.

U.S. Department of Agriculture (USDA) and U.S. Department of Health and Human Services (DHHS). Dietary Guidelines for Americans, 2020–2025. 9th Edition. December 2020. Available at DietaryGuidelines.gov.

U.S. Department of Health and Human Services (DHHS) (2012). *Preventing tobacco use among youth and young adults: A report of the surgeon general*. Atlanta, GA: U.S. Department of Health and Human Services, Centers for Disease Control and Prevention, National Center for Chronic Disease Prevention and Health Promotion, Office on Smoking and Health.

U.S. Department of Health and Human Services (DHHS) (2014). *The health consequences of smoking—50 years of progress*. Atlanta, GA: U.S. Department of Health and Human Services, Centers for Disease Control and Prevention, Office on Smoking and Health.

U.S. Department of Health and Human Services (DHHS) (2018). *Physical activity guidelines for americans*. Washington, DC: US Department of Health and Human Services. Available from: https://health.gov/sites/default/files/2019-09/Physical_Activity_Guidelines_2nd_edition.pdf

U.S. Department of Health and Human Services (DHHS) (2020). *Smoking cessation: A report of the surgeon general*. Atlanta, GA: U.S. Department of Health and Human Services, Centers for Disease Control and Prevention, National Center for Chronic Disease Prevention and Health Promotion, Office on Smoking and Health.

U.S. Preventive Services Task Force (USPST) (2014). *Guide to clinical preventive services*. Rockville, MD: Agency for Healthcare Research and Quality.

U.S. Preventive Services Task Force (USPST) (2024). Screening for breast cancer: US preventive services task force recommendation statement. *Journal of the American Medical Association, 331*(22), 1918–1930.

Valaitis, R., Meagher-Stewart, D., Martin-Misener, R., Wong, S. T., MacDonald, M., & O'Mara, L. (2018). Organizational factors influencing successful primary care and public health collaboration. *BMC Health Services Research, 18*(1), 420.

van den Berg, A., Nielsen, A., Akhavan, N., Pulido, C. L., Basu, S., Hussaini, A., Jovanovic, C., Janda, K., Denis, L., & Ranjit, N. (2019). Design and evaluation of a coalition-led obesity initiative to promote healthy eating and physical activity in low-income, ethnically diverse communities: The Go! Austin/Vamos! Austin initiative. *Archives of Public Health, 77*(25), 1.

van Empelen, P., & Kok, G. (2008). Action—specific cognitions of planned and preparatory behaviors of condom use among Dutch adolescents. *Archives of Sexual Behavior, 37*(4), 626–640.

van Keulen, H. M., Otten, W., Ruiter, R. A. C., Fekkes, M., van Steenbergen, J., Dusseldorp, E., & Paulussen, T. W. G. M. (2013). Determinants of HPV vaccination intentions among Dutch girls and their mothers: A cross-sectional study. *BMC Public Health, 13*(111).

World Health Organization (WHO) (1948). *Preamble to the Constitution of the World Health Organization as adopted by the International Health Conference*, New York, 19–22 June, 1946. Geneva, Switzerland. p. 2.

Workowski, K. A., & Bolan, G. A. (2015). Sexually transmitted diseases treatment guidelines. *Morbidity and Mortality Weekly Report (MMWR), 64*(3), 1–135.

Zullig, L. L., Shaw, R. J., Shah, B. R., Peterson, E. D., Lindquist, J. H., Crowley, M. J., et al. (2015). Patient-provider communication, self—reported medication adherence, and race in a postmyocardial infarction population. *Patient Preference and Adherence, 9*, 311.

CHAPTER 7

INTERVENTION MAPPING STEP 3

Methods and Practical Applications

INTERVENTION MAPPING STEP 3 TASKS

1. Generate intervention ideas with the planning group
2. Choose theory- and evidence-based change methods
3. Select and design practical applications to deliver change methods

Background

In Step 3, planners work from the logic model of change (established in Step 2) begin to conceptualizing and designing the intervention. The final product of Step 3 is a series of concrete intervention ideas that are informed by theories about behavior and environmental change methods (theories of change, see Chapters 3 and 4). The main tasks in Step 3 are to brainstorm with the planning group potential interventions that could be feasible within the intervention setting, identify theory- and evidence-based behavior and environmental change methods that match with the identified personal determinant or environmental conditions, and translate these methods into practical applications that cover the change objectives, show adequate fit with the characteristics of the priority populations at the different ecological levels, and are feasible in the context in which the intervention will be implemented.

Most planning groups will have ideas about the program aspects as soon as they begin working through Intervention Mapping and will want to explore these ideas further at the start of Step 3. These might include ideas about how to best reach their priority populations as well as the practical applications and program materials that will be culturally congruent and can garner the attention of the participants.

The design task should be fun and creative, with scientific rigor going hand in hand. Regardless of the work style of the planning team, it is essential that within all program ideas, there are change methods that will be effective to influence the objectives in the change matrices developed in Step 2. Further, the team will want to keep in mind the parameters of the methods—the conditions under which the change methods have been shown effective—so that there is effective translation from change method to practical application to intervention program. For example, the health promoter who likes the idea of a nonsmoking contract should be aware that commitment is only effective as a method for increasing self-efficacy when the act of commitment has been made public (parameter for use). Therefore, contracts that individuals make in private settings may have positive effects as reminders, but they do not have the strong effect of public commitment (Ajzen et al., 2009).

In selecting change methods and practical applications, health promoters may take any of several routes based on their experience with theory and practice. Some will begin with the less abstract ideas about their program (delivery, themes, scope, and sequence) and then move to matching methods and their applications to change objectives and embedding the same in the program components. Others will move from change objectives to change methods and then to applications. Still others will move from objectives to applications and then back to the underlying change methods or will brainstorm methods and applications simultaneously. Referring to the previous example, a health promoter may think of public commitment as a theoretical method of change for increasing self-efficacy of adolescents to remain nonsmokers and then brainstorm about practical applications to apply that method. Another health promoter may think of a nonsmoking contract as a practical application for improving self-efficacy, later finding out from the literature that the underlying theoretical method is commitment. While reading about theory, the health promoter might also find alternatives to a nonsmoking contract that may have the same, or even better, results.

Change Methods and Practical Applications

The Intervention Mapping steps enable planners to develop a solid foundation for their program or intervention based in theory and evidence. Planners must find a balance between preliminary ideas for programs on the one hand and theory- and evidence-informed decisions for change methods, applications, and programs on the other hand. What planners think about the effectiveness of methods is not always congruent with the scientific evidence. For example, mass media campaigns may be useful for changing social norms, but probably seldom useful for increasing self-efficacy and skills. Fear-arousing messages may be popular with the representatives of the at-risk population and intermediates, but they often are not effective at influencing behavior (Kok et al., 2018; Peters et al., 2013).

In this chapter, we present various change methods for influencing different determinants, starting with methods for determinants that are related to change in the individual behavior of the priority population. Then we discuss methods for changing environmental conditions at the level of groups, organizations, communities, and public policy. We describe only a sample of methods that can be used to address change objectives, based on frequency in health promotion publications; there are many more. *A theory- and evidence-based change method* is a general technique for influencing the determinants of behaviors and environmental conditions. A *practical application* refers to the delivery of the change method in ways that fit the intervention population and the context in which the intervention will be conducted. For example, a change objective for an intervention might be to increase adolescents' self-efficacy to resist social pressure to use drugs. For the change objective of increasing self-efficacy, an intervention program might include the change methods of role modeling, skill training, guided practice with feedback, and reinforcement. One practical application for modeling could be a videotaped step-by-step demonstration by adolescents of how to resist peer pressure in situations they commonly encounter.

In another example, an environmental condition of adolescent drug use could be the availability of drugs for sale in neighborhoods where adolescents live, with a performance objective of the mayor getting police to actively enforce laws against neighborhood drug dealers. A change objective for this might be to increase the mayor's positive outcome expectations—for example, that this enforcement will save children's lives, be popular with constituents, be positively received by powerful groups in the city, and increase tourism to the city. The primary change method for this could be advocacy, which includes methods of information, persuasion, negotiation, and coercion. One application might be for influential neighborhood activists to hold a breakfast meeting with the mayor, neighborhood constituents, and key city opinion leaders. The activists might present detailed case histories of neighborhood teens, along with pictures of open drug dealing on the street. If the mayor does not respond to this application, the group might undertake, as additional practical applications, media advocacy with an exposé story calling for action by the mayor on the local television channel or a local social media platform (e.g., next door).

As shown in Figure 7.1, planners choose methods and applications to influence change objectives. *Change objectives* describe the desired changes in the determinants of performance objectives for health behavior and

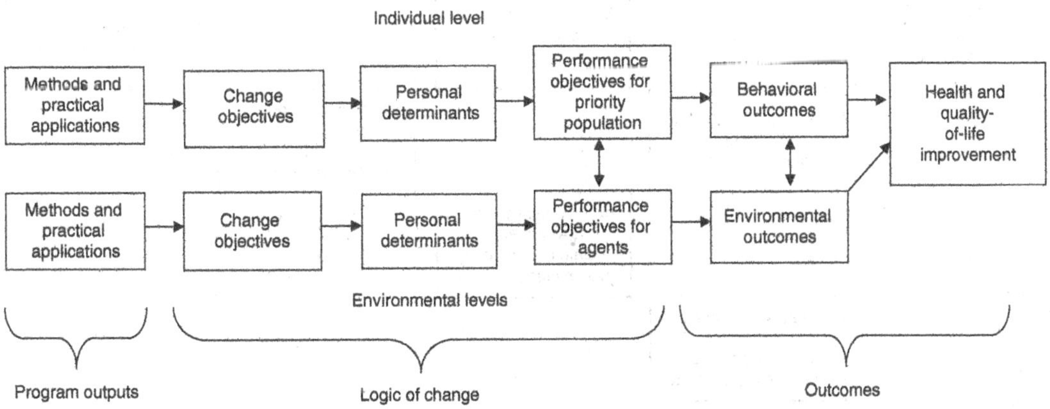

Figure 7.1 Intervention Logic Model

environmental conditions, at both individual and higher environmental levels. A change method may change individual health behavior, but the same change method could also be applied to influence the behavior of change agents in the individual's environment. For example, persuasive communication can be used to change attitudinal beliefs of the priority population and can also be used to convince line managers of the advantages of introducing a physical activity program for employees during work hours. Change agents, in turn, may apply that same or another change method to influence the behavior of the priority population. For example, an organization manager may incorporate the change method of positive reinforcement via providing incentives to influence employee behavior to increase physical activity. The same procedure of choosing change methods applies for the training of those who deliver the intervention to influence the priority population (see Chapter 9 on program implementation). Also, their behavior is influenced by personal determinants and environmental conditions. Figure 7.2 illustrates this cyclic process of environmental conditions being under the control of personal determinants and again environmental conditions (a process that then repeats again). Identified personal determinants are the endpoints of the causal chain and serve as targets for change methods at different environmental levels.

Parameters of Use

The difference between theoretical methods and practical applications can be confusing. Modeling is a method; use of role-model stories is an application; and demonstrations are applications. The point is that change methods should always be considered, and practical applications should never be

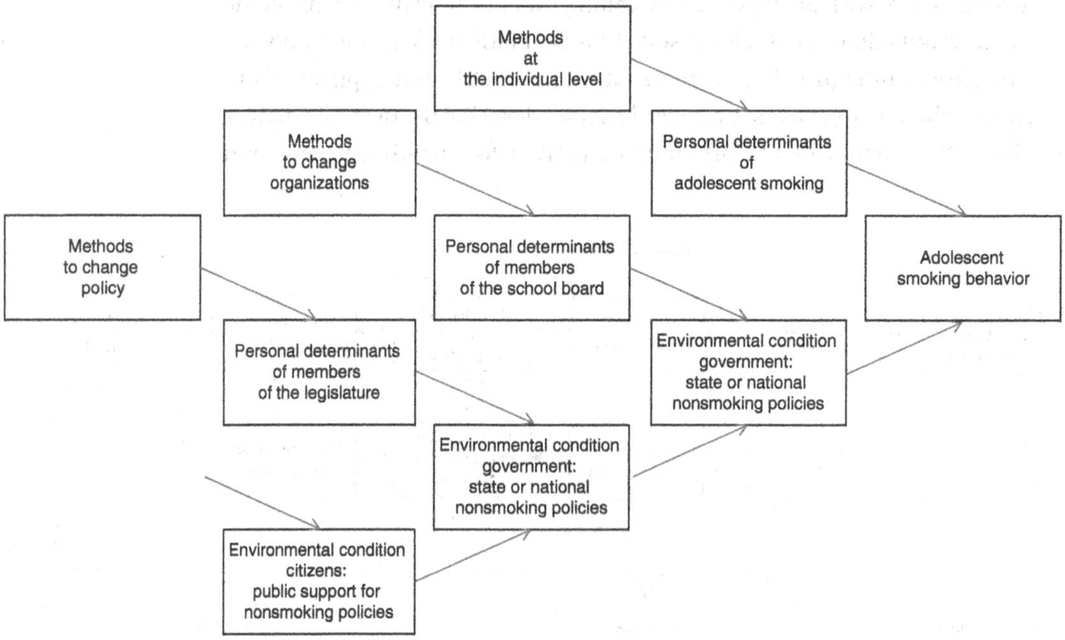

Figure 7.2 Schematic Representation of Shift in Environmental Levels

devoid of the effective component, that is, the change method. Yet methods are easy to overlook because health promoters often think in terms of concrete program components, such as a mobile phone app or a website, versus the more abstract concept of the theoretical method (e.g., providing information) that informs the practical application. Identifying the theoretical method, however, is important as it allows us to broaden our understanding of the active ingredients that may influence behavioral and environmental change by connecting to theory, which can provide a conceptual map to guide understanding and change for health promotion (see Chapters 3 and 4 on individual and organizational level theories).

There is no reason why planners cannot start with applications and then think about theoretical change methods. However, the essential question here is: Why would the particular application work? For every creative idea, there needs to be a theoretical process describing why the expected effects are going to happen. The central challenge in translating change methods into practical applications is to adhere to *parameters of use* within which the methods can be expected to be effective. These parameters describe the theoretical conditions under which the change methods have been shown effective (Kok et al., 2016).

In a recent example of an intervention promoting continued adherence to COVID-19 guidelines among students at Maastricht University in the Netherlands, the university's management team designed a New Year's message with the help of behavior scientists. The New Year's message to students targeted determinants of students' adherence to guidelines, and specific behaviors, in this case specifically keeping distance from others during the Christmas break, as most students go visiting their families and friends. Embedded in the New Year's message was a short documentary in which students who have had COVID-19 share what this disease has done and was still doing to them (Varol et al., 2021).

The New Year's message was carefully crafted combining the outcomes of a qualitative and quantitative determinants study, expertise on behavior change in the members of the planning group, and the available literature on effective methods for behavior change organized by determinant (Kok et al., 2016). Based on the observed risk behaviors from the survey and their determinants, the main focus was on (1) the limited group of students who indicated that they are "not afraid of contracting COVID-19 because I am young"; (2) students who feel responsible for telling other people "to adhere to the guidelines"; (3) students who "become tired of the whole situation"; and (4) students who indicate that the "prevention guidelines are difficult to adhere to." These four determinants were targeted by change methods that matched with the targeted determinants.

Figure 7.3 presents the New Year's message, with the change methods that were used indicated in the text and described below the text. For example, scenario-based risk information was used to target the determinant risk perception and was applied by including the message: "It is a well-established fact that young people can transmit COVID-19 without experiencing any

Good preparation for a better 2021

For most of us, 2020 has not been easy. People became seriously ill from COVID-19. Some lost loved ones to the virus. And our social lives were largely put on hold[a]. Many of you have taken responsibility, for yourselves and for others. You have consistently followed the government guidelines both on and off the UM campus[b]. That makes us proud and grateful[c].

Unfortunately, the end of the pandemic is not yet in sight[a]. That is why we are looking ahead to the upcoming holiday period and the beginning of 2021. Our message: please stay the course so that 2021 will be a better year for all of us[c].

Even if you are young!

It is a well-established fact that young people can transmit COVID-19 without experiencing any symptoms themselves[d]. So, even if you are young and think you are protected against the effects of COVID-19, you can still be a danger to others[d]. Imagine how you would feel if someone else who is vulnerable were to become infected with COVID-19 because of you[e]. This could happen while you are visiting your family during the Christmas holidays, as well as if you stay in Maastricht and fail to follow the safety protocols[f]. Therefore, however healthy and strong you may feel, make sure you keep your distance and follow the guidelines as long as the pandemic persists[g]. This is how you can help to ensure that society returns to normal[h].

Sometimes young people do not feel sick if they have COVID-19. But often they do[i]. In this short documentary, students who have had COVID-19 share what this disease has done and is still doing to them[j,k]. They also let us know what they think of the measures[l,m].

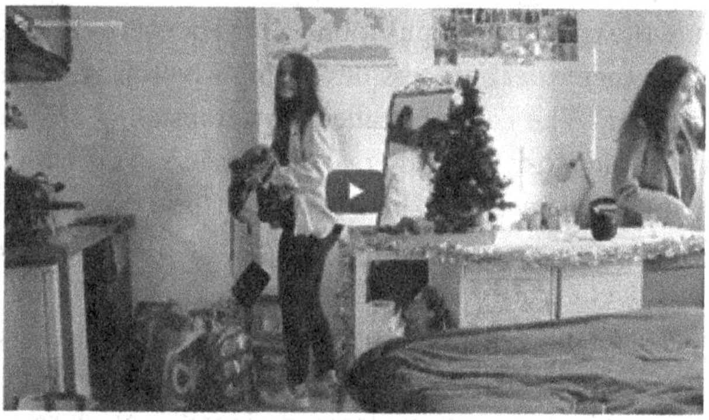

Good preparation...

Nobody underestimates how difficult it is—keeping your distance, few social contacts, not celebrating the holidays with your entire family and all your friends[a]. You can make it easier on yourself by thinking about it now. Prepare in advance, so you know what you are going to do to stay healthy and safe during the holiday period[n]. That way, you know what lies ahead. For example, you could follow these tips:

- Discuss in advance with your family and friends how to get through the holidays safely. For instance, create a top-10 list of safe activities that you can do together and make agreements on how to protect each other[n].
- Head outdoors and take a walk in nature while staying 1.5 meters away from each other[n].
- Keeping a physical distance doesn't mean you can't have social contacts. Celebrate New Year's via Zoom or another platform[n]. If we all do it, this will hopefully be the first and last time it needs to be done[o].
- Organize social gatherings in such a way that it is easy to keep your distance[n].
- If you have friends who don't want to follow the guidelines, don't invite them[p]. Also, don't visit people who are breaking the rules[p]. That might sound strict, but by doing this, you are helping a huge group of people[c]. Remember, the more people and the closer together they are, the faster the virus spreads[a,d].
- Very important: don't go to a social gathering if you have symptoms of COVID-19[a,d]. You can always call for a quick and easy test and stay at home until you have the results[n]. Of course, don't visit anyone if you have any symptoms, even if they are mild[n].

...makes for a better 2021!

A vaccine will be available in 2021. It will take a while before everyone gets their turn, but then we can move on to a new normal[c]. Until then, as a UM community, we will also follow the guidelines. It is a question of perseverance, however difficult it may be, but we are doing it for our friends, our families, the vulnerable in our society, and for ourselves[c]. Together, we will overcome[h,l].

Happy holidays and come back healthy!

a: Consciousness raising
b: Feedback
c: Reinforcement
d: Scenario-based risk information
e: Anticipated regret
f: Punishment
g: Goal setting
h: Environmental re-evaluation
i: Personalize risk
j: Modeling
k: Cultural similarity
l: Mobilizing social support
m: Information about others' approval
n: Planning coping responses
o: Environmental re-evaluation
p: Resistance to social pressure

Figure 7.3 New Year's message for the students, plus identification of underlying behavior change methods, adapted from Varol et al. (2021)

symptoms themselves. So, even if you are young and think you are protected against the effects of COVID-19, you can still be a danger to others." This was then followed by using the change method of anticipated regret to counter potential denying of the personal risk and change perspective: "Imagine how you would feel if someone else who is vulnerable were to become infected with COVID19 because of you." Those students who have difficulty adhering to guidelines were acknowledged so by using consciousness raising: "Nobody underestimates how difficult it is—keeping your distance, few social contacts, not celebrating the holidays with your entire family and all your friends." In line with the parameters of the effective use of consciousness raising, the message continued with providing tips on how to deal with high-risk situations in the upcoming Christmas/New Year break, applying the method of planning coping responses. As Varol et al. (2021) explain, it was possible to identify high-risk situations and communicate those to students in combination with a number of practical tips on what to do. However, actual practicing of coping responses was left to the responsibility of students, which shows that translation of a method into a practical application can be constrained by choices related to format and delivery of the intervention messages (in this case an email with a New Year's message).

The Case of the Missing Methods

Unfortunately, articles presenting interventions in the health education literature often do not report the causal chain from determinants to objectives to change methods to applications. Without this description, the reader may not be able to judge the theory and evidence base for what the planners have chosen to include in the intervention. Most publications on health education interventions, often evaluation studies, lack clear information about how the authors expected to cause a change. They often present the application and the program—for example, a tailored letter to encourage mammography or a videotape to discourage tobacco use. However, they may not be explicit about what change methods they used in the letter or how the videotape discouraged the risk behavior. Tailoring can be considered a general method, but the letter must also use specific methods that would, according to theory, "cause" a woman to obtain a mammogram. Did the researchers use persuasion, modeling with vicarious reinforcement, a cue to action, or some other method? In the Mapping process, all program theory- and evidence-based methods are linked to the personal determinants identified in Step 2 and then translated into practical applications that accommodate the change objectives and are suited to reach the priority population.

Using Methods Correctly

One source of confusion about change methods may be that the same concept, such as modeling or reinforcement, can be used to describe both determinants and methods. The double use of these concepts suggests that the theory explains both behavior and behavior change. The difference for health promoters is that modeling as a determinant refers to what happens in the actual situation, which is in line Fishbein and Ajzen's (2010) operationalization of a descriptive norm. Modeling as a change method is part of a well-designed program and describes the use of role models to influence people's decision-making. For instance, with respect to condom use, modeling that occurs on social media platforms that adolescents see may be negative (modeling as determinant illustrating a practice of having unsafe sex), whereas health promoters may use positive role models in their interventions to compensate for those negative counterparts in the media thus using modeling as change method to curb a negative descriptive norm toward condom use with a favorable injunctive norm message (Schaalma et al., 2004).

Translating change methods into practical applications demands a sufficient understanding of the theory behind the method, especially the theoretical parameters that are necessary for the change process to be effective (de Bruin et al., 2015; Kok et al., 2004; Peters et al., 2015). For example, modeling can be a strong method but only when certain parameters are met, such as reinforcement of the modeled behavior. People or environmental decision-makers do not usually imitate behavior simply because a model demonstrates that behavior; they behave comparably to the model only when the model exhibits certain characteristics, such as being reinforced for that particular behavior and when they expect to be reinforced in a similar way. Translating the change method of modeling to a practical application includes taking care that, in the actual program, from the perspective of the program participants, the model is reinforced. As a second example, goal setting can be a very effective method to enhance performance, but only when the goal is challenging as well as acceptable for the actor (Epton & Armitage, 2020; Locke & Latham, 2019). People often choose goals outside those parameters. A third classic example is provided by the method implementation intentions. While very effective when properly applied, violation of its main parameter of use (a preexisting intention to perform the behavior) greatly reduces or eliminates this effectiveness (Keller et al., 2020).

Using Different Methods at Different Levels of Intervention

Change methods at the individual level can be directed toward agents at higher ecological levels. See again Figure 7.2. The theoretical process behind the method is the same; however, often the application of the method is somewhat different, depending on the target. For instance, in a review of interventions to change environmental conditions, persuasion was found to be applied at various ecological levels (Kok et al., 2008). For example, in a project to decrease carbon dioxide transmission, the health promoter reported a persuasive communication approach that illustrated to businesses the advantages of approaching and dealing with the issue of carbon dioxide emissions. The health promoter showed them how reducing carbon dioxide is profitable and made it clear to companies that being environmentally friendly is good for company image. The potential effect on the company's image and profitability are typical organizational-level arguments.

In another example, smoking by adolescents is influenced by personal determinants but also by a supportive school environment. When the school environment is not supportive enough, the health promoter will want to change this environmental condition by urging the school management to develop and implement a nonsmoking school policy. So, the focus of the health promoter will shift, in this instance, to the behavior of agents related to the school (e.g., school management, parents). However, there are environmental influences on the school management's decision-making as well, in the form of state and national regulations related to nonsmoking policies in schools. When those regulations are lacking, the health promoter might want to change this environmental condition by urging state, provincial, or national agencies to declare stricter rules banning smoking in schools. The health promoter will use the method of political advocacy to influence this policy-making process. Even a government will be influenced by external factors, such as public support with calls for the use of approaches that can influence public opinion, such as social action. Refer again back to Figure 7.2 for a schematic representation of this chain of events.

In building from the examples above, two broad categories of environmental change methods are those focused on engaging and/or influencing environmental agents to make an environmental change (e.g., participatory problem-solving, organizational diagnosis, media advocacy to influence legislators to enact gun control legislation) and those focused specifically on changing the environment—for example through structural redesign (e.g., redesigning the cafeteria serving line to promote healthier options) or facilitation (e.g., bringing COVID-19 vaccination facilities to vulnerable communities with a truck), robust methods to change aspect of the environment to support individual behavior. Other examples of change methods at the community and societal (policy) levels that aim to change or harness the environment to support individual-level behavior change include "joint use/shared use agreements" in which school yards are opened up to the community as a place to do physical activity on the weekends, "health in all policies" in which a health focus is inserted into policy process, and "environmental print" in which health messaging is interwoven into the information environment (e.g., physical activity messaging inserted into electric bills).

Combining Change Methods

Planners frequently bundle together methods at the individual level to create a change method at a higher ecological level. This is because environmental agents along with organization and community members are also individuals, and the determinants of their behaviors are similar to determinants of behavior at the individual level. The change target and the overall method, however, are specific to the environmental change level. For example, community organization can include the individual methods of persuasion, modeling, skills training, and public commitment; however, these methods are bundled together to accomplish a change in a community-level problem and to increase community capacity. Organizational development, in fact, has been defined as the transfer of behavioral science knowledge to increase organizational effectiveness, and the process resembles behavioral self-regulation applied to the organizational level (see McLean, 2005).

There may be different approaches for targeting a level or being targeted from a level (Kok et al., 2012). On the one hand, organizations may apply methods for improving the health of their employees, such as to reduce prolonged sitting behavior and increase physical activity (Berninger et al., 2020). Those methods might include tailoring, goal setting, and monitoring. The activities are initiated by the management and are directed at the employees. On the other hand, health promoters and health-promoting organizations may apply methods to get organizations to start health-promoting activities. A national voluntary heart organization may try to encourage companies to facilitate physical activity programs for their employees. Methods that are used include persuasive communication, advocacy and lobbying, and organizational modeling and facilitation. These activities are initiated outside the organization, usually by a health promoter, and are directed at the organization, often the management.

A Taxonomy of Behavior and Environmental Change

There is increasing interest in systematic descriptions of health promotion interventions, the theory- and evidence-based change methods they contain, and the determinants that are targeted for change. For instance, Michie and colleagues provide a theory-linked coding taxonomy generally applicable to health behavior change techniques (BCTs), all directed at individual change (Abraham & Michie, 2008; Marques et al., 2023; Michie et al., 2011, 2013, 2015). Some of those techniques are linked with determinants of behavior, an approach comparable to what is presented in Intervention Mapping (Marques et al., 2023). Other authors combined the original taxonomy by Abraham and Michie (2008) with the Intervention Mapping approach to develop a checklist for coding methods in patient education interventions (de Bruin et al., 2010; van Achterberg et al., 2011) and HIV prevention programs (Godin et al., 2007). Addressing the need for a socio-ecological approach in health promotion, Ruiter et al. (2020) describe the use of behavior change methods at the interpersonal, organization, community, and societal levels (Ruiter et al., 2020). By connecting the socio-ecological approach with systems thinking theory, they discuss recent claims for whole system approaches in health promotion. Linking up with (complex) systems thinking theory, whole system approaches emphasize the need for multi-level actions across multiple sectors (life domains) while allowing for continuous program adaptation in response to change in the complex intervention contexts (Sawyer et al., 2021). For other descriptions of change methods at the individual and higher environmental levels, we refer the reader to behavioral science texts, particularly those with explicit applications to health promotion (Glanz et al., 2015; Hagger, Cameron, et al., 2020; Minkler & Wakimoto, 2021).

Step 3 Tasks

The three primary tasks for conducting Step 3 are presented in Box 7.1 and described below.

BOX 7.1. INTERVENTION MAPPING STEP 3 TASKS

1. Generate intervention ideas with the planning group
2. Choose theory- and evidence-based change methods
3. Select and design practical applications to deliver change methods

Task 1: Generate Intervention Ideas with the Planning Group

The first task in Step 3 is to generate intervention ideas with the planning group.

The planning group, established in Step 1 of Intervention Mapping, should include both members of the potential program participants and implementers to make sure the group has a good forum for balancing ideas on applications and programs, theoretical and empirical input on change methods, and limitations and potentials of the program context.

The product of the first part of this step is an initial plan that describes the program. The program plan should account for the contacts with each group of program participants. For example, in a program for patients, three contacts might be a video presentation followed by a discussion with a nurse and a reminder by a physician. The overall program might also include contacts to train the health care provider. Health promoters might already have ideas about the amount of the program that is expected to be delivered and the way the program should look at each interface with participants. They might also discuss the general outline of the components and materials that will be delivered. The format for the initial program ideas will vary from program to program, but it should include a description of who the priority population is for the intervention, how the priority population will be reached, and by whom. In developing the program plan, it is also important to consider the available financial and other resources such as time and personnel, as well as the community resources and environmental assets identified in Step 1 that can be harnessed or activated for the intervention (e.g., existing community organizations that can support the intervention). This planning process can be helpful to further guide the selection of theoretical methods and their translation to practical applications, tasks 2 and 3, respectively, of Step 3.

Generating Intervention Ideas

A central problem plagues planners in every profession—how to have a good idea ... how to "think outside of the box." In generating good ideas, we embrace the scientist Linus Pauling's famous saying that "The best way to a good idea is to have a lot of ideas." And the key to having a lot of ideas is to generate them without editing and without adhering to a strictly logical process. Prior to considering real-world constraints, de Bono suggests a lateral process that creates movement from one idea to another, breaks up current thinking, and disrupts reliance on the status quo (de Bono, 2015). At this point, planners can dismiss all preconceived notions and program constraints. They can ask themselves, "What would we do if we could do anything that comes to mind?" The diversity of the planning group will allow for the generation of unique ideas and innovative concepts.

Looking for empirical and theoretical support by using Core Processes (Chapter 2) can also be useful to generate ideas but should not take the place of brainstorming and lateral thinking. A literature review can identify the types of practical applications and programs others have used and the evidence for success using such approaches. Using behavior change theory will help in generating thoughts about methods and ways to use them. Finally, going to the potential participants (formative research) and continuing to fuel the process with their ideas is imperative. Focus groups can be used for this purpose and are particularly suited, because stimulus materials can be created from the change objectives, change methods, and practical applications and will generate discussion regarding acceptability and potential effectiveness. Sample questions include "If you were trying to figure out how to [change objective X], what would you do?" For example: "If you were going to increase the confidence of parents in discussing hormonal contraceptives with their teenage daughters, what would you do?"

Task 2: Choosing Theory- and Evidence-Based Change Methods to Address Program Objectives

The next task is to choose theory- and evidence-based change methods to address program objectives.

Theory- and evidence-based change methods are general techniques for influencing changes in determinants of behaviors of the at-risk group or environmental agents. To match a method with a change objective, the linking concept is the determinant involved. For example, take the following change objective: adolescents (the population) demonstrate skills (the determinant) in communicating with a partner about condom use (the performance objective). The method to reach this objective can be identified by considering methods for the determinant: skills. Of course, within the various methods for skills training, the planner will need to also consider the population and the performance objectives. Adolescents can be reached through the schools, and teachers may have ideas on what skills training methods they would want to apply with the topic of condom use.

To get from the matrices with change objectives as a result of Step 2 to the selection of methods in Step 3, planners reorganize the change objectives by determinants. They make a list of all change objectives related to increasing knowledge, another list of all change objectives related to changing outcome expectations, and so forth. They then match change methods to the determinants. Often, they have multiple change methods for a determinant as well as multiple objectives to be influenced by each method. For example, modeling is often used for skills-related change objectives, but for training some skills, it may also be necessary to use guided practice.

In the development of Long Live Love+, a Dutch online program to promote sexual health in senior high school students (Mevissen et al., 2018), methods were identified for different personal determinants and then matched with the change objectives, or the more specific "determinants" that created by combining the determinants with the performance objectives. Table 7.1 shows four change objectives for two performance objectives, as well as proposed methods for changing the personal determinants that underlie the change objectives. The planners of this intervention elected to use persuasive communication and discussion as a method for changing attitude, shifting perspective to communicate norms regarding gender differences in sexual desire and arousal, and planning coping

Table 7.1 Example of Selecting Methods for Changing Personal Determinants Organized by Change Objectives

Performance Objectives and Change Objectives	Change Methods (Determinant)
A. Performance objective: Formulate their own relationship-related as well as their sexual wishes and boundaries	
Change objectives (determinant): A.1. Mention differences and similarities between men and women regarding (expressions of) wishes and boundaries in (sexual) relationships (awareness). A.2. Mention that desire and sexual arousal differ between genders and people (attitude, norms).	Persuasive communication (awareness, attitude) Shifting perspective (norms)
B. Performance objective: Decide on using contraception to prevent pregnancy when (becoming) sexually active	
Change objectives: B.1. Express positive attitudes regarding the use of contraception other than and next to condom use (referred to as "double dutch") (attitude). B.2. Demonstrate ways to use contraception correctly and consistently (e.g., reminders for timing) (self-efficacy, skills).	Discussion (attitude) Planning coping responses (self-efficacy, skills)

Adapted from Mevissen et al., 2018.

response to increase self-efficacy and skills in promoting consistent contraceptive use, respectively.

Environmental Agents, Personal Determinants, and Change Methods for Environmental Conditions

Environmental conditions are not likely to be under the direct control of the individuals at risk for the health problem. They are controlled by external agents, such as parents, peers, teachers, managers, decision-makers such as a city council, and other gatekeepers. Therefore, performance objectives for environmental outcomes are formulated by referring to an environmental agent, who is the person or group of people who will implement a given performance objective. For example, implementing a school policy to prevent e-cigarette use in high school students may require various steps, or performance objectives, with different environmental agents leading the different performance objectives (e.g., a school principal may lead the performance objective (PO) of convening an interdisciplinary group of school partners and health promotion experts to develop the policy; teachers may lead the PO of informing their students about the policy). Or in the Me & You Study (see Chapter 6), there are matrices for the priority population (children) and important stakeholders (parents and teachers) environment.

The same method can be applied at any ecological level; however, methods at the higher levels often take a different form than similar methods at the individual level. Persuasive communication with individuals in a counseling context is different from persuasive communication as a part of political advocacy in a meeting between politicians and a lobbying group or in a meeting between company managers and union representatives. The determinant may be the same (i.e., outcome expectations), but the content and the vehicle for delivering a selected method—in this case persuasive communication—are different. Therefore, when addressing the behavior of agents in the environment, planners will most often select methods for individual change by determinant, and then follow up by higher level methods for environmental change that are directed at the same determinants. For example, as shown in Table 7.2, in the Me & You study, there were several change objectives for skills and self-efficacy related to using effective communication strategies—at the individual level (middle school students) to communicate effectively with their peers and dating partners (Table 6.6), and at the interpersonal level (parents) to communicate effectively with their child about healthy relationships (see Table 6.8). Modeling is a useful method for changing skills and self-efficacy and can easily be applied for students with reinforcement of the model as an essential parameter (a condition under which the method is effective). Modeling can also be applied for the parent, but the content will be different. In this case, the parents are responsible for the healthy development of their child, so verbal persuasion may be another very effective method to change their skills. For example,

Table 7.2 Examples of Change Methods at Various Ecological Levels for the Determinants Skills and Self-Efficacy Organized by Change Objective

Performance Objectives and Change Objectives (determinant)	Change Methods
A. *Individual level performance objective:* Students use effective communication strategies to foster healthy peer and dating relationships (e.g., conflict resolution, problem-solving, and active consent)	
Change objective: Express confidence in ability to use effective communication strategies to foster healthy relationships (self-efficacy)	Modeling Reinforcement
B. *Interpersonal level performance objective:* Parents use effective communication strategies when talking with their child (e.g., active listening, being nonjudgmental)	
Change objective: Demonstrate ability to use effective communication strategies when talking with their child about healthy relationships (skills)	Modeling Verbal persuasion Resistance to social pressure

they have to realize how their behavior influences the health of their children. If that method was not effective, planners could move to methods for other determinants, such as resistance to social pressure by providing parents with tip cards (de Decker et al., 2014).

Using Core Processes

Two of the core processes presented in Chapter 2 are essential for identifying and selecting change methods: reviewing existing empirical evidence in the literature and reviewing theories of change. With the topic approach to finding and using theory, the health promoter goes back to the literature on the problem. For example, when searching the topic drug abuse, the health promoter will discover what change methods others have used to influence various program objectives including the specific performance objective of resisting social pressure. Unfortunately, many articles are vague about change methods and more forthcoming about practical applications. The health promoter can then use the construct approach to find methods targeted toward specific determinants. For example, if a change objective is stated as "resist social pressure (determinant) to use drugs," a planner will look for methods specifically about resisting social pressure to use drugs, resisting social pressure to other risk behaviors such as smoking, and resisting social pressure in general. The health promoter may find that this literature cites theories on conformity and nonconformity and on social comparison (Cialdini, 2008). The health promoter may also use the general theories approach to explore those theories that address behavior change in general—for example, Social Cognitive Theory (Luszczynska & Schwarzer, 2020), and discover what those general theories have to offer about accomplishing this particular objective.

There may be several change methods for one personal determinant as well as one method for multiple personal determinants. In cases in which available information is extremely sparse, such as reducing fear of social contact with people with AIDS (attitude), planners may have to develop more insight on appropriate methods through a third core process: additional research with the intervention group (see Stigma in Chapter 3 and in Table 7.11).

Methods for Changing Behavior

This section describes theoretical change methods, summarized in tables. The first part presents change methods geared toward changing certain personal determinants (e.g., attitude and skills) in members of the priority population (Tables 7.3–7.12). As individuals are part of larger ecological and environmental systems, we also need change methods that can both influence the people within different ecological levels to implement an environmental change that can support individual- and population-level health (e.g., forming a coalition to advocate for a specific health policy) and the methods that directly harness or change the environment (e.g., redesigning the school cafeteria serving line to promote healthier options). The second part, therefore, presents change methods geared toward changing personal determinants of agents within the various ecological levels as well as directly changing environments (Tables 7.13–7.18).

In each change method table, we include a definition, description, example of use, and parameter for effectiveness of a given change method. As described above, parameters for use are the conditions under which the theory-based method will be effective. We developed the tables of behavior change methods in a conceptual analysis that was repeated over time with the four editions of this book (Bartholomew et al., 2001, 2006, 2011, 2016). We derived most of the definitions of intervention methods directly from the theories within which they are described from textbooks, reviews, and meta-analysis of theories of (health) behavior and change.

How to Use the Tables To effectively use the tables with change methods, planners will have created change objectives by clearly stating the behavioral or environmental outcomes, identifying who will be expected to perform the behavior, and naming determinants to create change objectives (Chapter 6). To select methods, they will do the following:

1. Check the table for each relevant determinant from the matrices.
2. For each potential method, inspect the definition and the parameters to determine whether the method is applicable given the situation.
3. Use the references included in the tables to study the relevant literature for ideas about how the method has been used. Use bibliographic databases, such as Google Scholar, to locate more recent studies.
4. Repeat these steps for all determinants, until methods have been identified to address all the determinants. Then translate these methods into practical applications.

The tables have some complexities. The various determinants are not independent of each other. For example, knowledge is the basis for many other determinants, such as risk perception, attitude, and skill. Risk perception in turn is a specific part of attitude. Change methods described for one determinant may sometimes be used for other determinants as well. The tables combine comparable determinants when they appear in more than one theory—for example, attitudes, beliefs, and outcome expectations. Further, the planner should always consider change methods that may be applied to almost any determinant. These are described in the table of "Basic Methods." See Chapters 3 and 4 for the theoretical foundations of the change methods.

Basic Methods for Behavior Change Some methods for change at the individual level are useful for all determinants and at various levels. The members of the intervention group, for example, must pay attention to the intervention message, understand the content, and process the information carefully. Table 7.3 lists these basic requirements of health education and promotion at the individual level: participation, belief selection, persuasive communication, active learning, tailoring, individualization, modeling, feedback, reinforcement and punishment, motivational interviewing, facilitation, and nudging.

Table 7.3 Basic Methods at the Individual Level

Method (Related Theories and References)	Definition	Parameters	Examples
Participation (Diffusion of Innovations Theory; Theories of Power; Organizational Development Theories; Models of Community Organization: Brownson et al., 2015; Cummings & Worley, 2014; McCullum et al., 2004; Rogers, 2003)	Assuring high-level engagement of the participants' group in problem-solving, decision-making, and change activities; with highest level being control by the participants' group.	Requires willingness by the health promoter or convener to accept the participants as having a high level of influence; requires participants' group to possess appropriate motivation and skills.	A health promoter includes representatives of students in the project group that is developing a new sex education program for schools.
Belief selection (Theory of Planned Behavior; Reasoned Action Approach: Ajzen & Schmidt, 2020; Fishbein & Ajzen, 2010)	Using messages designed to strengthen positive beliefs, weaken negative beliefs, and introduce new beliefs.	Requires investigation of the current attitudinal, normative, and efficacy beliefs of the individual before choosing the beliefs on which to intervene.	In a program for HIV prevention for Hispanic men, the men's belief that condoms were unclean needed to be changed; the importance of family values needed to be reinforced; and the belief that condoms could prevent HIV infection needed to be introduced.

(continued)

Table 7.3 (*Continued*)

Method (Related Theories and References)	Definition	Parameters	Examples
Persuasive communication (Communication-Persuasion Matrix; Elaboration Likelihood Model; Diffusion of Innovations Theory: McGuire, 2001; Petty et al., 2009; Rogers, 2003)	Guiding individuals and environmental agents toward the adoption of an idea, attitude, or action by using arguments or other means.	Messages need to be relevant and not too discrepant from the beliefs of the individual; can be stimulated by surprise and repetition; will include arguments.	Viewing a television broadcast on the health consequences to children from environmental tobacco smoke and the benefits of protecting children from smoke may influence a mother to declare her home smoke-free.
Active learning (Elaboration Likelihood Model; Social Cognitive Theory: Luszczynska & Schwarzer, 2020; Petty et al., 2009)	Encouraging learning from goal-driven and activity-based experience.	Time, information, and skills.	Getting individuals to search for answers to questions they pose as a result of some stimulus leads to better information processing and learning than passive learning and to increased change in determinants and behavior.
Tailoring (Trans-Theoretical Model; Precaution Adoption Process Model; Protection Motivation Theory; Communication-Persuasion Matrix: DiClemente & Graydon, 2020; McGuire, 2001; Orbell et al., 2020; Weinstein et al., 2008)	Matching the intervention or components to previously measured characteristics of the participant.	Tailoring variables or factors related to behavior change (such as stage) or to relevance (such as culture or socioeconomic status).	A patient educator motivates her patients to engage in vigorous physical activity by giving different messages based on the stage of change of each patient, for example providing information that physical activity will reduce their cardiovascular risk and increase their stamina to patients who are precontemplators.
Individualization (Trans-Theoretical Model: Bartholomew, Czyzewski, et al., 2000; Bartholomew, Gold, et al., 2000; DiClemente & Graydon, 2020)	Providing opportunities for learners to have personal questions answered or instructions paced according to their individual progress.	Personal communication that responds to a learner's needs.	An AIDS services organization provides a phone facility for young gay people to ask questions about their sexual identity and coming-out.
Modeling (Social Cognitive Theory; Theories of Learning: Kazdin, 2012; Luszczynska & Schwarzer, 2020)	Providing an appropriate model; being reinforced for the desired action.	Attention, remembrance, self-efficacy and skills, reinforcement of model; identification with model; coping model instead of mastery model.	The health promoter finds a role model from the community or at-risk group who will encourage identification and serve as a coping model: "I tried to quit smoking several times and was not successful, then I tried… Now I have been off cigarettes for…"

Table 7.3 (*Continued*)

Method (Related Theories and References)	Definition	Parameters	Examples
Feedback (Theories of Learning; Goal-Setting Theory, Social Cognitive Theory: Kazdin, 2012; Locke & Latham, 2019; Luszczynska & Schwarzer, 2020)	Giving information to individuals and environmental agents regarding the extent to which they are accomplishing learning or performance, or the extent to which performance is having an impact.	Feedback needs to be individual, follow the behavior in time, and be specific.	A physical activity counselor informs a client that her body mass index has decreased by 4% since she has begun her physical activity program.
Reinforcement (Theories of Learning; Social Cognitive Theory: Bouton, 2014; Gneezy et al., 2020; Kazdin, 2012; Luszczynska & Schwarzer, 2020; McSweeney & Murphy, 2014)	Providing reinforcement: linking a behavior to any consequence that increases the behavior's rate, frequency, or probability.	Reinforcement needs to be tailored to the individual, group, or organization, to follow the behavior in time, and to be seen as a consequence of the behavior.	An elementary school teacher praises a student for selecting a healthful dessert.
Punishment (Theories of Learning: Bouton, 2014; Gneezy et al., 2020; Kazdin, 2012; McSweeney & Murphy, 2014)	Providing punishment: linking a behavior to any consequence that decreases the behavior's rate, frequency, or probability.	Punishment needs to be tailored to the individual, group, or organization, to follow the behavior in time, and to be seen as a consequence of the behavior. Punishment should be avoided because of negative side effects. If used, emphasis should be on positive reinforcement.	In the framework of behavior modification (e.g., with tantrums or aggression), one method that is applied is the so-called timeout: a period of time in a less reinforcing environment, made contingent on a behavior.
Motivational interviewing, MI (Self-Determination Theory; Theories of Self-Regulation: Berman et al., 2020; de Ridder, Feitsma, et al., 2020; Hagger, Hankonen, et al., 2020; Hofmann et al., 2020; Miller & Rollnick, 2012; Ryan & Deci, 2017)	Providing a collaborative, goal-oriented style of communication with particular attention to the language of change; designed to strengthen personal motivation for and commitment to a specific goal by eliciting and exploring the person's own reasons for change within an atmosphere of acceptance and compassion.	A supportive relationship between client and professional combined with the evocation of patient change talk. Professionals must recognize that MI involves collaboration not confrontation, evocation not education, autonomy rather than authority, and exploration instead of explanation.	A practitioner supports the autonomy of an adolescent with a chronic medical condition by valuing of the patient's perspective (e.g., reflecting ambivalence about treatment), minimizing pressures and demands (e.g., asking for permission before providing information), and offering choices wherever possible (e.g., providing a menu of self-care options).

(*continued*)

Table 7.3 (*Continued*)

Method (Related Theories and References)	Definition	Parameters	Examples
Facilitation (Social Cognitive Theory: Bandura, 1986)	Creating an environment that makes the action easier or reduces barriers to action.	Requires real changes in the environment instead of in the perceptions of the environment. Requires the identification of barriers and facilitators and the power for making the appropriate changes. Facilitating conditions on one environmental level are usually dealt with by intervening on a higher environmental level.	A program that targets improvement in drug users' self-efficacy for using clean needles must also facilitate accessibility of clean needles.
Nudging (Theories of Automatic, Impulsive, and Habitual Behavior: de Ridder, 2014; Thaler & Sunstein, 2008)	Simple changes in the presentation of choice alternatives that make the desired choice the easy, automatic, or default choice.	Requires autonomy: freedom of choice, a sense of awareness, and the healthy choice being default: easy and attractive.	In a university building, orange colored footsteps on the floor stimulate students and faculty to take the stairs instead of the elevator.

Methods to Promote Information Exchange

Table 7.4 gives an overview of the methods and parameters for promoting effective information exchange and increasing knowledge. Knowledge is a necessary (though not sufficient) prerequisite for most other determinants, such as risk perception, attitudinal beliefs, perceived norms, and skills. Conventional wisdom has long held that increasing knowledge by giving people information could change their behavior, and thereby solve health and social problems. However, just providing knowledge does seldom lead directly to behavior change (nor is assuring that the priority population attains knowledge necessarily an easy task). Also, knowledge is often confused with beliefs that people hold with regard. For example, expected risks and outcomes of behavior, skills and barriers to perform the behavior, and experienced social pressure and support. Information that describes how to say no to friends or state the negative consequences of not using a condom relates to the determinants skills and risk perception, respectively, rather than being mere information that has the same objective meaning across people and is not further evaluated. We therefore prefer the term information exchange instead of increasing knowledge to identify methods that can help in informing priority population and environmental agents. Theories of Information Processing provide several concepts that suggest methods for successfully conveying information. In practice, these methods should be applied in combination with one or more other methods that address more proximal determinants of behavior and are listed in this chapter, to result in behavior change (Brownson et al., 2015).

Methods to Change Awareness and Risk Perception Table 7.5 presents methods that may help people perceive their risk. Before they become motivated to make a health-promoting behavior change, people need to be aware of a risk. Most of these methods are derived from theories on risk perception and risk communication; others come from stages of behavioral change theories that start with an awareness stage.

Methods to Change Habitual, Automatic, and Impulsive Behaviors Table 7.6 summarizes methods for changing habitual and automatic behaviors, as well as methods to promote action control over impulsive behaviors. Many behaviors are automatic and habitual. Even when people make reasoned and planned behavioral intentions, they may fail to follow up on those intentions. There is evidence that executive training tasks can change people's evaluations of and preferences for products such as food items, smartphone applications and smoking cues (Chen et al., 2016; Johannes et al., 2021; Najberg et al., 2021; Scholten et al., 2019; Tzavella & Chambers, 2023), and body weight (Lawrence et al., 2015; Stice et al., 2017). For example, during go/no-go training participants may consistently respond to some products (e.g., healthy food items) and inhibit responses to other products (e.g., unhealthy food items) depending on the presentation of respectively a go or no-go cue. These cues are presented shortly after presentation of the products. This training reduces attractiveness of the products paired with no-go cues and creates preferences for products paired with go cues over products paired with no-go cues, and effects of a single training session last for at least a week (Veling et al., 2022).

Methods to Change Attitudes, Beliefs, and Outcome Expectations Table 7.7 lists methods that may be used to change people's attitudes toward health. Attitudes are a positive or negative reaction to something; however, they can include the more specific constructs of beliefs, outcome expectations, assessments of advantages and disadvantages, perceptions of benefits and barriers, self-evaluations, and motivations to act. Social psychology has devoted much attention to attitude change, and the table represents a very brief summary of this work here (for a more in-depth review, see Crano & Prislin, 2011; Petty & Cacioppo, 2012).

Methods for Changing Social Influence Table 7.8 presents methods for changing social influence. The influence of the social environment is an important determinant of many behaviors and as such occurs frequently in change objectives. The Theory of Planned Behavior (TPB) and its successor the Reasoned Action Approach (Fishbein & Ajzen, 2010; Montaño & Kasprzyk, 2015) explain social influence. In these theories, behavior is determined by intention, and that intention is determined by attitudes, perceived norms, and perceived behavioral control (self-efficacy).

Social influence in this theory is described as perceived expectations of "people who are important to me" and perceived behavior of "people like me" (comparable to modeling). Social influence through modeling is a central construct in Social Cognitive Theory, which explicates intervention methods that change the social environment as well as perceived social influence (Bandura, 1986; Kelder et al., 2015). Social influence may also occur as upward and downward social comparison: Facilitating the observation of nonexpert others in order to evaluate one's own opinions and performance abilities (Suls et al., 2002).

Methods to Influence Skills, Capability, and Self-Efficacy and to Overcome Barriers Table 7.9 presents change methods to enhance skills and self-efficacy. Constructs addressed in this section are self-efficacy, perceived behavioral control, perceived barriers, skills, and perceived skills. Self-efficacy is often a crucial determinant in changing health behavior.

When people are motivated, the remaining question is whether they are able and feel confident to change their behavior. Self-efficacy is a determinant for the precursors of behavior—intention, preparation to act, and decision to act—but it also can directly influence implementation and maintenance of behavior change. Self-efficacy and related concepts are all personal determinants, but there is a distinction between perceptions (e.g., perceived skills) and reality (e.g., real skills). Even with sufficient real skills, people may not try the new behavior when their perceived skills are low. And people with high perceived skills may fail because they have insufficient real skills. Methods to improve self-efficacy are therefore often methods that also improve real skills.

Methods to Reduce Public and Self Stigma The last three tables on changing individual behavior, Tables 7.10–7.12, present methods to reduce public stigma, self-stigma, and structural stigma, respectively. Stigma is very difficult to change (Paluck & Green, 2009), but there are methods that may be successful under certain circumstances. Therefore, sticking to the parameters is especially crucial.

Table 7.4 Methods to Promote Information Exchange

Method (Related Theories and References)	Definition	Parameters	Examples
Chunking (Theories of Information Processing: Gobet, 2005; Gobet et al., 2001)	Using stimulus patterns that may be made up of parts but that one perceives as a whole.	Labels or acronyms are assigned to material to aid memory.	Children in the asthma self-management program learned a rap song with the words "watch, discover, think, and act" for the stages of self-management.

Table 7.4 (*Continued*)

Method (Related Theories and References)	Definition	Parameters	Examples
Advance organizers (Theories of Information Processing: Kools, 2012; Kools et al., 2006)	Presenting an overview of the material that enables a learner to activate relevant schemas so that new material can be associated.	Schematic representations of the content or guides to what is to be learned.	In a brochure for children with asthma, graphic organizers were placed on the top of every page, with the relevant concepts addressed on that page highlighted by means of thick lines and shadings.
Using imagery (Theories of Information Processing: Wright, 2012)	Using artifacts that have a similar appearance to some subject.	Familiar physical or verbal images as analogies to a less familiar process.	A patient educator helps a learner memorize a long self-care process by attaching the steps in the procedure to landmarks on a familiar daily route.
Discussion (Elaboration Likelihood Model: Petty et al., 2009)	Encouraging consideration of a topic in open informal debate.	Listening to the learner to ensure that the correct schemas are activated.	A classroom teacher has students discuss what they learned in a video about defusing a bullying situation.
Elaboration (Theories of Information Processing; Elaboration Likelihood Model: Petty et al., 2009)	Stimulating the learner to add meaning to the information that is processed.	Individuals with high motivation and high cognitive ability; messages that are personally relevant, surprising, repeated, self-pacing, not distracting, easily understandable, and include direct instructions; messages that are not too discrepant and cause anticipation of interaction.	A classroom teacher has students discuss the safe sex message: "When you want to get pregnant, use a condom"; stimulating adolescents to discover that Chlamydia can cause infertility: "If you want to get pregnant *later*, use a condom *now*."
Providing cues (Theories of Information Processing; Nudging: de Ridder, Feitsma, et al., 2020; Unsworth et al., 2013)	Assuring that the same cues are present at the time of learning and the time of retrieval.	Cues work best when people are allowed to select and provide their own cues.	For teens who are learning to negotiate condom use, the cues present during learning, such as what the partner says, should be as similar as possible to what teens will actually encounter in real life.

Table 7.5 Methods to Change Awareness and Risk Perception

Method (Related Theories and References)	Definition	Parameters	Examples
Consciousness raising (Health Belief Model; Precaution-Adoption Process Model; Trans-Theoretical Model: DiClemente & Graydon, 2020; Orbell et al., 2020; Weinstein et al., 2008)	Providing information, feedback, or confrontation about the causes, consequences, and alternatives for a problem or a problem behavior.	Can use feedback and confrontation; however, raising awareness must be quickly followed by increase in problem-solving ability and (collective) self-efficacy.	An HIV counselor reminds a person of recent episodes of failure to use condoms when having sex and the potential consequences of that behavior on significant others.
Personalize risk (Precaution-Adoption Process Model: Weinstein et al., 2008)	Providing information about personal costs or risks of action or inaction with respect to target behavior.	Present messages as individual and undeniable, and compare them with absolute and normative standards.	Individuals receive personal risk feedback on their fat intake, indicating whether it is higher than their self-rated level.
Scenario-based risk information (Precaution-Adoption Process Model: Mevissen et al., 2009, 2012)	Providing information that may aid the construction of an image of the ways in which a future loss or accident might occur.	Plausible scenario with a cause and an outcome; imagery. Most effective when people generate their own scenario or when multiple scenarios are provided.	Peer models in an HIV-prevention program present a series of scenarios in which they describe how they found themselves in risky situations, e.g., a sexual relationship over the summer holidays.
Framing (Protection Motivation Theory: Orbell et al., 2020; Van't Riet et al., 2014; Werrij et al., 2012)	Using gain-framed messages emphasizing the advantages of performing the healthy behavior; or loss-framed messages, emphasizing the disadvantages of not performing the healthy behavior.	Requires high self-efficacy expectations. Gain frames are more readily accepted and prevent defensive reactions.	Missing early detection of cancer by not getting a Pap test every year can cost you your life (loss frame). Getting a Pap test every year may enable you to live to see your grandchildren grow up (gain frame).
Self-reevaluation (Trans-Theoretical Model: DiClemente & Graydon, 2020)	Encouraging the combination of both the cognitive and affective assessments of one's self-image with and without an unhealthy behavior.	Stimulation of both cognitive and affective appraisal of self-image. Can use feedback and confrontation; however, raising awareness must be quickly followed by increase in problem-solving ability and self-efficacy.	A person can compare his or her image as a sedentary person to a possible image as an active person.
Dramatic relief (Trans-Theoretical Model: DiClemente & Graydon, 2020)	Encouraging emotional experiences, followed by reduced effect or anticipated relief if appropriate action is taken.	Preferably should be done in counseling context so that emotions can be aroused and subsequently relieved.	A counselor encourages a client to role-play a traumatic experience so that the emotion can be experienced and then relieved.

Table 7.5 (*Continued*)

Method (Related Theories and References)	Definition	Parameters	Examples
Environmental reevaluation (Trans-Theoretical Model: DiClemente & Graydon, 2020)	Encouraging the combination of both the affective and cognitive assessments of how the presence or absence of a personal behavior affects one's social environment.	May include awareness about serving as a role model for others.	In a smoking cessation class, participants describe how their family members feel about their smoking.
Fear arousal (Protection Motivation Theory; Extended Parallel Process Model: Kok et al., 2018; Orbell et al., 2020; Peters et al., 2013; Ruiter et al., 2001, 2014; van't Riet & Ruiter, 2013)	Arousing negative emotional reactions in order to promote self-protective motivation and action.	Requires high self-efficacy expectations rather than high outcome expectations alone; is rarely effective.	A health promoter shows in an emotionally moving way how a child is hurt by fireworks before demonstrating techniques for safer firework handling.
Self-affirmation (Self-Affirmation Theory: Cohen & Sherman, 2014; Epton et al., 2015; Harris et al., 2020)	Increasing people's self-image by having them elaborate on their relevant values or desirable characteristics.	Must be tailored to individual self-image.	A stress management class includes a writing exercise in which people record as many of their desirable characteristics as they can think of.

Table 7.6 Methods to Change Habitual, Automatic, and Impulsive Behaviors

Method (Related Theories and References)	Definition	Parameters	Examples
Counterconditioning (Theories of Automatic, Impulsive and Habitual Behavior: Custers & Aarts, 2010; Qin et al., 2021; Wood & Neal, 2007)	Encouraging the learning of healthier behaviors that can substitute for problem behaviors.	Availability of substitute behaviors.	When they feel the urge to smoke, smokers in a cessation program are instructed to do other behaviors than smoking, such as taking a short walk, chewing gum, or making a positive self-statement.
Implementation intentions (Theories of Goal Directed Behavior; Theories of Automatic, Impulsive and Habitual Behavior: Gollwitzer & Sheeran, 2006; Hagger et al., 2016; Keller et al., 2020; Rhodes et al., 2020)	Prompting making if-then plans that link situational cues with responses that are effective in attaining goals or desired outcomes.	Existing positive intention.	You are more likely to go for a cervical smear if you decide when and where you will go. Please write in below when, where, and how you will make an appointment.
Cue altering (Theories of Goal Directed Behavior; Theories of Automatic, Impulsive and Habitual Behavior: Gardner et al., 2020; Orbell & Verplanken, 2020; Rhodes et al., 2020; Verplanken & Aarts, 1999)	Teaching people to change a stimulus that elicits or signals a behavior.	Existing positive intention.	Dieters change the places they keep snack food in order to prevent taking the snack automatically.

(*continued*)

Table 7.6 *(Continued)*

Method (Related Theories and References)	Definition	Parameters	Examples
Stimulus control (Theories of Automatic, Impulsive and Habitual Behavior; Dual-Systems Models: Custers & Aarts, 2010; Deutsch & Strack, 2020; DiClemente & Graydon, 2020; Friese et al., 2011; Gardner et al., 2020)	Encouraging removing cues for unhealthy habits and adding prompts for healthier alternatives.	Needs insight in the behavioral chain leading to the automatic response.	Interventions to break habits should be directed at people when they are in new environments. For example, smokers are encouraged to remove all smoking paraphernalia (e.g., ashtrays, matches) from their houses and cars.
Planning coping responses (Attribution Theory and Relapse Prevention Theory; Theories of Goal Directed Behavior: de Ridder, Feitsma, et al., 2020; Epton & Armitage, 2020; Hofmann et al., 2020; Marlatt & Donovan, 2005; Rhodes et al., 2020)	Getting the person to identify potential barriers and ways to overcome these.	Identification of high-risk situations and practice of coping response.	The HIV nurse and the patient define the causes of nonadherence as caused by habits. Then the HIV nurse and the patient formulate solutions to solve or avoid the causes for nonadherence.
Early commitment (Theories of Learning: Robbins et al., 2001)	Having people choose a (larger) delayed reward far in advance.	Making the choice may be forced but the choice for the delayed reward needs to be voluntary.	A designated driver who voluntarily refrains from alcohol (immediate reward) during a party to bring friends safely home feels good about his role and will use a friend's service as designated driver at the next party (delayed reward).
Public commitment (Theories of Automatic, Impulsive and Habitual Behavior: Ajzen et al., 2009)	Stimulating pledging, promising, or engaging oneself to perform the healthful behavior, and announcing that decision to others.	Most effective when publicly announced; may include contracting.	A patient trying to get more exercise makes a private commitment to self and then announces her decision to others in the social environment.
Training executive functioning (Theories of Automatic, Impulsive and Habitual Behavior; Dual Systems Models: Deutsch & Strack, 2020; Diamond, 2013; Friese et al., 2011; Wiers et al., 2013)	Improving the top-down mental control processes that are used when going on automatic or relying on instinct or intuition would be ill-advised, insufficient, or impossible.	The task has to be challenging and substantial repetition is required to sufficiently train the executive functions.	A child will engage in computerized working memory training, such as Cogmed.
Go/no-go training (Theories of automatic, Impulsive and Habitual Behavior: Berkman et al., 2017; Veling et al., 2022)	Cues to respond (go cues), or not respond (no-go cues) are presented in temporal proximity of attractive products in a cognitive training task.	Products should preferably be tailored to match preferences of individuals. The go and no-go cues should be presented shortly after presentation of the products.	Computerized online training that consistently pairs healthy foods with go cues and unhealthy foods with no-go cues

Table 7.7 Methods to Change Attitudes, Beliefs, and Outcome Expectations

Method (Related Theories and References)	Definition	Parameters	Examples
Classical conditioning (Theories of Learning: Bouton, 2014; Kazdin, 2012)	Stimulating the learning of an association between an unconditioned stimulus (UCS) and a conditioned stimulus (CS).	Most effective when the time interval is short and the CS precedes the UCS.	Women with high body concern completed a conditioning procedure in which pictures of their bodies were selectively linked to positive social feedback: smiling faces.
Self-reevaluation (Trans-Theoretical Model: DiClemente & Graydon, 2020; Prochaska et al., 2015)	Encouraging the combination of both the cognitive and affective assessments of one's self-image with and without an unhealthy behavior.	Stimulation of both cognitive and affective appraisal of self-image. Can use feedback and confrontation; however, raising awareness must be quickly followed by increase in problem-solving ability and self-efficacy.	A person can compare his or her image as a sedentary person to a possible image of themselves as an active person.
Environmental reevaluation (Trans-Theoretical Model: DiClemente & Graydon, 2020; Prochaska et al., 2015)	Encouraging the realization of both the negative impact of the unhealthy behavior and the positive impact of the healthful behavior.	Stimulation of both cognitive and affective appraisal to improve appraisal and empathy skills.	Empathy training, viewing of documentaries or testimonials, or family interventions.
Shifting perspective (Theories of Stigma and Discrimination: Batson et al., 2002)	Encouraging taking the perspective of the other.	Initiation from the perspective of the learner; needs imaginary competence.	Parents instructing small children to cross the street kneel down to see traffic from the child's height.
Arguments (Kok, 2021)	Using a set of one or more meaningful premises and a conclusion.	For central processing of arguments, they need to be in the right direction, relevant, valid, and new to the message receiver.	Hearing for the first time about the benefits of protecting children from smoke may influence a mother to declare her home smoke-free.
Direct experience (Theories of Learning: Maibach & Cotton, 1995)	Encouraging a process whereby knowledge is created through the interpretation of experience.	Rewarding outcomes from the individual's experience with the behavior or assurance that the individual can cope with and reframe negative outcomes.	Rehabilitation counselors in training try taking a trip while in a wheelchair. This may change their attitudes about what it is like to use a wheelchair.

(*continued*)

Table 7.7 *(Continued)*

Method (Related Theories and References)	Definition	Parameters	Examples
Central information processing (Elaboration Likelihood Model: Petty et al., 2009)	Stimulating the learner to add meaning to the information that is processed.	Individuals with high motivation and high cognitive ability; messages that are personally relevant, surprising, repeated, self-pacing, not distracting, easily understandable, and include direct instructions; messages that are not too discrepant and cause anticipation of interaction.	*Sex, Games, and Videotapes*, an HIV-prevention program for homeless mentally ill men in a New York shelter, made messages personally relevant, surprising, and repeated by embedding them in playing competitive games, storytelling, and watching videos, activities that were salient pastimes in the shelter.
Anticipated regret (Theory of Planned Behavior; Reasoned Action Approach: Brewer et al., 2016; Richard et al., 1995)	Stimulating people to focus on their feelings after unintended risky behavior, before any losses actually materialize.	Stimulation of imagery; assumes a positive intention to avoid the risky behavior.	A sex educator asks people to imagine how they would feel after risky behavior such as having had unsafe sex.
Repeated exposure (Theories of Learning: Bouton, 2014; Zajonc, 2001)	Making a stimulus repeatedly accessible to the individual's sensory receptors.	Neutrality of original attitude.	Adolescents may be shown condoms repeatedly in classroom HIV-prevention education.
Cultural similarity (Communication-Persuasion Matrix: Kreuter & McClure, 2004; McGuire, 1985)	Using characteristics of the target group in source, message, and channel.	Using surface characteristics of the target group enhances receptivity. Using social-cultural characteristics leads to a more positive reception of the message.	Trained members of the Latino community give culturally relevant messages for cancer prevention and screening trials.

Table 7.8 Methods to Change Social Influence

Method (Related Theories and References)	Definition	Parameters	Examples
Information about others' approval (Theory of Planned Behavior; Reasoned Action Approach; Social Comparison Theory; Self-Determination Theory: Forsyth, 2018; Gerber et al., 2018; Hagger, Hankonen, et al., 2020; Mollen et al., 2010)	Providing information about what others think about the person's behavior and whether others will approve or disapprove of any proposed behavior change.	Positive expectations are available in the environment.	University students are given data showing the percentage of students who drink on campus, which usually is less than the students predict.

Table 7.8 *(Continued)*

Method (Related Theories and References)	Definition	Parameters	Examples
Resistance to social pressure (Inoculation Theory: Compton et al., 2016; McGuire, 1964)	Stimulating building skills for resistance to social pressure.	Commitment to earlier intention; relating intended behavior to values; psychological inoculation against pressure.	Young women learn effective refusal skills to use when a partner does not want to use a condom.
Shifting focus (Theory of Planned Behavior; Reasoned Action Approach: Ajzen & Schmidt, 2020; Fishbein & Ajzen, 2010)	Prompting hiding of the unpopular behavior or shifting attention away from the behavior.	Preferably shift focus to a new reason for performing the behavior.	Young women tell a partner that they want to use a condom to prevent pregnancy (instead of preventing STI/HIV).
Mobilizing social support (Diffusion of Innovations Theory; Theories of Social Networks and Social Support; Self-Determination Theory: Brownson et al., 2015; Hagger, Hankonen, et al., 2020; Holt-Lunstad and Uchino 2015; Valente, 2015)	Prompting communication about behavior change in order to provide instrumental and emotional social support.	Combines caring, trust, openness, and acceptance with support for behavioral change; positive support is available in the environment.	An exercise in a sex education program has students talk about safe sex and using condoms to make the positive expectations for using condoms more visible.
Provide opportunities for social comparison (Social Comparison Theory: Gerber et al., 2018)	Facilitating observation of nonexpert others in order to evaluate one's own opinions and performance abilities.	Upward comparison may help setting better goals; downward comparison may help feeling better or more self-efficacious.	A breast cancer patient may have had a lumpectomy, but sees herself as better off than another patient who lost her breast (downward comparison).

Table 7.9 Methods to Change Skills, Capability, and Self-Efficacy and to Overcome Barriers

Method (Related Theories and References)	Definition	Parameters	Examples
Guided practice (Social Cognitive Theory; Theories of Self-Regulation; Goal Setting Theory: Ajzen & Schmidt, 2020; de Ridder, Gillebaart, et al., 2020; Luszczynska & Schwarzer, 2020)	Prompting individuals to rehearse and repeat the behavior various times, discuss the experience, and provide feedback.	Subskill demonstration, instruction, and enactment with individual feedback; requires supervision by an experienced person; some environmental changes cannot be rehearsed.	The trainer first models the target behavior a number of times and then asks the trainees to do the same a number of times. The trainer gives brief comments on the trainees' performances, emphasizing aspects done well.

(continued)

Table 7.9 *(Continued)*

Method (Related Theories and References)	Definition	Parameters	Examples
Enactive mastery experiences (Social Cognitive Theory; Theories of Self-Regulation and Self Control: de Ridder, Gillebaart, et al., 2020; Hofmann et al., 2020; Luszczynska & Schwarzer, 2020)	Providing increasingly challenging tasks with feedback to serve as indicators of capability.	Requires willingness to accept feedback.	After the students are taught the necessary know-how of intervening in bullying situations, they perform the new skills in a simulated setting in order to experience their mastery at handling bullying class mates.
Verbal persuasion (Social Cognitive Theory; Theories of Self-Regulation: de Ridder, Feitsma, et al., 2020; Luszczynska & Schwarzer, 2020)	Using messages that suggest that the participant possesses certain capabilities.	Credible source.	Teachers were shown a videotape on which teachers like them discussed their successful experiences in the regular classroom using the intervention with difficult-to-teach children.
Improving physical and emotional states (Social Cognitive Theory: Luszczynska & Schwarzer, 2020; Weiner, 2018)	Prompting interpretation of enhancement or reduction of physiological and affective states, to judge own capabilities.	Must carefully interpret and manage emotional states.	Students in a public speaking class are taught to breathe deeply and relax prior to their presentation. They label the anxiety they feel as excitement. Reduce stress and depression while building positive emotions—as when fear is labeled as excitement.
Reattribution training (Attribution Theory and Relapse Prevention Theory; Theories of Self-Regulation: de Ridder, Gillebaart, et al., 2020; Mann et al., 2013; Marlatt & Donovan, 2005; Weiner, 1986, 2018)	Helping people reinterpret previous failures in terms of unstable attributions and previous successes in terms of stable attributions.	Requires counseling or bibliotherapy to make unstable and external attributions for failure.	The counselor suggests that a smoker's relapse was due to a temporary condition and that she can learn from this experience to stay off cigarettes.
Self-monitoring of behavior (Theories of Self-Regulation and Self Control: Creer, 2000; de Ridder, Gillebaart, et al., 2020; Hofmann et al., 2020; Mann et al., 2013)	Prompting the person to keep a record of specified behavior(s).	The monitoring must be of the specific behavior (that is, not of a physiological state or health outcome). The data must be interpreted and used. The reward must be reinforcing to the individual.	Patients keep a diary on their therapy adherence in order to find out when and why medication is missed.

Table 7.9 (*Continued*)

Method (Related Theories and References)	Definition	Parameters	Examples
Provide contingent rewards (Theories of Learning; Theories of Self-Regulation and Self Control; Self-Determination Theory: Bandura, 1986; de Ridder, Gillebaart, et al., 2020; Hagger, Hankonen, et al., 2020; Hofmann et al., 2020; Mann et al., 2013)	Praising, encouraging, or providing material rewards that are explicitly linked to the achievement of specified behaviors.	Rewards need to be tailored to the individual, group or organization, to follow the behavior in time, and to be seen as a consequence of the behavior.	Smokers who are trying to quit smoking receive monetary vouchers for breath samples with carbon monoxide (CO) levels of 8 ppm or less.
Cue altering (Theories of Automatic, Impulsive, and Habitual Behavior; Theories of Self-Regulation: Achtziger et al., 2008; Mann et al., 2013)	Teaching people how to change a stimulus, either consciously or unconsciously perceived, that elicits or signals a behavior.	Existing positive intention.	Dieters change the route they take walking to work in order to avoid easy access to snack shops.
Public commitment (Theories of Automatic, Impulsive, and Habitual Behavior: Ajzen et al., 2009)	Stimulating pledging, promising, or engaging oneself to perform the healthful behavior and announcing that decision to others.	Needs to be a public announcement; may include contracting.	High school students sign individual contracts not to smoke, which are then placed on the classroom wall for all to see.
Goal setting (Goal-Setting Theory; Theories of Self-Regulation: Locke & Latham, 2019; Mann et al., 2013)	Prompting to plan what the person will do, including a definition of goal-directed behaviors that result in the target behavior.	Commitment to the goal; goals that are difficult but available within the individual's skill level.	Dietician and patient discuss the goal for the next meeting, deciding on a goal that is acceptable to the patient and to the dietician.
Set graded tasks (Social Cognitive Theory; Theories of Self-Regulation and Self Control: de Ridder, Gillebaart, et al., 2020; Epton & Armitage, 2020; Hofmann et al., 2020; Mann et al., 2013)	Setting easy tasks and increase difficulty until target behavior is performed.	The final behavior can be reduced to easier but increasingly difficult sub-behaviors.	Physiotherapist and patient discuss increasingly intensive exercises for the patient in order to gradually build up the patient's condition.
Planning coping responses (Attribution Theory and Relapse Prevention Theory; Theories of Self-Regulation: Mann et al., 2013; Marlatt & Donovan, 2005)	Prompting participants to list potential barriers and ways to overcome these.	Identification of high-risk situations and practice of coping response.	The HIV nurse and the patient define the causes of nonadherence (lack of understanding, lack of motivation, insufficient action plan, barriers). Then the HIV nurse and the patient formulate solutions to solve or avoid the causes for nonadherence.

Table 7.10 Methods to Reduce Public Stigma

Method (Related Theories and References)	Definition	Parameters	Examples
Interpersonal contact (Contact theory: Allport, 1954; Maunder & White, 2019)	Bringing people with and without the stigmatized identity or condition in contact with one another. Contact can be direct or indirect (vicarious, extended, or imagined contact).	Requires positive experiences. Most effective when status is equal, contact is intensive; contact is externally sanctioned, and there are common or shared goals.	*Direct contact*: People with a stigmatized identity or condition give a presentation to people who have had no previous or very little contact with people with that identity or condition. *Indirect contact*: Mass media campaign showcasing, normalizing, and humanizing people with a stigmatized identity or condition.
Empathy induction (Perspective-Taking: Batson et al., 2002; Todd et al., 2012)	Stimulating people to empathize with another person, i.e., imagining how the other person feels.	Requires being willing and able to identify with the other, being able to imagine how the other would feel (rather than imagining how you would feel as this can lead to empathy but also distress).	An exercise in which intervention participants imagine or experience some form of exclusion followed by a reflection on how a person with a stigmatized condition or identity would feel if stereotyped and stigmatized.
Provision of stereotype-inconsistent information (Theories of Stigma and Discrimination: Bos et al., 2008)	Providing positive examples of people with a stigmatized identity or condition.	Require multiple examples (to avoid subtyping) and the examples cannot be too discrepant from original stereotype.	Positive portrayals of stigmatized individuals in mass media or leaflets.
Cooperative learning (Theories of Stigma and Discrimination: Aronson, 2015)	Engineering lessons in a way that students must learn from one another.	Requires careful organization of lesson information distribution.	Teachers give each student one piece of the lesson plan, so that they have to collaborate in order to understand the lesson plan.
Conscious regulation of impulsive stereotyping and prejudice (Theories of Stigma and Discrimination: Bos et al., 2008)	Forcing oneself to control negative reactions to people with a stigmatized identity or condition.	Mere suppression almost always leads to counterproductive effects and is not advisable. Conscious self-regulation of automatic stereotyping can be used effectively.	Participants practice saying "Stop thinking this way" to themselves as they watch videos of people with a stigmatized identity or condition.
Changing attitudes	*See methods for attitude change (Table 7.7)*		Direct experience, arguments, elaboration, self-reevaluation, environmental reevaluation, anticipated regret, repeated exposure, cultural similarity

Table 7.11 Methods to Reduce Self-Stigma

Method (Related Theories and References)	Definition	Parameters	Examples
Cognitive restructuring (Cognitive Behavioral Therapy: Beck, 2011)	Process by which people identify and change negative thinking patterns.	Requires ability to identify thoughts that generate negative feelings, as well as inconsistencies between perception and reality.	People with a stigmatized identity or condition are asked to write down stereotypes about their identity and condition. They then reflect on the extent to which they have internalized those stereotypes, and are challenged to question whether they are actually a reflection of those stereotypes.
Psychological flexibility (Acceptance and Commitment Therapy: Hayes et al., 1999)	Being able to stay in contact with the present moment regardless of unpleasant thoughts, feelings, and bodily sensations, while choosing one's behaviors based on the situation and personal values.	Requires awareness of emotions, sensations, and thoughts, and ability to reflect.	People with a stigmatized identity or condition think mindfully about their experiences with stigma, and the (difficult) emotions, sensations, and thoughts that accompany those experiences, and then are encouraged to explore their goals and values in life and to link the accomplishment of desired goals to values rather than to automatic thoughts and feelings.
Planning coping responses (Attribution Theory and Relapse Prevention Theory; Theories of Goal Directed Behavior: de Ridder, Gillebaart, et al., 2020; Epton & Armitage, 2020; Hofmann et al., 2020; Marlatt & Donovan, 2005; Rhodes et al., 2020)	Identifying potential negative situations and planning how to deal with them.	Ability to identify negative situations and practice of coping response	In a group context, people with a stigmatized identity or condition share personal experiences of stigmatization and exchange behavioural strategies for dealing with those experiences (e.g., disengagement, confrontation).
Seeking social support (Stress and Coping Social Support Theory; Relational Regulation Theory: Cohen & Wills, 1985; Lakey & Orehek, 2011)	Seeking out instrumental, emotional, and/or informational assistance and care.	Requires a social network and the ability to ask for support.	People with a stigmatized identity or condition identify and reach out to people in their environment that would be able to offer them one or more forms of support and/or come together in person or online to support one another.

(*continued*)

Table 7.11 *(Continued)*

Method (Related Theories and References)	Definition	Parameters	Examples
Building resilience (Theory of Resilience and Resiliency: Richardson, 2002)	Adapting positively to adversity in ways that result in the identification, fortification, and enrichment of resilient qualities or protective factors.	Requires the ability to engage in introspection.	People with a stigmatized identity or condition are asked to discuss the myths and realities surrounding their identity or condition, and then identify protective factors that they can access to deal with stigmatization.
Empowerment (Empowerment Theory: Linhorst et al., 2002; Rappaport, 1981)	Creating experiences that foster the activation and utilization of motivational forces in individuals and groups so that they can gain mastery over their lives and assert their rights.	Requires time, trust, respect, and the ability to develop (decision-making) skills and a sense of agency.	People with a stigmatized identity or condition develop their own anti-stigma intervention.

Table 7.12 Methods to Reduce Structural Stigma

Method (Related Theories and References)	Definition	Parameters	Examples
Reducing inequalities of class, race, gender and sexuality (Theories of Stigma and Discrimination: Hatzenbuehler et al., 2013)	*See methods for changes at higher environmental levels (Tables 13–18).*		Mobilizing social support, community organizing, empowerment of stigmatized persons, agenda setting, creating and enforcing laws and regulations, and threatening with coercion.
Media advocacy (Models of Community Organization: Dorfman & Krasnow, 2014; Wallack, 2008; Wallack et al., 1993)	Foreground stigma and its effects in media to draw attention to the problem of stigmatization. A type of advocacy.	Requires the media to approve the news value of the message and accept the message without changing its essential content.	An HIV patient organization contacts a reputable newspaper and invites them to do an article on experiences of stigma and its effects among people with HIV, and how stigmatization can best be tackled.
Agenda setting (Multiple Streams Theory, Advocacy Coalition Theory, Theories of Power: Clavier & de Leeuw, 2013; Sabatier, 2003; Weible, 2008; Weible et al., 2009)	Process of moving an issue to the political agenda for action; may make use of broad policy advocacy coalitions and media advocacy.	Requires appropriate timing (see policy window) and collaboration of (media) gatekeepers. Will often include persuasive communication and consciousness raising.	Transgender activists develop a position paper on the legal recognition of transgender identity. They release the report to the media and hold meetings with key state legislators on the recommendations put forth in the report.

Table 7.12 (*Continued*)

Method (Related Theories and References)	Definition	Parameters	Examples
Timing to coincide with policy windows (Multiple Streams Theory: Kingdon, 2003; Zahariadis, 2007)	Advocating policy when politics, problems, and policy solutions are aligned to be receptive to a policy issue.	Requires an astute policy advocate who is well prepared.	Advocates of same-sex marriage develop coalitions and release position papers shortly before the elections of a politician known to be supportive of same-sex marriage.
Creating and enforcing laws and regulations (Multiple Streams Theory, Theories of Power: Clavier & de Leeuw, 2013; Kingdon, 2003; Longest, 2006)	Forcing compliance or dictating or precluding choices. Sometimes implementing existing laws to accomplish change. Laws and regulations may also provide incentives.	Requires unequal power and availability of control and sanctions.	LGBTIQ+ non-discrimination laws are revised and enforced in employment contexts.

Methods for Changing Environmental Conditions

This section first lists basic methods for change that can be applied at all environmental levels and then methods related to environmental conditions at each ecological level. These tables refer the reader back to earlier tables of methods for both individual and general determinants, indicating that these methods can be used to change the environmental condition or that the individual-level methods are embedded in the environmental change methods. Planners should note that some change methods at the individual level are also useful at most environmental levels. Skills training by guided practice (see Table 7.9 for example) can be applied in almost any method directed at changing an environmental agent's behavior, even though the form and content of the training may be different when this method is applied at the strictly individual level.

Basic Methods for Change of Environmental Conditions Table 7.13 lists basic methods at the environmental level for the health promoter: systems change, participatory problem-solving, coercion, advocacy and lobbying, modeling, and technical assistance. Intervention planners should always consider these methods when identifying promising methods for change at all environmental levels. See Chapter 4 for the theoretical and empirical background for these basic methods.

Methods to Change Social Norms Table 7.14 presents methods for changing social norms. Chapter 4 presented social norms theory as a community-level theory. However, social norms are influential at all levels. In Table 7.8, we summarized the methods to change social influence, of which social norms are a relevant form. There, the focus was on the individual's perception of, and coping with, social norms, whereas here the focus is on changing the norms themselves.

Methods to Change Social Support and Social Networks Table 7.15 describes methods at the interpersonal level:

1. to change social networks so that they offer social support more effectively to their members,
2. to help members mobilize support from their networks, and
3. to link members with other networks.

Networks can engage in participatory problem-solving processes aimed at finding ways to solve specific problems of individuals, families, or communities. We highlight the use of lay health workers specifically. These are natural helpers (community members to whom other persons turn for advice, emotional support, and tangible aid) who receive special training to support others, including linking them to the formal service delivery system (Mokhele et al., 2022).

Methods to Change Organizations Table 7.16 presents methods from organizational change theories, including organizational development, the Stage Theory of Organizational Change, Diffusion of Innovations Theory (DIT), and Stakeholder Theory. These include organizational processes, such as participatory problem-solving and team building, which can create changes in organizational norms and practices. DIT and the Stage Theory of Organizational Change provide methods that can influence the adoption, implementation, and continuation innovations such as health promotion programs. Methods from Stakeholder Theory focus on using influence from external agents to promote organizational change.

Methods to Change Communities Table 7.17 summarizes methods to promote community change. These include problem-posing education or conscientization, community assessment, community development, social action, forming coalitions, social planning, and framing to shift perspectives (See Chapter 3). The skillful community organizer selects methods that fit the context of the community and the key issues to be addressed. These often shift over time. The community methods relate to two types of interventions: (1) those implemented by the health promoter with the community to develop empowerment and community capacity, and (2) those implemented by the community toward the environmental agent. For example, the health promoters carry out a facilitated community intervention designed to assist the community in understanding the issues it must face, setting priorities, and developing and implementing action plans to address the key issues. Then the community implements the action plan, using methods of change appropriate to the environmental agent and desired change. This may involve individuals, organizations, and government. We discuss specific methods for political change in the next section.

Methods to Change Policy Political change takes place using many of the methods for individual, organizational, and community change in the earlier tables. However, these methods should be applied in the context of theories that explain how policy is formulated, implemented, and modified. In Chapter 3, we discussed the Multiple Streams Theory and the Advocacy Coalition Framework. These theories provide insight into when to use various individual and community influence methods, such as media advocacy, agenda setting, timing to coincide with policy windows, and creating and enforcing laws and regulations (see Table 7.18).

Table 7.13 Basic Methods for Change of Environmental Conditions

Method (Related Theories and References)	Definition	Parameters	Examples
Systems change (Systems Theory: Lambe et al., 2020; Luna Pinzon et al., 2022; Mkhitaryan et al., 2020)	Interacting with the environment to change the elements and relationship among elements of a system at any level, especially through dialogue with stakeholders, action, and learning through feedback.	Methods and actors depend on the level of the system.	A city's transportation department created bicycle lanes on streets to encourage people to ride bicycles to work as a result of a stakeholder advisory committee's recommendations. The committee monitored the use of the bicycle lanes and held a focus group of bicyclists about their experiences.
Participatory problem-solving (Organizational Change Theories; Social Capital Theory; Models of Community Organization: Butterfoss & Kegler, 2022; Cummings & Worley, 2018; Minkler et al., 2022)	Diagnosing the problem, generating potential solutions, developing priorities, making an action plan, and obtaining feedback after implementing the plan.	Requires willingness by the health promoter or convener to accept the participants as equals and as having a high level of influence; requires target group to possess appropriate motivation and skills. Will often include goal setting, facilitation, feedback and consciousness raising.	A health promotion consultant assists employees of a small company to identify the level of perceived work stress and sources of work stress, to develop a plan with management support to address sources of stress and provide coping strategies, to implement the plan, and to monitor perceived work stress.

(*continued*)

Table 7.13 (*Continued*)

Method (Related Theories and References)	Definition	Parameters	Examples
Coercion (Theories of Power: Freudenberg & Tsui, 2014; Popay et al., 2021; Turner, 2005)	Attempting to control others against their will.	Requires or creates a power differential.	Health promotion activists organize a consumer boycott of a company that sells formula in developing countries.
Advocacy and lobbying (Stage Theory of Organizational Change; Models of Community Organization; Agenda-Building Theory; Multiple Streams Theory: Christoffel, 2000; Galer-Unti et al., 2004; Kingdon, 2003; Wallack et al., 1993; Weible et al., 2009)	Arguing and mobilizing resources on behalf of a particular change; giving aid to a cause; active support for a cause or position.	Form of advocacy must match style and tactics of the people, communities or organizations represented, and the nature of the issue; includes policy advocacy; often tailored to a specific environmental agent. Will often include persuasive communication, information about others' approval, and consciousness raising.	Members of the American Public Health Association use the organization's action alert system to contact their legislators to urge them to vote for pending health care reform legislation.
Modeling (Social Cognitive Theory; Organizational Development Theories; Diffusion of Innovations Theory; Empowerment Theory: Bandura, 1997; Luszczynska & Schwarzer, 2020; Rogers, 2003)	Providing an appropriate model being reinforced for the desired action.	Appropriate models will vary by level, including group members and organizational, community, and policy change agents.	An article in the state medical journal highlights the experience of a city hospital emergency department that has instituted routine HIV testing, found new cases of HIV that would have gone undetected, and received recognition from the state's HIV Community Planning Group.
Technical assistance (Organizational Development Theories, Diffusion of Innovations Theory, Social Capital Theory, Models of Community Organization: Flaspohler et al., 2008; Mitchell & LaGory, 2002)	Providing technical means to achieve desired behavior.	Nature of technical assistance will vary by environmental level, but must fit needs, culture, and resources of the recipient.	A health department liaison helps a community health center design recruitment procedures, training, and supervisory guidelines as they establish a new lay health worker program.

Table 7.14 Methods to Change Social Norms

Method (Related Theories and References)	Definition	Parameters	Examples
Mass media role-modeling (Diffusion of Innovations Theory; Social Cognitive Theory; Social norm theories: Bandura, 1997; Chung & Rimal, 2016; Cislaghi & Heise, 2018; Rimal & Lapinski, 2015; Rogers, 2003)	Providing appropriate models being reinforced for the desired action through the mass media.	Conditions for modeling; conditions for persuasive communication (see Table 7.3).	A feature story about mammography screening on the news includes a woman who caught the cancer early by having routine mammogram. The cancer was removed by lumpectomy.
Entertainment education (Diffusion of Innovations Theory; Social norm theories: Moyer-Gusé, 2008; Petraglia, 2007; Shen & Han, 2014; Sood et al., 2017)	Providing a form of entertainment designed to educate (about health behavior) as well as to entertain.	Consideration of source and channel; balance of media professionals and health promoter's needs.	A soap opera has a storyline about a lead character's being arrested for drinking and driving.
Behavioral journalism (Diffusion of Innovations Theory; Social Cognitive Theory; Social norm theories: McAlister, 2017; van Empelen et al., 2003)	Using by the mass and local media of appropriate role-model stories of behavior change based on authentic interviews with the target group.	Adequate role models from the community and elicitation interviews to describe the behavior and the positive outcome.	Baseball card-size cards with a picture and a short story concerning how a woman got her boyfriend to willingly use a condom are part of a sex education program for runaway teens.
Mobilizing social networks (Theories of Social Networks and Social Support; Social norm theories: He et al., 2020; Minkler & Wakimoto, 2022; Valente, 2015)	Encouraging social networks to provide informational, emotional, appraisal, and instrumental support.	Availability of social network and potential support givers. Will often include information about others' approval, facilitation, and persuasive communication.	Parents are coached on how to make their negative views about smoking clear to their children as part of a tobacco prevention program.

Table 7.15 Methods to Change Social Support and Social Networks

Method (Related Theories and References)	Definition	Parameters	Examples
Enhancing network linkages (Theories of Social Networks and Social Support: Holt-Lunstad and Uchino 2015; Valente & Pitts, 2017)	Training network members to provide support and members of the target group to mobilize and maintain their networks.	Available network.	A patient educator helps a patient who has had a stroke and her family members to make plans for the patient to return home. The plans include linking to a patient support group and community day care.

(*continued*)

Table 7.15 *(Continued)*

Method (Related Theories and References)	Definition	Parameters	Examples
Developing new social network linkages (Theories of Social Networks and Social Support: Holt-Lunstad, 2022, 2023; Valente & Pitts, 2017)	Linking members to new networks by mentor programs, buddy systems, and self-help groups.	Willingness of networks to reach out; availability of networks that can provide appropriate support and linkage agents.	Volunteers who are breast cancer survivors are linked to newly diagnosed patients to provide emotional and informational support.
Use of lay health workers; peer education (Theories of Social Networks and Social Support; Models of Community Organization: Mokhele et al., 2022)	Mobilizing members of the target population to serve as boundary spanners, credible sources of information, and role models.	Natural helpers in community with opinion leader status and availability to volunteer for training.	*Promotoras* from a local clinic provide information and outreach to community members at risk for diabetes.

Table 7.16 Methods to Change Organizations

Method (Related Theories and References)	Definition	Parameters	Examples
Sense-making (Organizational Development Theory: Weick & Quinn, 1999)	Leaders reinterpret and relabel processes in organization, create meaning through dialogue, and model and redirect change.	Used for continuous change, including culture change.	A supervisor in a hospital talks to his staff about the positive aspects of finding and correcting mistakes in documentation of medication administration.
Organizational diagnosis and feedback (Organizational Development Theory: Cummings & Worley, 2018)	Assessing of organizational structures and employees' beliefs and attitudes, desired outcomes, and readiness to take action, using surveys and other methods.	Methods appropriate to organizational characteristics, e.g., size and information technology. Will often include feedback and consciousness raising.	An organizational consultant conducts a survey of employees' health behaviors and determinants and holds focus groups of employees to review the results and plan for health promotion programs.
Team building and human relations training (Organizational Development Theory: Cummings & Worley, 2018)	Grouping development activities based on the values of human potential, participation, and development.	Compatible with the culture.	Participants in a retreat work interdependently to solve a puzzle.
Structural redesign (Organizational Development Theory: Cummings & Worley, 2018)	Change organizational elements such as formal statements of organizational philosophy, communication flow, reward systems, job descriptions, and lines of authority.	Management authority and agreement.	A health promotion consultant works with an organization to renew the organizational vision statement to include the health of employees.

Table 7.16 (*Continued*)

Method (Related Theories and References)	Definition	Parameters	Examples
Increasing stakeholder influence (Stakeholder Theory: Brown et al., 2003; Kok et al., 2015; Mitchell et al., 1997)	Increase stakeholder power, legitimacy, and urgency, often by forming coalitions and using community development and social action to change an organization's policies.	The focal organization perceives that the external organization or group is one of its stakeholders.	A community group uses media advocacy to highlight the groundwater pollution by gas storage tanks located in the community and to demand that the tanks be moved by the gas company that owns them.

Table 7.17 Methods to Change Communities

Method (Related Theories and References)	Definition	Parameters	Examples
Problem-posing education (Conscientization Theory; Empowerment Theory: Freire, 1973a, 1973b; Wallerstein et al., 2015)	Participatory analysis using critical reflection, self-disclosure, and dialogue regarding the social forces underlying a problem and a commitment to change self and community.	A safe environment for participation and disclosure; a critical stance.	In facilitated small-group discussion, adolescents share the effects of their own and others' alcohol abuse on their lives. They reflect on what this means both personally and to their community. They ask, "What can we do about this?" and take action.
Community assessment (see also task 1.2 on asset assessment, Chapter 5) (Models of Community Organization: Minkler et al., 2022)	Assessing a community's assets and needs, with feedback of results to the community.	Requires expert assistance and possibilities for feedback.	Community members, with technical assistance from the health department, used surveys, door-to-door interviewing, and community asset mapping to conduct a community assessment. The findings were presented and discussed at a community-wide meeting.
Community development (Models of Community Organization; Theories of Power: Minkler et al., 2022; Wallerstein et al., 2015)	A form of community organization, based on consensus, in which power is shared equally and members engage together in participatory problem-solving.	Starting where the community is; may be grassroots or professional driven. Will often include consciousness raising, facilitation, goal setting, and information about others' approval.	A community organizer convenes a task force of representatives of the school board, the mayor's office, the disenfranchised community, and the city council member representing the community to discuss the findings of a report documenting inequities in the schools and to make plans to address them.

(*continued*)

Table 7.17 *(Continued)*

Method (Related Theories and References)	Definition	Parameters	Examples
Social action (Theories of Power; Stakeholder Theory: Kok et al., 2015; Rivera-Rodriguez et al., 2025; Wallerstein et al., 2015)	A form of community organization, based in conflict, in which disenfranchised people wrest power from the official power.	Starting where the community is; may be grassroots or professional driven. Will often include consciousness raising, persuasive communication, information about others' approval, and modeling.	A community organizer works with a low-income community that has identified a need to improve educational resources available to their children. They document the inequities in the schools and extracurricular programs across the city, present their findings, and challenge the school board to act on them in a press conference. They organize community members to attend the next school board meeting to demand that this inequality be redressed.
Forming coalitions (Models of Community Organization; Social Capital Theory: Butterfoss & Kegler, 2022; Claridge, 2018; Clavier & de Leeuw, 2013)	Forming an alliance among individuals or organizations, during which they cooperate in joint action to reach a goal in their own self-interests.	Requires collaboration across various agendas; requires attention to stages of partnership development. Will often include persuasive communication, consciousness raising, goal setting, facilitation, and information about others' approval.	A grant application requires that a community develop a tobacco prevention coalition with representatives from public health, education, voluntary health associations, law enforcement, businesses, the health care sector, and other community groups to address the issue of youth smoking.
Social planning (Models of Community Organization: Minkler & Wakimoto, 2022)	Using information based on research to address issues.	Requires credible source of the information.	The health department planner presented epidemiological data on HIV/AIDS prevalence and trends to the Prevention Planning Group as they selected priority populations for programs.
Framing to shift perspectives (Models of Community Organization: Dorfman et al., 2022; Dorfman & Krasnow, 2014)	Assigning meaning and interpretation to relevant events and conditions in order to mobilize potential constituents, gain bystander support, and demobilize antagonists.	Match with culture.	Community organizers in tobacco prevention frame youth smoking as the result of heavy targeted advertising by the tobacco industry rather than as an individual decision.

Table 7.18 Methods to Change Policy

Method (Related Theories and References)	Definition	Parameters	Examples
Media advocacy (Models of Community Organization: Dorfman et al., 2022; Dorfman & Krasnow, 2014)	Expose environmental agents' behaviors in the mass media to order to get them to improve health-related conditions. A type of advocacy.	Requires the media to approve the news value of the message and accept the message without changing its essential content.	A public-interest group holds a press conference to focus attention on the serving sizes of and fat and calories in foods served in fast food restaurants; how that contributes to the obesity epidemic; and what the restaurants, as responsible community businesses, should do.
Agenda setting (Multiple Streams Theory, Advocacy Coalition Theory, Theories of Power: Clavier & de Leeuw, 2013; Kingdon, 2003)	Process of moving an issue to the political agenda for action; may make use of broad policy advocacy coalitions and media advocacy.	Requires appropriate timing (see policy window) and collaboration of (media) gatekeepers. Will often include persuasive communication and consciousness raising.	A state child health advocacy group developed a position paper on the expansion of the child health insurance program. They released the report to the media and held meetings with key state legislators on the recommendations.
Timing to coincide with policy windows (Multiple Streams Theory: Clavier & de Leeuw, 2013; Kingdon, 2003)	Advocating policy when politics, problems, and policy solutions are aligned to be receptive to a policy issue.	Requires an astute policy advocate who is well prepared	Health care reform advocates in the United States began to develop coalitions and position papers with the election of a president known to be supportive of that issue.
Creating and enforcing laws and regulations (Multiple Streams Theory, Theories of Power: Clavier & de Leeuw, 2013; Kingdon, 2003; Longest, 2006)	Forcing compliance or dictating or precluding choices. Sometimes implementing existing laws to accomplish change. Laws and regulations may also provide incentives.	Requires unequal power and availability of control and sanctions.	Based on a citizen group's request the police department began to enforce the loitering ordinance to reduce drug-related activity in the community.

Task 3: Moving from Methods to Applications

The third task in Step 3 is to select or design practical applications to operationalize change methods.

One change method may be accomplished by many applications, and the planner must decide which applications best fit the situation's context. The Web-based case studies give examples of the links between objectives, methods, applications, and programs (see Publisher's website www.wiley.com/go/bartholomew4e). The first challenge of this task for most health promoters is how to come up with creative practical applications. Some planning groups may feel less than creative at this point because they have been grappling with the science of intervention—describing the problem and gathering theory and evidence on which to base the intervention. This task, along with the first task in this step, requires stepping back from the details of program planning to freely discuss all the ideas that have been bubbling up for intervention applications.

How to Think About Applications

After working on the first two tasks of this step, planners will have a sense of how they will deliver their program and a sense of what theory- and evidence-based methods the program will contain. They can think about the change methods as the program's *active ingredients*, and the active ingredients need to be presented in practical applications. For example, the method of modeling might be presented as a role model story in print, or as a personal testimonial in person or online—or in any number of creative applications. The core of an application is the messages that will be processed by the target group for that application. Spending time with members of the intervention populations and potential program implementers will be a great help for thinking about applications and for writing the messages in the applications in Step 4 (see Chapter 8). Suitable applications will depend greatly on to whom and where the program is being delivered. For example, the Cystic Fibrosis Family Education Program (CF FEP) (Bartholomew et al., 1991) included many Social Cognitive Theory (SCT) constructs, so the planning team might logically have thought of applications that included a lot of interaction, such as group sessions and role playing for modeling. However, the team knew from having met with parents and adolescents during the needs assessment that they could reach only about 25% of the parent intervention group and almost none of the adolescents in a group setting. They therefore used applications such as role-model stories in newsletters, and they integrated delivery into families' clinical encounters. These types of application decisions, based on formative work, are very important.

Stick to the Theoretical Parameters of Change Methods

The methods tables presented earlier provided considerations for effective use of the change methods. These considerations include theoretical parameters and, particularly at the environmental levels, characteristics of the context that program planners must take into account. The challenge for health-promotion program planners is to design creative intervention applications that fit the context and characteristics of the program participants while ensuring that these applications also address the parameters of the selected methods.

For example, modeling from Social Cognitive Theory (see Chapter 3) is a method with the potential to increase self-efficacy (the determinant in the change objective). Bandura (1997) and Luszczynska and Schwarzer (2020) are sources for understanding the method and for discovering that modeling is effective under specific conditions or parameters (Bandura, 1997; Luszczynska & Schwarzer, 2020).

1. The learner identifies with the model
2. The model demonstrates feasible subskills
3. The model receives reinforcement
4. The observer perceives a coping model, not a mastery model

Using modeling in the program would be effective only when the parameters for this method are applied in the method's practical application. Modeling can be combined with other change methods, for instance, active learning. Active learning may be effective in almost any change method, as long as the situation provides sufficient motivation, information, time for elaboration, and skills-related advice. Skills-related advice is also essential for effective risk communication, particularly when using fear appeals.

Theories of fear-arousing communication and recent meta-analyses suggest that although fear arousal may enhance the motivation to avert the threat, acceptance of health recommendations is mainly dependent on people's outcome expectations regarding the recommendations (What will happen if I follow the recommendations?) and their self-efficacy (How confident am I that I can do the recommendations?). In addition, high levels of fear may easily inhibit persuasion through processes of denial and defensive avoidance, especially when response efficacy or self-efficacy is low (Kok et al., 2018; Peters et al., 2013; Ruiter et al., 2014; Tannenbaum et al., 2015). Thus, when using fear arousal, program developers should always provide coping methods for reducing the perceived threat and teach the skills for applying these coping methods.

Methods and Applications at Different Levels

Translating methods into applications for interventions to change environmental conditions, such as those directed toward social networks, organizations, communities, and policy makers, brings in some special considerations. At each of these levels, the environmental agent is influenced by methods addressing change objectives derived from the person's role. For example, outcome expectations for legislators related to voting to fund mammograms for low-income women might relate to constituent response or to expectations of improved constituent health.

The use of methods and practical applications to change determinants vary with ecological level. Health promoters can use the same methods with environmental agents that they direct toward individuals to increase knowledge, awareness, attitudes, skills, and social influence. However, at the environmental level these methods are often packaged into broader methods or processes that take into account the level and context of the situation. These broader methods include participatory problem-solving, advocacy, or organizational development. For example, participatory problem-solving as an environmental change method includes basic individual methods and those specific to knowledge change, attitude change, skills building, self-efficacy and collective efficacy, and other individual-level determinants. It includes diagnosing the problem, generating potential solutions, developing priorities, making an action plan, and obtaining feedback after implementing the plan. At the social network level, the application might take the form of calling together the family, friends, and helpers of an older person living alone for a meeting to discuss what the situation is and how they can come together to handle increasing needs for activities of daily living. At the organizational level, an intervention to improve employee morale might include conducting a survey of employee attitudes, giving feedback on the findings to employees and managers, holding small-group discussions of what the findings mean and how to address them, discussing the importance and changeability of the proposed activities, setting priorities, putting the changes into place, and getting feedback concerning their effectiveness through focus groups and surveys. At the community level, the application might be a workshop to develop a strategic plan for a community problem, such as obesity. Persons representing government and other organizations in the community meet with residents with a stake in the issue to discuss data concerning the problem, possible solutions, and available community resources. They brainstorm and evaluate applications for solutions, prioritize them, and develop action plans using committees for different community sectors.

Where Have All the Objectives Gone?

At the end of Intervention Mapping Step 3, the planner has moved from objectives to program ideas, methods, parameters, and applications. During that process, the planner has made many decisions, from theoretical and practical perspectives. The planner has estimated the strength of the evidence of methods and the feasibility of applications. The planner has anticipated issues in implementation by program users. At this point, it is necessary to ensure that all the objectives that were selected for the program are still matched in the current list of applications. If that is the case, the planner may continue to the next step of planning program production; if not, the planner has to decide whether to leave some objectives out or to go back and develop methods and applications to cover the neglected objectives.

Planning for Process Evaluation

The choice of appropriate change methods and practical applications for a program will have a lot to do with whether the program is effective or not.

However, the direct implications for evaluation of the methods and application choices are in the process evaluation. The process evaluation includes whether the theoretical methods that have been chosen are based on evidence and theory to support that they can produce changes in the determinants and change objectives from the matrices. Another question is whether the methods have been operationalized in ways that adhere to the parameters or the assumptions inherent in the use of the proposed theoretical change methods. Finally, a process evaluation question that relates to this step is whether the correct methods and parameters are apparent in the applications that are ultimately delivered to participants.

FOR OUR CHILDREN EXAMPLE: STEP 3

In Step 3, the planning group is tasked with building upon their previous work from Steps 1 and 2 to begin designing the intervention. This includes brainstorming intervention ideas for an initial program plan and selecting theory- and evidence-based change methods and applications to reach the behavioral and environmental objectives identified.

Task 1: Generate Ideas with the Planning Group

Once the tasks for Step 2 were completed for the ***For Our Children*** or, in Spanish, ***Por Nuestros Hijos* (PNH)** project (discussed in Chapter 6), the project planning group set up periodic planning meetings to generate potential ideas for the intervention based on the logic model of change developed in Step 2. With initial ideas for the intervention established during the grant writing process (i.e., a multi-component, multimedia web-based program), the planning group then assessed further the feasibility of these components for the intervention goals established in Step 1 and the alignment of the components with the behavioral and environmental outcomes, POs, and determinants identified in Step 2. As indicated in Step 1, the initial setting planned for intervening with parents and providers was within community health centers in the Greater Houston metropolitan area, with the intention of making the intervention available within the county safety net system (Harris Health System), federally qualified community health centers, and private and community clinics throughout Texas. This was an important consideration while assessing the feasibility of proposed components as well as during the grant writing process when the planners initially generated ideas about the potential intervention.

Task 2: Choose Theory- and Evidence-Based Change Methods and Task 3: Select and Design Practical Applications

After re-confirming that their initial intervention ideas were still feasible and appropriate, building on previous work (Kreuter, 2012), the PHN planning group set out to develop a program that would deliver clear messages about HPV, the HPV vaccine, and HPV-associated cancers to parents and providers, utilizing multiple intervention delivery vehicles, including interactive multimedia content delivered via a web-based application (parents and providers) and visual, print-based materials parents could review outside of the clinic.

The PHN planners began by generating a list of possible theory-based change methods expected to drive change in determinants identified in Task 2. They also considered methods shown in the literature to be effective at motivating parents to vaccinate their adolescent children (Holmes et al., 2007; Auger, 2007; Kreuter et al., 2000; Schmid et al., 2008; Van't Riet et al., 2016; Gerend et al., 2008; Kelder et al., 2015) and motivating healthcare providers to recommend/administer the HPV vaccine for their adolescent patients (Grandahl et al., 2017; Krawczyk et al., 2015; Moss et al., 2016; Brewer et al., 2017). They matched possible methods with relevant determinants and selected the final methods based on their feasibility and fit with the intervention context. Considering specific change objectives within the parent and provider matrices, the planners designed practical applications that would operationalize selected change methods, while ensuring that parameters critical to effective method translation were met.

Tables 7.19 and 7.20 provide a partial list of change methods selected and practical applications designed to target parent and provider determinants and change objectives identified in Task 2. For example, two theory-informed change methods selected for the parent component of the PNH intervention were *tailoring and modeling,* which both have roots in Social Cognitive Theory (Bandura, 1998). To operationalize the change method of *tailoring*, the planning group incorporated *self-tailoring and automatic-tailoring pause points* within an interactive web-based application developed for parents (practical applications), which would deliver tailored information. At these pause points, parents would select the types of information they were interested in viewing. For example, at one self-tailoring pause point, the app would display a list of common questions about the HPV vaccine and ask parents to select from this list all the questions they have about the vaccine. The app would then tailor subsequent content based on parents' selections. Using automatic tailoring pause points, the app would ask parents questions based on determinants identified in Task 2, then display different messages depending on parents' response to these questions (Rodriguez et al., 2018). To operationalize the *modeling* change method, the planning group planned to deliver program content within the web-based app featuring bilingual (English & Spanish), Hispanic actors that the priority population could identify with. These relatable actors would model actions the planners wanted parents to emulate, which aligned with performance objectives identified in Task 2 (e.g., a scene with a Hispanic mother initiating a conversation about the HPV vaccine with her child's healthcare provider) and fulfils the condition to have a coping model demonstrating the sub-behaviors rather than a mastery model that simply obtains the required behavioral outcome. It also fulfills the condition of the model being rewarded for completing the desired behavior rather than being punished for undesirable behavior.

Table 7.19 Partial Table of Methods and Applications for Parents from Por Nuestros Hijos Project

Behavioral Outcome	Determinant and Targeted Change Objectives	Method	Parameters for Use	Practical Application	Program Component
Parents will obtain the HPV vaccine for their adolescent children	State that they may have to initiate a conversation about the HPV vaccine with their son's/daughter's physician (K.2.a) Express confidence in and demonstrate ability to initiate a discussion even if it is not mentioned. (SSE.2.a) and ask questions about the HPV vaccine for son/daughter (SSE.2.b) Express belief that their child could be at risk of HPV infection at some point in their life (PS.2.a)	Modeling; Tailoring	Modeling: Attention, remembrance, self-efficacy and skills, reinforcement of model; identification with model; coping model instead of mastery model. Tailoring: Variables or factors related to behavior change (such as stage) or to relevance (such as culture or socioeconomic status)	• Self-tailoring pause point: slide to select information either for sons or daughters • Scene with mother from similar cultural background initiating conversation with the physician; • Scene with parent having an open discussion with child's physician; • Scene with doctor giving personalized, age applicable information to parent & child	Interactive multimedia/ Fotonovela
	State that they can get the vaccine for their child during the same appointment (K.4a.a.) Express belief that: vaccinating their sons/daughters during the same appointment could be beneficial and time/cost-effective (A.4a.a); and that it is important to make an appointment to obtain the vaccine (A.4b.a) Express confidence in and demonstrate ability to: request the vaccine while at the doctor's office (SSE.4a.a); make the appointment (SSE.4b.a.); and keep child's appointment (SSE.4b.b)	Modeling; Tailoring	Modeling: Attention, remembrance, self-efficacy and skills, reinforcement of model; identification with model; coping model instead of mastery model. Tailoring: Variables or factors related to behavior change (such as stage) or to relevance (such as culture or socioeconomic status).	• Scene with mother using resource list • Automatic-tailoring pause point: slide to select whether the parent would feel that making and keeping HPV vaccine appointments would be a problem for them • Scene with mother and teenage son/daughter at doctor's office • Scene with mother and son/daughter at doctor's office making appointment • Scene with mother and friend encouraging her to make appointment • Scene with parent calling clinic on resource list and making an appointment • Scene with parent traveling to clinic with son/daughter • Scene with parents discussing how they vaccinated their sons/daughters during same visit • Scene with mothers/parents discussing how they made and kept HPV vaccination appointments	Interactive multimedia/ Fotonovela

Table 7.20 Partial Table of Methods and Applications for Healthcare Providers from Por Nuestros Hijos Project

Environmental Outcome	Determinant and Targeted Change Objectives	Method	Parameters for Use	Practical Application	Program Component
Healthcare providers will vaccinate all eligible patients against HPV in accordance with Advisory Committee on Immunization Practices (ACIP) guidelines.	Describe CDC recommendation that providers deliver strong "bundled and unqualified" HPV vaccine recommendation for all eligible patients (K.2.a); and with Tdap and MCV (K.2.b.) Describe that receiving a strong "bundled and unqualified" recommendation for the HPV vaccine is a significant predictor of vaccine uptake (K.2.c.) Express confidence in and demonstrate ability to deliver a strong HPV vaccine recommendation to all eligible patients (SSE.2.a.); and to deliver a bundled vaccine recommendation to patients due for other vaccines (SSE.2.b.) Express belief that delivering a bundled recommendation will increase HPV vaccination in clinic (OE.2.c.); and reduce parental or patient hesitancy and refusal of the HPV vaccine (OE.2.d.)	Information; Persuasive communication; Modeling	Information: Informative arguments supported by data; trustworthy source Persuasive Communication: Messages need to be relevant and not too discrepant from the beliefs of the individual; can be stimulated by surprise and repetition; will include arguments. Modeling: Attention, remembrance, self-efficacy and skills, reinforcement of model; identification with model; coping model instead of mastery model.	• Mobile app—information from CDC and other respected agencies on a strong HPV recommendation is shared. • Mobile app – physician actor shares relevant data from scientific journals and credible websites on impact of a strong bundled HPV recommendation. • Mobile app—physician actor demonstrates how to give a strong HPV recommendation at different scenarios (by age) • Mobile app—physician actor demonstrates how to give age-appropriate bundling recommendations during a visit for other adolescent vaccines options. • Mobile app—skills-based exercises/puzzle to practice giving recommendation by answering correctly different scenarios (by age) for recommendation. • Mobile app—physician actor cites data highlighting that provider recommendations plays a significant role in HPV vaccination. • Mobile app—physician actor reinforces the role that the provider plays in increasing HPV vaccination.	MiApp (Module#2)

Summary

This chapter explained creative, theory- and evidence-based program design. We discussed the importance of all program components having theoretical behavior change and environmental change methods as well as practical applications at both the individual level and the environmental level. Planners first generate program ideas with the planning group. They discuss the rough outlines of a possible intervention program. Then they choose theory-based change methods to address program objectives, applying the core processes provided in Chapter 2. Tables of methods in this chapter provided definitions, parameters for application, and examples at individual and environmental levels. In the last task planners select or design practical applications of change methods. The chapter emphasized the importance of applying the methods correctly using the parameters for use.

Discussion Questions and Learning Activities

1. Explain the characteristics that distinguish theoretical methods from practical applications. Give examples of theoretical methods and related practical applications.
2. Discuss why it is important to review program ideas with intended program participants before making decisions on what methods and practical applications will be used to plan the interventions.
3. Describe how core processes can be used to choose theoretical methods. Give an example of a question that can be asked to guide the use of core processes to choose theoretical methods.
4. Discuss examples of basic methods that can be applied at the individual level and examples that can be applied at environmental levels of intervention.
5. For each of the following categories of personal determinants or environmental change, select one method and describe the parameters for use that are critical for the method to influence a change: knowledge, awareness and risk perception, habits and automatic behavior, attitudes, social influence, skills and self-efficacy, social norms, organizational change, community change, and policy change.
6. For each of the theoretical methods selected for the intervention, discuss the parameters that would have to be considered to ensure that the application of the methods would likely be effective in changing the determinants of behavior and environmental outcomes.

References

Abraham, C., & Michie, S. (2008). A taxonomy of behavior change techniques used in interventions. *Health Psychology, 27*, 379–387.

Achtziger, A., Gollwitzer, P. M., & Sheeran, P. (2008). Implementation intentions and shielding goal striving from unwanted thoughts and feelings. *Personality & Social Psychology Bulletin, 34*(3), 381–393. doi:10.1177/0146167207311201

Ajzen, I., Czasch, C., & Flood, M. G. (2009). From intentions to behavior: Implementation intention, commitment, and conscientiousness. *Journal of Applied Social Psychology, 39*(6), 1356–1372.

Ajzen, I., & Schmidt, P. (2020). Changing behavior using the theory of planned behavior. In M. Hagger, L. Cameron, K. Hamilton, N. Hankonen, & T. Lintunen (Eds.), *The handbook of behavior change* (pp. 17–31). Cambridge University Press. doi:10.1017/9781108677318

Allport, G. W. (1954). *The nature of prejudice*. Addison-Wesley.

Aronson, E. (2015). Jigsaw classroom. http://www.jigsaw.org/

Auger, S., & Verbiest, S. (2007). Lay health educators' roles in improving patient education. *North Carolina Medical Journal, 68*(5), 333–335.

Bandura, A. (1986). *Social foundations of thought and action: A social cognitive theory*. Prentice-Hall.

Bandura, A. (1997). *Self-efficacy: The exercise of control*. W. H. Freeman & Co.

Bandura, A. (1998). Health promotion from the perspective of social cognitive theory. *Psychology and Health, 13*(4), 623–649.

Bartholomew, K. L., Czyzewski, D. I., Swank, P. R., McCormick, L., & Parcel, G. S. (2000). Maximizing the impact of the cystic fibrosis family education program: Factors related to program diffusion. *Family & Community Health, 22*(4), 27–47.

Bartholomew, L. K., Gold, R. S., Parcel, G. S., Czyzewski, D. I., Sockrider, M. M., Fernandez, M., Shegog, R., & Swank, P. (2000). Watch, discover, think, and act: Evaluation of computer-assisted instruction to improve asthma self-management in inner-city children. *Patient Education and Counseling, 39*(2), 269–280.

Bartholomew, L. K., Markham, C. M., Parcel, G. S., Kok, G., Gottlieb, N. H., & Fernandez, M. E. (2016). *Planning health promotion programs: An intervention mapping approach* (Vol. 4). Jossey-Bass.

Bartholomew, L. K., Parcel, G. S., Kok, G., & Gottlieb, N. H. (2001). *Planning health promotion programs: An intervention mapping approach* (Vol. 1). Jossey-Bass.

Bartholomew, L. K., Parcel, G. S., Kok, G., & Gottlieb, N. H. (2006). *Planning health promotion programs: An intervention mapping approach* (Vol. 2). Jossey-Bass.

Bartholomew, L. K., Parcel, G. S., Kok, G., & Gottlieb, N. H. (2011). In M. E. Fernandez (Ed.), *Planning health promotion programs: An intervention mapping approach* (Vol. 3). Jossey-Bass.

Bartholomew, L. K., Parcel, G. S., Seilheimer, D. K., Czyzewski, D., Spinelli, S. H., & Congdon, B. (1991). Development of a health education program to promote the self- management of cystic fibrosis. *Health Education & Behavior, 18*(4), 429–443.

Batson, C. D., Chang, J., Orr, R., & Rowland, J. (2002). Empathy, attitudes, and action: Can feeling for a member of a stigmatized group motivate one to help the group? *Personality and Social Psychology Bulletin, 28*(12), 1656–1666.

Beck, J. S. (2011). *Cognitive behavior therapy: Basics and beyond* (2nd ed.). The Guilford Press.

Berkman, E. T., Berkman, E. T., Hutcherson, C. A., Livingston, J. L., Kahn, L. E., & Inzlicht, M. (2017). Self-control as value-based choice. *Current Directions in Psychological Science, 26*(5), 422–428. doi:10.1177/0963721417704394

Berman, A., Beckman, M., & Lindqvist, H. (2020). Motivational interviewing interventions. In M. Hagger, L. Cameron, K. Hamilton, N. Hankonen, & T. Lintunen (Eds.), *The handbook of behavior change*. Cambridge University Press. doi:10.1017/978110867731

Berninger, N. M., ten Hoor, G. A., Plasqui, G., Kok, G., Peters, G.-J. Y., & Ruiter, R. A. C. (2020). Sedentary work in desk-dominated environments: A data-driven intervention using intervention mapping. *JMIR Formative Research, 4*(7), e14951. doi:10.2196/14951

Bos, A. E., Schaalma, H. P., & Pryor, J. B. (2008). Reducing AIDS-related stigma in developing countries: The importance of theory- and evidence-based interventions. *Psychology, Health & Medicine, 13*, 450–460.

Bouton, M. E. (2014). Why behavior change is difficult to sustain. *Preventive Medicine, 68*, 29–36. doi:10.1016/j.ypmed.2014.06.010

Brewer, N. T., DeFrank, J. T., & Gilkey, M. B. (2016). Anticipated regret and health behavior: A meta-analysis. *Health Psychology, 35*(11), 1264–1275. doi:10.1037/hea0000294

Brewer, N. T., Hall, M. E., Malo, T. L., Gilkey, M. B., Quinn, B., & Lathren, C. (2017). Announcements versus conversations to improve HPV vaccination coverage: A randomized trial. *Pediatrics, 139*(1).

Brown, L. D., Bammer, G., Batliwala, S., & Kunreuther, F. (2003). Framing practice-research engagement for democratizing knowledge. *Action Research, 1*(1), 81–102.

Brownson, R., Glanz, K., Tabak, R., & Stamatakis, K. (2015). Implementation, dissemination and diffusion of public health interventions. In K. Glanz, B. K. Rimer, & K. Viswanath (Eds.), *Health behavior: Theory, research, and practice* (Vol. 5, pp. 544–592). Jossey-Bass.

Butterfoss, F. D., & Kegler, M. C. (2022). Community coalition action theory: Designing and evaluating community collaboratives. In F. D. Butterfoss & M. C. Kegler (Eds.), *Community organizing and community building for health and social equity* (4th ed., pp. 307–324). Rutgers University Press.

Chen, Z., Veling, H., Dijksterhuis, A., & Holland, R. W. (2016). How does not responding to appetitive stimuli cause devaluation: Evaluative conditioning or response inhibition? *Journal of Experimental Psychology: General, 145*(12), 1687–1701. doi:10.1037/xge0000236

Christoffel, K. K. (2000). Public health advocacy: Process and product. *American Journal of Public Health, 90*(5), 722–726.

Chung, A. C. A., & Rimal, R. N. (2016). Social norms: A review. *Review of Communication Research, 4*, 01–28. doi:10.12840/issn.2255-4165.2016.04.01.008

Cialdini, R. B. (2008). *Influence: Science and practice.* Allyn & Bacon.

Cislaghi, B., & Heise, L. (2018). Theory and practice of social norms interventions: Eight common pitfalls. *Globalization and Health, 14*(1), 83. doi:10.1186/s12992-018-0398-x

Claridge, T. (2018). Functions of social capital–bonding, bridging, linking. *Social Capital Research, 20*(1), 1–7. doi:10.5281/zenodo.7993853

Clavier, C., & de Leeuw, E. (2013). *Health promotion and the policy process.* Oxford University Press.

Cohen, G. L., & Sherman, D. K. (2014). The psychology of change: Self-affirmation and social psychological intervention. *Annual Review of Psychology, 65,* 333–371.

Cohen, S., & Wills, T. A. (1985). Stress, social support, and the buffering hypothesis. *Psychological Bulletin, 98*(2), 310–357. doi:10.1037/0033-2909.98.2.310

Compton, J., Jackson, B., & Dimmock, J. A. (2016). Persuading others to avoid persuasion: Inoculation theory and resistant health attitudes. *Frontiers in Psychology, 7*(122). doi:10.3389/fpsyg.2016.00122

Crano, W. D., & Prislin, R. (2011). *Attitudes and attitude change.* Psychology Press.

Creer, T. L. (2000). Self-management of chronic illness. In M. Boekaerts, P. R. Pintrich, & M. Zeidner (Eds.), *Handbook of self-regulation* (pp. 601–629). Academic Press.

Cummings, T. G., & Worley, C. G. (2014). *Organization development and change* (Vol. 10). South-Western Cengage Learning.

Cummings, T. G., & Worley, C. G. (2018). *Organization development and change* (11th ed.). Cengage Learning.

Custers, R., & Aarts, H. (2010). The unconscious will: How the pursuit of goals operates outside of conscious awareness. *Science, 329*(5987), 47–50. doi:10.1126/science.1188595

de Bono, E. (2015). *Lateral thinking: Creativity step by step.* Harper Colophon.

de Bruin, M., Crutzen, R., & Peters, G.-J. Y. (2015). Everything should be as simple as possible, but this will still be complex: A reply to various commentaries on IPEBA. *Health Psychology Review, 9*(1), 38–41.

de Bruin, M., Viechtbauer, W., Schaalma, H. P., Kok, G., Abraham, C., & Hospers, H. J. (2010). Standard care impact on effects of highly active antiretroviral therapy adherence interventions: A meta-analysis of randomized controlled trials. *Archives of Internal Medicine, 170*(3), 240–250.

de Decker, E., de Craemer, M., de Bourdeaudhuij, I., Verbestel, V., Duvinage, K., Iotova, V., Grammatikaki, E., Wildgruber, A., Mouratidou, T., & Manios, Y. (2014). Using the intervention mapping protocol to reduce European preschoolers' sedentary behavior, an application to the ToyBox-Study. *International Journal of Behavioral Nutrition and Physical Activity, 11*(1), 1–18.

de Ridder, D. (2014). Nudging for beginners: A shortlist of issues in urgent need of research. *European Health Psychologist, 16*(1), 2–6.

de Ridder, D., Feitsma, J., van den Hoven, M., Kroese, F., Schillemans, T., Verweij, M., Venema, T., Vugts, A., & de Vet, E. (2020). Simple nudges that are not so easy. *Behavioural Public Policy, 8,* 154–172. doi:10.1017/bpp.2020.36

de Ridder, D., Gillebaart, M., & Friese, M. (2020). Self-control interventions. In M. S. Hagger, L. D. Cameron, K. Hamilton, N. Hankonen, & T. Lintunen (Eds.), *The handbook of behavior change* (pp. 586–598). Cambridge University Press. doi:10.1017/9781108677318

Deutsch, R., & Strack, F. (2020). Changing behavior using the Reflective-Impulsive Model. In M. S. Hagger, L. D. Cameron, K. Hamilton, N. Hankonen, & T. Lintunen (Eds.), *The handbook of behavior change* (pp. 164–177). Cambridge University Press.

Diamond, A. (2013). Executive functions. *Annual Review of Psychology, 64*, 135.

DiClemente, C. C., & Graydon, M. M. (2020). Changing behavior using the transtheoretical model. In M. Hagger, L. Cameron, K. Hamilton, N. Hankonen, & T. Lintunen (Eds.), *The handbook of behavior change* (pp. 136–149). Cambridge University Press. doi:10.1017/9781108677318

Dorfman, L., Gonzales, P., & Cuestas, S. M. (2022). Media advocay: A potent strategy for engaging communities in the fight for equitable public policy. In M. Minkler & P. Wakimoto (Eds.), *Community organizing and community building for health and social equity* (4th ed., pp. 416–428). Rutgers University Press.

Dorfman, L., & Krasnow, I. D. (2014). Public health and media advocacy. *Annual Review of Public Health, 35*(1), 293–306. doi:10.1146/annurev-publhealth-032013-182503

Epton, T., & Armitage, C. J. (2020). Goal setting interventions. In M. S. Hagger, L. D. Cameron, K. Hamilton, N. Hankonen, & T. Lintunen (Eds.), *The handbook of behavior change* (pp. 554–571). Cambridge University Press. doi:10.1017/9781108677318

Epton, T., Harris, P. R., Kane, R., van Koningsbruggen, G. M., & Sheeran, P. (2015). The impact of self-affirmation on health-behavior change: A meta-analysis. *Health Psychology, 34*(3), 187–196. doi:10.1037/hea0000116

Fishbein, M., & Ajzen, I. (2010). *Predicting and changing behavior: The reasoned action approach*. Taylor & Francis Group.

Flaspohler, P., Duffy, J., Wandersman, A., Stillman, L., & Maras, M. A. (2008). Unpacking prevention capacity: An intersection of research-to-practice models and community-centered models. *American Journal of Community Psychology, 41*(3), 182–196.

Forsyth, D. R. (2018). *Group dynamics*. Cengage Learning.

Freire, P. (1973a). *Education for critical consciousness*. Seabury Press.

Freire, P. (1973b). *Pedagogy of the oppressed*. Seabury Press.

Freudenberg, N., & Tsui, E. (2014). Evidence, power, and policy change in community-based participatory research. *American Journal of Public Health, 104*(1), 11–14.

Friese, M., Hofmann, W., & Wiers, R. W. (2011). On taming horses and strengthening riders: Recent developments in research on interventions to improve self-control in health behaviors. *Self and Identity, 10*(3), 336–351. doi:10.1080/15298868.2010.536417

Galer-Unti, R. A., Tappe, M. K., & Lachenmayr, S. (2004). Advocacy 101: Getting started in health education advocacy. *Health Promotion Practice, 5*(3), 280–288.

Gardner, B., Rebar, A. L., & Lally, P. (2020). Habit interventions. In M. S. Hagger, L. D. Cameron, K. Hamilton, N. Hankonen, & T. Lintunen (Eds.), *The handbook of behavior change* (pp. 599–616). Cambridge University Press.

Gerber, J. P., Wheeler, L., & Suls, J. (2018). A social comparison theory meta-analysis 60+ years on. *Psychological Bulletin, 144*(2), 177–197. doi:10.1037/bul0000127

Gerend, M. A., Shepherd, J. E., & Monday, K. A. (2008). Behavioral frequency moderates the effects of message framing on HPV vaccine acceptability. *Annals of Behavioral Medicine, 35*(2), 221–229.

Glanz, K., Rimer, B. K., & Viswanath, K. (2015). *Health behavior: Theory, research, and practice* (5th ed.). John Wiley & Sons.

Gneezy, U., Kajackaite, A., & Meier, S. (2020). Incentive-based interventions. In M. S. Hagger, L. D. Cameron, K. Hamilton, N. Hankonen, & T. Lintunen (Eds.), *The handbook of behavior change* (pp. 523–536). Cambridge University Press. doi:10.1017/9781108677318

Gobet, F. (2005). Chunking models of expertise: Implications for education. *Applied Cognitive Psychology, 19*(2), 183–204. doi:10.1002/acp.1110

Gobet, F., Lane, P. C., Croker, S., Cheng, P. C., Jones, G., Oliver, I., & Pine, J. M. (2001). Chunking mechanisms in human learning. *Trends in Cognitive Sciences, 5*(6), 236–243.

Godin, G., Gagnon, H., Alary, M., Levy, J., & Otis, J. (2007). The degree of planning: An indicator of the potential success of health education programs. *Promotion & Education, 14*(3), 138–142.

Gollwitzer, P. M., & Sheeran, P. (2006). Implementation intentions and goal achievement: A meta-analysis of effects and processes. *Advances in Experimental Social Psychology, 38*, 69–119.

Grandahl, M., Tydén, T., Westerling, R., Nevéus, T., Rosenblad, A., Hedin, E., et al. (2017). To consent or decline HPV vaccination: A pilot study at the start of the national school-based vaccination program in Sweden. *Journal of school health, 87*(1), 62–70.

Hagger, M., Hankonen, N., Chatzisarantis, N., & Ryan, R. (2020). Changing behavior using self-determination theory. In M. Hagger, L. Cameron, K. Hamilton, N. Hankonen, & T. Lintunen (Eds.), *The handbook of behavior change* (pp. 104–119). Cambridge University Press. doi:10.1017/9781108677318

Hagger, M., Luszczynska, A., de Wit, J., Benyamini, Y., Burkert, S., Chamberland, P.-E., ... Gollwitzer, P. M. (2016). Implementation intention and planning interventions in health psychology: Recommendations from the Synergy Expert Group for research and practice. *Psychology & Health, 31*(7), 814–839. doi:10.1080/08870446.2016.1146719

Hagger, M. S., Cameron, L. D., Hamilton, K., Hankonen, N., & Lintunen, T. (2020). *The handbook of behavior change*. doi:10.1017/9781108677318

Harris, P. R., Jessop, D. C., & Harris, P. S. (2020). Self-affirmation and health. In *The wiley encyclopedia of health psychology* (pp. 587–595). John Wiley & Sons. doi:10.1002/9781119057840.ch109

Hatzenbuehler, M. L., Phelan, J. C., & Link, B. G. (2013). Stigma as a fundamental cause of population health inequalities. *American Journal of Public Health, 103*(5), 813–821. doi:10.2105/AJPH.2012.301069

Hayes, S. C., Strosahl, K. D., & Wlison, K. G. (1999). *Acceptance and commitment therapy: An experiential approach to behavior change.* Guilford Press.

He, S., Ojo, A., Beckman, A. L., Gondi, S., Gondi, S., Betz, M., Faust, J. S., Choo, E., Kass, D., & Raja, A. S. (2020). The story of #GetMePPE and GetUsPPE.org to mobilize health care response to COVID-19: Rapidly deploying digital tools for better health care. *Journal of Medical Internet Research, 22*(7), e20469. doi:10.2196/20469

Hofmann, W., Dohle, S., & Diel, K. (2020). Changing behavior using self-control theory. In M. S. Hagger, L. D. Cameron, K. Hamilton, N. Hankonen, & T. Lintunen (Eds.), *The handbook of behavior change* (pp. 150–163). Cambridge University Press. doi:10.1017/9781108677318

Holt-Lunstad, J. (2022). Social connection as a public health issue: The evidence and a systemic framework for prioritizing the "social" in social determinants of health. *Annual Review of Public Health, 43*(1), 193–213. doi:10.1146/annurev-publhealth-052020-110732

Holt-Lunstad, J. (2023). 2023 national health guidelines for social connection: What is the evidence in support and what might the guidelines say? *Policy Insights From the Behavioral and Brain Sciences, 10*(1), 41–50. doi:10.1177/23727322221150204

Holt-Lunstad, J., & Uchino, B. N. (2015). Social suppport and health. In K. Glanz, R. Rimer & K. Viswanath (Eds.), *Health behavior and health education: Theory, research and practice* (5th ed., pp. 183–204). Jossey-Bass.

Holmes, M., Bacon, T. J., Dobson, L. A., McGorty, E. K., & Silberman, P. (2007). *North Carolina Medical Journal, 68*(5), 319–326.

Johannes, N., Buijzen, M., & Veling, H. (2021). Beyond inhibitory control training: Inactions and actions influence smartphone app use through changes in explicit liking. *Journal of Experimental Psychology: General, 150*, 431–445. doi:10.1037/xge0000888

Kazdin, A. (2012). *Behavior modification in applied settings* (7th ed.). Waveland Press.

Kelder, S., Hoelscher, D., & Perry, C. (2015). How individuals, environments, and health behaviour interact: Social Cognitive Theory. In K. Glanz, B. Rimer, & K. Viswanath (Eds.), *Health behavior: Theory, research, and practice* (5th ed., pp. 285–325). Jossey-Bass.

Keller, L., Gollwitzer, P., & Sheeran, P. (2020). Changing behavior using the model of action phases. In M. Hagger, L. Cameron, K. Hamilton, N. Hankonen, & T. Lintunen (Eds.), *The handbook of behavior change* (pp. 77–88). Cambridge University Press. doi:10.1017/9781108677318

Kelder, S., Hoelscher, D., & Perry In, C. (2015). In K. Glanz, B. Rimer, & K. V. Jossey-Bass (Eds.), *Health behavior: Theory, research, and practice* (5th ed.).

Kingdon, J. W. (2003). *Agenda, alternatives, and public policies* (2nd ed.). Longman.

Kok, G. (2021). Novelty as a parameter for using arguments in persuasive communication. *Health Psychology Bulletin, 5*(1), 12. doi:10.5334/hpb.13

Kok, G., Gottlieb, N., Commers, M., & Smerecnik, C. (2008). The ecological approach in health promotion programs: A decade later. *American Journal of Health Promotion, 22*(6), 437–442.

Kok, G., Gottlieb, N., Panne, R., & Smerecnik, C. (2012). Methods for environmental change: An exploratory study. *BMC Public Health, 12*, 1037.

Kok, G., Gottlieb, N., Peters, G.-J., Mullen, P., Parcel, G., Ruiter, R., Fernandez, M., Markham, C., & Bartholomew, L. (2016). A taxonomy of behavior change methods: An intervention mapping approach. *Health Psychology Review, 10*(3), 297–312. doi:10.1080/17437199.2015.1077155

Kok, G., Gurabardhi, Z., Gottlieb, N. H., & Zijlstra, F. R. H. (2015). Influencing organizations to promote health: Applying stakeholder theory. *Health Education & Behavior, 42*(1_suppl), 123S–132S. doi:10.1177/1090198115571363

Kok, G., Peters, G.-J., Kessels, L., ten Hoor, G., & Ruiter, R. (2018). Ignoring theory and misinterpreting evidence: The false belief in fear appeals. *Health Psychology Review, 12*(2), 111–125. doi:10.1080/17437199.2017.1415767

Kok, G., Schaalma, H., Ruiter, R., van Empelen, P., & Brug, J. (2004). Intervention mapping: Protocol for applying health psychology theory to prevention programmes. *Journal of Health Psychology, 9*(1), 85–98.

Kools, M. (2012). Making written materials easy to use. In C. Abraham & M. Kools (Eds.), *Writing health communication: An evidence-based guide* (pp. 43–62). Sage.

Kools, M., van de Wiel, M., Ruiter, R., Cruts, A., & Kok, G. (2006). The effect of graphic organizers on subjective and objective comprehension of a health education text. *Health Education & Behavior, 33*(6), 760–772.

Krawczyk, A., Knäuper, B., Gilca, V., Dubé, E., Perez, S., Joyal-Desmarais, K., et al. (2015). Parents' decision-making about the human papillomavirus vaccine for their daughters: II. Qualitative results. *Human Vaccines & Immunotherapeutics, 11*(2), 322–329.

Kreuter, M., & McClure, S. (2004). The role of culture in health communication. *Annual Review of Public Health, 25*, 439–455.

Kreuter, M. W., Fernandez, M. E., Brown, M., Cofta-Woerpel, L., Pfeiffer, D., Adams-Piphus, B., Krebill, H., Gonzalez, D. A., Campos, D. M., Kirklin, G. T., Betsworth, S., Casey, C., & Luke, D. (2012 Jan-Mar). Increasing information-seeking about human papillomavirus vaccination through community partnerships in African American and Hispanic communities. *Fam Community Health, 35*(1), 15–30. doi:10.1097/FCH.0b013e3182385d13

Kreuter, M., Farrell, D., Olevitch, L., & Brennan, L. (2000). *Tailoring health messages: Customizing communication with computer technology*. Lawrence Erlbaum Associates Publishers.

Lakey, B., & Orehek, E. (2011). Relational regulation theory: A new approach to explain the link between perceived support and mental health. *Psychological Review, 118*(3), 482–495. doi:10.1037/a0023477

Lambe, F., Ran, Y., Jürisoo, M., Holmlid, S., Muhoza, C., Johnson, O., & Osborne, M. (2020). Embracing complexity: A transdisciplinary conceptual framework for understanding behavior change in the context of development-focused interventions. *World Development, 126*, 104703. doi:10.1186/s12966-022-01267-3

Lawrence, N. S., O'Sullivan, J., Parslow, D., Javaid, M., Adams, R. C., Chambers, C. D., & Verbruggen, F. (2015). Training response inhibition to food is associated with weight loss and reduced energy intake. *Appetite, 95*, 17–28.

Linhorst, D. M., Hamilton, G., Young, E., & Eckert, A. (2002). Opportunities and barriers to empowering people with severe mental illness through participation in treatment planning. *Social Work, 47*(4), 425–434. doi:10.1093/sw/47.4.425

Locke, E. A., & Latham, G. P. (2019). The development of goal setting theory: A half century retrospective. *Motivation Science, 5*(2). doi:10.1037/mot0000127

Longest, B. B. (2006). *Health policymaking in the United States* (4th ed.). Health Administration Press.

Luna Pinzon, A., Stronks, K., Dijkstra, C., Renders, C., Altenburg, T., Den Hertog, K., Kremers, S. P. J., Chinapaw, M. J. M., Verhoeff, A. P., & Waterlander, W. (2022). The ENCOMPASS framework: A practical guide for the evaluation of public health programmes in complex adaptive systems. *International Journal of Behavioral Nutrition and Physical Activity, 19*(1), 33. doi:10.1186/s12966-022-01267-3

Luszczynska, A., & Schwarzer, R. (2020). Changing behavior using social cognitive theory. In M. Hagger, L. Cameron, K. Hamilton, N. Hankonen, & T. Lintunen (Eds.), *The handbook of behavior change* (pp. 32–45). Cambridge University Press. doi:10.1017/9781108677318

Maibach, E., & Cotton, D. (1995). Moving people to behavior change: A staged social cognitive approach to message design. In E. Maibach & R. Parrott (Eds.), *Designing health messages: Approaches from communication theory and public health practice* (pp. 41–64). Sage.

Mann, T., de Ridder, D., & Fujita, K. (2013). Self-regulation of health behavior: Social psychological approaches to goal setting and goal striving. *Health Psychology: Official Journal of the Division of Health Psychology, American Psychological Association, 32*(5), 487–498. doi:10.1037/a0028533

Marlatt, G., & Donovan, D. (2005). In G. Marlatt & D. Donovan (Eds.), *Relapse prevention: Maintenance strategies in the treatment of addictive behaviors* (2nd ed.). Guilford Press.

Marques, M. M., Wright, A. J., Corker, E., Johnston, M., West, R., Hastings, J., Zhang, L., & Michie, S. (2023). The behaviour change technique ontology: Transforming the behaviour change technique taxonomy v1. *Wellcome Open Research, 8*, 308. doi:10.12688/wellcomeopenres.19363.1

Maunder, R. D., & White, F. A. (2019). Intergroup contact and mental health stigma: A comparative effectiveness meta-analysis. *Clinical Psychology Review, 72*, 101749. doi:10.1016/j.cpr.2019.101749

McAlister, A. (2017). Behavioral journalism in health and risk messaging. In M. Powers (Ed.), *Oxford research encyclopedia of communication* (online ed.). Oxford Academic, New York, NY. doi:10.1093/acrefore/9780190228613.013.326, accessed 20 Apr. 2026

McCullum, C., Pelletier, D., Barr, D., Wilkins, J., & Habicht, J. P. (2004). Mechanisms of power within a community-based food security planning process. *Health Education & Behavior, 31*(2), 206–222. doi:10.1177/1090198103259163

McGuire, W. J. (1964). Inducing resistance to persuasion. Some contemporary approaches. In W. O. Kaelber & C. C. Haaland (Eds.), *Self and society: An anthology of readings* (pp. 192–230). Ginn Custom Publishing.

McGuire, W. J. (1985). Attitude and attitude change. In E. Aronson & G. Lindzey (Eds.), *The handbook of social psychology* (pp. 233–346). Random House.

McGuire, W. J. (2001). Input and output variables currently promising for constructing persuasive communications. In R. Rice & C. Atkin (Eds.), *Public communication campaigns* (3rd ed., pp. 22–48). Sage.

McLean, G. (2005). *Organizational development: Principles, processes, performance.* Berrett-Koehler.

McSweeney, F., & Murphy, E. (2014). *The Wiley Blackwell handbook of operant and classical conditioning.* John Wiley & Sons.

Mevissen, F. E. F., Meertens, R. M., Ruiter, R. A. C., Feenstra, H., & Schaalma, H. P. (2009). HIV/STI risk communication: The effects of scenario-based risk information and frequency-based risk information on perceived susceptibility to Chlamydia and HIV. *Journal of Health Psychology, 14*, 78–87.

Mevissen, F. E. F., Meertens, R. M., Ruiter, R. A. C., & Schaalma, H. P. (2012). Bedtime stories: The effects of self - constructed risk scenarios on imaginability and perceived susceptibility to sexually transmitted infections. *Psychology & Health, 27*(9), 1036–1047.

Mevissen, F. E. F., van Empelen, P., Watzeels, A., van Duin, G., Meijer, S., van Lieshout, S., & Kok, G. (2018). Development of Long Live Love +, a school-based online sexual health programme for young adults. An intervention mapping approach. *Sex Education, 18*(1), 47–73. doi:10.1080/14681811.2017.1389717

Michie, S., Ashford, S., Sniehotta, F., Dombrowski, S., Bishop, A., & French, D. (2011). A refined taxonomy of behaviour change techniques to help people change their physical activity and healthy eating behaviours: The CALO-RE taxonomy. *Psychology & Health, 26*(11), 1479–1498.

Michie, S., Richardson, M., Johnston, M., Abraham, C., Francis, J., Hardeman, W., Eccles, M., Cane, J., & Wood, C. (2013). The behavior change technique taxonomy (v1) of 93 hierarchically clustered techniques: Building an international consensus for the reporting of behavior change interventions. *Annals of Behavioral Medicine, 46*(1), 81–95. doi:10.1007/s12160-013-9486-6

Michie, S., Wood, C. E., Johnston, M., Abraham, C., Francis, J. J., & Hardeman, W. (2015). Behaviour change techniques: The development and evaluation of a taxonomic method for reporting and describing behaviour change interventions (a suite of five studies involving consensus methods, randomised controlled trials and analysis of qualitative data). *Health Technology Assessment, 19*(99), 1–888. doi:10.3310/hta19990

Miller, W. R., & Rollnick, S. (2012). *Motivational interviewing: Helping people change* (3rd ed.). Guilford Press.

Minkler, M., & Wakimoto, P. (2021). *Community organizing and community building for health and social equity* (4th ed.). Rutgers University Press.

Minkler, M., & Wakimoto, P. (2022). Introduction to community organizing and community building in a new era. In M. Minkler & P. Wakimoto (Eds.), *Community organizing and community building for health and social equity* (4th ed., pp. 7–25).

Minkler, M., Wallerstein, N., & Hyde, C. A. (2022). Improving health through community organizing and community building: Perspectives from health education and social work. In M. Minkler & P. Wakimoto (Eds.), *Community organizing and community building for health and social equity* (4th ed., pp. 35–52). Rutgers University Press.

Mitchell, C., & LaGory, M. (2002). Social capital and mental distress in an impoverished community. *City & Community, 1*(2), 199–222.

Mitchell, R., Agle, B., & Wood, D. (1997). Toward a theory of stakeholder identification and salience: Defining the principle of who and what really counts. *Academy of Management Review, 22*(4), 853–886.

Mkhitaryan, S., Giabbanelli, P. J., de Vries, N. K., & Crutzen, R. (2020). Dealing with complexity: How to use a hybrid approach to incorporate complexity in health behavior interventions. *Intelligence-Based Medicine, 3–4,* 100008. doi:10.1016/j.ibmed.2020.100008

Mokhele, I., Sineke, T., Vujovic, M., Fox, M. P., Ruiter, R. A. C., & Onoya, D. (2022). Using intervention mapping in motivational interviewing training to improve ART uptake in Gauteng, South Africa. *Journal of Health Psychology, 27*(3), 589–600.

Mollen, S., Ruiter, R., & Kok, G. (2010). Current issues and new directions in psychology and health: What are the oughts? The adverse effects of using social norms in health communication. *Psychology & Health, 25*(3), 265–270.

Montaño, D. E., & Kasprzyk, D. (2015). Theory of reasoned action, Theory of planned behavior, and the integrated behavioral model. In K. Glanz, B. K. Rimer, & K. Viswanath (Eds.), *Health behavior: Theory, research, and practice* (Vol. 5, pp. 168–222). Jossey-Bass.

Moss, J. L., Reiter, P. L., Rimer, B. K., & Brewer, N. T. (2016). Collaborative patient-provider communication and uptake ofadolescent vaccines. *Social Science & Medicine, 159,* 100–107.

Moyer-Gusé, E. (2008). Toward a theory of entertainment persuasion: Explaining the persuasive effects of entertainment-education messages. *Communication Theory, 18*(3), 407–425.

Najberg, H., Rigamonti, M., Mouthon, M., & Spierer, L. (2021). Modifying food items valuation and weight with gamified executive control training. *Royal Society Open Science, 8*(5), 191288.

Orbell, S., & Verplanken, B. (2020). Changing behavior using habit theory. In M. S. Hagger, L. D. Cameron, K. Hamilton, N. Hankonen, & T. Lintunen (Eds.), *The handbook of behavior change* (pp. 178–192). Cambridge University Press.

Orbell, S., Zahid, H., & Henderson, C. (2020). Changing behavior using the health belief model and protection motivation theory. In M. Hagger, L. Cameron, K. Hamilton, N. Hankonen, & T. Lintunen (Eds.), *The handbook of behavior change* (pp. 46–59). Cambridge University Press. doi:10.1017/9781108677318

Paluck, E., & Green, D. (2009). Prejudice reduction: What works? A review and assessment of research and practice. *Annual Review of Psychology, 60,* 339–367.

Peters, G.-J., de Bruin, M., & Crutzen, R. (2015). Everything should be as simple as possible, but no simpler: Towards a protocol for accumulating evidence regarding the active content of health behaviour change interventions. *Health Psychology Review, 9*(1), 1–14.

Peters, G.-J., Ruiter, R., & Kok, G. (2013). Threatening communication: A critical re-analysis and a revised meta-analytic test of fear appeal theory. *Health Psychology Review, 7,* S8–S31.

Petraglia, J. (2007). Narrative intervention in behavior and public health. *Journal of Health Communication, 12*(5), 493–505.

Petty, R., & Cacioppo, J. (2012). *Communication and persuasion: Central and peripheral routes to attitude change.* Springer Science & Business Media.

Petty, R. E., Barden, J., & Wheeler, S. C. (2009). The Elaboration Likelihood Model of persuasion: Developing health promotions for sustained behavioral change. In R. J. DiClemente, R. A. Crosby, & M. Kegler (Eds.), *Emerging theories in health promotion practice and research* (2nd ed., pp. 185–214). Jossey-Bass.

Popay, J., Whitehead, M., Ponsford, R., Egan, M., & Mead, R. (2021). Power, control, communities and health inequalities I: Theories, concepts and analytical frameworks. *Health Promotion International, 36*(5), 1253–1263. doi:10.1093/heapro/daaa133

Prochaska, J. O., Redding, C. A., & Evers, K. E. (2015). The transtheoretical model of stages of change. In K. Glanz, B. K. Rimer, & K. Viswanath (Eds.), *Health behavior: Theory, research, and practice* (Vol. 5, pp. 168–222). Jossey-Bass.

Qin, K., Marien, H., Custers, R., & Aarts, H. (2021). Environmental control of human goal pursuit: Investigating cue-based forced responses in a Pavlovian-to-instrumental transfer paradigm. *Motivation Science.* doi:10.1037/mot0000219

Rappaport, J. (1981). In praise of paradox: A social policy of empowerment over prevention. *American Journal of Community Psychology, 9*(1), 1–25. doi:10.1007/BF00896357

Rhodes, R., Grant, S., & de Bruijn, G.-J. (2020). Planning and implementation intention interventions. In M. Hagger, L. Cameron, K. Hamilton, N. Hankonen, & T. Lintunen (Eds.), *The handbook of behavior change* (pp. 572–585). Cambridge University Press. doi:10.1017/9781108677318

Richard, R., Pligt, J., & de Vries, N. (1995). Anticipated affective reactions and prevention of AIDS. *British Journal of Social Psychology, 34*(1), 9–21.

Richardson, G. E. (2002). The metatheory of resilience and resiliency. *Journal of Clinical Psychology, 58*(3), 307–321. doi:10.1002/jclp.10020

Rimal, R. N., & Lapinski, M. K. (2015). A re-explication of social norms, ten years later. *Communication Theory, 25*(4), 393–409. doi:10.1111/comt.12080

Rivera-Rodriguez, A., Mercado, E., Tropp, L. R., & Dasgupta, N. (2025). When social hierarchy, power, and collective autonomy motivate social movement and counter-movement mobilization among disadvantaged and advantaged groups. *Personality and Social Psychology Review, 30*(1), 3–28. doi:10.1177/10888683241305662

Robbins, S., Schwartz, B., & Wasserman, E. (2001). *Psychology of learning and behavior* (5th ed.). Norton.

Rodriguez, S. A., Roncancio, A. M., Savas, L. S., Lopez, D. M., Vernon, S. W., & Fernandez, M. E. (2018 Jun). Using Intervention Mapping to Develop and Adapt Two Educational Interventions for Parents to Increase HPV Vaccination Among Hispanic Adolescents. *Front Public Health, 15*(6), 164. doi:10.3389/fpubh.2018.00164

Rogers, E. M. (2003). *Diffusion of innovations.* Free Press.

Ruiter, R., Kessels, L., Peters, G.-J., & Kok, G. (2014). Sixty years of fear appeal research: Current state of the evidence. *International Journal of Psychology, 49*(2), 63–70.

Ruiter, R. A. C., Abraham, C., & Kok, G. (2001). Scary warnings and rational precautions: A review of the psychology of fear appeals. *Psychology and Health, 16*, 613–630. doi:10.1080/08870440108405863

Ruiter, R. A. C., Crutzen, R., de Leeuw, E., & Kok, G. (2020). Changing behavior using theories at the interpersonal, organizational, community, and societal levels. In M. S. Hagger, L. D. Cameron, K. Hamilton, N. Hankonen, & T. Lintunen (Eds.), *The handbook of behavior change* (pp. 251–266). Cambridge University Press. doi:10.1017/9781108677318

Ryan, R. M., & Deci, E. L. (2017). *Self-determination theory: Basic psychological needs in motivation, development, and wellness.* Guilford Press.

Sabatier, P. (2003). Policy change over a decade or more. In P. Lee, C. Estes, & F. Rodriguez (Eds.), *The nation's health* (pp. 143–174). Jones and Bartlett.

Sawyer, A., den Hertog, K., Verhoeff, A. P., Busch, V., & Stronks, K. (2021). Developing the logic framework underpinning a whole-systems approach to childhood overweight and obesity prevention: Amsterdam Healthy Weight Approach. *Obesity Science & Practice, 7*, 591–605. doi:10.1002/osp4.505

Schaalma, H., Abraham, C., Gillmore, M., & Kok, G. (2004). Sex education as health promotion: What does it take? *Archives of Sexual Behavior, 33*(3), 259–269.

Scholten, H., Granic, I., Chen, Z., Veling, H., & Luijten, M. (2019). Do smokers devaluate smoking cues after go/no-go training? *Psychology & Health, 34*(5), 609–625.

Schmid, K. L., Rivers, S. E., Latimer, A. E., & Salovey, P. (2008). Targeting or tailoring? *Marketing Health Services, 28*(1), 32.

Shen, F., & Han, J. (2014). Effectiveness of entertainment education in communicating health information: A systematic review. *Asian Journal of Communication, 24*(6), 605–616.

Sood, S., Riley, A. H., & Alarcon, K. C. (2017). *Entertainment-education and health and risk messaging.* Oxford University Press. doi:10.1093/acrefore/9780190228613.013.245

Stice, E., Yokum, S., Veling, H., Kemps, E., & Lawrence, N. S. (2017). Pilot test of a novel food response and attention training treatment for obesity: Brain imaging data suggest actions shape valuation. *Behaviour Research and Therapy, 94*, 60–70.

Suls, J., Martin, R., & Wheeler, L. (2002). Social comparison: Why, with whom, and with what effect? *Current Directions in Psychological Science, 11*(5), 159–163.

Tannenbaum, M. B., Hepler, J., Zimmerman, R. S., Saul, L., Jacobs, S., Wilson, K., & Albarracín, D. (2015). Appealing to fear: A meta-analysis of fear appeal effectiveness and theories—A message-behavior-audience framework. *Psychiatric Bulletin, 141*(6), 1178–1204. doi:10.1037/a0039729

Thaler, R., & Sunstein, C. (2008). *Nudge.* Yale University Press.

Todd, A. R., Galinsky, A. D., & Bodenhausen, G. V. (2012). Perspective taking undermines stereotype maintenance processes: Evidence from social memory, behavior explanation, and information solicitation. *Social Cognition, 30*(1), 94–108. doi:10.1521/soco.2012.30.1.94

Turner, J. C. (2005). Explaining the nature of power: A three-process theory. *European Journal of Social Psychology, 35*(1), 1–22.

Tzavella, L., & Chambers, C. D. (2023). Explicit and implicit devaluation effects of food-specific response inhibition training. *Journal of Cognition, 6*(1), 10.

Unsworth, N., Brewer, G. A., & Spillers, G. J. (2013). Working memory capacity and retrieval from long-term memory: The role of controlled search. *Memory & Cognition, 41*(2), 242–254. doi:10.3758/s13421-012-0261-x

Valente, T. W. (2015). Social networks and health behavior. In K. Glanz, B. K. Rimer, & K. Viswanath (Eds.), *Health behavior: Theory, research, and practice* (5th ed., pp. 205–222). Jossey-Bass.

Valente, T. W., & Pitts, S. R. (2017). An appraisal of social network theory and analysis as applied to public health: Challenges and opportunities. *Annual Review of Public Health, 38*(1), 103–118. doi:10.1146/annurev-publhealth-031816-044528

van Achterberg, T., Huisman-de Waal, G., Ketelaar, N., Oostendorp, R., Jacobs, J., & Wollersheim, H. (2011). How to promote healthy behaviours in patients? An overview of evidence for behaviour change techniques. *Health Promotion International, 26*(2), 148.

van Empelen, P., Kok, G., van Kesteren, N. M., van den Borne, B., Bos, A. E., & Schaalma, H. P. (2003). Effective methods to change sex-risk among drug users: A review of psychosocial interventions. *Social Science & Medicine, 57*(9), 1593–1608. doi:10.1016/s0277-9536(02)00557-9

van't Riet, J., & Ruiter, R. A. C. (2013). Defensive reactions to health-promoting information: An overview and implications for future research. *Health Psychology Review, 7*. doi:10.1080/17437199.2011.606782

van't Riet, J., Cox, A. D., Cox, D., Zimet, G. D., de Bruijn, G. J., Van den Putte, B., de Vries, H., Werrij, M. Q., & Ruiter, R. A. C. (2014). Does perceived risk influence the effects of message framing? A new investigation of a widely held notion. *Psychology & Health, 29*(8), 933–949.

Van't Riet, J., Cox, A. D., Cox, D., Zimet, G. D., De Bruijn, G. J., Van den Putte, B., et al. (2016). *Psychology & Health, 29*(8), 933–949.

Varol, T., Crutzen, R., Schneider, F., Mesters, I., Ruiter, R. A. C., Kok, G., & ten Hoor, G. A. (2021). Selection of determinants of students' adherence to COVID-19 guidelines and translation into a brief intervention. *Acta Psychologica, 219*, 103400. doi:10.1016/j.actpsy.2021.103400

Veling, H., Becker, D., Liu, H., Quandt, J., & Holland, R. W. (2022). How go/no-go training changes behavior: A value-based decision-making perspective. *Current Opinion in Behavioral Sciences, 47*, 101206. doi:10.1016/j.cobeha.2022.101206

Verplanken, B., & Aarts, H. (1999). Habit, attitude, and planned behaviour: Is habit an empty construct or an interesting case of goal-directed automaticity? *European Review of Social Psychology, 10*(1), 101–134.

Wallack, L. (2008). Media advocacy: A strategy for empowering people and communities. In M. Minkler (Ed.), *Community organizing and community building for health* (2nd ed., pp. 419–432). Rutgers University Press.

Wallack, L., Dorfman, L., Jernigan, D., & Themba, M. (1993). *Media advocacy and public health: Power for prevention*. Sage.

Wallerstein, N., Minkler, M., Carter-Edwards, L., Avila, M., & Sanchez, V. (2015). Improving helath through community engagement and community building. In K. Glanz, B. Rimer, & K. Viswanath (Eds.), *Health behavior: Theory, research, and practice* (5th ed.). Jossey-Bass.

Weible, C. (2008). Expert-based information and policy subsystems: A review and synthesis. *Policy Studies Journal, 36*(4), 615–635.

Weible, C., Sabatier, P., & McQueen, K. (2009). Themes and variations: Taking stock of the Advocacy Coalition Framework. *Policy Studies Journal, 37*(1), 121–140.

Weick, K. E., & Quinn, R. E. (1999). Organizational change and development. *Annual Review of Psychology, 50*(1), 361–386.

Weiner, B. (1986). *An attributional theory of motivation and emotion.* Springer-Verlag.

Weiner, B. (2018). The legacy of an attribution approach to motivation and emotion: A no-crisis zone. *Motivation Science, 4*(1). doi:10.1037/mot0000082

Weinstein, N. D., Sandman, P. M., & Blalock, S. J. (2008). The precaution adoption process model. In K. Glanz, F. M. Lewis, & B. K. Rimer (Eds.), *Health behavior and health education: Theory, research, and practice* (Vol. 4, pp. 123–165). Jossey-Bass.

Werrij, M. Q., Ruiter, R. A. C., Riet, J. V. T., & de Vries, H. (2012). Message framing. In C. Abraham & M. Kools (Eds.), *Writing health communication: An evidence-based guide* (pp. 134–143). Sage.

Wiers, R. W., Gladwin, T. E., Hofmann, W., Salemink, E., & Ridderinkhof, K. R. (2013). Cognitive bias modification and cognitive control training in addiction and related psychopathology: Mechanisms, clinical perspectives, and ways forward. *Clinical Psychological Science, 1*(2), 192–212. doi:10.1177/2167702612466547

Wood, W., & Neal, D. (2007). A new look at habits and the habit-goal interface. *Psychological Review, 114*(4), 843–863.

Wright, P. (2012). Using graphic effectively in text. In C. Abraham & M. Kools (Eds.), *Writing health communication: An evidence-based guide* (pp. 62–82). Sage.

Zahariadis, N. (2007). The multiple streams framework: Structure, limitations, prospects. In P. Sabatier (Ed.), *Theories of the policy process* (2nd ed., pp. 65–92). Westview Press.

Zajonc, R. (2001). Mere exposure: A gateway to the subliminal. *Current Directions in Psychological Sciene, 10*(6), 224–228.

CHAPTER 8

INTERVENTION MAPPING STEP 4

Intervention Design and Production

INTERVENTION MAPPING STEP 4 TASKS

1. Define Intervention Structure (Themes, Components, Scope, and Sequence)
2. Plan Intervention Messages, Materials and Activities
3. Produce Intervention Materials, Activities, and Protocols
4. Pretest, Refine and Finalize Materials, Activities, and Protocols

Overview

The purpose of this chapter is to enable intervention planners to produce creative and effective materials, activities, and protocols for health promotion interventions as part of Step 4 of Intervention Mapping (IM). Interventions will often be multicomponent, addressing the needs of both target group and environmental agents, with each part of the intervention being supported by materials, activities, and protocols. The goal is for these to be creative, effective pieces that promote and support key messages of the planned intervention. In this step, the methods and practical applications selected in Step 3 are translated into concrete materials, activities, and protocols that are effectively operationalized and meet the change objectives (from the matrices in Step 2).

The planning steps completed to this point have created the foundation for the production of creative materials, activities, and protocols. These are based on the thinking captured in the matrix of change objectives in Step 2 and the selection of change methods and practical applications in Step 3. In particular, planners should design intervention materials, activities, and protocols considering and applying the parameters that pertain to the selected change methods (see Chapter 7). For example, if planners decide to use modeling (method), they must ensure that their role-model stories (practical application) include models that participants can identify with (parameter) and which are reinforced for their positive health behavior (parameter). The end product of Step 4 should be materials, activities, and protocols that are consistent with the planning in Steps 1, 2, and 3.

Step 4 also aims to ensure that the final intervention "fits" with both the populations for whom it is intended and within the context in which it will be delivered. Engagement with potential participants, as well as adopters and implementers, is key for this step. At the end of this step, planners will have an intervention plan for the target group and the environmental agents. The next step (Step 5) focuses on the development of implementation strategies for adopters and implementers to ensure adoption, implementation, and maintenance of the intervention (see Chapter 9).

Throughout this chapter, we encourage adherence to the plans from the previous steps to create engaging and culturally relevant materials, activities, and protocols. The intervention should be feasible to implement and should fit within the intervention context. A crucial aspect to take into account is the (health) literacy level of potential participants and adherence to health communication principles in general. The key tasks in Step 4 are first to define intervention structure and how to reach intervention participants, and second to plan, produce, pretest, refine and finalize intervention materials, activities, and protocols.

Using Steps 1, 2, and 3

Steps 1, 2, and 3 will inform the work to be completed in the tasks of Step 4. In Step 1, the planners conducted a needs and assets assessment to thoroughly explore the health problem and describe priority populations. In Step 2, they developed matrices of change objectives for the target group and environmental agents. In Step 3, they identified change methods and practical applications for each matrix. In Step 4, the planners will design the intervention plan, which includes intervention themes, components, scope and sequence, as well as the messages, materials, and activities that will bring these ideas to life.

There are multiple strategies for moving forward depending on budget and time frame. Sometimes planners will be able to locate existing materials that match the objectives, methods, and practical applications identified in previous steps; other times planners will produce original material. Such production always requires plans, often specified in design documents, to ensure that intervention messages and materials meet the intervention specifications. Production sometimes requires design and technical consultants such as copywriters, graphic designers, computer programmers, videographers, and app developers. Working with these design consultants will require guidance from detailed design documents.

Designing for Implementation

As planners design intervention materials, activities, and protocols, they should continue to consider the intervention context. Importantly, building from community-based participatory research principles (Collins et al., 2018) and the guidelines for collaboration cited in Chapter 5 (Step 1), they will want to involve potential participants in the intervention design. Also, if potential adopters and implementers have not been involved in the planning group to this point, planners will need to recruit them to understand aspects of the implementation context important to the intervention design. These individuals can help planners understand what materials can be delivered feasibly and to further explore the preferences of potential participants, adopters, and implementers. They can also help planners make sure that intervention materials, activities, and protocols are easily usable and include the characteristics of an intervention that makes them more likely to be used, such as low complexity, good fit with organizational routines, values, and mission, resource conserving, and easy to attempt (see Chapter 9). Seeing characteristics of materials and activities from the viewpoint of potential adopters and implementers is important for both the initial implementation of an intervention and the later wide-scale dissemination. This is also known as "designing for dissemination" (Chambers, 2020; Huebschmann et al., 2019).

Step 4 Tasks

The four primary tasks for conducting Step 4 are presented in Box 8.1 and described below.

BOX 8.1. INTERVENTION MAPPING STEP 4 TASKS

1. Define Intervention Structure (Themes, Components, Scope, and Sequence)
2. Plan Intervention Messages, Materials and Activities
3. Produce Intervention Materials, Activities, and Protocols
4. Pretest, Refine and Finalize Materials, Activities, and Protocols

Task 1: Define Intervention Structure (Themes, Components, Scope, and Sequence)

The first task in Step 4 is to define the intervention structure and think about how to reach intervention participants. At this point, planners have to make decisions about various practical aspects of the intervention. For example, some questions to be answered include:

- What is the extent of the intervention and its duration (scope)?
- In what order will practical applications and their corresponding materials and activities be delivered (sequence)?
- Are there certain components (units or modules) with an identifiable scope and sequence?
- Will the intervention have a theme, more than one theme, and/or a title?

Some planning groups will have ideas about some of these aspects of the intervention as soon as they begin working through IM. Others will begin thinking about the interventions aspects as they work through Step 4. Given the iterative nature of IM, it is crucial to complete Steps 1, 2, and 3 before developing materials and activities for the intervention. The products of the previous steps often inform the work to be completed in Step 4, anticipating the adoption and implementation of the intervention. This might encourage a reconsideration of ideas raised in earlier steps regarding intervention aspects. In other words, the iterative nature implies that work on Step 4 can start, but never finish, before completing earlier steps.

Generating Themes, Components, Scope, and Sequence

Generating intervention themes, components, scope, and sequence is a participatory process, and it is imperative to discuss these intervention aspects and ways to use them with the planning group. Building from the linkage system concept cited in Step 1, the planning group ideally will include stakeholders who know the context of the intervention and who have an understanding of the implementation context (e.g., teachers in a school setting, healthcare providers in a clinic setting).

The product of the first part of Step 4 is the *intervention structure*: an *initial intervention plan* that describes the intervention and when there is contact with each group of intervention participants. For example, in an intervention for patients, three contacts might be, a video presentation delivered in the waiting room, followed by a discussion with a nurse, and lastly a reminder from a physician. The intervention structure might also include training for the personnel implementing the intervention, such as the nurse or health care provider. In these next tasks, the *intervention plan* is completed with the messages, materials, and activities that will bring these ideas to life.

Exploring Intervention Ideas In initiating the design process, planners first need to explore creative and impactful ideas for the intervention. In doing so, a central problem plagues planners in every profession—how to have a good idea ... how to "think outside of the box." The key to having a good idea is to have more than one idea—maybe even hundreds (De Bono, 2015). And the key to having a hundred ideas is to generate them without editing and without adhering to a strictly logical process. This is similar to the idea of brainstorming—one of the core processes (see Chapter 2)—to be as open as possible and not being limited before planning begins. Prior to considering real-world constraints, De Bono suggests a lateral process that creates movement from one idea to another, breaks up current thinking, and disrupts reliance on the status quo. At this point, planners can dismiss all preconceived notions and intervention constraints. They can ask themselves, "What would we do if we could do anything that comes to mind?" The diversity of the planning group will allow for the generation of unique ideas and innovative concepts. To successfully allow for creative brainstorming, it is encouraged for planners to explore all thoughts and ideas that are within the planning group before deciding on intervention themes, components, scope, and sequence.

Innovative thinking is a way to come up with new or significantly improved ideas (Barak et al., 2020; Cropley, 2015). There are four consistent behaviors through which novel ideas are most likely obtained: Observing, Exploring, Questioning, and Idea Networking (Dyer et al., 2019). These innovative thinking skills, which are expressed in behavior, are the catalyst for identifying new ideas (Barak et al., 2020; Dyer et al., 2019) and can be defined as: "First, Observing refers to intensely observing the world around while seeking new ideas. Second, Exploring refers to engaging in active experimentation to explore options and generate novel designs. Third, Questioning refers to asking questions that challenge the status quo. Fourth, Idea Networking refers to creating networks of individuals with diverse backgrounds and perspectives that could lead to new ideas and insights" (Barak & Yuan, 2021). The latter stresses once again the importance of the diversity of the planning group and involving them in the process of generating ideas. There are multiple ways to do this, besides brainstorming, such as mind mapping, stream-of-consciousness writing, and six thinking caps, which are described in more detail elsewhere (Walesh, 2016).

Themes A *theme* is a general organizing construct or idea for an intervention. Themes, together with several recurring visual and linguistic subthemes or ideas, can support the delivery of the health message. Both themes and recurring subthemes can be based on the health topic, such as the themes for the TLL Temple Foundation Stroke Project, "Call 911" and "Is there treatment for stroke?" (Morgenstern et al., 2002). Heinen and colleagues developed a self-management intervention to increase physical activity and reduce wound days in leg ulcer patients called "Lively Legs" (Heinen et al., 2006, 2012).

Themes also may be based on performance objectives. For example, the *Watch, Discover, Think, and Act* theme of intervention for asthma was based on the self-regulatory processes taught in the computer program, informed by Bandura's theory of self-regulation. This primary message became the intervention title and a structure in recurring visuals and messaging (Bartholomew et al., 2000a, 2000b). In the Me & You intervention, "select, detect, protect" was a theme. "Select (knowing your personal rules to have healthy relationships), detect (watching for signs that could challenge your personal rules), protect (avoid or use refusal skills to get out of a risky situation where rules are being challenged)" followed a self-regulation decision-making paradigm that could help youth play by their personal rules and build healthy relationships (Peskin et al., 2018).

Themes may also derive from characteristics of target groups, cultures, or preferred learning styles identified through formative research. In an

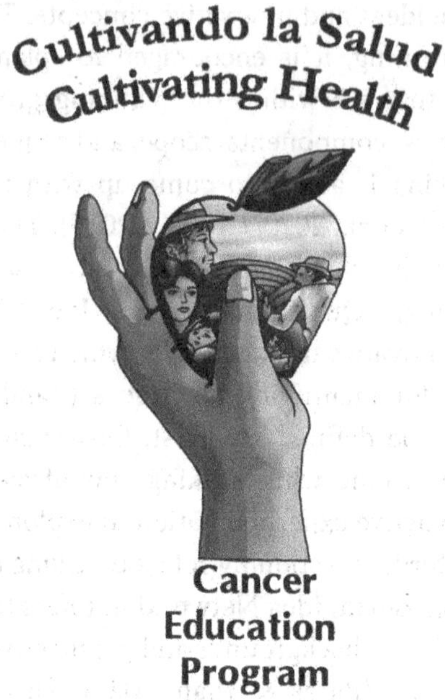

Figure 8.1 Cultivando La Salud. National Center for Farmworker Health,Inc. / U.S. Department of Health and Human Services / Public domain

intervention to increase breast and cervical cancer screening for US Hispanic farm-working women, the intervention theme was "Cultivando La Salud" ("Cultivating Health"), which expressed a culturally significant message for the target group (Fernández et al., 2005) (Figure 8.1). The overarching message that a theme can deliver may reach not only intervention participants, but also a broader audience (e.g., parents, peers, and community members). For example, "Don't mess with Texas" was the theme of an intervention that was initially targeted at men under 25 and aimed to reduce littering on Texas roadways, but became "an identity statement, a declaration of Texas swagger" (Fernandez, 2013).

Components, Scope, and Sequence A *component* is a discrete identifiable intervention unit or module that forms a part of the larger intervention. Components may be defined by the priority population (a parent component and a child component), by setting (a cafeteria component, classroom component, and afterschool program component), at the environmental level (policy-level component, organizational-level component, and the individual-level component), or by delivery vehicle (physicians and local newspaper). These all can include one or more applications in the intervention as well. Interventions overall are often combinations of components. An intervention might consist, for example, of a component comprised of messages that neighborhood volunteers deliver one-on-one to the priority population and another component consisting of mass media messages delivered in public service announcements (PSAs) and billboards, both being tied together with a theme. In the Me & You intervention there were three components: a youth component (consisting of sixth-grade lessons), a parent component (consisting of parent-student take-home activities), and a school staff component (Peskin et al., 2018). In order to identify and describe components, planners might ask themselves "If you had to give an elevator speech to describe your intervention, how would you 'chunk' your intervention into easily describable components?" Health promotion interventions have components with an identifiable scope and sequence.

The *scope* is the breadth and amount of an intervention and defines what is and what is not in the intervention. For example, when developing an intervention to interrupt periods of prolonged sitting among office employees, both the interpersonal (e.g., support by colleagues and managers) and the individual (e.g., office workers) levels were taken into account when planning the intervention. Higher levels (e.g., organization and community) were outside the scope of this intervention out of concern for the cost-effectiveness of the intervention (Berninger et al., 2020). The key question to ask when defining the scope of an intervention is, what is feasible given the available resources? This involves checking budget and time constraints for development as well as implementation. Within these constraints, it is crucial that the scope of an intervention targets the most important outcomes and agents. However, less important outcomes or agents must be kept in the project when possible. Given the iterative nature of IM, it requires going back to Step 2 as changes in outcomes and agents that are included might lead to changes in what can be expected from an intervention given these constraints. Therefore, it is encouraged to have a clear view on any constraints as early as possible when moving through the steps of IM. Changes later steps are often more expensive in terms of the effort and time required to update.

The *sequence* is the order in which components are delivered across time as well as the duration of each component. The questions to ask are: Who will get what part of this intervention? When will they get it? How will they get it? How long will it last overall? How long will each interaction be? Table 8.1 presents an example of a scope and sequence for the Me & You intervention. It is important to note that the scope and sequence only encompasses intervention components and are distinct from a project timeline. The latter might also include other aspects relevant to the project, such as a recruitment period and measurement time points that are part of the evaluation plan in Step 6.

Selecting Delivery Channels and Vehicles to Reach Intervention Participants

Intervention materials and activities are what the participants see, do, read, hear, and feel when participating in the intervention. It is important to think ahead about how to reach intended intervention participants to stimulate their interaction with the intervention materials and activities. The importance of reach is captured in the RE-AIM framework which focuses on five key dimensions of an intervention: reach (R), effectiveness (E),

Table 8.1 Scope and Sequence for *Me & You*

	Youth Component	
Lesson Number	**Sixth Grade Lessons**	**Vehicle**
1	**Me & You** • Describe the goals of the curriculum • List agreements for classroom discussion • Describe different types of relationships • Describe how people in their lives can support them	Classroom
2	**Healthy Friendships** • Demonstrate the ability to evaluate friendships • Feel confident in the ability to have healthy friendships • Recognize that peers can have healthy friendships • Resist social pressure to have an unhealthy friendship	Computer
3	**Playing by Your Rules** • Describe the three steps necessary for playing by your rules (SELECT, DETECT, PROTECT) in the context of healthy friendships and relationships • Define the meaning of a "personal rule" • Identify situations that may challenge personal rules • Identify actions to help stick with personal rules	Classroom
4	**Protecting Your Rules about Relationships** • Identify situations that may challenge personal rules about healthy relationships • Identify actions to help stick with personal rules about healthy relationships • List characteristics of a "clear NO" statement • Distinguish between ineffective and effective approaches to using "clear NO" statements • Use "clear NO" statements effectively • Avoid unhealthy relationships	Classroom-Computer Blended
5	**Healthy Dating Relationships** • Demonstrate the ability to evaluate dating relationships • Recognize that teens can be in healthy dating relationships • Recognize the importance of respecting other people's rules in dating relationships • Resist pressure to have an unhealthy dating relationship • Evaluate healthy and unhealthy dating relationships	Computer
6	**The Thoughts and Emotions Link** • Recognize that "a healthy relationship starts with you" • Identify different emotional responses • Describe the connection between thoughts and feelings • Describe types of damaging thoughts, stinkin' thinkin', that may influence emotional responses • Describe the three steps to managing emotional responses: Relax, Rewind, Replay • Personalize how they can manage their emotions in challenging situations	Computer
7	**Communication for Healthy Relationships** • State the importance of effective communication (with family/friends, and future dating partners) • Describe effective negotiation (speaking and listening) skills • Demonstrate the ability to effectively communicate with others in order to protect personal rules about healthy relationships	Classroom-Computer Blended

Table 8.1 *(Continued)*

Youth Component		
Lesson Number	**Sixth Grade Lessons**	**Vehicle**
8	**Tech Protect** • Identify unhealthy friendship and dating relationship behaviors that occur in the context of technology • Describe ways to protect personal rules about online communication and behavior • Demonstrate the ability to protect personal rules about online communication and behavior within the context of relationships, including how they behave toward others	Computer
9	**Unhealthy Dating Relationships** • List types of violence (emotional, physical, and sexual) • Recognize signs of an unhealthy dating relationship • Recognize that domestic violence (DV) can be in person or through technology • Understand the importance of active consent in relationships • Personalize what is important to them in a dating relationship	Computer
10	**Consequences of Unhealthy Dating Relationships** • Understand the importance of active consent in relationships • Recognize warning signs of an unhealthy dating relationship • Identify physical, social, and emotional consequences of unhealthy dating relationships for victims and perpetrators • Understand the importance of establishing rules about healthy relationships • Identify the influence of gender stereotypes and power differentials in relationships	Classroom
11	**Getting Out of Unhealthy Dating Relationships** • Recognize the importance of getting out of unhealthy friendships and dating relationships • Recognize that disclosing an unhealthy relationship can lead to support from others to get out of the relationship • Identify resources and social support sources for getting out of unhealthy relationships • Recognize how they can help friends who are in unhealthy relationships • Demonstrate the ability to manage unavoidable relationships that are unhealthy	Classroom-Computer Blended
12	**Keeping Your Relationships Healthy** • Distinguish between situations that have active consent vs. situations in which there is no consent • Describe various strategies for keeping relationships healthy • Demonstrate the ability to manage emotions and use effective communication to keep their relationships healthy • Identify the influence of gender roles and power differentials in relationships	Classroom
13	**Wrap-Up** • Describe what they learned from the curriculum • Describe how they will use what they learned in the future	Classroom

Parent Component		
Lesson Number	**Parent-Student Take-Home Activities**	**Vehicle**
5	**Healthy Relationships** • Characteristics of healthy friendships and dating relationships • Dating rules and expectations	Worksheet group debriefing
7	**Talking Together** • Communication and negotiation skills	Worksheet group debriefing
11	**My Escape Plan** • Getting out of unhealthy relationships	Worksheet group debriefing

(continued)

Table 8.1 *(Continued)*

Lesson Number	Parent-Student Take-Home Activities	Vehicle
	Parent Component	
	Parent Newsletter	
1	• Overview of *Me and You* • Tips for how parents can be involved with *Me and You* • Tips for talking with your child • Importance and tips for increasing parent-child connectedness	Newsletter
9	• Review of *Me and You* • Setting and sticking to rules for healthy relationships • Tech Protect: Helping kids stay safe online • Tips for effective parent-child communication • Warning signs of an unhealthy dating relationship	Newsletter
	School Staff Component	
Prior to 1	**School Teacher Training** • Overview of *Me and You* • Facilitation skills and teaching with fidelity • Exploring values and attitudes • Answering sensitive questions • What you can do as a member of the school staff (recognize, respond, refer) • Importance of confidentiality • Lesson demonstration and practice	Training
1	**School Newsletter** • Overview of *Me and You* • Unhealthy relationship behaviors • Why bullying and DV are issues for schools • What you can do as a member of the school staff (recognize, respond, refer)	Newsletter

adoption (A), implementation (I), and maintenance (M) (Glasgow et al., 2019). In order for an intervention to have an impact, it should not only be effective, but also be adopted, implemented, and maintained (see Chapter 9). And, before an intervention is used in the first place, it should reach the intended intervention participants. Glasgow et al. (2019) define *reach* as "the absolute number, proportion, and representativeness of individuals who are willing to participate in a given initiative, intervention, or program" (Glasgow et al., 2019).

Reaching participants is a multifaceted issue. In Step 1, there is a task dedicated to exploring settings where the priority population may be reached. The current task builds upon that and deals with selecting appropriate delivery channels and vehicles that are and can be used by participants. Reach is also related to the extent to what participants see, do, read, hear, and feel resonates with them (e.g., in terms of cultural sensitivity). A useful tool to cover this during the design process is McGuire's Persuasion-Communication matrix (McGuire, 2001). In this matrix, input variables (e.g., message, channel) are linked to output variables (e.g., exposure, attention). For all aspects of reaching participants, it is crucial to conduct formative research in line with the participatory approach of IM.

This participatory approach is not limited to target group members and environmental agents, but also concerns implementers (e.g., teachers, nurses, physicians, and outreach workers). Implementers have to perform one or more behaviors to enable implementation. This often means that the intermediate intervention materials, activities, and protocols must be developed as well. The same would apply to adopters and maintainers. This development should be in line with the results from Step 5, emphasizing the iterative nature of IM. It is important to identify these stakeholders as early as possible to enable discussing the intervention with them and make adjustments if necessary. This concerns the intervention structure in general, but also plans for materials and activities that are prepared for these stakeholders specifically.

Channels and Vehicles Plans for materials and activities demand decisions about how to deliver intervention messages.

A *channel* is the method used to deliver intervention messages. This can be either interpersonal (delivered by an individual) or mediated (all other ways to deliver intervention messages). A *vehicle* is how a message is actually packaged and delivered. These vehicles are constantly changing—for example, with the adoption of technology via smartphones (Fakih El Khoury et al., 2019) and new social media platforms (Plackett et al., 2020). Technological solutions are often presented as the solution to a problem increasing the trend of techno-optimism. An example of techno-optimism is the introduction of digital contact tracing to control the COVID-19 pandemic. The use of a contact-tracing app could slow the virus's spread by reducing the time between infection and quarantine, and it could inform people who are infected but not yet symptomatic (Ferretti et al., 2020). This idea behind a contact-tracing app is fairly simple, from a technological point of view, and was met with a lot of enthusiasm. The technological potential of contact tracing via smartphones also led to public debate about the legal (e.g., data protection, privacy) and ethical (e.g., proportionality, accessibility) ramifications of using the technology (Morley et al., 2020). However, the pilot study in the Netherlands showed that the more important challenges—from a behavior change point of view—were at an organizational level. For example, if a citizen gets an alert from a contact-tracing app, does the health service employee then know what to do? And can all citizens who receive an alert get tested? So, technological possibilities offered by certain vehicles should be seen as a tool, not a panacea (Bandura, 2004). See Table 8.2 for examples of channels and vehicles and their use. This table summarizes advantages and disadvantages of various vehicles, which is helpful when generating thoughts on possible delivery channels and vehicles.

Generating thoughts on channels and vehicles is a participatory process. Most interventions incorporate multiple channels and vehicles, often having a primary delivery mode and a secondary mode that may focus on

Table 8.2 Examples of Channels and Vehicles

Vehicles	Typical Uses, Methods, and Practical Applications	Advantages	Disadvantages
Interpersonal Delivery Channels			
Community leaders Peer leaders Community health workers (promotoras)	Skill training Social reinforcement Modeling Tutoring Small-group discussion	Powerful source of influence and persuasion Can be inexpensive Involve community and enhance capacity Cultural connectivity	Difficult to train and motivate individuals to deliver one-on-one or small-group messages Expert involvement needed for delivery of specific content and reinforcement
Teachers	Mastery learning Tutoring Small-group discussion Lecture Modeling	Expert in didactic teaching techniques Fit organizational context of school Sustainable model for school setting and integration for dissemination and implementation	Can be resistant to interactive techniques Can be limited by curriculum and administrative constraints Content may need approval from decision makers
Health care providers	Skill training Social reinforcement Counseling Tutoring	Powerful source of influence and persuasion Expert in patient assessment and counseling Captive audiences interested in personal health issues Content expertise and ability to integrate evidence-based messages	Can be difficult to train and motivate Lack of time Can have difficulty integrating counseling techniques if they are used to a more direct "medical model" Can be perceived as too dissimilar from the patient Certification may be needed as incentive for continuing education
Mediated Delivery Channels			
Newspapers	Letters to the editor Editorial commentary Role-model stories Information Persuasion	Inexpensive Positive consumer attitudes about vehicle Narratives focused on community needs Fast and timely dissemination	Depends on reading literacy Short life span Many newspapers on the market compete for attention Require cultivation of relationship with gatekeepers such as health reports at the newspaper Require to capitalize on short media attention span for issues
Magazines	Information Persuasion Role-model stories	Good audience segmentation High audience receptivity Credibility and prestige Targeted cultural sensitivity	Depends on reading literacy Short life span Many magazines on the market compete for attention Lack of flexibility Lack of control of distribution
Newsletters	Information Persuasion Role-model stories	Good audience segmentation High audience receptivity Strong possibility to target Control of distribution Multiple messages with ongoing reach	Require high degree of novelty Access to subscribers and continued reach to subscriber population

Table 8.2 (*Continued*)

Vehicles	Typical Uses, Methods, and Practical Applications	Advantages	Disadvantages
Billboards, posters	Attention Awareness Cue to action	Can be very effective in calling attention to a campaign Direct messages Use of novel images and language	Can only target limited change objectives (such as knowledge and awareness) Limited view time
Brochures	Skill training Modeling Information with extensive detail Persuasion Vicarious reinforcement	Can target a variety of change objectives Entry into households Used to reinforce messages and delivery of key messages Lend to multilanguage formatting	No standard distribution routes Use for specific project
Radio (news items, interviews)	Information Awareness Persuasion	Good audience segmentation High audience receptivity Language specific reach	Short life span Clutter (many vehicles on the market compete for attention) Require cultivation of relationship with gatekeepers such as health reports at the newspaper Require to capitalize on short media attention span for issues
Radio (public service announcement)	Information Awareness Persuasion Role-model stories	Good audience segmentation Language specific reach Messaging with key words and taglines for branding	Require high degree of novelty Role-model stories not supported by visuals Repeated exposure/messages needed
Television (news stories, interviews)	Information Awareness Persuasion	Wide distribution Possibility for segmentation Language specific reach	Short life span Many television programs on the market compete for attention Require cultivation of relationship with gatekeepers such as health reports at the newspaper Require to capitalize on short media attention span for issues
Television (public service announcement)	Information Awareness Persuasion Role-model stories	Wide distribution Possibility for segmentation Language specific reach Messaging with key words and taglines for branding	Require high degree of novelty Repeated exposure/messages needed
Computer- and internet-based interventions (tailored messaging; decision support; serious gaming)	Skill training Information with extensive detail Modeling Vicarious reinforcement	Interactive Tailored to user profile Availability (24/7) Can include many combinations of change methods	Competitive market for programming skills Requires constant updating to meet technological standards
Smartphones (mobile applications)	Skill training Information with extensive detail Vicarious reinforcement	Interactive Tailored to user profile Availability (24/7) Can include many combinations of change methods	Competitive market for programming skills High variety in devices raises technological challenges

(*continued*)

Table 8.2 *(Continued)*

Vehicles	Typical Uses, Methods, and Practical Applications	Advantages	Disadvantages
Wearables	Self-monitoring Vicarious reinforcement	Sensors can be used to provide contextual information and feedback Tailored to user profile Availability (24/7)	High variety in devices raises technological challenges Interoperability of data
Social media	Information Awareness Persuasion Role-model stories Vicarious reinforcement	Microtargeting is possible (language, socio-demographics) Messaging with key words and taglines for branding	Lack of control over comments and sharing of information Need to monitor comments and interact Repeated exposure/messages needed

reinforcement of key change behaviors and the intervention theme. It is imperative to discuss channels and vehicles within the participatory planning group. These discussions should be open and not limited to a specific vehicle beforehand ("let's build a mobile app"). Choices regarding vehicles should not dictate the possibilities to deliver intervention messages, but they should be chosen because they offer the possibilities that are needed for a specific intervention. Moreover, planners must ascertain the preferred and most accepted vehicles used by the intended audiences to increase their effectiveness.

Choosing vehicles is a matter of balancing the needs and preferences of the intended intervention participants and how to reach them, taking into account logistics, budget constraints, team skills, and sustainability. With children, planners often look to school-based education, using teachers and peer leaders; to magazines, radio, and television addressed to children; and to computer and video games. Keep in mind that these vehicles may also help reach a secondary audience, caregivers, family, or friends, who are influential in motivating and promoting change objectives.

Reviewing Intervention Structure

Before starting to plan intervention messages, materials, and activities (the second task of Step 4), it is crucial to check whether alignment between methods, applications, parameters, and change objectives has not shifted or been lost in translation. The preliminary plans for intervention structure can be reconsidered (e.g., to rearrange the order of presentation). In fact, this alignment is something that needs to be continuously re-evaluated throughout the planning process. It is even more important at this stage, however, because once planners go from plans to production (the third task within Step 4), it becomes harder (and possibly very expensive) to make major changes.

Task 2: Plan Intervention Messages, Materials, and Activities

At this point, planners should have preliminary plans for the overarching theme or themes of the intervention, intervention components, the scope and sequence of the components, and the change methods and practical applications. Issues that have to be dealt with at this stage, within the constraints of resources discussed in the previous task, are best summarized as considering feasibility and fit. If part of an intervention will be incorporated into a school curriculum, what materials are needed for a teacher to effectively and efficiently deliver the curriculum? In Task 2, planners review existing material and activities, write intervention messages, and develop design documents.

Reviewing Existing Materials and Activities

When preparing plans for materials and activities, planners will want to consider using existing materials and activities, or parts of them, rather than "reinventing the wheel." The planning group may want to start the review of existing materials and activities with the following questions:

- Do existing materials and activities enable the relevant change objectives to be met?
- Do they deliver the intended change methods and practical applications?
- Do they fit into the planned scope and sequence of the intervention?

To determine whether the available materials and activities are appropriate, the planners review them by checking their correspondence with the matrices (from Step 2) and lists of methods and practical applications (from Step 3). The review of existing materials and activities cannot start before previous steps are completed.

The match between existing materials and activities and the results from previous steps should be aligned and any gaps in addressing all change objectives should be clearly identified. Materials and activities can cover multiple change objectives. Similar change objectives can be covered in multiple materials and activities. If gaps exist, the planners will have to determine whether the gaps can be filled either by adapting the existing material and activities or by creating additional materials and activities for the intervention. Chapter 11 (IM Adapt) provides in-depth guidance on how to review and adapt existing material and activities.

Prior to the full review and evaluation of identified intervention materials, planners should determine whether the materials are available in the quantity needed, in the appropriate time frame, and at an acceptable cost. Some materials may be available in electronic form and can be downloaded for reproduction. Moreover, before deciding to use parts of existing interventions, a more fine-grained analysis is needed regarding (health) literacy of the priority population.

Paying Attention to (Health) Literacy A crucial aspect when reviewing existing materials and creating new materials is to pay attention to (health) literacy. Literacy is defined as "understanding, evaluating, using and engaging with written texts to participate in society, to achieve one's goals, and to develop one's knowledge and potential" (OECD, 2019). People with lower literacy levels experience lower physical and mental health, make more use of health care, and are less able to adequately engage in self-management (Van der Heide & Rademakers, 2015). While there is large variety between countries in the percentage of adults scoring at each proficiency level in literacy, low literacy levels are a global phenomenon (OECD, 2019).

Almost all adults with low literacy levels have a basic knowledge of print vocabulary (i.e., they are able to identify the printed word corresponding to a concrete object from a set of four alternatives). However, reading multi-paragraph, continuous prose texts and maintaining attention and persistence can be a challenge to people with low literacy (Grotlüschen et al., 2016). The National Institutes of Health recommends that the reading level of intervention material should not exceed a sixth-grade level. However, all patient information of the American Urogynecologic Society (AUGS) and International Urogynecological Association (IUGA) in English documents scored above this level. Spanish documents were written at a lower reading level than their English counterparts (Haller et al., 2019). Studies on materials from other topics, such as oncology pharmaceutics (Van Ballegooie, 2020), atrial fibrillation (Siddiqui et al., 2020), and ophthalmology (Williams et al., 2016), show similar findings. Therefore, two issues should be addressed: What should the reading level be for an intervention's intended audience? What is the actual reading level of the material?

The website of the Programme for the International Assessment of Adult Competencies (PIAAC) provides a wealth of information related to the first issue: reading level of people around the world (OECD, n.d.). This website presents, for example, the results on adults' proficiency in key information-processing skills—literacy, numeracy, and problem-solving—in over 40 countries. It also provides detailed information on how these data can be collected among an intervention's intended audience. The second issue is how to assess the reading level of a document. Many tools are available with most being based on formulas that assess the average number of words in a sentence and the average number of syllables in a word. The former is used as a measure of complexity and the latter as a measure of vocabulary level. There are guidelines available for assessing (and rewriting) materials as well as valuable additional resources (Harvard T.H. Chan School of Public Health, n.d.). Common assessment tools are available as well and include SMOG, a tool for assessing the reading level of material in sentence and paragraph format, which is very useful for field work (McLaughlin, 1969); PMOSE/IKRISCH, a tool focusing on materials in the form of lists, charts, and graphs, (Mosenthal & Kirsch, 1998); and SAM, which focuses on other aspects of materials such as organization format, design, and culture (Doak et al., 1996).

However, reading level assessments are focused on literacy, not health literacy. Rademakers and Heijmans (2018) provide more details on the assessment of health literacy. Literacy should be addressed and recognized as necessary to consider, but planners should focus as heavily on the interpretation and use of information within the context of proposed change objectives. The concept of "health literacy" refers to the personal and relational factors that affect a person's ability to acquire, understand, and use information about health and health services (Batterham et al., 2016). It "entails people's knowledge, motivation and competences to access, understand, appraise, and apply health information in order to make judgments and take decisions in everyday life concerning healthcare, disease prevention and health promotion to maintain or improve quality of life during the life course" (Sørensen et al., 2012).

Lower health literacy is associated with poorer health outcomes and use of health care services (Berkman et al., 2011), and higher health system costs (WHO, 2013). In fact, health literacy mediates the relationship between socioeconomic status and quality of life, health outcomes, and health behaviors. It is a modifiable risk factor of socioeconomic disparities in health, whereby educational attainment is the most important determinant of health literacy (Stormacq et al., 2019). A review indicated that health literacy interventions increase both health literacy and treatment adherence outcomes (Miller, 2016).

Writing Intervention Messages

Messages are focused attempts to effectively promote and accomplish a change objective. They are the verbal or visual elements of the intervention that target the specific change objectives. In Step 3, planners decide on methods that would be included in each intervention component to address specific change objectives. Each method will be operationalized with multiple health messages and activities and delivered through a variety of channels and vehicles. In all cases, messages need to be written. Abraham and Kools (2012) provide detailed guidance on writing health messages. Key points are summarized in the next section.

The messages developed to address and promote the change objectives are informed specifically by data and information from Steps 1–3. The community assessment information identified in Step 1 will allow for an understanding of demographic and clinical characteristics as well as specific clinical information including incidence and prevalence of illness and risk that will allow for writing specific messages to influence determinants of behavior. Messages may promote an individual's understanding and knowledge of a specific issue, deliver information to determine an individual's level of susceptibility to the illness, identify the severity of the illness or exposure, or promote intentions to engage in a specific behavior (e.g., exercise or the use of condoms).

Many health promotion intervention materials contain two types of messages: focused messages to enable change objectives and contextual messages. For example, in the Me & You intervention, a virtual role-play activity script was developed to ensure students could develop skills related to using avoidance and refusal strategies (Peskin et al., 2018). Messages were developed to address change objectives and these messages used appropriate models and remediation (see example script in Figure 8.2). The second type of messages, contextual messages, might set up a scenario, provide information about the intervention, or provide an engaging narrative. In the Me & You intervention, for example, the script also specified the

Lesson #: 8, **Activity #:** 5
Change Objectives:
(1) Increase self-efficacy for effective negotiation via skills practice,
(2) Demonstrate ability to communicate personal limits to friends and partners, and
(3) Use appropriate refusal skills to keep from doing things you don't want to do
Timing: 5:00
Description/Script/Audio: In this activity the learner chooses one scenario to complete. Three scenarios are provided. Each is a video-based simulation. The camera takes the learner's point of view (POV). The learner interacts with a video model by selecting a negotiation line from available options and seeing this played out. After the video model responds the video freezes until the learner makes his/her next selection.

Mia VO: Here are three important rules. Protecting these rules will require open and honest negotiation. Scroll over each rule to see the situation that you will need to negotiate through. Choose the rule that is most right for you.

Three rule options are displayed with titles and explanations. Text on screen reads:
SELECT your rule

1. Choosing not to look at explicit material online:
You are choosing to not look at explicit pictures or material online.
(*Freeze frame setting – in a living room doing homework with a friend.*)
2. Choosing not to get involved in cyber-bullying: *[Example script provided below]*
You have decided that you will not participate in any form of bullying.
(*Freeze frame setting – in a driveway*).
3. Choosing not participate in sexting:
You have decided that you will not send explicit pictures of any kind.
(*Freeze frame setting – in your bedroom*)

Actor: "Check out my post and comment on it! I wrote something about "you know who" that's going to have everyone laughing at him. You should repost it too, so all your friends see it."
Learner:
a. No, that's not cool.
b. I don't want to have anything to do with that. I'll just mind my own business.
c. Really? As soon as I get a chance, I'll check it out.

IF learner selects C, THEN remediation
Mia or Derek VO: *Sorry! You are opening the door for your friend to think you might be ok with this later. Try again!*

Actor: "Why? I thought you didn't like him either."
Learner:
a. Ugh…what is it you want me to say?
b. That's not the point. I'm not comfortable talking about people, especially online.

Figure 8.2 Virtual Role-Play Script (Lesson 8, Student Curriculum in *Me & You*)

c. No, I'm telling you I don't want to get involved.

IF learner selects A, THEN remediation
Mia or Derek VO: *This is not a clear or strong enough response to protect your rule. You are not stating your position at all. Try again!*

Actor: "So what are you saying? You're too good to just comment?"
Learner:
a. I'm saying that I don't want to get involved. Saying mean things online is the same as doing it in person.
b. No, not at all. Maybe I'll just like the post?
c. You're turning this around. Honestly, I feel that we're *both* too good.

IF learner selects B, THEN remediation
Mia or Derek VO: *Sorry! You are not sticking to your rules... "liking" the post is also bullying. There is a better response.*

Actor: "I don't get it...not even a simple LOL?"
Learner:
a. I'll do it this time, but don't ask me to do something like this again.
b. No, not even LOL.
c. Saying LOL *is* getting involved, and I really would like if you respect my decision to stay out of it.

IF learner selects A, THEN remediation
Mia or Derek VO: *Don't give in that easy. Make sure to stick to your rule and repeat your NO message if you have to. Try again!*

Actor: "Ok, well can you log onto someone else's account and comment then?"
Learner:
a. I don't even know how to get on anyone else's account and I wouldn't do that anyway. Maybe you should delete the post.
b. If I'm not going to comment from mine, then I'm not going to comment from someone else's. I really think you should take it down.
c. You're killing me...whose account do you have in mind?

IF learner selects C, THEN remediation
Mia or Derek VO: *Wow, you're going to give up that easily? This won't protect your rule. Select a better response.*

Actor: "Ok, I understand what you're saying...I'll take it down."
[GO TO Mia OUTRO]

Figure 8.2 *(Continued)*

self-tailoring options available. Specifically, students could select a partner based on gender preference and could choose the most relevant scenario for themselves.

The following steps can assist in focusing the planners through message development:

1. Consider the change methods and practical applications that planners have decided on for a particular set of objectives. Identify those that will "fit" together for presentation in a particular vehicle, such as a newspaper story.
2. Draft messages matched to each change objective or combinations of change objectives.
3. Draft contextual messages that will be incorporated into the vehicle.

Writing to Enhance Cognitive Processing The capacity of an individual's working memory is limited. Therefore, message writers should promote more cognitive processing and use of information by doing the following (Abraham & Kools, 2012):

- Carefully plan (and limit) the number of concepts introduced.
- Match graphics to messages.
- Recognize the prior knowledge of the recipient: use the prior knowledge and fill gaps.
- Help the recipient make inferences with stimulation of active processes.
- Follow an explicit logic in the order of topics, sessions, and sentences within materials.
- Make links between sections explicit to the reader, viewer, or listener.
- Match the reading level of the intended audience.
- Write in the active voice.
- Make lists understandable without introductory sentences (e.g., in a list of things people should not do, every item should begin with "Do not").
- Write as clearly as possible (e.g., if the meaning is "do not," copywriters should not use the term avoid).
- Present the material in the order in which the reader will need it.
- Include only messages in support of the change objectives; remove superfluous material unless it provides an appropriate context.
- Use subheadings to break up or chunk the text.
- Use a careful hierarchy to support comprehension.
- Tell the recipient how the material is structured (use advance organizers, see Chapter 7).
- Use sentences and designs that encourage interaction, such as checklists with boxes that readers can check.
- Use one- and two-syllable words and short, simple sentences with definitions of more difficult words in appositional phrases and parenthetical statements.
- Provide visual cues.
- Use strong topic sentences for paragraphs.

Also when writing messages, it is warranted to build on available theory and evidence. The Elaboration Likelihood Model, for example, explains different ways of processing stimuli and why they are used (Cacioppo et al., 1986). Such theoretical insights can be used to address people's need for cognition in health promotion interventions (Nikoloudakis et al., 2018). Parrott (2017) edited a comprehensive theoretically guided work in health and risk message design and processing.

Translation Translation of intervention materials and messages into another language is not a trivial matter. A good translation is usually aimed at symmetry: a translation that is loyal to the meaning of the source language while ensuring equal familiarity and colloquiality in both languages. Another term for this symmetry is decentering (from the source language). Decentering implies a de-emphasis of the developer's language in such a way that the system of symbols supersedes a single culture. At best, decentering eliminates the distinction between source and target language. Decentering requires a multistage translation that allows for paraphrasing the meaning of the source materials and of the translation before deciding on a translated version. The translation is then translated back to the original language, and the versions are compared. The process of translation and back translation continues until the two versions are acceptable. The goal is a dynamic equivalence in which a cultural symbol in the source language is translated into a cultural symbol in the target language that evokes the same functional response from the reader or listener. A classic example by Werner and Campbell (1973) concerns the problem of finding a Navajo word for measles, where presenting a list of symptoms might have evoked a more meaningful response than trying to find one word that did not originally exist in a language. They relate an even more significant problem of meaning when they explain that the literal translation of the word meningitis into Navajo would be "the covering of the brain is getting red." The translation period is another good time to work with interviews and focus groups to understand the words used to describe certain phenomena. A Dutch study revealed that meanings children assign to weight-related words are shaped by their experiences in the broader social context, especially at school and with healthcare professionals (Stuij et al., 2020).

Visual Elements The focus of the previous sections has been mainly on writing "verbal" messages. Most interventions also include visual elements. Just like verbal messages are made up of words, grammar, and syntax, visual elements are also made up of several basic elements, such as shape, texture, and dimensions. These elements can be combined to build a strong and clear message and to ease interpretation (Costa et al., 2020). Social media demonstrates the power of visual elements in self-representation and storytelling (Pearce et al., 2020). Visual elements also play a crucial role in evaluations of and willingness to share messages (Farace, 2019). Costa et al. (2020) provide guidelines for directing the design of visual elements by considering how people process visuospatial information (Castro-Alonso et al., 2019). These guidelines are based on the results of experimental research on cognitive load theory and the cognitive theory of multimedia:

- Visual elements should be designed according to cognitive principles rather than just on engagement variables. In other words, the processing advantages of visual elements, such as providing scaffolds for textual information, should be utilized.

- Visual elements should not be designed with their information separated but integrated spatially. For example, visual elements and their text labels should follow the spatial contiguity principle and be placed near each other.
- Visual elements should be designed with auditory descriptions, rather than too much information on screen. By providing narrations, auditory processing is used and visuospatial processing is left to manage the key visual elements and not also written explanations.
- Extra information that is not fundamental to the message should be deleted from visual elements.
- Visual elements are more effective when they have cues to direct the receiver to the most important parts.
- Long dynamic visual elements whose pace cannot be controlled should be changed to pace control formats, shorter versions, or static visual elements.

A Cultural Perspective on Writing Messages Many cultural characteristics directly influence how people communicate and how they understand and respond to the health messages they receive. As with the design of other materials, the message writers will want to understand the preferred communication styles of the intended intervention recipients and will want to involve representatives from the community to increase appropriateness. Many aspects of cultural preferences can affect message writing. For example, the structure of arguments (with the main point first or with a buildup to the climax), the use of words, and the standards used to judge credibility.

Planners must be particularly careful to clearly understand a cultural communication method before using it. Airhihenbuwa (1994) gives a classic example of the pitfalls of superficial use of oral culture (ear-to-mouth) versus visual culture (eye-to-object) storytelling methods. He points out that stories are a reciprocal vehicle that depends on the listeners' interaction with the teller to create the learning. Any adaptation that makes this vehicle a one-way street loses the method's power (Airhihenbuwa, 1994). This is also highly relevant in today's media landscape. The ephemeral nature of instant-messaging applications, such as Snapchat, applies an oral paradigm. While online discourse of computer-mediated communication shares many qualities with oral communication, ephemeral applications implement orality on highly visual contents. The technology that is used fades visual contents as if they were spoken words fading in the air after utterance (Soffer, 2016). The use of a delivery vehicle from outside the culture has different pitfalls. For example, if text-based messages are used to convey information in an oral culture, learners will face problems with attention, comprehension, and memory because the learner will first have to learn to use this novel source of information. However, some vehicles may be used in conjunction with others to build a stronger intervention and reinforce specific messages. In general, culture-sensitive health communication strategies are needed to close the gap in the social determinants of health and risk (Iwelunmor & Airhihenbuwa, 2017).

Aiming at Cultural Sensitivity In following IM, from the intervention's inception and through each step, the planning group will have involved intended intervention participants throughout the planning process. The planning group will have taken into account culture by fully describing the causes of health problems in specific groups (Step 1), suggesting what should change among members of the target group and in their environments (Step 2), and thinking about change methods and practical applications with the potential intervention participants (Step 3). However, the issues of cultural sensitivity resurface when planners begin to prepare plans for materials and activities.

The two-dimensional theory of cultural sensitivity defines the construct as "the extent to which ethnic/cultural, characteristics, experience, norms, values, behavioral patterns and beliefs of a target population as well as relevant historical, environmental, and social forces are incorporated in the design, delivery, and evaluation of targeted health promotion materials and programs" (Resnicow et al., 1999). In addition to ethical considerations of developing interventions that are culturally sensitive, a growing body of evidence indicates that enhancing cultural sensitivity strengthens the effectiveness of health promotion interventions (Ballard et al., 2020; Huang & Shen, 2016). Moreover, cultural sensitivity is closely related to the principle of participation in intervention development—a key guiding principle for community engagement (Collins et al., 2018) and the guidelines for collaboration cited in Chapter 5 (Step 1) and integral for all steps in IM.

The structure of culturally sensitive materials and activities has two dimensions, which were coined and popularized by Noam Chomsky: deep structure and surface structure (Singelis et al., 2018). Deep structure refers to the factors that influence the health behavior of the intervention's intended participants. For example, empowerment, collectivism, and privacy are sociocultural constructs relevant to African-Americans in colorectal cancer screening (Sanders Thomposn et al., 2015). This example shows that culture concerns more aspects than ethnic identity only. In the process of planning interventions with IM, these aspects are usually addressed in earlier steps because they can influence what behaviors, environmental conditions, performance objectives, and determinants become the intervention focus. If planners have not characterized these factors correctly to this point, attention to the cultural sensitivity of materials and activities is unlikely to be effective because the intervention will not have salience to the intended cultural group.

Assuming that the planning group has brought to bear the insights of the cultural group to the behaviors and determinants and the methods that can change them, they can turn their attention to surface structure and the creation of materials and activities. Surface structure comprises the superficial but still important characteristics of a cultural group such as familiar people, language, music, clothing, and so on.

There are various categories of mechanisms by which planners can work to achieve attention to both surface and deeper aspects of culture in their intervention planning (Brand et al., 2019; Kreuter et al., 2003).

- Peripheral processes match materials' characteristics to the culture's surface characteristics. This attempt to make materials familiar and comfortable to the intended audience relies heavily on visual aspects of production (O'Donovan et al., 2020).
- Evidential strategies remind the cultural group of the health problem's significance to them. For example, by providing national and local prevalence data related to the obesity and health behaviors of ethnic minority youth (Messiah et al., 2017).
- Linguistic strategies provide materials and activities in the language of the cultural group. For example, Turkish and Moroccan women in the Netherlands expressed the need for materials regarding cervical cancer screening participation in their mother tongue, because some of them lack a good command of the Dutch language (Hamdiui et al., 2021).
- Constituent-involving approaches cover several strategies for involving the intended intervention participants, including hiring staff from the cultural group, using lay health workers from the group, and continuing to work with the group as members of the planning group.
- Sociocultural strategies embed health promotion in the context of broader cultural values and issues. For example, to enhance relevance for Black and Hispanic youth, Me & You embedded surface (e.g., music, clothing) and deep (e.g., respect for family) structure sociocultural features (Peskin et al., 2018).

Conducting Formative Research Formative research is a type of research conducted in the early stages of a project or design process to gather insights, understand user needs, and inform decision-making. In intervention design, formative research can be both preproduction research as well as production testing. Preproduction research elucidates characteristics of the intended participants' needs, cultural preferences, knowledge, attitudes, beliefs, and health literacy that relate to message, medium, and situation. Production testing (pretesting—see Task 4 below) is a process in which prototypes of intervention materials are tested for audience reaction (Elsbernd et al., 2018; Larsson et al., 2018). Regardless of the population's demographic, cultural, or clinical background, the conduct of formative research is an important step in the design of effective materials and activities.

In the *preproduction research phase*, the team may explore interpersonal as well as media channels to identify the best methods for intervention delivery to the participant population. Preproduction testing can include both informal feedback and ratings of sources, messages, themes, persuasive arguments, and stylistic devices. Focus groups and interviews are widely used methods for preproduction testing (Wyatt et al., 2008). For example, Shafer and colleagues (2011) demonstrated how both methods can be used in preproduction message research to develop messages that would motivate racially diverse mothers of preteen girls for human papillomavirus (HPV) vaccination (Shafer et al., 2011). Personas are often constructed to represent specific segments of intervention participants by a fictional character (Wray et al., 2019). In general, formative research should include specific exploration of cultural issues (Bentley et al., 2014).

Methods that are used in the preproduction research phase have one aspect in common; they are not a one-way street. Involvement of and interaction with intended intervention participants is key and it is often an iterative process that results in design documents guiding the production process. Over the years, many approaches have been developed to shape this involvement of and interaction with intended intervention participants. Approaches such as co-creation (Halvorsrud et al., 2019) and human-centered design (Chen et al., 2020) have gained in popularity.

In health and social sciences, *co-creation principles* are promoted to include more experience-near forms of knowledge and ensure that interventions are relevant to priorities and needs of interested parties (Halvorsrud et al., 2019). The rationale for this spirit of participation relates to voice and engagement (those with lived experience should be engaged in processes of development, redesign, and improvements), empowerment (engagement has positive individual and societal benefits), and advancement (quality of life and other health outcomes for everyone involved should improve as a result) (Palmer et al., 2019). *Human-centered design* is a creative approach to problem-solving that brings together what is desirable from a human POV with what is technologically feasible and economically viable (Chen et al., 2020).

These approaches align well with this phase in IM. As mentioned in this and earlier chapters, participation in health promotion planning is a key perspective used throughout IM. *Agile methods* are often used when applying these approaches. Agile methods have in common that designs for materials and activities start almost immediately based on a first rough draft. These drafts are then evaluated and adjusted in cycles that quickly succeed each other (Peters, 2019). This also fits with the iterative nature of IM. These agile methods might therefore be a useful addition when preparing plans for materials and activities but cannot replace the work to be completed in Steps 1, 2, and 3 that should inform these plans in the first place.

Develop Design Documents for Materials and Activities

Whether the planning group hires design consultants (see Task 3 of Step 4) or produces materials and activities themselves, they will need documents to convey the intent of materials and activities in detail to those who write or select content from available resources and design graphics and other communications. These documents, called "design documents," will guide production to ensure that intervention materials and activities are culturally relevant, meet the intervention objectives, and follow the parameters for use of their selected methods and practical applications. There are two basic types of design documents:

- A set of design documents from the planning group to the production team. The production team can be a member of the planning group or design consultants who are new to the project at this stage.
- A series of production design documents from the production team to the planning group showing details about the creative translation of plans into materials and activities.

The first design documents the planning group will share with the production team are a *project prospectus* that gives the length of the product, a brief description of the audience, the way that the user will interact with the product, the purpose of the piece (the intended impact), the central messages, and the expected budget. A second design document from the planning group is *the set of matrices from Step 2.* Some teams highlight each set of change objectives as they pertain to each material or activity. A variety of highlighter colors are good for this purpose. The design documents then become more specific with one document for each material. Preparing design documents for materials, activities, and messages that are mediated by interactive technology, such as computer-tailored web-based interventions, may be more complex than for other types of materials. It requires, for example, flowcharts depicting the sequence of content and branching logic depending on the user's input (what the user will experience and its order), screen maps depicting how the screen contents are arrayed with functional definitions of screen components (what the user will see and do), and scripts (see Figure 8.2 for an example of a virtual role-play script used in Me & You) and storyboards (a written list of audio and visuals of each embedded animation, video, quiz, or other interactive activity).

The production design documents that flow from the production team to the planning group are usually more than written words. They might be written, as in a concept for a videotape, or they might be a combination of words and pictures, as in a storyboard or a rough sketch of a layout. They also might be illustrations or photographs in a layout or rough-cut videotape. These documents are all elements of conveying the creative person's image of the final product as it is developed first in the mind of that person and then in some medium. Figure 8.3 presents sample screenshots from intervention materials used in Me & You.

Readers who are planning an intervention that includes such methods and practical applications as policy development, coalition building, and media advocacy may be thinking: "All this discussion about design documents doesn't refer to me! I won't be developing traditional materials." However, design documents are needed to guide intervention components that are not products, such as videotapes, PSAs, and the like. Products can be activities such as advisory board and committee meeting structure and function, coalition development and maintenance, and lobbying. Each of these activities needs a design document and sometimes more than one.

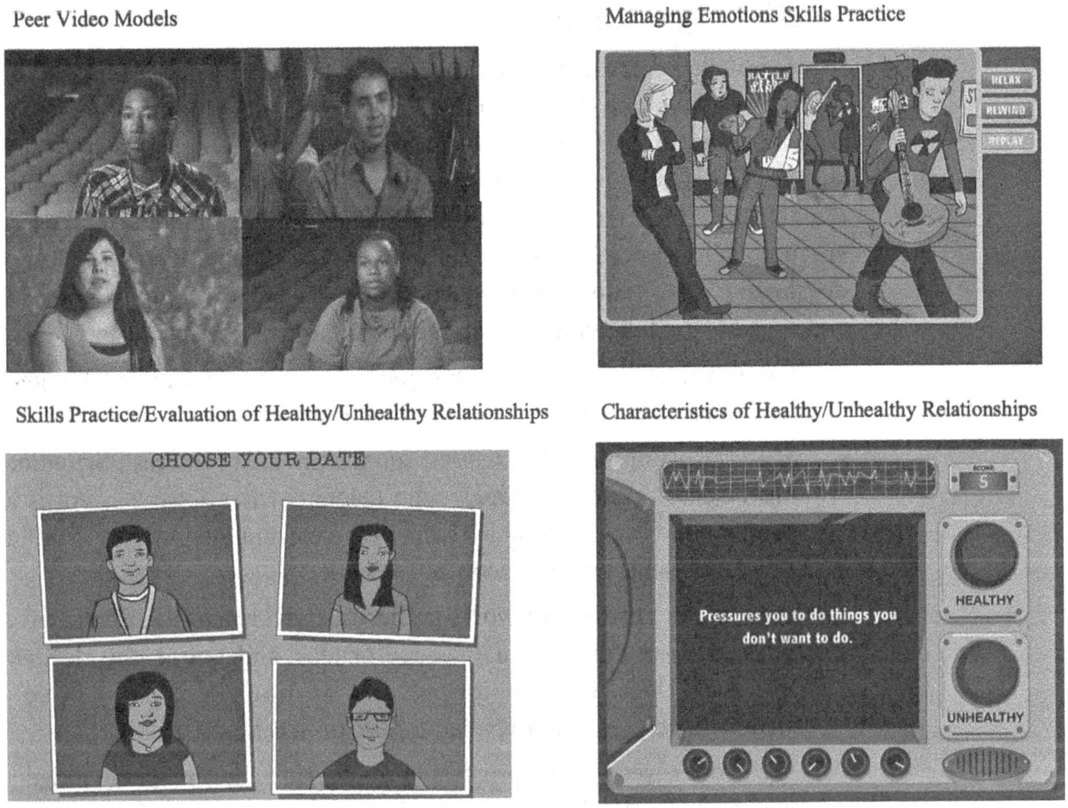

Figure 8.3 Sample Screenshots from *Me & You*

Coalitions, for example, need a design document that specifies how coalition members will be recruited, how meetings will be run, and how minutes or meeting summaries will be constructed and delivered. A coalition might also need training for membership, and the training session will require a design document. Not only can such documents prevent breakdowns in communication but they can also make the processes smooth, productive, and reinforcing for the participants. A synthesis of existing studies on the community coalition approach identified seven, partly overlapping, aspects that are important when applying the approach in urban areas: the diverse expertise of the members, the clarity of the goal, the member's interest and motivation, the leadership, the trust and cohesion of the coalition members, the clarity of the members' roles, and understanding the norm and the culture of the target community (Sokang et al., 2020). These aspects should be specified in a design document when applying this approach.

Task 3: Produce Intervention Materials, Activities, and Protocols

The design documents are key to go from intervention design to the production of intervention materials, activities, and protocols—the third task in Step 4. This results in prototype materials and protocols for activities that need to be pretested, refined, and finalized (the final task of Step 4).

Hiring Design Consultants

In an ideal budgetary world, planners should take the advice of Balderman (1996), who says that if you weren't trained to do something, don't do it. A design consultant should be hired when the planners do not have the specific skill needed to create a component of the intervention (Balderman, 1996). Commonly used design consultants include copywriters, graphic designers, computer programmers, videographers, and app developers. The seminal work by Balderman (1996) is still highly relevant and suggests the following ways to recruit talent to a project:

- Put together a synopsis of the job including approximate budget, length, purpose, concept, and producing agency.
- Send the synopsis with a request for statements of interest. Schedule meetings with the individuals who respond. Interviewing talent is a good way not only to look for help on the current job but also to build a file of possible resources for future work.
- Look at the portfolio of work. Is there any evidence that this person has conveyed the type of message needed and gotten the desired response? Does the range of previous work of the creative person include the type of work needed for the project?
- Ask about several of the projects in the portfolio. Is a range of budgets represented? Ask the person to talk about each project. If the type of product the team wants is not represented in the portfolio (which is the best of the best), then it is probably not available from this vendor.

Remember that in the circumstance the planners hire one or more design consultants, these people will be designing and creating the material, activities, and protocols. Planners should not have to take over the creative process assuming that they have communicated the intent of the materials and activities well enough that the design consultant can bring skills to the team and create materials and activities that are congruent with the ideas of the planning group. This scenario implies that the design consultants should not only be creative but also willing to thoroughly understand the team's intent. The planners should pay close attention when they interview design consultants: *How do they present themselves? As salespeople or as people who want to understand the project? Are they too quick to assume that the project is "just like other projects" they have done? Do they seem sensitive to the planning group's needs and find the design documents helpful?*

Planners should effectively give their creative contractors an easy-to-understand background of the project. The creative additions should bring to life rather than override or misinterpret the planning group's understanding of the problem and its solution.

Working with Design Consultants

To get started with a design consultant, planners usually invite him or her to a team meeting to talk about the project once the planning group can give a fairly consistent message. If possible, a planner takes the design consultant to visit with members of the community. Sometimes the design consultant can go to focus groups or interviews. In an ideal situation, the design consultant can work with the planning group from the beginning of planning, offering ideas as to format, and serving as an expert witness on what is, and what is perhaps not, doable. The next best approach is to bring the design consultants in when the matrices, methods, and practical applications have been hammered out but before the team has decided on intervention messages. The earlier the design consultant can enter the process, the more his or her skills will enrich it.

Regardless of whether the messages are verbal, visual, or a combination of both, or which vehicles are used to deliver them, there are certain aspects that need to be considered at the beginning of the production process. The importance of various aspects differs per project, but it is worthwhile to consider, for example:

- What are the costs and how are they charged (e.g., per product delivered, per hour invested, a lump sum)?
- What are arrangements regarding copyrights and credits? Do they relate to the project at hand or does it also allow for scale-up in the future? Will these items need to be updated in the future, and if so by whom? What standards are used (e.g., format for graphics and videos, file types, color schemes)?
- What process will be used to review initial ideas, preliminary sketches, or other proposed work?

Often, these aspects are not only agreed upon within the planning group but also by means of contracts with design consultants.

After agreeing on these aspects and possibly signing contracts, the actual production process starts. On the one hand, the planning group should try not to interfere with the creativity during this process. Design documents should have been created in such a way that it is clear what the planning group intends. However, design consultants can sometimes take creative liberties that can jeopardize intervention effectiveness, for example where they consider changes that lead to omission of change objectives or messages or the violation of the parameters of use. It is therefore important to stay vigilant and direct the design consultants when necessary. The design documents can support supervision during this process to ensure that all change objectives remain addressed and all parameters for use remain respected.

This process is iterative in nature, as sometimes changes are warranted and design consultants need to take one step back before being able to move forward in the production process. More in general, this is also something to consider when discussing, for example, contracts with design consultants or thinking about the planning of the project at large. It is crucial to distinguish between the duration of the production itself and the duration of the production process. The production itself might take, for example, six weeks, but more time might be needed to go back and forth with the planning group for review and possible changes. The latter is also important with regard to finalizing materials, activities, and protocols. Before doing so, time for pretesting and refining needs to be included in the planning.

Task 4: Pretest, Refine, and Finalize Materials, Activities, and Protocols

Pretesting is trying out the specific messages and other characteristics of the intervention materials, activities, and protocols with the intended participants before final production. This is crucial to determine whether planning has resulted in appealing and understandable materials, activities, and protocols that adhere to the parameters specified in Step 3. Sometimes planners do not conduct pretesting because they are behind schedule. No matter how big the hurry, planners must make time for trying out materials, activities, and protocols. Sometimes planners object to taking time to pretest by pointing out that the planning group already comprises representatives of the potential intervention participants and implementers. However, representatives who have been involved in the planning have probably come to value the intervention that they have developed in a way that biases their objectivity. This step requires going back out into the communities to receive and integrate new feedback.

Define Pretest Objectives

Pretesting starts by defining pretest objectives. The pretest objectives can cover many aspects, such as:

- Concept testing (e.g., to test the key phrases and visuals that portray the main ideas)
- Readability testing (e.g., to estimate school-grade level required to read text)
- Message execution (e.g., to assess whether intervention materials and messages are attended to, comprehended, appealing, and culturally relevant)
- Impact (e.g., to estimate impact of messages on determinants)
- Adoption/implementation characteristics (e.g., to assess perceptions of implementers about complexity, trialability, observability, and relative advantage of materials)

In addition, the planners will want to make sure that the parameters for operationalizing the methods and practical applications are met. These parameters are a useful source to help in defining pretest objectives. Chapter 7 presented parameters under which each change method will be most effective. In Step 3, the planners made decisions about methods and practical applications. For instance, in the development of It's Your Game ... Keep It Real the developers selected scenario-based risk information as one method for improving skills and self-efficacy for evaluating dating relationships (Shegog et al., 2014). For the practical application, the developers created a computer-based, mock TV dating game show in which students had to evaluate the healthy and unhealthy characteristics of potential dating situations. In this example, the parameters for the use of scenario-based risk information were that students would find these scenarios plausible and that multiple scenarios would be provided (Mevissen et al., 2009). Pretesting should provide assurance that these assumptions are met. The developers tested the mock TV show with potential participants and found that all of the scenarios were plausible and believable to the youth.

It is important to get an overview of all assumptions underlying the intervention materials, activities, and protocols and use them to define pretest objectives. However, there are often insufficient resources to pretest everything, and therefore, it is important to select which objectives to pretest. To make such a selection, it is required to select methods for pretesting. Please note that certain objectives can be pretested by various methods and certain methods can be used to pretest various objectives. In other words, there is not a one-on-one relationship between pretest objectives and methods for pretesting.

Selecting Methods for Pretesting

Table 8.3 presents various pretesting methods linked to pretest objectives. This is a brief overview, and other sources of information on pretesting will be helpful (Whittingham et al., 2008; Whittingham et al., 2009; Willoughby & Brickman, 2020). Table 8.3 lists various examples of pretest objectives that can be addressed including intervention participants' responses to messages and materials and perceptions of material characteristics by adopters and implementers (see Chapter 9). For each pretest objective that the planners define, at least the following aspects should be considered:

- Have you selected the method to use for this pretest objective? Most pretest objectives can be addressed with a number of different methods.
- Who is the target group for the pretest? This can be potential participants, adopters, and implementers, but also other groups, such as parents of children.
- Have you determined the procedure of the pretest?
- Have you selected the operationalization(s) that will be used in the pretest? An operationalization is what is used to measure or manipulate the variable of interest.

Considering all these aspects is also helpful to make decisions regarding what is feasible to pretest (e.g., in terms of resources). If certain parts of the intervention are not pretested, which is not recommended, it is important to document this decision. This contributes to the summative evaluation, which includes a later assessment of how the audience received the

Table 8.3 Examples of Pretesting Objectives and Methods

	Concept Testing	Readability Testing	Message Execution	Impact	Adoption/ Implementation Characteristics
Objectives	To test whether the key phrases portray the main idea of the intervention; to discover vernacular regarding intervention topic	To estimate school-grade level required to read text	To assess whether intervention materials are attended to; to assess whether messages are comprehended	To estimate impact of messages on determinants	To assess complexity and relative advantage of materials
Methods	Interviews, focus groups	Text and readability formula/tools	Interviews, focus groups, cognitive interviewing	Experimental pretesting	Interviews, focus groups, observations
Procedures	Use key phrases as stimulus material; ask people to freely talk about the intervention topic	Apply formula to each intervention message	Show different versions of materials; ask what participants "got" from messages	Compare different versions of messages and assess changes in determinants	Ask for review by naïve potential implementers; observe implementers when they work with material
Limitations	Isolated setting lacking the broader context of the intervention	Readability is a prerequisite but not a guarantee of message comprehension	Only outcome variables on top of persuasion-communication matrix (McGuire, 2001)	Requires adequate sample size to accurately estimate changes (Peters & Crutzen, 2021)	Isolated setting lacking the broader context of the intervention

materials during implementation and whether the methods and practical applications were operationalized effectively enough to have an impact on the change objectives (see Chapter 10).

In addition to the guiding questions above, a major question at this stage is how to get materials in final-enough form to be good stimulus material while keeping an eye on the budget. For example, videotapes can be presented in storyboard format, radio PSAs can be read aloud, and newsletters can be produced with a word processing program. In general, as much of the final product as possible should be included: illustrations, photographs, and graphics for newsletters rather than just the words, for example. It is also important to evaluate individual aspects of materials, activities, and protocols rather than just the whole.

Making Sense of Pretest Data

At every step of pretesting, there is the likelihood of obtaining a lot of information and possibly conflicting opinions. The planning group will want to have a plan about how to display data and keep track of recommended changes. For example, a table of pretesting data might include the unit of material, activities and protocols being tested, the questions being asked, and an enumeration of the answers. The team will want to know what intervention participants and implementers think about the intervention materials, activities and protocols, how they respond to them, and how strongly they hold their opinions. Different types of feedback may lead to different team responses. For example, the team might ask potential implementers of a patient education intervention to review the materials and find that while the intervention was being developed, treatment guidelines changed—an obvious need to modify the materials for accuracy.

But what happens when reviewers disagree on design characteristics, cultural sensitivity, or suitability? The planning group will have to have a plan for adjudicating recommendations for changes. Furthermore, when decisions are made to change something, the planning group will need to make sure that the change has not disrupted or eliminated an important element of the intervention such as a change method.

Making appropriate use of pretest data requires working back through messages, practical applications, and methods to matrices to ensure that changes in the intervention materials do not leave gaps in the intervention chain of causation (i.e., the logic model resulting from Steps 2 and 3). This is required for refining material, activities, and protocols. Sometimes multiple iterations are needed to end up with versions of materials, activities, and protocols that can be pushed to the final production. The final production of the intervention is where Step 4 ends.

FOR OUR CHILDREN EXAMPLE: STEP 4

In Step 4, the program planning group fully fleshes out the intervention plan including the program themes, components, and scope and sequence. They translate the methods and practical applications identified in Step 3 into concrete messages, materials, and activities and develop intervention materials, activities, and protocols that align with the intervention content planned. The planning group also pre-tests, refines, and finalizes the intervention materials, activities, and protocols.

Task 1: Define Intervention Structure (Themes, Components, Scope, and Sequence)

After generating and reconfirming initial ideas for the intervention in Step 3, the ***For Our Children*** or, in Spanish, ***Por Nuestros Hijos (PNH)*** planning group brainstormed about a title and theme for the intervention. Research staff conducted focus groups with parents from the priority population and interviews with healthcare providers to ensure that program ideas would be relevant. For example, parents advised against overusing fear-based messaging or messages that promoted sexual activity in adolescence, as it often turned parents off, ultimately hindering action. They instead emphasized their overwhelming desire to protect their children from harm. It was from these conversations that the planning group developed the overall program theme and subsequent title, *Por Nuestras Hijos (For Our Children)*. The intent of this theme was to convey a message of protection that was interwoven throughout the program by consistently highlighting that the HPV vaccine protects daughters and sons from HPV and that parents protect their children from cancer by obtaining the HPV vaccine for them. The planning group determined that the intervention components targeting parents would follow the story of a mother gathering information about the HPV vaccine and making the decision to vaccinate her child to protect them against cancer (one version features a daughter while another version features a son). The planning group determined that this protective framework would be effective for this population. Messages that specifically frame mothers as protectors and the HPV vaccine as the best way to protect their children against a potential threat (the HPV virus), increase Hispanic mothers' intentions to vaccinate their children (McGlone, 2017).

From the in-depth interviews conducted with healthcare providers, the planning team learned that there were knowledge gaps regarding HPV and the HPV vaccine among different types of healthcare providers. For example, physicians had different ways they typically recommended the HPV vaccine and did not always recommend it strongly. This aligned with existing literature that indicates that one of the most common reasons for poor uptake of HPV vaccine is lack of a provider recommendation or a weak recommendation (Beavis and Levinson, 2016). The providers recommended that the planning group design the intervention content using modules or flashcards because these are commonly used formats in training apps for residents and medical students. Additionally, they suggested separate modules for providers versus medical assistants and that the length of the training be kept to a minimum given that providers have limited time. Learnings from these interviews informed the overall focus of the provider intervention, motivating and training providers to give a strong, bundled HPV vaccine recommendation to parents of adolescents. The training program was subsequently titled, *HPVCancerCoach App*.

As proposed in the grant and reconfirmed in Step 3, the group determined that the PNH intervention (parent and provider components) would utilize multiple communication channels (interpersonal and mediated) and multiple delivery vehicles including tailored interactive multimedia content delivered via web-based applications and print materials. Next, they developed a program scope and sequence for the parent (Table 8.4) and provider (Table 8.5) components of the intervention to illustrate the breadth and amount of content (scope) within the intervention and the order in which the content would be delivered (sequence).

The parent intervention consisted of two components, a tailored interactive multimedia intervention (TIMI) and a print fotonovela, delivered in a single education session by a program facilitator (e.g., community health worker, promotora, and healthcare professional). The TIMI is an interactive web-based application designed to provide parents with information about HPV, HPV-related cancers, and the HPV vaccine. Using video vignettes, it follows the story of a mother who decides to vaccinate her child against HPV. It also incorporates video presentations by a health professional and graphic design, illustrations, and animation with voiceover narration to provide parents with information and encourage them to vaccinate their children. In addition, the content presented is tailored based on parents' answers to a series of questions about HPV and the vaccine. The fotonovela, a printed brochure commonly used in Hispanic communities, is similar to a comic book and uses photographs and dialogue boxes to present information. They often employ theory and evidence-based methods such as social modeling and vicarious learning, and have been shown to be effective in helping individuals personalize health issues, identify with and internalize the information being presented, and engage in positive health behaviors (Auger and Verbiest, 2007; Holmes et al., 2007). For the PNH intervention,

Table 8.4 Partial Scope and Sequence for Parent Components of Por Nuestros Hijos Project

Module	Description	Vehicle
Component: Tailored Interactive Multimedia Intervention (TIMI)		
Module 0/tailoring[a] [H1]	Language selection (**English** or Spanish) Healthcare provider introduces the For Our Children/Por Nuestros Hijos program Gender tailoring (**daughter** or son)	Video embedded within tablet-based app
Module 1.1 [S1]	Mother watching TV, receives information about HPV vaccine on the TV. Mother looks curious and interested in the information that she saw.	Video vignette embedded within tablet-based app
Module 1.2 [H2]	Healthcare provider shares information about HPV and HPV-related cancers. She shares information about HPV vaccine, including information that is approved for both boys and girls between 9 and 26 years.	Video vignette embedded within tablet-based app
Tailoring[a]	Parent is asked to indicate whether child (son or daughter) could be at risk of getting an HPV infection, either now or in the future (perceived risk)? [Yes/No/**I'm not sure**][a]	Video vignette embedded within tablet-based app
Module 2.1 [P1]	Information presented visually on how common the virus is, highlighting cervical and oropharyngeal cancers and warts.	Text/graphic illustrations with voiceover narration embedded within tablet-based app
Module 2.2 [P2]	General facts about HPV, cancers, and the vaccine	Text/graphic illustrations with voiceover narration embedded within tablet-based app
Testimonials	Female cancer survivor shares her experience of beating cervical cancer.	Video testimonials embedded within tablet-based app
Tailoring[a]	Parent is asked to indicate benefits of vaccinating against HPV-related cancers. [Yes/No/**I'm not sure**]	Text/graphic illustrations with voiceover narration embedded within tablet-based app
Module 3.1 [P3]	Information presented visually on HPV vaccine, its efficacy and effectiveness, and that it is safe.	Text/graphic illustrations with voiceover narration embedded within tablet-based app
Tailoring[a]	Parent asked to select common questions other parents have about the HPV vaccine [select ONE or **ALL concerns**][a]	Text/graphic illustrations with voiceover narration embedded within tablet-based app
Component 2: Fotonovella		
Cover page/introduction	Introduces the For Our Children/Por Nuestros Hijos program Includes link/QR code to TIMI	Text-based content and still photos illustrated in print brochure
Scene 1	Two friends meet after a long time.	Still photos with relevant dialogue box illustrated in print brochure
Scene 2	Mother 1 shares that she was at the clinic to get her daughter and her son vaccinated. Mother 2 is surprised to know that the HPV vaccine is also available for boys.	Still photos with relevant dialogue box illustrated in print brochure

(*continued*)

Table 8.4 *(Continued)*

Module	Description	Vehicle
Scene 3	Mother 2 shares that her doctor did not share this information, but she will make a list of questions to ask the doctor at her next visit.	Still photos with relevant dialog box illustrated in print brochure
Scenes 4-6	Mother 2 asks doctor about HPV vaccine for boys. Doctor explains that HPV vaccine can also be given to boys, and that both boys and girls need to complete the HPV vaccine series.	Still photos with relevant dialogue box illustrated in print brochure
FAQ	Information and resources provided related to the following questions: 1. Why should I be worried about my son/daughter getting HPV? 2. How can I get help paying for my child's vaccine? 3. Where can I go to get my child vaccinated?	Text-based content included in print brochure
Component 3: HPV Vaccination Reminders		
Initiation (1st dose)—Four weeks before child is age-eligible to receive vaccine	An initial text message and reminder text messages sent to parents to encourage them to schedule an appointment to initiate the HPV vaccine series for their age-eligible child.	Free text messaging web-based platform
Initiation follow-up—Every week after the initial text reminder (up to eight reminders)		
Completion (2nd dose)—Four weeks before next dose of vaccine is due	An initial text message and reminder text messages sent to parents to encourage them to schedule an appointment for their child's next dose of the HPV vaccine series.	
Completion Follow-up—Every week after the initial text reminder (up to eight reminders)		

Note: Full scope and sequence not presented. Fotonovellas are brief print stories with pictures and dialog, popular among Hispanic populations for conveying health information. Full scope and sequence not presented. Version for parents of boys is presented here.
[H] = Host, [S] = Scene, [P] = Slideshow/animation.
[a] Bolded text in brackets indicates the tailoring option illustrated in the table, which is the most comprehensive sequence option.

the fotonovela follows the same story as the TIMI and addresses common barriers to HPV vaccination. To deliver the parent intervention, if the parent has 20 minutes or more, the facilitator delivers the education session using the TIMI, then gives the fotonovela to the parent to review on their own at home. If the parent has less than 20 minutes, the program facilitator delivers the education session using the fotonovela, and then provides parents with the link to view the TIMI on their own at home.

The provider intervention consisted of a single component, an interactive web-based training application, the HPVCancerCoach App. The app uses narrated, graphically designed presentations and video testimonials to educate healthcare providers on topics related to HPV, the HPV vaccine, providing a strong HPV vaccination recommendation, and mitigating parental concerns about the vaccine. Similar to the TIMI for parents, the content presented is tailored based on providers' answers to a series of questions.

Table 8.5 Partial Scope and Sequence for Healthcare Provider Component of Por Nuestros Hijos Project

***HPVCancerCoach*: Healthcare Provider HPV Education App**		
Module	**Description**	**Vehicle**
Introduction and welcome message	Healthcare provider (e.g., physician/nurse) introduces the app, explains the purpose of the information covered in the app and why it is important.	Stock images and graphic illustrations with voiceover narration embedded within mobile app
Providers have the power to prevent cancer	Healthcare provider describes different HPV-related cancer types in men and women and the importance of the healthcare provider's role and recommendation in cancer prevention.	Stock images and graphic illustrations with voiceover narration embedded within mobile app
Dose schedule and recommended guidelines	Healthcare provider describes CDC recommended guidelines for HPV vaccination and reviews dose schedule for 11-, 12-, 13-, and 17-year-olds.	Stock images and graphic illustrations with voiceover narration embedded within mobile app
Hear from cancer survivors	Healthcare provider suggests to watch testimonial videos that personalize reasons to protect children from HPV vaccine (tailored section).	Testimonial videos embedded within mobile app
How to provide a strong HPV vaccine recommendation	Healthcare provider describes difference between presumptive and optional recommendation, bundled recommendation, and how to provide strong and effective HPV vaccine recommendation. They introduce Mad Lib exercise for viewers to practice giving strong and effective HPV vaccine recommendation (tailored section).	Stock images and graphic illustrations with voiceover narration and *Mad Lib* exercise embedded within mobile app
Learn how your peers recommend	Healthcare provider suggests to watch videos of other healthcare providers on how and why they recommend HPV vaccine (tailored section).	Stock images and graphic illustrations with voiceover narration and testimonial videos embedded within mobile app
Strategies to address concerns of parents	Healthcare provider (e.g., physician/nurse) describes strategies to mitigate and address concerns of hesitant parents' individual strategies to address concerns—(1) take time to listen, (2) acknowledge risks and benefits, (3) solicit and welcome questions, (4) share facts and stories (tailored section).	Stock images and graphic illustrations with voiceover narration embedded within mobile app
Your recommendation matters!	Healthcare provider summarizes presumptive and bundled strong recommendation and provides examples of motivational statements to understand and address parental concerns.	Stock images and graphic illustrations with voiceover narration embedded within mobile app

Task 2: Plan Intervention Messages, Materials, and Activities

To ensure that they had methods and applications to cover all the change objectives identified in Step 2 and that all applications generated in Step 3 contained well-translated methods, the planning group developed design documents to flesh out in detail the program content and flow as described in Task 1. Once complete, these documents are shared with the creative teams to guide program production for the TIMI and HPVCancerCoach App, including detailed flowcharts with branching logic at tailoring points and information on content placement (Figures 8.4 and 8.5), mockups of all informational presentations, and scripts for the video vignettes and presentations translated into English and Spanish with simple, direct sentences free of jargon (Figures 8.6 and 8.7).

Design documents indicated the targeted change objectives, methods, and applications; estimated duration; and a detailed description of characters and setting. The planners wrote content (messages) for all activities (i.e., videos, presentations, and print materials) to operationalize the specific methods and applications and ensured that the parameters of the specified methods were met. For example, the HPVCancerCoach used the method of *modeling*; thus, the planners made sure that each module started and ended with the main character (either a physician or nurse) reinforcing the message of how powerful a provider recommendation is for parents to make an informed decision. Patient-provider scenarios were created to simulate clinic settings. Two in-office (during healthcare visit) role-playing scenarios were presented to healthcare providers to demonstrate (model) how to give a strong recommendation based on the child's age (one scenario based on guidelines for adolescents 11–12 years old and the other for adolescents 15 years or older). Providers were then asked to practice giving a strong recommendation based on two training techniques, *Announcement* vs *Conversation*, shown by Brewer et al. (2017), to improve uptake of the vaccine in a randomized control trial (Brewer et al., 2017).

For the fotonovella, the planning group developed storyboards that conveyed similar messages as those covered in the TIMI but in a simplified, comic book-like format. The storyboards included still images from the TIMI video vignettes with relevant dialogue boxes to convey desired messages. It also included additional HPV and vaccination information and resources for parents to address barriers to vaccination. Once complete, the planning group shared design documents with creative teams to guide program production for the TIMI, fotonovella, and HPVCancerCoach App.

Task 3: Produce Intervention Materials, Activities, and Protocols

For the production of the TIMI, the PNH planning team hired creative consultants (video production agency, video editors, photographer, graphic designer, application design team, talent consultant and agency, and actors) to produce the video vignettes and presentations. Actors were bilingual Hispanic actors with experience in health-related productions. Preproduction tasks for video development included casting talent, securing locations, collecting props, and scheduling video shoots. Postproduction tasks included working with video editors to include special effects such as voiceovers, music, and graphics, and to ensure that the messages and methods were presented as intended. The planners worked iteratively with the application design team and conducted alpha testing to ensure that all parameters, tailoring, and other specifications outlined in the design documents were met. A similar production process was followed for the HPVCancerCoach App, excluding video production. Instead, the application design team embedded stock images and text-based/graphic illustrations with voiceover narration as well as publicly available video testimonials to cover the desired content. For the fotonovella, a graphic designer was contracted to produce it using the storyboards developed by

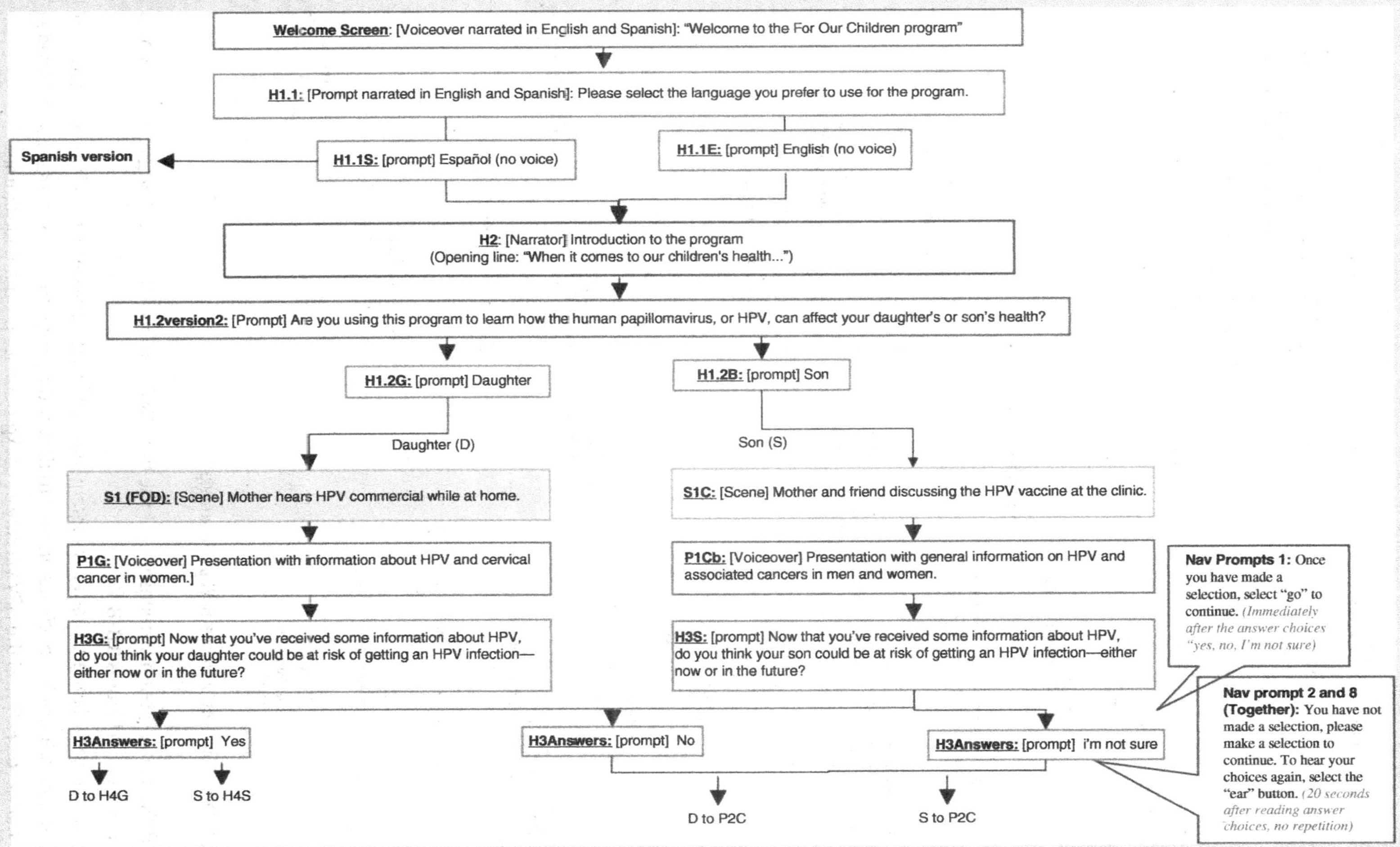

Figure 8.4 Partial Flowchart for Parent TIMI

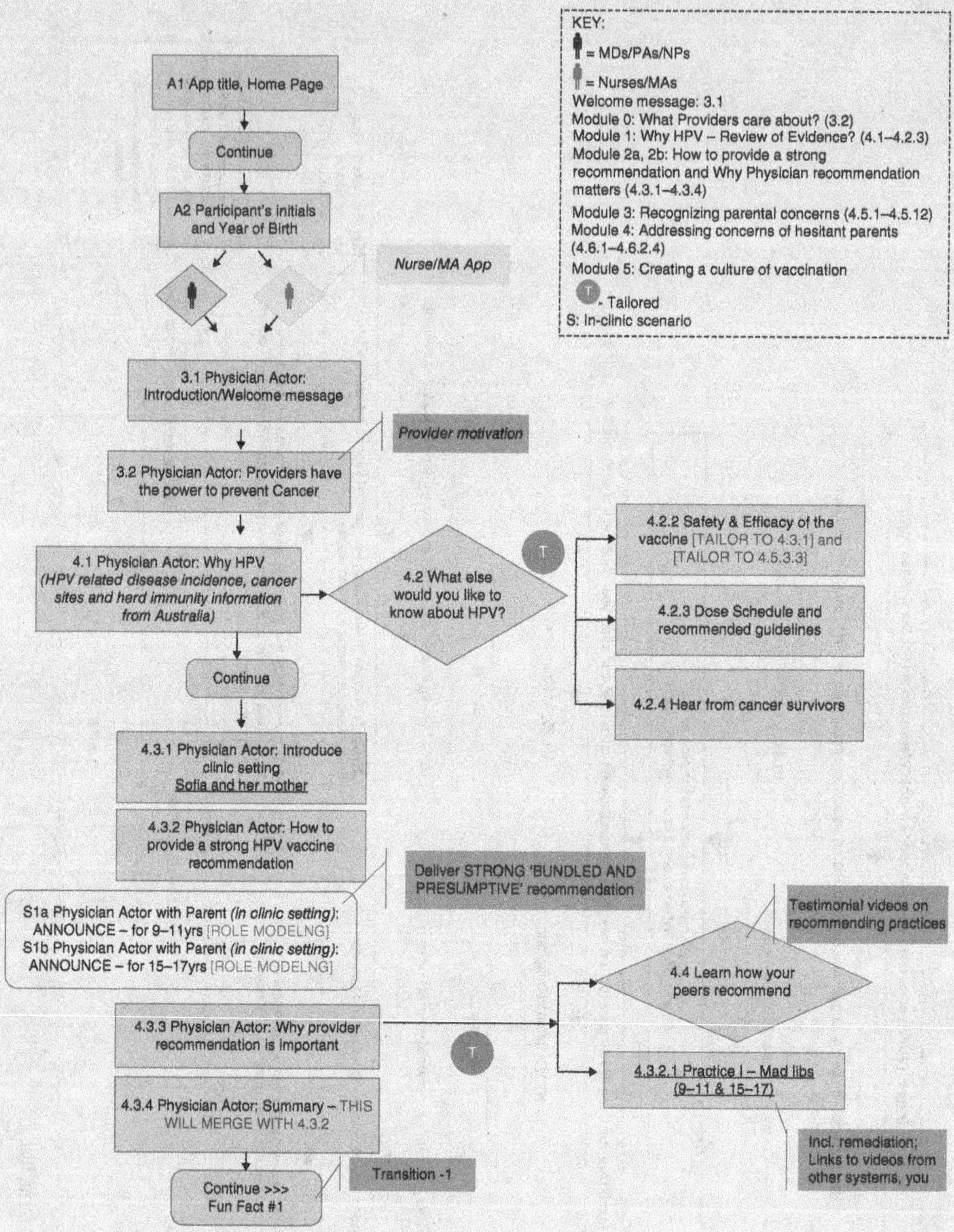

Figure 8.5 Partial Flowchart for Provider HPVCancerCoach App

the PNH planning team. Screenshots of the final TIMI, fotonovella, and HPVCancerCoach App are presented in Figures 8.8–8.10.

Finally, the planners drafted program manuals that provide a step-by-step guide for organizations, agencies, or clinics on how to deliver the program components. It also provides information on HPV and the HPV vaccine as background for program facilitators.

<u>SIC</u> Mom in clinic waiting room (sitting layout preferred in a corner, L-shape)
Mom and Friends talking about the vaccine (available for boys too/talk to MD about recommendation)

Mom is sitting on a chair reading an HPV pamphlet she picked up at the clinic. She hears someone come into the waiting room and looks up and sees her friend Elena with her daughter. Elena waves and sits across from Isabel.

Isabel: Hi, Elena! I haven't seen you in a long time. How are you?

Elena: We're doing good. I'm bringing Teresa in to get her last dose of the HPV vaccine.

Isabel: Oh. That's the vaccine for the Human Papilloma Virus (glancing at the pamphlet) right? I was just reading about it. (smiles at Teresa)

Elena: Yes. This is Teresa's last shot. I also vaccinated Mario last year. He is done with his doses.

Isabel: Really?! I didn't know that vaccine was available for boys.

Elena: Yes. When the vaccine first came out it was recommended for girls, but a few years later it was recommended for boys too.

Isabel: I didn't know that. I need more information about the vaccine. Maybe I should talk to David's doctor about it.

Elena: Sounds good.

<u>S8B.</u> Mom and doctor – initiating doses

Doctor and Isabel and David are already in the middle of their appointment. Music at beginning of scene and doctor and Isabel talking. Music fades out and scene starts on Isabel's line.

Isabel: Dr. Gómez, I've been thinking about the HPV vaccine. I talked to a friend who vaccinated her daughter and son. But, I wanted to find out more about it for David. I wrote down some questions that I have about the vaccine. Can I ask them now?

Doctor: Of course! It is good that you wrote them down.

Isabel: *(Smiles, relieved. She looks down at her questions and begins.)* First, is the vaccine safe for David?

Doctor: Yes. The HPV vaccine is as safe as all the other vaccines that children David's age receive. The most common side effect is a little bit of pain on the arm at the injection site.

Isabel: And why is the vaccine recommended at such a young age?

Doctor: Well, the HPV vaccine produces a higher immune response in younger adolescents so it is best to have your child vaccinated at 11 or 12 years old. Also, the types of HPV that cause cancer and genital warts are transmitted by sexual contact. The HPV vaccine can help protect against HPV, but ideally, if the boy or girl is vaccinated before becoming sexually active.

Isabel: Okay, I see. My last question is about the doses. Why does David need more than one dose of the vaccine?

Figure 8.6 Sample Scripts for TIMI Video Vignettes

Section 5.2—What is a strong recommendation for HPV vaccine?

PO3: Deliver strong 'bundled and unqualified' HPV vaccination recommendation to parents of all eligible patients at time of visit

Section #: A5.2

Objectives: Providers will get a quick review of:

- **Scenario 1 HPV vaccine is optional**
- **Scenario 2 Explain all**
- **Scenario 3 Less is more**

Timing: ~3–4min

Narrator: *"Select the way you would introduce the vaccines to Sophia and her mom."*

Script + Image (VO): Scenarios (Scenario 1 and 2):

Scenario 1 (image + text only) – HPV Vaccine is Optional:

"Sophia is due for HPV, meningococcal and Tdap vaccines. We can discuss the HPV vaccine, if you like."

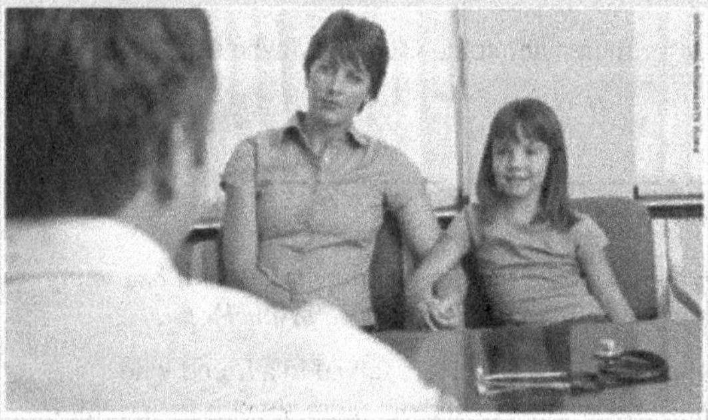

Problem with this scenario (VO):

Research shows that when providers start with a presumptive statement, such as "Sophia is due for shots today, let's go ahead and vaccinate her, " 90% of parents agree to have their child vaccinated during that visit. When providers offer vaccines as optional, saying something like, "what do you want to do about the shots she should get today?" only 17% of parents get their child vaccinated that day [Opel, 2012]

We often announce childhood vaccines, so let's do the same for adolescent vaccines to normalize the process?

Figure 8.7 Partial Mockup of Video Presentation for HPVCancerCoach App

Task 4: Pretest, Refine and Finalize Materials, Activities, and Protocols

In the final task of Step 4, the PNH planning group pretested aspects of the intervention materials in focus groups with parents and providers from the target population to ensure that the language, characters, scenarios, and settings were relevant, realistic, and engaging. For example, the planners played select video clips embedded within the TIMI for parents and asked them to describe what they learned from the content shared, what they liked and disliked, and how it could be improved. They also reviewed several text messages that could be sent as a reminder to parents to initiate or complete HPV vaccination for their child, and planners asked them to indicate which of the messages made them think more about vaccination, made them more concerned, made them feel like HPV vaccination was important, and would make them

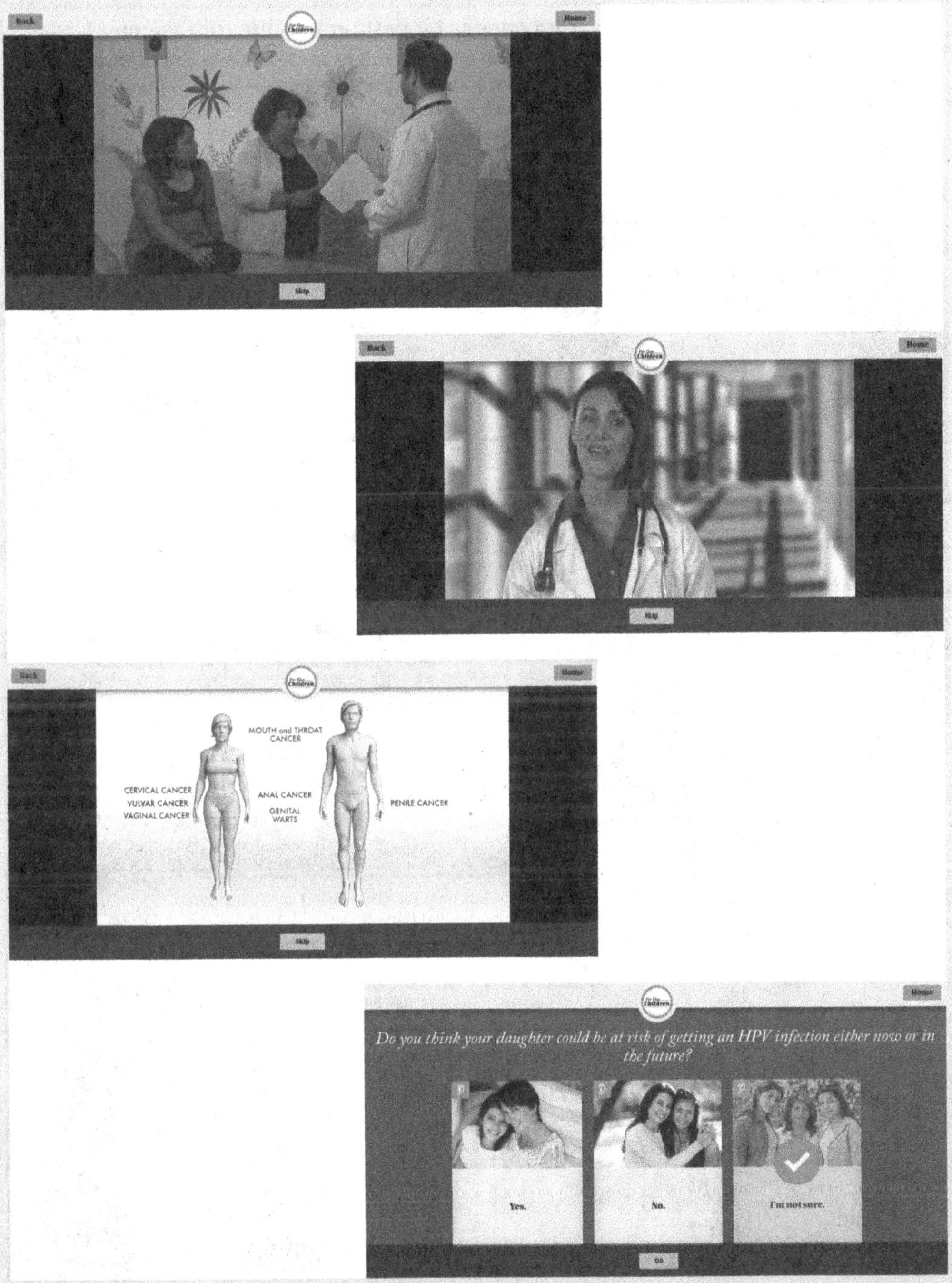

Figure 8.8 Screenshots of Modules from TIMI (Version for Parents of Girls)

more likely to take action. The planners also pretested prototypes, or near-final versions, of each intervention component with individual parents to solicit feedback on usability parameters, including ease of use, credibility, understandability, and acceptability.

Overall, parent feedback on the TIMI was positive. Usability parameters were highly rated with a majority rating that the app was easy to use, the characters were relatable, the content

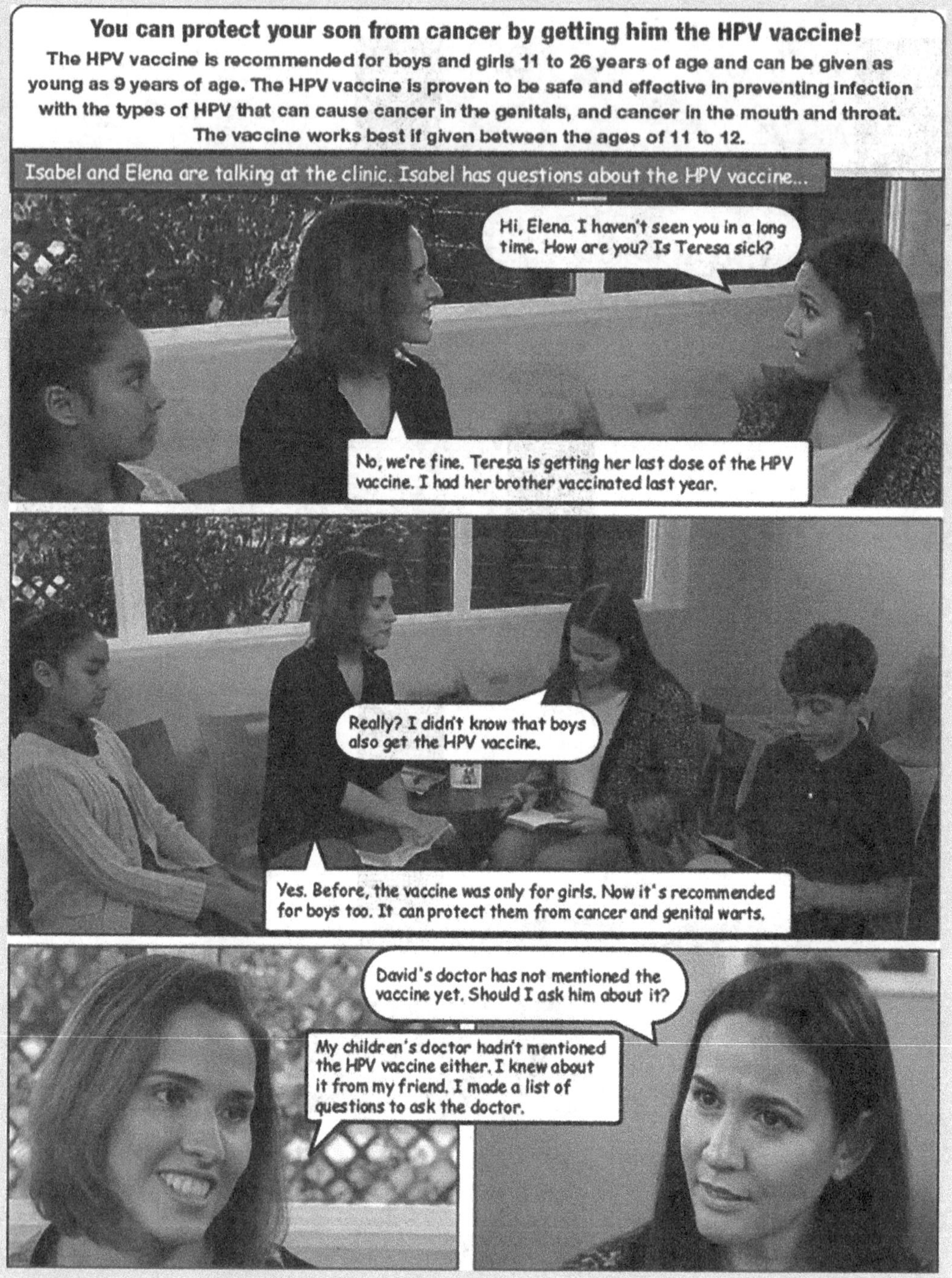
You can protect your son from cancer by getting him the HPV vaccine!
The HPV vaccine is recommended for boys and girls 11 to 26 years of age and can be given as young as 9 years of age. The HPV vaccine is proven to be safe and effective in preventing infection with the types of HPV that can cause cancer in the genitals, and cancer in the mouth and throat. The vaccine works best if given between the ages of 11 to 12.
Isabel and Elena are talking at the clinic. Isabel has questions about the HPV vaccine...
Hi, Elena. I haven't seen you in a long time. How are you? Is Teresa sick?
No, we're fine. Teresa is getting her last dose of the HPV vaccine. I had her brother vaccinated last year.
Really? I didn't know that boys also get the HPV vaccine.
Yes. Before, the vaccine was only for girls. Now it's recommended for boys too. It can protect them from cancer and genital warts.
David's doctor has not mentioned the vaccine yet. Should I ask him about it?
My children's doctor hadn't mentioned the HPV vaccine either. I knew about it from my friend. I made a list of questions to ask the doctor.

Figure 8.9 Screenshot from Fotonovella (Version for Parents of Boys)

was correct and trustworthy, most words used were understandable, and the tone, messages, and strategies used to deliver the content were appealing, appropriate, and informative. Parents also largely reacted favorably to the fotonovella and text message reminders; however, some parents in the Spanish-speaking focus groups indicated that some of the translations needed to

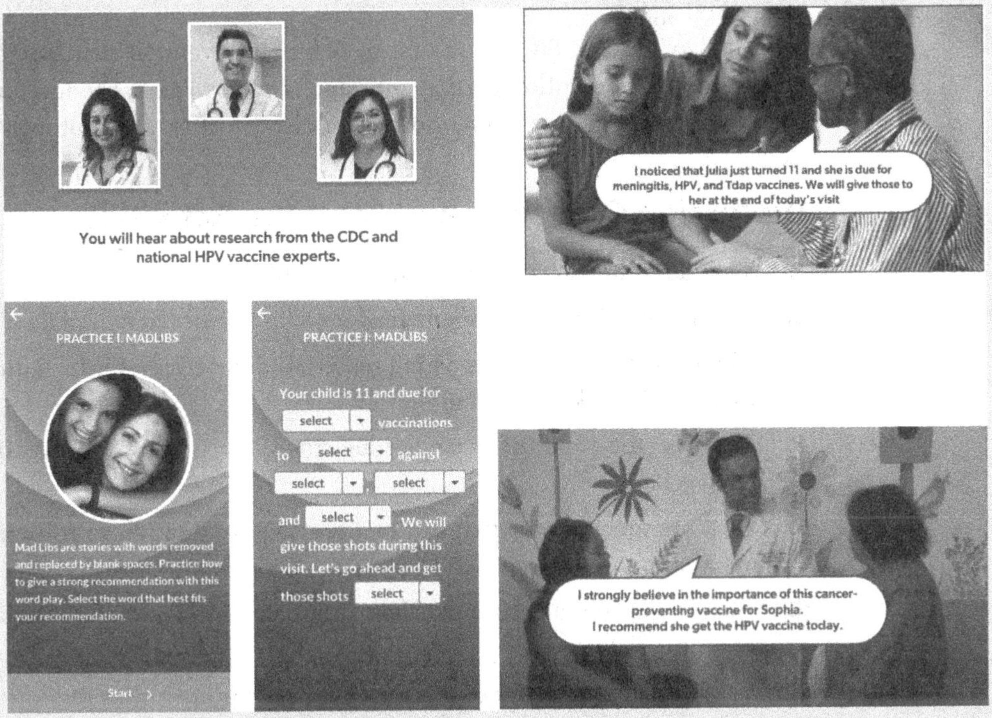

Figure 8.10 Screenshots of Modules from HPVCancerCoach App

be improved. They also found in psychometric testing that text messages that framed HPV transmission as a result of the predatory nature of the HPV virus, led mothers to perceive HPV as more severe and their daughters as more susceptible than messages that presented their daughters as the transmission mode (McGlone, 2017).

The planning team reviewed the feedback collected for each component, and due to budget and time constraints, prioritized revisions expected to be the most impactful and that were feasible to adjust prior to the final production of program materials.

Summary

Chapter 8 presents the process of producing creative and effective materials, activities, and protocols for health promotion interventions as part of Step 4 of IM. Interventions will often be multicomponent, addressing the needs of both target groups and environmental agents. In this step, the methods and practical applications selected in Step 3 are translated into concrete materials, activities, and protocols that are effectively operationalized and meet the change objectives (from the matrices in Step 2).

Step 4 also aims to ensure that the final intervention "fits" with both the populations for whom it is intended and within the context in which it will be delivered. Engagement with potential participants, as well as adopters and implementers, is key for this step. At the end of this step, planners will have an intervention plan for the target group and the environmental agents.

The key tasks in Step 4 are first to define intervention structure and how to reach intervention participants, and second to plan, produce, pretest, refine, and finalize intervention materials, activities, and protocols.

Discussion Questions and Learning Activities

1. What does the intervention structure entail?
2. How are decisions about scope made?
3. When you are reviewing existing materials and activities, which questions should be kept in mind?
4. What is the role of change objectives in writing intervention messages?
5. What are mechanisms that can be used to pay attention to culture in intervention planning?
6. What is the role of planners when producing intervention materials, activities, and protocols?
7. Which aspects need to be considered for each pretest objective?

References

Abraham, C., & Kools, M. (2012). *Writing health communication: An evidence—based guide*. London, UK: Sage.

Airhihenbuwa, C. O. (1994). Health promotion and the discourse on culture: Implications for empowerment. *Health Education Quarterly, 21*(3), 345–353.

Auger, S., & Verbiest, S. (2007). Lay health educators' roles in improving patient education. *North Carolina Medical Journal, 68*(5), 333–335.

Balderman, B. (1996). *Buying creative services* (pp. 1996). Lincolnwood, IL: NTC Publishing Group.

Ballard, A. M., Davis, A., & Hoffner, C. A. (2020). The impact of health narratives on persuasion in African American women: A systematic review and meta-analysis. *Health Communication*. doi:10.1080/10410236.2020.1731936

Bandura, A. (2004). Health promotion by social cognitive means. *Health Education & Behavior, 31*(2), 143–164.

Barak, M., & Yuan, S. (2021). A cultural perspective to project-based learning and the cultivation of innovative thinking. *Thinking Skills and Creativity, 39*, 100766.

Barak, M., Watted, A., & Haick, H. (2020). Establishing the validity and reliability of a modified tool for assessing innovative thinking of engineering students. *Assessment and Evaluation in Higher Education, 45*, 212–223.

Bartholomew, L. K., Gold, R. S., Parcel, G. S., Czyzewski, D. I., Sockrider, M. M., Fernandez, M., et al. (2000a). Watch, discover, think, and act: Evaluation of computer—assisted instruction to improve asthma self—management in inner—city children. *Patient Education and Counseling, 39*(2), 269–280.

Bartholomew, L. K., Shegog, R., Parcel, G. S., Gold, R. S., Fernandez, M., Czyzewski, D. I., et al. (2000b). Watch, discover, think, and act: A model for patient education program development. *Patient Education and Counseling, 39*(2), 253–268.

Batterham, R. W., Hawkins, M., Collins, P. A., Buchbinder, R., & Osborne, R. H. (2016). Health literacy: Applying current concepts to improve health services and reduce healthinequalities. *Public Health, 132*, 3–12.

Beavis, A. L., & Levinson, K. L. (2016). Preventing cervical cancer in the United States: Barriers and resolutions for HPV vaccination. *Frontiers of Oncology*, (6), 19. doi:10.3389/fonc.2016.00019.

Bentley, M. E., Johnson, S. L., Wasser, H., Creed-Kanashiro, H., Shroff, M., Fernandez Rao, S., et al. (2014). Formative research methods for designing culturally appropriate, integrated child nutrition and development interventions: An overview. *Annals of the New York Academy of Sciences, 1308*, 54–67.

Berkman, N. D., Sheridan, S. L., Donahue, K. E., Halpern, D. J., & Crotty, K. (2011). Low health literacy and health outcomes: An updated systematic review. *Annals of Internal Medicine, 155*(2), 97–107.

Berninger, N. M., Ten Hoor, G. A., Plasqui, G., Kok, G., Peterts, G.-J. Y., & Ruiter, R. A. C. (2020). Sedentary work in desk-dominated environments: A data-driven intervention using intervention mapping. *JMIR Formative Research, 4*, e14951.

Brand, T., Barbek, R., Gencer, H., Samkange-Zeeb, F., & Zeeb, H. (2019). Socioculturally sensitive disease prevention and health promotion: Development of a theoretical framework and results of a survey of physical activity promotion projects. *Gesundheitswesen, 82*, 202–208.

Brewer, N. T., Hall, M. E., Malo, T. L., Gilkey, M. B., Quinn, B., & Lathren, C. (2017). Announcements versus conversations to improve HPV vaccination coverage: A randomized trial. *Pediatrics, 139*(1), e20161764. doi:10.1542/peds.2016-1764

Cacioppo, J. T., Petty, R. E., Kao, C. F., & Rodriguez, R. (1986). Central and peripheral routes to persuasion: An individual difference perspective. *Journal of Personality and Social Psychology, 51*, 1032–1043.

Castro-Alonso, J. C., Ayres, P., & Sweller, J. (2019). Instructional visualizations, cognitive load theory, and visuospatial processing. In J. C. Castro-Alonso (Ed.), *Visuospatial processing for education in health and natural sciences* (pp. 111–143). Cham: Springer.

Chambers, D. A. (2020). Sharpening our focus on designing for dissemination: Lessons from the SPRINT program and potential next steps for the field. *Translational Behavioral Medicine, 10*, 1416–1418.

Chen, E., Leos, C., Kowitt, S. D., & Moracco, K. E. (2020). Enhancing community-based participatory research through human-centered design strategies. *Health Promotion Practice, 21*, 37–48.

Collins, S. E., Clifasefi, S. L., Stanton, J., Board, T. L. A., Straits, K. J. E., Gil-Kashiwabara, E., et al. (2018). Community-based participatory research (CBPR): Towards equitable involvement of community in psychology research. *The American Psychologist, 73*, 884–898.

Costa, A. C., Bakker, J., & Plucinska, G. (2020). How and why it works: The principles and history behind visual communication. *Medical Writing, 29*, 16–21.

Cropley, D. H. (2015). Promoting creativity and innovation in engineering education. *Psychology of Aesthetics, Creativity, and the Arts, 9*, 161–171.

De Bono, E. (2015). *Lateral thinking: Creativity step by step* (pp. 2015). New York, NY: Harper Colophon.

Doak, C. C., Doak, L. L., & Root, J. H., (1996). *Teaching patients with low literacy skills* (2nd ed.). J. B. Lippincott Company.

Dyer, J., Gregersen, H., & Christensen, C. M. (2019). *The innovator's DNA* (pp. 2019). Brighton, MA: Harvard Business Review Press.

Elsbernd, A., Hjerming, M., Visler, C., Halgrim, L. L., Nieman, C. U., Boisen, K. A., et al. (2018). Using cocreation in the process of designing a smartphone app for adolescents and young adults with cancer: Prototype development study. *JMIR Formative Research, 2*, e23.

Fakih El Khoury, C., Karavetian, M., Halfens, R., Crutzen, R., Khoja, L., & Schols, J. M. G. A. (2019). The effects of dietary mobile apps on nutritional outcomes in adults with chronic diseases: A systematic review. *Journal of the Academy of Nutrition and Dietetics, 4*, 626–651.

Farace, S. (2019). *The power of narrative images: A visual semiotic analysis of consumer and brand messages in social media* (pp. 2019). Maastricht: Maastricht University.

Fernandez, M. (2013). Not to be, um, trifled with, Texas guards its slogans. The New York Times.

Fernández, M. E., Gonzales, A., Tortolero-Luna, G., Partida, S., & Bartholomew, L. K. (2005). Using intervention mapping to develop a breast and cervical cancer screening program for Hispanic farmworkers: Cultivando La Salud. *Health Promotion Practice, 6*, 394–404.

Ferretti, L., Wymant, C., Kendall, M., Zhao, L., Nurtay, A., Abeler-Dörner, L., et al. (2020). Quantifying SARS-CoV-2 transmission suggests epidemic control with digital contact tracing. *Science, 368*, eabb6936.

Glasgow, R. E., Harden, S. M., Gaglio, B., Rabin, B., Smith, M. L., Porter, G. C., et al. (2019). RE-AIM planning and evaluation framework: Adapting to new science and practice with a 20-year review. *Frontiers in Public Health, 7*, 64.

Grotlüschen, A, Mallows, D., Reder, S., Sabatini, J. (2016). Adults with low proficiency in literacy or numeracy: OECD education working papers no. 131.

Haller, J., Keller, Z., Barr, S., Hadden, K., & Oliphant, S. S. (2019). Assessing readability: Are urogynecologic patient education materials at an appropriate reading level. *Female Pelvic Medicine & Reconstructive Surgery, 25*, 139–144.

Halvorsrud, K., Kucharska, J., Adlington, K., Rüdell, K., Brown Hajdukova, E., Nazroo, J., et al. (2019). Identifying evidence of effectiveness in the co-creation of research: A systematic review and meta-analysis of the international healthcare literature. *Journal of Public Health*. doi:10.1093/pubmed/fdz126

Hamdiui, N., Marchena, E., Stein, M. L., Steenbergen, J. E. V., Crutzen, R., Keulen, H. M. V., et al. (2022). Decision-making, barriers, and facilitators regarding cervical cancer screening participation among Turkish and Moroccan women in the Netherlands: A focus group study. *Ethnicity & Health. 27*, 1147–1165. doi:10.1080/13557858.2020.1863921

Harvard T.H. Chan School of Public Health. (n.d.). *Health literacy studies*. https://hsph.harvard.edu/fellowship-special-program/takemi/international-health-literacy/health-literacy-studies/

Heinen, M. M., Bartholomew, L. K., Wensing, M., van de Kerkhof, P., & van Achterberg, T. (2006). Supporting adherence and healthy lifestyles in leg ulcer patients: Systematic development of the Lively Legs program for dermatology outpatient clinics. *Patient Education and Counseling, 61*, 279–291.

Heinen, M., Borm, G., van der Vleuten, C., Evers, A., Oostendorp, R., & van Achterberg, T. (2012). The Lively Legs self-management programme increased physical activity and reduced wound days in leg ulcer patients: Results from a randomized controlled trial. *International Journal of Nursing Studies, 49*, 151–161.

Holmes, A. E., Widén, S. E., Erlandsson, S., Carver, C. L., & White, L. L. (2007). Perceived hearing status and attitudes toward noise in young adults. *American Journal of Audiology, 16*(2), S182–S189. doi:10.1044/1059-0889(2007/022)

Huang, Y., & Shen, F. (2016). Effects of cultural tailoring on persuasion in cancer communication: A meta-analysis. *Journal of Communication, 66*, 694–715.

Huebschmann, A. G., Leavitt, I. M., & Glasgow, R. E. (2019). Making health research matter: A call to increase attention to external validity. *Annual Review of Public Health, 40*, 45–63.

Iwelunmor, J., & Airhihenbuwa, C. (2017). Culture, a social determinant of health and risk: Considerations for health and risk messaging. In R. L. Parrott (Ed.), *The Oxford encyclopedia of health and risk message design and processing*. New York, NY: Oxford University Press.

Kreuter, M. W., Lukwago, S. N., Bucholtz, R. D. D. C., Clark, E. M., & Sanders-Thompson, V. (2003). Achieving cultural appropriateness in health promotion programs: Targeted and tailored approaches. *Health Education & Behavior, 30*, 133–146.

Larsson, I., Staland-Nyman, C., Svedberg, P., Nygren, J. M., & Carlsson, I.-M. (2018). Children and young people's participation in developing interventions in health and well-being: A scoping review. *BMC Health Services Research, 18*, 507.

McGuire, W. J. (2001). Input and output variables currently promising for constructing persuasive communications. In R. E. Rice & C. K. Atkin (Eds.), *Public communication campaigns* (3th ed., pp. 22–48). Thousand Oaks, CA: SAGE Publications.

McGlone, M. S., Stephens, K. K., Rodriguez, S. A., & Fernandez, M. E. (2017). Persuasive texts for prompting action: Agency assignment in HPV vaccination reminders. Vaccine, *35*(34), 4295–4297. https://doi.org/10.1016/j.vaccine.2017.06.080

McLaughlin, G. H. (1969). SMOG grading: A new readability formula. *Journal of Reading, 12*(8), 639–646.

Mosenthal, P. & Kirsch, I. (1998). A new measure for assessing document complexity: The PMOSE/IKIRSCH document readability formula. *Journal of Adolescent and Adult Literacy, 41*, 638–657.

Messiah, S. E., Lebron, C., Moise, R., Mathew, M. S., Sardinas, K., Chang, C., et al. (2017). Healthy caregivers-healthy children (HC2) phase 2: Integrating culturally sensitive childhood obesity prevention strategies into childcare center policies. *Contemporary Clinical Trials, 53*, 60–67.

Mevissen, F. E. F., Meertens, R. M., Ruiter, R. A. C., Feenstra, H., & Schaalma, H. P. (2009). HIV/STI risk communication: The effects of scenario-based risk information and frequency-based risk information on perceived susceptibility to Chlamydia and HIV. *Journal of Health Psychology, 14*, 78–87.

Miller, T. A. (2016). Health literacy and adherence to medical treatment in chronic and acute illness: A meta-analysis. *Patient Education and Counseling, 99*, 1079–1086.

Morgenstern, L. B., Staub, L., Chan, W., Wein, T. H., Bartholomew, L. K., King, M., et al. (2002). Improving delivery of acute stroke therapy: The TLL temple foundation stroke project. *Stroke, 33*, 160–166.

Morley, J., Cowls, J., Taddeo, M., & Floridi, L. (2020). Ethical guidelines for COVID-19 tracing apps. *Nature, 582*, 29–31.

Nikoloudakis, I. A., Crutzen, R., Vandelanotte, C., Quester, P., Dry, M., Skuse, A., et al. (2018). Can you elaborate on that? Addressing participants' need for cognition in computer-tailored health behavior interventions. *Health Psychology Review, 12*, 437–452.

O'Donovan, J., Thompson, A., Stiles, C., Opintan, J. A., Kabali, K., Willis, I., et al. (2020). Participatory approaches, local stakeholders and cultural relevance facilitate an impactful community-based project in Uganda. *Health Promotion International*. doi:10.1093/heapro/daz127

Organisation for Economic Co-operation and Development (OECD). (2019). *Technical report of the survey of adult skills (PIAAC)* (3rd ed.). https://www.oecd.org/content/dam/oecd/en/about/programmes/edu/piaac/technical-reports/cycle-1/PIAAC_Technical_Report_2019.pdf.

Organisation for Economic Co-operation and Development (OECD). (n.d.). *Survey of adult skills (PIAAC)*. https://www.oecd.org/en/about/programmes/piaac.html

Palmer, V. J., Weavell, W., Callander, R., Piper, D., Richard, L., Maher, L., et al. (2019). The participatory zeitgeist: An explanatory theoretical model of change in an era of coproduction and codesign in healthcare improvement. *Medical Humanities, 45*, 247–257.

Parrott, R. L. (2017). *The Oxford encyclopedia of health and risk message design and processing* (pp. 2017). New York, NY: Oxford University Press.

Pearce, W., Özkula, S. M., Greene, A. K., Teeling, L., Bansard, J. S., Omena, J. J., et al. (2020). Visual cross-platform analysis: Digital methods to research social media images. *Information, Communication & Society, 23*, 161–180.

Peskin, M. F., Markham, C. M., Gabay, E. K., Shegog, R., Cuccaro, P. M., Temple, J. R., et al. (2018). Using intervention mapping to develop "Me & You: Building Healthy Relationships," a healthy relationship intervention for early middle school students. In D. A. Wolfe & J. R. Temple (Eds.), *Adolescent dating violence* (pp. 467–501). San Diego: Academic Press.

Peters, G. –J. Y. (2019). The hare and the turtle: Why agile approaches are often not feasible in applied psychology.

Peters, G.-J. Y., & Crutzen, R. (2021). Knowing how effective an intervention, treatment, or manipulation is and increasing replication rates: Accuracy in parameter estimation as a partial solution to the replication crisis. *Psychology & Health, 36*, 59–77.

Plackett, R., Kaushal, A., Kassianos, A. P., Cross, A., Lewins, D., Sheringham, J., et al. (2020). Use of social media to promote cancer screening and early diagnosis: Scoping review. *Journal of Medical Internet Research, 22*, e21582.

Rademakers, J., & Heijmans, M. (2018). Beyond reading and understanding: Health literacy as the capacity to act. *International Journal of Environmental Research and Public Health, 15*, 1676.

Resnicow, K., Baranowski, T., Ahluwalia, J. S., & Braithwaite, R. L. (1999). Cultural sensitivity in public health: Defined and demystified. *Ethnicity & Disease, 9*(1), 10–21.

Sanders Thomposn, V. L., Harris, J., Clark, E. M., Purnell, J., & Deshpande, A. D. (2015). Broadening the examination of sociocultural constructs relevant to African-American colorectal cancer screening. *Psychology, Health & Medicine, 20*, 47–58.

Shafer, A., Cates, J. R., Diehl, S. J., & Hartmann, M. (2011). Asking mom: Formative research for an HPV vaccine campaign targeting mothers of adolescent girls. *Journal of Health Communication, 16*, 988–1005.

Shegog, R., Peskin, M. F., Markham, C., Thiel, M., Karny, E., Addy, R. C., et al. (2014). It's your game-tech: Toward sexual health in the digital age. *Creative Education, 5*, 1428–1447.

Siddiqui, E., Shah, A. M., Sambol, J., & Waller, A. H. (2020). Readability assessment of online patient education materials on atrial fibrillation. *Cureus, 12*, e10397.

Singelis, T. M., Garcia, R. I., Barker, J. C., & Davis, R. E. (2018). An experimental test of the two-dimensional theory of cultural sensitivity in health communication. *Journal of Health Communication, 2018*(23), 321–328.

Soffer, O. (2016). The oral paradigm and snapchat. *Social Media + Society, 2*. doi:10.1177/2056305116666306

Sokang, Y. A. (2020). *A starting mark of health promotion in Jakarta: Voicing the community's perspective*. Maastricht: Maastricht University. https://doi.org/10.26481/dis.20200528asp

Sørensen, K., Van den Broucke, S., Fullam, J., Doyle, G., Pelikan, J., Slonska, Z., et al. (2012). Health literacy and public health: A systematic review and integration of definitions and models. *BMC Public Health, 12*, 80.

Stormacq, C., Van den Broucke, S., & Wosinski, J. (2019). Does health literacy mediate the relationship between socioeconomic status and health disparities? Integrative review. *Health Promotion International, 34*, e1–e17.

Stuij, M., van Maarschalkerweerd, P. E. A., Seidell, J. C., Halberstadt, J., & Dedding, C. (2020). Youth perspectives on weight-related words used by healthcare professionals: A qualitative study. *Child: Care, Health and Development, 46*, 369–380.

Van Ballegooie, C. (2020). Assessment of Canadian patient education material for oncology pharmaceutics. *Journal of Oncology Pharmacy Practice*. doi:10.1177/1078155220960823

Van der Heide, I., & Rademakers, J. (2015). *Literacy and health: State of the art* (pp. 2015). Utrecht, The Netherlands: NIVEL.

Walesh, S. G. (2016). *Introduction to creativity and innovation for engineers* (pp. 2016). London, UK: Pearson Education.

Werner, O., & Campbell, D. T. (1973). Translating, working through interpreters, and the problem of decentering. In R. Naroll & R. Cohen (Eds.), *A handbook of methods in cultural anthropology* (pp. 398–422). New York, NY: Columba University Press.

Whittingham, J. R. D., Ruiter, R. A. C., Castermans, D., Huiberts, A., & Kok, G. (2008). Designing effective health education materials: Experimental pretesting of a theory-based brochure to increase knowledge. *Health Education Research, 23*, 414–426.

Whittingham, J. R. D., Ruiter, R. A. C., Bolier, L., Lemmers, L., Van Hasselt, N., & Kok, G. (2009). Avoiding counterproductive results: An experimental pretest of a harm reduction intervention on attitude toward party drugs among users and nonusers. *Substance Use & Misuse, 44*, 532–547.

World Health Organization (WHO). (2013). *Closing the health equity gap: Policy options and opportunities for action*. Contract No.: 27 May 2013.

Williams, A. M., Muir, K. W., & Rosdahl, J. A. (2016). Readability of patient education materials in ophthalmology: A single-institution study and systematic review. *BMC Ophthalmology, 16*, 133.

Willoughby, J. F., & Brickman, J. (2020). Adding to the message testing tool belt: Assessing the feasibility and acceptability of an EMA-style, mobile approach to pretesting mHealth interventions. *Health Communication*. doi:10.1080/10410236.2020.1750748

Wray, T. B., Kahler, C. W., Simpanen, E. M., & Operario, D. (2019). User-centered, interaction design research approaches to inform the development of health risk behavior intervention technologies. *Internet Interventions, 15*, 1–9.

Wyatt, T. H., Krauskopf, P. B., & Davidson, R. (2008). Using focus groups for program planning and evaluation. *The Journal of School Nursing, 24*, 71–82.

CHAPTER 9

INTERVENTION MAPPING STEP 5

Implementation Mapping

Overview

The ultimate impact of any intervention depends on both its effectiveness and its reach in the population. No matter how effective a health promotion program (or any intervention) is, it will have little impact if it is not fully adopted, rarely or incompletely used, discontinued prematurely, or never disseminated (Guerin et al., 2022; Holtrop et al., 2018; Rowbotham et al., 2019; Sacca et al., 2022). Without a plan for how a health promotion program will be put into practice, it may stay on the developers' shelf and never be adopted—or on the organization's shelf if the program is adopted but not fully implemented- (Rowbotham et al., 2019; Sacca et al., 2022). Even if a program is adopted and used, if it is not maintained over time, it may not produce or sustain the desired outcomes (Bodkin & Hakimi, 2020). To ensure that health promotion programs are adopted, implemented, and maintained, we must design powerful interventions (implementation strategies) that enable implementers to deliver the program effectively.

Step 5 of Intervention Mapping (IM)—planning implementation strategies—can be significantly enhanced by integrating concepts from implementation science. Indeed, the testing of implementation strategies is a central area of focus in the field of implementation science.

Implementation science is the study of methods that support the systematic adoption and integration of evidence-based interventions (EBIs), practices, and policies into routine public health and healthcare settings (Eccles & Mittman, 2006). It focuses on identifying determinants of intervention adoption, implementation, and sustainment, and on developing strategies that accelerate uptake and support long-term use.

INTERVENTION MAPPING STEP 5 TASKS

1. **Conduct an implementation needs and assets assessment and identify program implementers**
2. **Identify implementation performance objectives and determinants to create matrices of change objectives**
3. **Choose change methods and design implementation strategies**
4. **Produce implementation protocols and materials**
5. **Evaluate implementation outcomes**

Throughout this chapter and in the application of the processes described in Step 5, we rely heavily on implementation science concepts, definitions, and frameworks. We refer to interventions to increase program use (adoption, implementation, and/or maintenance) as **implementation strategies.** In earlier editions of this book, we had referred to them as "implementation interventions" primarily because multilevel health promotion programs require multiple strategies to be effectively implemented. This, however, caused some confusion between what was to be implemented (the health promotion program or intervention) and the approaches to ensure program use (implementation strategies).

To avoid confusion, we now use the term implementation strategies, which is aligned with the implementation science field and is defined as *methods or techniques used to accelerate and/or improve the adoption, implementation, and sustainability of a health promotion program or any health intervention (e.g., clinical program or practice, policy) within a particular setting* (Powell et al., 2012; Proctor et al., 2011). Proctor et al. (2011) underscores that the term implementation strategies can be used for single approaches to improve an implementation effort (e.g., audit and feedback) or multiple combined strategies, often required to implement multilevel interventions such as those designed with IM.

To provide clear and accessible language for distinguishing interventions (e.g., health promotion programs) from the strategies used to deliver them, Curran (2020) suggested simplified terms (see Figure 9.1).

Intervention vs. Implementation Strategy
The intervention, practice, or innovation (e.g., health promotion program) is **THE THING.**
Investigates whether **THE THING** actually works.
Explores how to best support people and places **DOING THE THING.**
These are the tools and actions we use to help people and places **DO THE THING.**
Measure how much and how well people and places **DO THE THING.**

Figure 9.1 Simple Language for Talking about Implementation. Adapted from Curran (2020)

The purpose of Step 5 is to create implementation strategies – including protocols, materials, and activities – that will support the successful adoption, implementation, and sustainment of the health promotion intervention (or other innovation). This step can be useful for two different scenarios: (1) to plan the initial implementation of a newly designed program to ensure that the original health promotion program plan includes details about how it should be adopted, implemented, and maintained, and (2) to provide guidance for the development or selection and tailoring of implementation strategies to increase use of existing EBIs (including policies, guidelines, and practices). For new programs, demonstration projects, and research projects, the focus of Step 5 is to plan for initial implementation to ensure that the program is used as intended during evaluation of efficacy or effectiveness. For programs that have already been implemented and evaluated, Step 5 can be used to improve implementation or for scale up and spread of interventions. In either case, we refer to this step as "Implementation Mapping" (Fernandez et al., 2019). Thus, Implementation Mapping can be helpful (1) to plan implementation the first time an intervention is used (during initial intervention design, implementation, and evaluation); (2) to optimize implementation of an existing EBI, that is, to accelerate and improve EBI adoption, implementation, and sustainment; or (3) to "scale-up" EBIs for wide-spread use.

In the field of health promotion, as in other fields, effective programs, policies, and practices are often available but not used to improve public health. Closing the gap between what we know works in health promotion and what is implemented in communities and clinical settings is critical to improving population health (Gabbert et al., 2023; Livingood et al., 2020; Towfighi et al., 2020). This chapter (Step 5 – Implementation Mapping) helps planners design (or select and tailor) implementation strategies to enable program uptake, use, and sustainment. To date, Implementation Mapping has been used in diverse settings, including community and primary care, specialty outpatient care, hospitals, community pharmacies, and rehabilitation settings, to facilitate the implementation of public health and clinical interventions and practices across an array of health topics (Warhurst et al., 2025). Step 5 results in the development of implementation strategies that will accelerate and improve adoption, implementation, and sustainment of a new intervention (or an existing evidenced-based intervention).

Designing Health Promotion Programs for Dissemination

Using the IM planning process (Steps 1–4) can contribute to the design of an intervention that is both effective and can be readily implemented. For example, the establishment of the planning group (from Step 1) that includes implementers from the beginning who can influence program planning decisions helps ensure that the resulting program is usable in the real-world settings in which they work or practice. The foundational processes of participatory planning increase the probability that the characteristics of the intervention will be compatible with the needs of the priority population and consistent with the context in which the program will be implemented (Adsul et al., 2024; Damschroder et al., 2022b; Holcomb et al., 2022; Turin et al., 2023).

Designing health promotion programs with the evidence- and theory-based approach of IM helps planners make decisions about program focus and content, including the behaviors, environmental conditions, and determinants that are most relevant for the priority population and environmental agents. It also guides the selection of change methods, practical applications, delivery channels, and materials that not only influence the priority population and environmental actors but also components that implementers find acceptable, feasible, and sustainable. Although planning for program use is positioned as Step 5 in IM, program planners should consider potential factors that will influence the adoption and implementation of the program at each of the preceding steps to ensure that the intervention will be a good fit for potential program participants and implementers. Rogers' Diffusion of Innovation Theory, for example, and the Consolidated Framework for Implementation research (CFIR) both describe characteristics of innovations that make them more likely to be adopted and used (e.g., compatibility, trialability, etc.) (Damschroder, 2022b; Rogers, 1983). If planners are considering these characters during Step 2 of program design, then they are essentially "designing for dissemination."

To facilitate implementation, descriptions of programs, including those within published studies, should provide information about the program logic, including goals, behaviors, environments, and determinants targeted, change methods selected, and practical applications used in evidence-based programs. When planners have used IM Steps 1–4, the logic of how an intervention is supposed to work is clearly laid out in the logic model of change. This makes interventions easier to adapt and implement because the way in which the program was designed to work is explicit and planners can see the potential impact of proposed changes. For EBIs that did not use IM nor explicitly describe the intervention logic, or "form and function" of the program (Fox et al., 2025; Hawe et al., 2004; Perez Jolles et al., 2019), using Evidenced-Based Intervention Mapping (EBI Mapping), described in Chapter 11, can help map the behaviors, environments, theoretical methods, and practical applications the intervention used to make the program logic more explicit (Szeszulski et al., 2022; Walker et al., 2022a).

Implementation Strategies

Once a program planner has progressed through IM Steps 1–4, they have designed a full multilevel intervention that will need to be adopted, implemented, and maintained to attain population health impact. Step 5 helps planners create implementation strategies to ensure this occurs. Program failure, both for new programs and the ones that have previously been tested, can often be traced to problems with inadequate program adoption and implementation. A review of more than 500 studies of prevention and health promotion programs demonstrated that the level of implementation affected program outcomes (Durlak & DuPre, 2008) a finding reinforced by subsequent empirical work (Berkel et al., 2018; Hartveit et al., 2022). Failure to implement the intervention as designed can result in a Type III error, where evaluators mistakenly assess the effectiveness of a program that was never properly delivered (Basch et al., 1985). This underscores the critical importance of robust implementation planning to ensure valid evaluation and meaningful conclusions. Thus, to be able to demonstrate effectiveness of a program, it must be successfully implemented; to do so, implementation strategies that address potential barriers to program use are required. For planners who are designing new programs, Implementation Mapping (Step 5) is a logical next step that helps complete the overall program plan. All interventions must be delivered before they can be evaluated. Step 5 helps the planner create implementation strategies containing protocols and materials that enable program implementers to deliver the program. For a comprehensive evaluation (as planned in Step 6) of the program including assessment of implementation and effectiveness outcomes, the implementation plan must already be in place.

Although planning for program use is positioned as Step 5 in IM, program planners should consider potential factors that will influence the adoption and implementation of the program at each of the preceding steps to ensure that the intervention will be a good fit for potential program participants and implementers. Existing EBIs, even when highly effective, are often not maintained over time or disseminated widely; this limits their potential impact on health and quality of life. Although there are efforts to make EBIs available through websites and other resources, such as the guide to Community Preventive Services (thecommunityguide.org) (see Chapter 11), these have traditionally been underutilized. Notable exceptions include the Coordinated Approach to Child Health (CATCH) that has been implemented successfully across populations and settings and has been disseminated globally (Kelder et al., 2003; Reis et al., 2016). This, however, is an exception and due to careful implementation planning (Cawley, 2010; Hoelscher et al., 2011).

Most programs, however, rely on passive diffusion of evidence-based programs (e.g., publications, mass mailings), which has been ineffective in promoting program use (Bero et al., 1998; Grimshaw et al., 2001; Vedel et al., 2018). Implementation strategies must align with the specific context in which interventions are delivered to ensure that evidence-based practices are not only adopted but also sustained over time. Strategies that are mismatched with the setting often fail to gain traction, regardless of the strength of the underlying intervention. As such, assessing contextual fit and feasibility is now considered a best practice in implementation planning (Collaborative for Implementation Practice (CIP) & National Implementation Research Network (NIRN), 2021).

A foundational contribution to the field of implementation science was the Expert Recommendations for Implementing Change (ERIC) project, led by Powell et al. (2015) and Waltz et al. (2015, 2019). This initiative produced a comprehensive taxonomy of 73 discrete implementation strategies, ranging from educational outreach to restructuring service delivery. The ERIC compilation has been instrumental in providing a shared language and framework for describing implementation efforts across diverse settings. However, while the ERIC taxonomy identifies what strategies exist, it does not provide guidance on *how* to design strategies to address specific factors influencing implementation or how to select or tailor them to specific implementation contexts.

Simply choosing strategies from the ERIC list without a structured planning process presents several challenges. First, the taxonomy was created primarily examining what was used to implement interventions in clinical settings, therefore the strategies listed may be less relevant for community or other settings. Additionally, the compilation is extensive and can be overwhelming, especially for practitioners or teams without formal training in implementation science. More critically, the ERIC strategies are not inherently linked to specific contextual determinants, such as those identified through frameworks like the CFIR. This disconnect can lead to the selection of strategies that are poorly aligned with the actual barriers and facilitators present in a given setting, reducing the likelihood of successful implementation. In fact, Waltz et al. (2019) conducted a study in which implementation experts were asked to match ERIC strategies to CFIR-based barriers. The results revealed substantial heterogeneity in responses: for each of the 39 CFIR barriers, an average of 47 different ERIC strategies were endorsed at least once as being among the top seven most appropriate. This lack of consensus underscores the difficulty of intuitively matching strategies to barriers and highlights the need for more systematic, theory-informed approaches to strategy selection.

This is where Implementation Mapping offers a valuable solution. Implementation Mapping is a systematic process that guides users through identifying implementation outcomes, performance objectives, and determinants, and then selecting and tailoring strategies that are theoretically and empirically linked to those determinants (Fernandez et al., 2019; Powell et al., 2017). Implementation Mapping integrates the participation of interested parties including implementers, theoretical and conceptual frameworks, and empirical evidence to design implementation strategies that include clearly defined mechanisms of action—that is, the processes through which these strategies are expected to lead to desired implementation outcomes (Fernandez et al., 2019). Unlike the ERIC list, which is descriptive, Implementation Mapping is prescriptive—it helps planners move from diagnosis to action by linking strategies (that contain methods and practical applications) to specific determinants of implementation behaviors and contextual factors. It proposes precise mechanisms of action through the Implementation Mapping Logic Model (see Figure 9.2). It also emphasizes stakeholder engagement and contextual fit, ensuring that strategies are not only evidence-based but also feasible and acceptable in the settings where they will be applied. In this way, Implementation Mapping complements the ERIC taxonomy by providing a structured pathway for either creating implementation strategies or selecting and operationalizing strategies that are most likely to succeed in real-world implementation efforts (Powell et al., 2015, 2017).

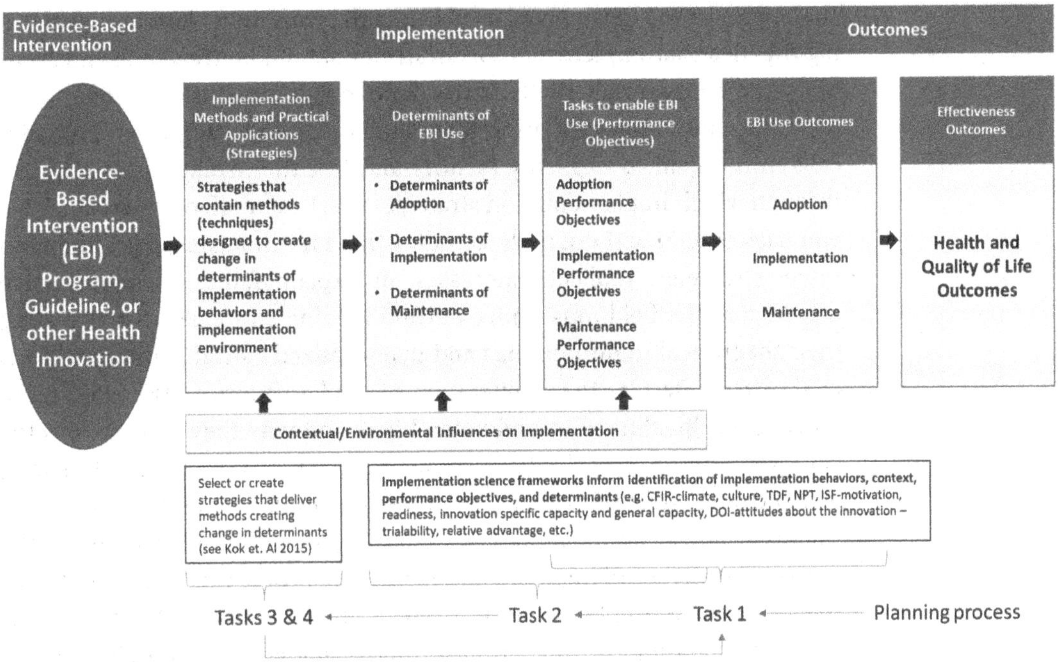

Figure 9.2 Implementation Mapping Logic Model

The Implementation Mapping Logic Model

Figure 9.2 depicts the Implementation Mapping Logic Model, a description of the causal pathway of how implementation strategies influence health outcomes by addressing determinants of program adoption, implementation, and maintenance (Fernandez et al., 2024; Walker et al., 2025a). The model also clearly distinguishes between the intervention to be implemented (i.e., the EBI) and the implementation strategies (i.e., the strategies used to promote the adoption, implementation, and maintenance of the EBI). We distinguish the Implementation Mapping Logic Model from the Intervention Logic Model that is described in other chapters, which is focused on the logic of the intervention itself.

Read from left to right, the Implementation Mapping Logic Model illustrates a causal pathway: the planning team selects or develops an intervention, then designs an implementation strategy to influence the determinants of program use—the behavioral, organizational, and contextual factors that affect whether and how the intervention is adopted and used (Figure 9.2). We note that when we talk about determinants of implementation outcomes, we include both intrapersonal factors (those that reside within the implementers), such as knowledge, attitudes, and skills, and factors at other "levels" including organizational and policy factors. These determinants, when changed, influence implementation performance objectives, which in turn affect implementation outcomes related to adoption, fidelity, and sustainability. If the intervention is implemented with fidelity, it is expected to lead to the desired health outcomes. This causal chain mirrors the logic model used in health promotion planning, reinforcing the idea that implementation strategies should be treated as interventions in their own right, with clearly defined mechanisms of action.

Use of the Implementation Mapping Logic Model aligns with broader calls in the field to explicitly identify and test the mechanisms of action through which implementation strategies exert their effects. Scholars have emphasized that without understanding these mechanisms, it is difficult to refine strategies, replicate successes, or explain failures. Authors have argued that the field must move beyond naming strategies to articulating their theoretical underpinnings and hypothesized causal pathways (Lewis et al., 2022). Despite the proliferation of implementation strategies, there remains a critical need to understand how and why they work in specific contexts. Without this clarity, implementation efforts risk being inefficient, ineffective, or unsustainable. The Implementation Mapping Logic Model can also be used to illustrate the use of Implementation Mapping in the prospective design of implementation strategies, or it can be used to retrospectively "map" implementation strategies that already exist to gain a better understanding of the components, implementation determinants targeted, and the mechanisms of action (Walker et al., 2026).

The Implementation Mapping Logic Model is a visual representation of the products of the Implementation Mapping tasks and can be used as a "short cut" for going through the tasks of Implementation Mapping and can be done prospectively or retrospectively. Walker et al. (2026) have highlighted the value of using Implementation Mapping Logic Models in both contexts. Their work demonstrates how the model can enhance transparency and better understanding of implementation strategy mechanisms in real-world settings—whether those strategies are newly developed or already in use.

When used prospectively, it helps planners explicitly link implementation strategies to their intended determinants and outcomes. This forward-looking approach is exemplified in the SEMM-DIA case, where the Implementation Mapping Logic Model was developed during strategy planning to support the implementation of Salud en Mis Manos, a cancer prevention program. The model was informed by Tasks 2 and 3 of Implementation Mapping, which identify performance objectives, determinants, and change methods, and was used to visualize how the strategy components were expected to influence implementation outcomes such as fidelity and reach. The Implementation Mapping Logic Model for SEMM-DIA can be found in Figure 9.3.

The Implementation Mapping Logic Model can also be constructed retrospectively to make sense of an existing implementation strategy. Walker et al. (2025a) present the case of the Strong Kids implementation strategy. In this case the logic model was used to describe the strategy after it had already been used in Boys & Girls Clubs. Researchers began by identifying the strategy components and outcomes, then worked backward to specify the underlying change methods and determinants. Their study

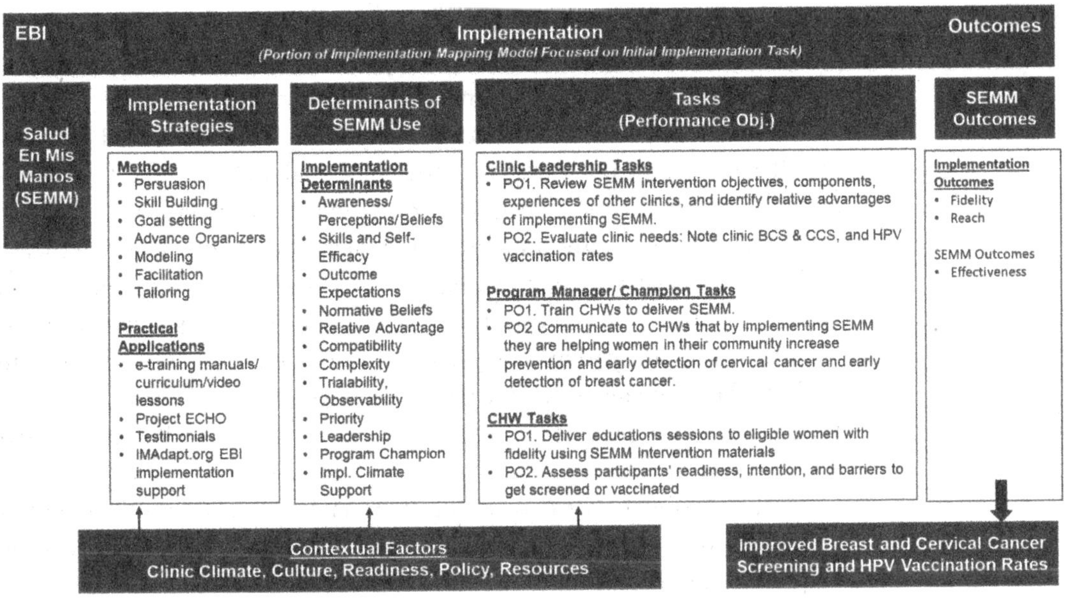

Figure 9.3 SEMM-DIA Implementation Mapping Logic Model

ultimately mapped strategies to specific determinants and mechanisms of action, revealing how even well-established implementation strategies can be better understood and refined through this structured approach. This retrospective use of the logic model helps clarify not only what strategies were used, but why they may have worked—or failed—based on their alignment with theoretical constructs and contextual factors. This approach enhances transparency and replicability in implementation research and supports more intentional strategy design in future efforts.

Using Theories and Frameworks from Implementation Science to Inform Step 5

A central contribution of implementation science to Step 5 is the use of theories, models, and frameworks (TMFs) to guide the development of implementation strategies. While the strength of evidence supporting an intervention is critical, successful implementation also depends on a deep understanding of the contextual, organizational, and behavioral factors that affect its uptake and sustainability (Fernandez et al., 2022; Moullin et al., 2020; Ridde et al., 2020; Stensland et al., 2022).

Implementing interventions in real-world healthcare and community settings requires navigating complex, multilevel systems involving diverse stakeholders. These stakeholders (or implementers) operate at various levels, including individual providers (interpersonal level), clinic directors and administrative staff (organizational level), and health system leaders or regulators (community or policy level). Each level contributes unique influences on the adoption, implementation, and sustainment of interventions. Not only are individual determinants (implementer's knowledge, beliefs, self-efficacy, etc.) important, but so are external influences (at multiple levels) that affect the willingness and ability of program adopters, implementers and sustainers to carry out implementation action.

Research findings underscore the importance of understanding these multilevel dynamics. For example, McGuier et al. (2024) found that *team-level factors* such as shared goals, communication quality, and adaptive functioning significantly influence implementation success in healthcare and human service settings. Similarly, a rapid review by Chapman et al. (2025) identified key barriers and facilitators across four levels—intervention, staff, patient, and system—in rural and regional healthcare settings. These included factors such as intervention complexity, staff attitudes and skills, patient engagement, and system-level leadership and resource availability.

Organizational characteristics also remain central to implementation outcomes. In Chapter 4, we describe organizations theories that can be helpful in understanding influences on those who will be responsible for delivering interventions. Kwok et al. (2024) found that agencies with strong leadership, a supportive organizational climate, and positive staff attitudes toward EBIs were more likely to build capacity for training and sustain implementation efforts. Using theories and frameworks that help identify and understand determinants of implementation at multiple levels such as CFIR can be useful during implementation planning. When applied through structured approaches like Implementation Mapping, these frameworks help planners identify relevant stakeholders, assess contextual determinants, and tailor strategies to address barriers and leverage facilitators at each level of the system.

TMFs from implementation science, as well as from behavioral, social, and organizational sciences, offer structured approaches to identifying multilevel determinants of implementation. While in Steps 1–4 we focus on "personal determinants" of the priority population and environmental agents, which refer to intrapersonal factors such as beliefs, self–efficacy and skills, in Step 5, we focus on "implementation determinants," which include not only personal determinants of adopters, implementers and sustainers, but also organizational, community, and policy-related factors. These include factors such as organizational readiness, leadership engagement, characteristics of the innovation and implementers, and the degree of contextual fit. By applying the determinants described in TMFs in Step 5, planners can design more targeted, theory-informed strategies that are better positioned to achieve effective and sustained implementation of EBIs in real-world settings.

Over several decades, foundational work by Rogers (1983, 1995, 2003) and Dearing (2009) laid the groundwork for understanding how and why innovations are adopted, implemented, and sustained over time. This body of work, often referred to as Diffusion of Innovations Theory (DOI), focuses on the spread of new ideas and practices, particularly emphasizing the early stages of adoption and initial use. Building on this foundation, implementation science has increasingly expanded its focus to include the full continuum of implementation, including effective delivery and long-term sustainment of EBIs in real-world settings (Hailemariam et al., 2019; Proctor et al., 2015; Shelton, 2020; Wiltsey Stirman et al., 2012).

Researchers have developed and refined a wide array of TMFs to guide implementation efforts. One of the most influential contributions in this area is the work of Tabak et al. (2012), who conducted a comprehensive review and classification of 61 dissemination and implementation models. Their framework organizes TMFs based on construct flexibility, focus on dissemination versus implementation, and the socio-ecological level at which the model operates (Tabak et al., 2012). More recently, the field has seen a proliferation of TMFs, with over 150 now cataloged and applied across diverse settings and populations. These frameworks range from broad process models like EPIS and Quality Implementation Framework) (Aarons et al., 2011; Meyers et al., 2012) to determinant frameworks like CFIR (Damschroder et al., 2022b) and outcome-focused models like the Reach, Effectiveness, Adoption, Implementation, and Maintenance (RE-AIM) framework and the Practical Robust Implementation and Sustainability Model (PRISM) (Glasgow et al., 2019; Trinkley et al., 2023). Updated versions of these models have emphasized the importance of adaptability, rapid-cycle learning, and equity-focused implementation (McNett et al., 2024; Shelton & Brownson, 2024).

Together, this expanding body of work provides a rich toolkit for implementation planners. When used in conjunction with structured approaches like Implementation Mapping, these TMFs can guide the selection of appropriate strategies, clarify mechanisms of change, and ensure alignment with both the phase of implementation and the multilevel context in which the intervention is being delivered.

Given the growing number and diversity of available TMFs, selecting the most appropriate one for a given implementation effort can be challenging. To help planners navigate this complexity, Nilsen (2015, 2025) proposed a widely used categorization that distinguishes among five types of TMFs: process models, determinant frameworks (including classic theories and implementation theories), and evaluation frameworks (Figure 9.4). Each type serves a distinct purpose in the implementation planning process and can be used to inform different aspects of strategy design. For example, process models can inform planning by taking into consideration the various phases of implementation and can inform the types of strategies that would be helpful at different phases. Determinant frameworks can be useful for understanding factors influencing implementation at multiple levels, while classic theories help understand individual (implementer) motivations. Evaluation frameworks can help describe expected implementation and effectiveness outcomes informing decisions about evaluation measures and designs.

A scoping review explored how TMFs have been used to advance implementation. Findings informed the Systematic Evaluation and Selection of Implementation Science Theories, Models and Frameworks

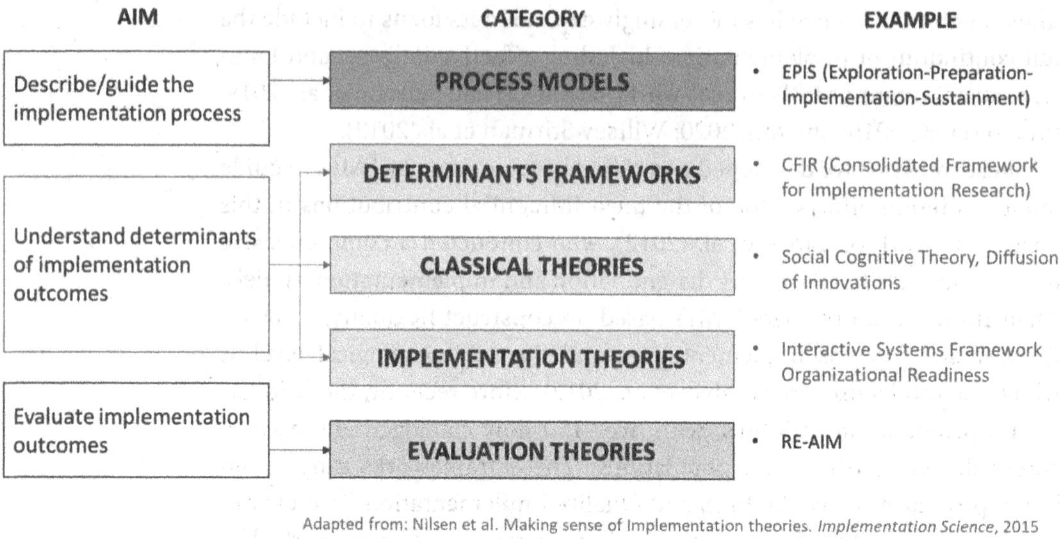

Figure 9.4 Types of Theories, Models, and Frameworks for Understanding Implementation and Guiding the Design and Evaluation of Implementation Strategies; Adapted from Nilsen (2015)

(SELECT-IT) meta-framework. This framework provides guidance for making decisions about what TMFs may be most useful and recommends the following steps: (1) determine the purpose(s) of using TMF(s); (2) identify potential TMFs; (3) evaluate short-listed TMFs against attributes; and (4) assess practical considerations of using TMF(s) within the project context (Fontaine et al., 2025).

There are good examples of the application of theory to inform implementation strategy development. Donaldson and Poulos (2014) applied Diffusion of Innovations Theory (Rogers, 2003) to guide the development of an implementation strategy for a neck-injury prevention program among sports coaches. Henderson et al. (2020) used the Integrated PRISM and Socio-Ecological Model (SEM) framework to guide development and implementation of a breast cancer screening program for underserved populations in the United States. Thackeray et al. (2022) leveraged CFIR to develop an implementation plan for a physical therapy intervention for older adults in the Netherlands, using Implementation Mapping to guide the process. The latter authors' use of Step 5 led to context-specific, theory-informed approaches that addressed adoption and implementation at multiple levels.

To illustrate how theory can inform planning during Step 5, we present the various examples of frameworks. The examples illustrate frameworks that can clarify outcomes of dissemination and implementation: RE-AIM (Glasgow et al., 1999); actors and behaviors related to implementation: Interactive Systems Framework) (Wandersman et al., 2008); and contextual and other factors influencing implementation: CFIR (Damschroder et al., 2022b).

Although these frameworks can help inform decisions about what may influence implementation, none of these provide guidance for how to design implementation strategies that specifically address the factors included in the models. Implementation Mapping can serve as an overarching implementation intervention planning framework that incorporates constructs from other frameworks to inform development decisions at each task (Fernandez et al., 2019). This is analogous to how IM is used to organize theoretical constructs from health behavior models when planning a health promotion program (Steps 1–4).

Process Models

Recent advancements in implementation science have refined our understanding of the phases of implementation and offer valuable guidance for planning implementation strategies using Implementation Mapping. Two particularly useful frameworks are the Exploration, Preparation, Implementation, and Sustainment (EPIS) model and the Quality Implementation Framework (QIF).

The EPIS framework (Aarons et al., 2011; Moullin et al., 2019) outlines four dynamic phases—exploration, preparation, implementation, and sustainment—and emphasizes the importance of both inner (e.g., organizational culture, leadership) and outer (e.g., policy, funding) contextual factors, as well as bridging factors that connect them such as partnerships and linkages. These insights are directly applicable to Step 5, where planners must identify and address multilevel determinants of implementation. For example, EPIS can help guide the selection of strategies that align with the current phase of implementation and the specific contextual barriers and facilitators identified in earlier IM steps.

The QIF (Meyers et al., 2012) complements EPIS by offering a detailed, step-by-step synthesis of 14 key steps across four phases of implementation. QIF is particularly useful in Step 5 for ensuring that selected strategies are not only theoretically sound but also practically executable. It emphasizes readiness assessment, capacity-building, and continuous quality improvement—elements that align closely with the logic model of change and performance objectives developed in earlier IM steps.

By integrating EPIS and QIF into Implementation Mapping, planners can:

- Align strategies with the appropriate phase of implementation (e.g., exploration vs. sustainment),
- Ensure contextual fit by considering inner and outer setting influences,
- Enhance strategy quality through structured planning and readiness-building steps,
- Support sustainability by embedding feedback loops and continuous improvement mechanisms.

Process Framework Example: Exploration, Preparation, Implementation, Sustainment

The Exploration, Preparation, Implementation, Sustainment (EPIS) Framework is a multilevel, four-phase model that identifies factors in both the inner and outer context key to implementation at each of its four phases (Aarons et al., 2011). It was initially designed to promote implementation of evidence-based practice (EBP) in the public service sectors, although it has since been applied to other health settings (Moullin et al., 2019). The first of the phases, exploration, is characterized by awareness of an issue or challenge that needs to be addressed. The adoption decision/preparation phase involves the adoption of EBPs by organizations, which may include organizations experimenting with the EBP prior to broad implementation. The third phase is active implementation of the EBP, followed by the fourth phase of sustainment, which highlights the factors critical to sustaining an EBP (Aarons et al., 2011). A systematic review of studies using the EPIS framework found that implementation planning could benefit from careful consideration of the exploration and preparation phases to lay the groundwork for successful implementation, and that implementation efforts should place sustainment at the forefront (Moullin et al., 2019). Perez Jolles et al. (2022) used the EPIS framework in conjunction with Implementation Mapping to guide strategy development for implementation of the Adverse Childhood Experiences (ACEs) Aware state policy in California to increase ACE screening in a system of federally qualified health centers. The researchers leveraged Implementation Mapping to engage a diverse set of community partners and guide them through the process, which resulted in the development of an implementation strategy, with the EPIS phases and consideration of the inner context, outer context, and bridging factors informing decisions throughout the mapping process (Perez Jolles et al., 2022).

Savas and colleagues (2023) used EPIS and Implementation Mapping to develop a multicomponent implementation strategy to increase uptake and use of a lay health worker-delivered intervention to increase breast and cervical cancer screening and HPV vaccination, Salud en Mis Manos Dissemination and Implementation Assistance (SEMM-DIA). They applied several theories and frameworks to understand determinants of implementers (Social Cognitive Theory; Bandura, 1986, 2001), perceptions of the intervention to be implemented (Diffusion of Innovations; Rogers, 2003), and to gain insight into important implementation actions (organizational change theories). This approach targeted both individual and organizational change processes, demonstrating how theory can inform the design of implementation strategies. The EPIS framework informed the development of the performance objectives in line with the phases, including (1) Exploration (prioritizing SEMM), (2) Preparation (assessing clinic readiness), (3) Preparation for implementation of SEMM, (4) Implementation, and (5) Sustainment (or maintenance).

Process Framework Example: Normalization Process Theory

Normalization Process Theory (NPT) offers a framework that explains how interventions become routinely embedded in daily practice through a set of sociologic tools that address three core problems: implementation, embedding, and integration (May & Finch, 2009; May et al., 2009). There are four main mechanisms within NPT: coherence (sense-making), cognitive participation (engagement), collective action (work done for the intervention to happen), and reflexive monitoring (appraisals of the costs and benefits of the intervention) (May & Finch, 2009; May et al., 2009). It recognizes that this process requires the continuous investments by adopters and implementers to guide the intervention to normalization (May et al., 2009). A systematic review of studies that used NPT to research implementation processes demonstrated NPT is a useful conceptual framework to identify factors influencing implementation processes and to inform implementation strategy design (McEvoy et al., 2014). As a framework for evaluation, it has been applied to a number of contexts, including implementation of case management for dementia patients (Bamford et al., 2014), shared decision-making (Lloyd et al., 2013), nurse-led clinics for heart failure treatment (May et al., 2007), and suicide prevention practices (Richards et al., 2021). The results of these studies enable researchers to address emergent barriers and facilitators to implementation and understand how the NPT mechanisms operate in different intervention contexts.

Determinants Frameworks

Other implementation theories and frameworks describe factors that influence implementation and the types of resources, capacity, and systems that influence intervention uptake and use (Wandersman et al., 2008; Baumann et al., 2022; Damschroder et al., 2009; Nilsen & Bernhardsson, 2019; Wang et al., 2023). These frameworks can support Step 5 by helping the planner to think carefully about implementation outcomes, consider who the adopters and implementers may be, what may influence their actions (personal and contextual factors) (Nilsen & Bernhardsson, 2019), what types of capacity building may be required, and outer context factors (Escoffery et al., 2023).

Determinants Framework Example: Interactive Systems Framework

The Interactive Systems Framework (ISF) for dissemination and implementation was developed to help address the gap between research and practice (Noonan et al., 2012). It was designed to help researchers and practitioners have a better understanding of the process of implementation, and the varying levels and actors involved (Wandersman et al., 2008). The ISF describes three systems that work together to advance the implementation of prevention programs. The Prevention Synthesis and Translation System supports summarization of evidence and packaging evidence-based programs so that they can be understood, accessible and easy to use. The Prevention Support System provides general and program-specific training, tools, and technical assistance to increase practitioner and organizational capacity to implement EBIs. The Prevention Delivery System emphasizes the activities to deliver EBIs and capacity building to make those activities possible (Wandersman et al., 2008). Fernandez et al. (2014) and Wangen et al. (2023) describe collaborative activities of the Cancer Prevention and Control Research Network (CPCRN) to increase adoption and implementation of evidence-based cancer control interventions guided by ISF. For example, to support EBI implementation, the NIH lists EBIs on its Evidence-Based Cancer Control Programs (EBCCP) website (synthesis and translation system); CPCRN provides ready-to-use tools, facilitate peer support and training, and provides technical assistance (support system); and community clinics adopt those EBIs (delivery system) (Wangen et al., 2023). ISF has also supported international dissemination and implementation strategies as well. To improve hand hygiene following a spike in neonatal sepsis, a multimodal change package of World Health Organization-recommended strategies were implemented at a tertiary hospital in Ghana (Kallam et al., 2018). The package included strategies to address each of the three levels including adapting WHO training materials (synthesis and translation system), testing for hand hygiene knowledge (support system), and reinforcement at staff meetings (delivery system). The implementation of the change package saw an increase in hand hygiene overall from 67 to 92%.

The ISF can help planners using Implementation Mapping as they identify actors in each of the three systems the ISF describes. It can also help planners identify performance objectives for implementation by thinking about what actions may be necessary to enhance general or innovation specific capacity to improve implementation.

Organizational readiness is highly related to implementation outcomes (Weiner et al., 2020). Drawing from the ISF, Wandersman, Scaccia, and others have described a heuristic to understand the components of organizational readiness, and it has been further defined through a tool to assess readiness (Domlyn et al., 2021; Scaccia et al., 2015; Scott et al., 2024; Walker et al., 2020; Wandersman, 2017). The organizational readiness heuristic is described as:

$$\text{Organizational readiness} = \text{Motivation} \times \text{general Capacity} \times \text{innovation specific Capacity}\left(R = MC^2\right)$$

Some authors have used this framework to assess and build organizational readiness for high-quality implementation of innovations: programs, policies, practices, or processes. For example, Watson and colleagues used the R = MC^2 heuristic together with Implementation Mapping to help identify readiness needs, define change objectives, and develop targeted, theory-driven strategies to address them and to evaluate and improve organizations' preparedness for implementing sexual assault prevention interventions (Watson et al., 2022).

The R = MC^2 framework was also used to assess organizational readiness for implementation of colorectal cancer screening EBIs using a readiness assessment tool (Dias et al., 2025; Walker et al., 2020). Community clinics were given readiness reports that helped identify areas of potential improvement to enhance implementation of EBIs. In another study, the R = MC^2 was used to better understand factors influencing implementation of school-based physical activity programs (Craig et al., 2024). The various factors (constructs) that are assessed through this framework represent factors influencing implementation and can inform decisions during implementation planning using IM Step 5.

Determinant Framework Example: Consolidated Framework for Implementation Research

Developers describe the CFIR as an "overarching framework" to support development of implementation theory and assessment of what promotes dissemination in different situations and why (Damschroder et al., 2022b; Zulman et al., 2013). To develop the consolidated framework, Damschroder et al. (2009) conducted a systematic review of 19 published theories, models, and frameworks to identify constructs that may influence implementation, have consistent meanings, and be measurable. Based on user feedback on the framework, Damschroder and colleagues (2022b) updated the framework and produced CFIR 2.0. The CFIR 2.0 constructs are categorized into the following five domains without specifying relationships between them: innovation (e.g., cost, complexity), outer setting (e.g., external policy and incentives, patient needs, and resources), inner setting (e.g., implementation climate, available resources), individuals (e.g., self-efficacy, knowledge, and beliefs about the intervention), and implementation process (e.g., planning, reflecting, and evaluating). Program planners can use the CFIR domains to identify contextual factors that may influence implementation. Thinking about these factors can stimulate identification of implementers and creation of performance objectives to influence the context for implementation. The CFIR also contains constructs found in other theories, such as DOI "characteristics of the innovation," which planners can think about when identifying determinants of implementation behaviors. For example, if an adopter or implementer perceives that the health promotion program has evidence of effectiveness, fits with existing values of the organization, and is better than what is currently being used, they will be more likely to use it. Damschroder and colleagues (2022a) offered conceptual distinctions among types of outcomes for use with the CFIR to aid in the selection of outcome measures in CFIR-based research.

Many studies have used CFIR constructs for identifying and intervening on factors that may influence implementation (Dickson et al., 2022; Hoskins et al., 2022; King et al., 2020; Lopez et al., 2024; Thackeray et al., 2022; Weir et al., 2019; Wu et al., 2022). Van Citters et al. (2021) used the themes of CFIR to explore determinants of implementing telehealth programs for cystic fibrosis (CF) during the COVID-19 pandemic. They conducted focus group discussions and in-depth interviews with program directors and coordinators (n = 12 programs). The determinants of implementation included perceived advantage over in-person care, cost, platform quality (telehealth characteristics), needs and resources of those served by the CF program (external influences), needs and resources of those served by the CF program (characteristics of the CF program), individual stage of change (characteristics of team members), and engaging patients and teams (processes of implementation). Sanchez et al. (2014) used grounded theory to identify factors influencing implementation of medication reconciliation within a large urban medical center and an affiliated VA hospital resulting in themes organized using CFIR. Chin and colleagues (2014), used CFIR to describe a health care community initiative to improve diabetes outcomes by mapping its components to the domains of CFIR. Findings from these types of studies can help implementation planners identify contextual factors that may influence implementation and either include them as intervention targets or measure them as possible moderating variables.

Evaluation Frameworks

Evaluation frameworks are essential tools for systematically assessing the design, implementation, and impact of health interventions and programs. They provide structured approaches to understanding not only whether an intervention works, but also how, for whom, and under what conditions it is most effective. By guiding researchers and practitioners through key dimensions such as RE-AIM, these frameworks help ensure that programs are both evidence-based and practically applicable. In the following section, we explore one such widely used framework, RE-AIM (Glasgow et al., 1999), as an example of how evaluation models can be applied.

Evaluation Framework Example: RE-AIM

RE-AIM is a framework designed to improve the quality, speed, and public health impact of prevention programs (Glasgow et al., 1999). It was originally developed to promote consistent reporting of research results and for evaluating the overall impact of health promotion programs (Glasgow et al., 2006). Since its initial development, researchers have provided multiple refinements and expansions of RE-AIM. Glasgow et al. (2019) provided Expanded RE-AIM/PRISM and further specified the conceptual implications, applications, and distinctions among various RE-AIM dimensions. They also provided practical guidance on how to handle potential issues when applying them to research and practice. Reilly et al. (2020) integrated Implementation Outcomes Frameworks into RE-AIM, expanded the constructs of RE-AIM, and offered guidance on how to examine scale-up activities. To address the dynamic nature of real-life implementation contexts and advance health equity, Shelton, Chambers, and Glasgow (2020) offered an extension of RE-AIM with a specific focus on improving sustainability. Harden et al. (2019) provided a summary of resources to help with the practical application of RE-AIM in research and practice, along with real-life examples. Additionally, Glasgow et al. (2020) highlighted the mischaracterization of RE-AIM in the field and offered tips on how to appropriately use this evolving framework.

RE-AIM has been used in program planning to guide decisions during development by helping planners define explicit targets for intervention impact and reach, thus creating a better balance between internal and external validity (Glasgow et al., 1999, 2001; Holtrop et al., 2021) and to assess program impact across many different behaviors and settings, and to understand the impact of implementation interventions (Ashcraft et al., 2024; Gaglio et al., 2013; Munch et al., 2020; Quinn et al., 2019). For example, Nordberg et al. (2024) evaluated the implementation and effectiveness of a digital behavioral healthcare model embedded within routine primary care that referred patients to a system of evidence-based digital mental-health interventions. The applied the RE-AIM framework to determine reach, effectiveness, adoption, implementation, and maintenance of the outcomes of the model (Nordberg et al., 2024). In another example, researchers applied the RE-AIM framework to compare implementation of telehealth delivered pulmonary rehabilitation versus standard pulmonary rehabilitation for patients of chronic pulmonary obstructive disease (Polo et al., 2023). They assessed (a) if the target population was able to be enrolled (reach), (b) Six months rehospitalization and death after the intervention (effectiveness), (c) proportion of people willing to initiate the program (adoption), (d) whether the program was able to be executed as intended (implementation), and (e) if it was continued (maintenance). For planners developing implementation strategies in Step 5, RE-AIM can help define the various implementation outcomes (Polo et al., 2023).

A Participatory Approach to Implementation Planning

Too often, program developers and evaluators see dissemination as just another step along the "discovery to delivery" continuum in which developers must "push" their products out into the community or clinical setting

(Wandersman et al., 2008; Brownson et al., 2013, 2018; Kwan et al., 2022; Rimer et al., 2001). This perspective may blind them to the need to involve community stakeholders in either the development or implementation of programs. In the case of implementation of tested programs, communities may perceive that the EBIs that were tested elsewhere are not necessarily appropriate for their context. The "push" perspective also fails to take into account the importance of market "pull" or demand and may not address questions of delivery capacity (Kwan et al., 2022; Shato et al., 2024). In comparison, community-centered approaches begin with a focus on community needs and capacity and use principles from community-based participatory research (CBPR) to improve program delivery and the translation of research into practice (Kang & Foster, 2022; Merrill et al., 2025; Rhodes et al., 2020).

Importantly, a systems perspective highlights the concept of emergence—the idea that when an intervention interacts with a specific context, it creates a new, dynamic system that may differ significantly from the original design. This view shifts the focus from simply transferring solutions to fostering community health improvement, where interventions evolve in response to local assets, needs, and environments. It also acknowledges that interventions may be diluted or transformed when implemented in new settings and that approaches such as *health promotion interweaving* and community improvement planning can lead to more impactful outcomes by starting with the community and leveraging contextual strengths (Springer et al., 2017).

Including potential program implementers in planning development and implementation of EBIs can help make programs easier to implement, and can improve the external validity of evaluation research findings (Breslau et al., 2015; Kallam et al., 2018; Miller & Shinn, 2005; Trickett, 2011; Wandersman et al., 2008). Importantly, including potential implementers in program planning holds promise to activate "indigenous knowledge" about a given setting or organization, recognizing that people within a given intervention context know that context better than outside planners and bring rich perspectives about opportunities for and feasibility of proposed organizational change (Miller & Shinn, 2005). In Step 1, we recommended that potential adopters, implementers, and maintainers of the program should participate in the planning group, and provide input into each aspect of the design and development of the intervention. Planners should not wait until Step 5 of IM to involve potential program adopters and implementers, but they should take time at this point to make sure that potential program users are well represented in the planning group (Peterson et al., 2007). At this step, when the planning group has designed the program and better understands the requirements for adoption and implementation, it may need to add new members who can represent fresh views from potential program implementers. These new members of the planning group can be seen as a linkage system.

A linkage system, originally described by Havelock (1971) and Orlandi (1986), assures collaborative communication between program developers and user groups to promote program use. A primary characteristic of a linkage system is the presence of change agents or program champions who bridge the gap between developers and users (de Jong et al., 2023; Orlandi, 1986; Robinson et al., 2005). Several examples of linkage systems suggest their usefulness in promoting program use. Robinson et al. (2005) examined the utility of linkage systems for the dissemination of the Canadian Heart Health Initiative and found that they resulted in increased health promotion program capacity, delivery, and sustainability in public health organizations. In another example, a linkage system for a trial of activity for adolescent girls (TAAG) facilitated communication between the development team and school and community agency personnel to increase feelings of local ownership of the program. The TAAG program champions also facilitated continuation of TAAG after research support ended (Elder et al., 2007).

Recent work continues to emphasize the importance of multilevel linkage structures in implementation, particularly in complex systems like public health and education (Whelan et al., 2023; Zamantakis et al., 2024). These studies highlight how linkage systems can support sustainability, equity, and local ownership by aligning implementation strategies with community and organizational contexts.

The linkage system should provide a means to exchange information and ideas between planners and implementers, ensure access to the planning process for program implementers, and facilitate the development of user-friendly programs (Ammerman et al., 2002; Durlak & DuPre, 2008; Havelock, 1971; Johnson et al., 2004; Mizuno et al., 2020; Orlandi, 1986; Robinson et al., 2005).

Step 5 Tasks

BOX 9.1. INTERVENTION MAPPING STEP 5 TASKS

1. Conduct an implementation needs and assets assessment and identify program implementers.
2. Identify implementation performance objectives and determinants to create matrices of change objectives.
3. Choose change methods and design implementation strategies.
4. Produce implementation protocols and materials.
5. Evaluate implementation outcomes.

In Step 5, planners do the tasks listed in Box 9.1. In a sense, the tasks of Step 5 are similar to Steps 2, 3, and 4 of IM. The difference in Step 5 is that rather than focusing on the priority population and environmental agents, we are concerned with the behaviors and environmental conditions of individuals or groups who adopt the program, those who will use it in everyday practice, and those who will maintain it by rolling it into the routine operations of the organization. Importantly, Step 5 also involves learning about and activating the context itself—not just the individuals or agents involved in implementation. This includes identifying and leveraging environmental assets such as communication channels (information assets), community organizations and leadership structures (social/organizational assets), policies and procedures (policy assets), and physical spaces (built-environment assets) that can support and sustain implementation. These contextual elements, when harnessed effectively, can enhance program fit, feasibility, and long-term impact. This reinforces the importance of conducting a thorough asset assessment as part of Step 1 and revisiting it during Step 5 to ensure alignment between the intervention and the setting in which it is delivered.

Task 1: Conduct an Implementation Needs and Assets Assessment and Identify Program Adopters and Implementers

A foundational principle of Implementation Mapping is that implementation strategies should be developed through a participatory process that actively involves those who will adopt, implement, and sustain the program. Participatory approaches, such as CBPR, are not only ethical and inclusive but also practical. They help ensure that implementation strategies are grounded in the lived realities of the settings in which they will be used. By engaging stakeholders early and consistently, planners can co-create strategies that are more likely to be feasible, acceptable, and sustainable (Holcomb et al., 2022; LeClair et al., 2020; Wallerstein & Duran, 2006, 2010).

This participatory ethos is embedded in the original IM approach and is especially critical in Task 1. Here, planners begin by conducting a comprehensive assessment of the implementation context—an effort that includes identifying the individuals and organizations who will be responsible for adopting, delivering, and maintaining the program, as well as understanding the barriers and facilitators that may influence their ability to do so.

While it may seem obvious that it is important to clearly specify who will be responsible for adoption, implementation and maintenance of interventions, this is often not carefully considered before planning or choosing implementation strategies. Although some health promotion programs may be self-selected and directed by the participants, most require someone to make them available to participants. Programs also require individuals to ensure their continued use and outcomes over time. By the end of Step 5 Task 1, planners should be able to answer the following questions:

1. Who will decide to adopt and use the program?
2. Which stakeholders will decision-makers need to consult?
3. Who will make resources available to implement the program?
4. Who will implement the program?
5. Will the program require different people to implement different components?
6. Who will ensure that the program continues as long as it is needed?

Often the person or persons who will decide to adopt, and those who will deliver and maintain the program over time will be different. For example, school principals may support adoption of a program but usually will not be the implementer. Once a principal adopts a health-promotion curriculum, program implementers might be teachers who present health education programs to students. In a clinical setting, managers might organize review and adoption of new patient education procedures, whereas nurses, dietitians, physicians, or other hands-on providers present the programs to patients. In contrast, some programs, such as those delivered online or via mass media, do not need anyone to implement intervention activities. However, these media-based or online programs still need to reach intended participants, and adopters may be the gatekeepers for mass-media or online distribution systems. For example, program managers at radio or television stations may not be directly involved in conducting mass-media campaigns, but their support is essential in making sure the program is broadcast. Interventions delivered through online or social media platforms may be better implemented if supported by media influencers.

As they begin Step 5, usually, program planners know the organization or setting in which a program will be adopted and implemented, and can immediately answer the questions above. In some cases, however, Step 5 must start with selecting implementation partners from among several possible venues and organizations. Planners will want to recruit organizations that have a good potential reach to intended program participants. Organizations, such as schools, churches, social service organizations, and clinical practice settings typically serve large numbers of individuals who may represent the priority populations intended for the health-promotion program.

Task 1 extends beyond identifying adopters, implementers, and maintainers—it involves understanding the broader context in which implementation will occur. Planners will need to understand the organizational structure of adopting agencies to correctly identify not only the individuals who will be making decisions about program use but also the contextual influences that may impact implementation. For example, programs developed for clinic settings to increase mammography screening that include both patient-level and provider-level components could be adopted by individual primary care clinics or by groups of affiliated clinics, such as Federally Qualified Health Centers, health service collaboratives, or Health Maintenance Organizations, that include multiple clinic locations. Before making a decision on the implementing organization, planners will ask how certain characteristics of the organizations, such as size, leadership, readiness for change, and general capacity, may influence implementation. For example, in a study of implementation barriers and facilitators to self-measured blood pressure (SMBP) to support hypertension care, the research team found that while SMBP was acknowledged as a valuable management tool, limited funds, staff capacity, and lack of policies for recommendation limited provider recommendations within community health centers (Rodriguez et al., 2025). Other elements, such as feasibility, fit with organizational goals and values, and quantity of information or change that an organization can absorb (absorptive capacity), can also be important. While the process of learning about a setting or organization may begin in Step 1 as part of the environmental asset assessment and identification of settings for the intervention, using the implementation theories and frameworks described above and/or organizational level theories described in Chapter 4 may also be helpful for considering potential characteristics of implementing organizations as well as the types of adopters and implementers that may be important.

Understanding who the leaders are in organizations and communities is important because these individuals are often responsible for adoption decisions and can be essential in ensuring proper implementation. Senior management buy-in and support are almost always required for adoption and implementation (Moullin et al., 2018; Park et al., 2025), in addition to the more focused roles of program champions and opinion leaders as described in classical diffusion theory and other frameworks (Bonawitz et al., 2020; Miech et al., 2018; Williams et al., 2020).

There are many published examples illustrating how information from an implementation needs and assets assessment informed the design of implementation strategies. In one study, Implementation Mapping was used to adapt a cancer screening navigation program for safety-net clinics. Researchers conducted interviews with clinic staff and leadership to identify workflow barriers, resource constraints, and cultural considerations that could affect implementation (Savas et al., 2023). In another example, Cabassa and Baumann (2013) used a collaborative planning approach that blended CBPR principles with IM to adapt a healthcare manager intervention for Hispanics with serious mental illness. Their process included stakeholder interviews, patient focus groups, and iterative adaptation of the intervention and implementation plan. Similarly, Kang and Foster (2022) used Implementation Mapping with CBPR to develop tailored implementation strategies for a rehabilitation goal-setting intervention, MyGoals, engaging occupational therapists, clients, and researchers to identify determinants and co-design strategies. Informal discussions with community members allowed the planning group to identify occupational therapists as the primary implementers for the goal-setting intervention, and identify key implementation factors that will influence the uptake of the intervention.

Although the formal identification of implementation performance objectives and determinants occurs in Task 2, the implementation needs and assets assessment conducted in Task 1 provides a critical foundation. Much of the information gathered here—such as who is responsible for implementation, what resources are available, and what contextual challenges exist—will directly inform the matrices of change objectives and the selection of implementation strategies in subsequent tasks.

By the end of Task 1, planners should have a clear understanding of who the adopters and implementers are, what their roles entail, and what contextual factors will influence their ability to carry out those roles. This understanding is not only critical for effective strategy design—it is essential for ensuring that the program is used, sustained, and ultimately successful.

Task 2: Stating Outcomes and Performance Objectives for Program Use and Creating Matrices of Change

The primary goals of Step 5, Task 2 is to clearly describe adoption, implementation, and sustainment outcomes, to break these down into implementation sub-tasks or performance objectives, to identify determinants (factors influencing implementation), and finally, to create matrices of change objectives. This task closely resembles Step 2 in IM. The difference here is that when planning implementation strategies, the planning group focuses on those who are adopting, implementing and sustaining the multilevel program.

In this task, the planning team determines *who has to do what* to ensure that the program is adopted, implemented, and maintained with acceptable completeness and fidelity. Here, we lay the groundwork for the design of implementation strategies for one of two possible scenarios: (a) a planning team is preparing for the first use of a newly developed program (i.e., has completed the first four steps of IM), or (b) a planning team has selected an EBI and is developing an implementation strategy to support EBI use in a new site or in multiple sites (scale-up).

Program use outcomes can be grouped into three phases:

1. **Adoption** is a decision to use a new program (an innovation to the adopting organization). At a basic level, adoption decisions require knowledge of the program, awareness of an unmet need, and the decisions to choose and try a certain innovation to meet the perceived need.
2. **Implementation** is the use of the program to a "fair trial point," a use that is long enough to allow evaluation about whether the innovation meets the perceived need.

3. **Maintenance** is the extent to which the program is continued and then becomes a part of the normal practices and policies of the adopting organization.

The program planner states program use outcomes and writes performance objectives for each of these phases. Program use outcomes are similar in concept to the program outcomes stated in Step 2. Instead of stating behavioral outcomes and environmental outcomes, the planners state the expected outcomes for program adoption, implementation, and maintenance. Examples for each are given in the following section.

Stating Outcomes and Performance Objectives for Adoption

An **innovation** is an idea, practice, or product that is new to the adopter. The adopter may be an individual, a group of people, an organization, or even a community represented by decision-makers. The program that health promoters plan with IM Steps 1–4, developed to promote behavior and environmental change, can be thought of as an innovation because it will be new and will require changes in what individuals and environmental agents do and how they do it.

The adoption of a health promotion program is the decision to use it. Adoption decision makers or "adopters" can be individuals making an independent decision, such as a clinic director, a school principal, the head of an agency, a mayor, or the leader of a community-based organization. Adopters can also be groups or organizations that make collective decisions, such as an executive board at a community clinic, a school board, or a patient advocacy group. Adoption in organizational settings may involve multiple levels and usually is a more complex event than adoption by individuals. Organizational change theories provide guidance about the types of individuals who may be involved in adoption decisions as well as the contextual influences on implementation.

Planning teams can benefit from information from theory and the empirical literature to inform responses to the following questions that will lead to clear performance objectives: "What do representatives of these agencies have to do to adopt this program?" "What stakeholders do they need to consult?" and "What levels of approval do they need?" For example, in a school setting, a teacher team leader may hear about a program at a professional meeting and discuss it with other teachers and staff. The team leader may then request the curriculum coordinator or superintendent (depending on the school district's size and personnel structure) to adopt the program. The decision maker may then share the decision with parent groups or other interested parties.

In clinic settings, a clinic director may need to seek the approval of board members and garner support from clinic managers before adopting a program. They may also need to consult with consumer stakeholders.

It is important to note that in clinical settings, adoption and implementation of new practices, programs, or policies are often referred to as "practice change." Examples of clinical practice changes are implementation of new procedures, diagnostic or treatment guidelines, or implementation of an educational program to increase patient uptake of a preventive service. While Implementation Mapping can be used for implementation of any innovation including clinical guidelines, here we focus primarily on programs (interventions) that have tangible components and materials such as what would be available having gone through Steps 1–4.

To create a program adoption outcome, use the following model: [someone/ group] adopts the [innovative program] as indicated by [the evidence or document to indicate adoption]. For example, a program to expand adoption and implementation of the National Diabetes Prevention Program (DPP) (Perkison et al., 2023) stated an adoption outcome as follows: *Clinic leadership adopts the National DPP to prevent diabetes among patients with prediabetes as indicated by approval of a signed agreement with the National DPP.* Essentially, the adoption outcomes state the action that is required to constitute program adoption broadly. Next, planners list adoption performance objectives by answering the question: "Who needs to do what to ensure that the program is adopted?" Box 9.2 provides an example of adoption performance objectives for DPP.

Planners might also include performance objectives to change contextual factors necessary for program adoption. For example, a study of the dissemination of physical activity programs by state health departments found four contextual factors associated with adoption of interventions by communities:

BOX 9.2. ADOPTION OUTCOME AND PERFORMANCE OBJECTIVES FOR NATIONAL DPP

Adoption Outcome: Clinic leadership adopts the National DPP to prevent diabetes among patients with prediabetes as indicated by the approval of a signed agreement with the National DPP.

Clinic leadership will:

1. Partner with a CDC-recognized national DPP.
2. Delineate the clinic's National DPP referral goals.
3. Approve legal agreement with National DPP.
4. Gain support from stakeholders' reaction to the program (care providers, decision makers, navigators/schedulers, patients).
5. Designate a clinic program champion to spearhead the implementation of the National DPP referral program.

Source: Adapted from Perkison et al., 2023

available funding, physical activity being a high priority, adequate staffing at the state level, and a supportive legislature at the policy level (Brownson et al., 2007). If program planners decide that these factors are critical in their local settings and can be addressed as part of their planning for program use, they could state performance objectives, such as the following:

- The state legislature will pass legislation to provide funding for physical activity programs in local communities.
- The director of the state health department will allocate staff to support communities in adopting and implementing physical activity programs.
- The executive committee for the health department will make physical activity programs a high priority.

Stating Outcomes and Performance Objectives for Implementation

Implementation refers to the active use of a program in practice. Whether implementing a program for the first time or adapting an existing EBI, planners must clearly define what implementation means in their context. This includes specifying what successful implementation looks like, how it will be measured, and who is responsible for carrying out each component of the program.

To address this gap, implementation science has developed a taxonomy of implementation outcomes—conceptually distinct indicators that help define and measure implementation. Proctor et al. (2011) proposed eight core outcomes: acceptability, adoption, appropriateness, feasibility, fidelity, implementation cost, penetration, and sustainability. These outcomes are widely used to evaluate whether and how an intervention is being implemented. A scoping review of over 400 studies found that while outcomes such as acceptability, fidelity, and feasibility are frequently assessed, there remains limited evidence linking specific implementation strategies to these outcomes, highlighting the need for more rigorous, theory-driven research (Proctor et al., 2023).

From an Implementation Mapping perspective, however, it is important to distinguish between implementation outcomes and determinants of implementation. Some constructs described as outcomes in Proctor's framework—such as perceived acceptability and feasibility—function more accurately as determinants in the Implementation Mapping process. That is, they are factors that influence whether implementation occurs, rather than indicators that implementation has occurred. For example, if implementers perceive a program as acceptable and feasible, they are more likely to adopt and use it. These perceptions are therefore important to assess and address, but they are not themselves evidence of implementation.

In Task 2 of Implementation Mapping, implementation outcomes are stated in general terms to guide the development of performance objectives. Rather than specifying determinants of implementation or how implementation might be measured in a research study, at this stage, planners articulate what implementation success should look like. An outcome might be: *The program will be implemented with fidelity, including use of all core components.* This general statement provides a foundation for identifying the specific actions (performance objectives) that implementers must take to achieve that outcome.

At this stage, planners will want to describe implementation outcomes using dimensions such as fidelity, completeness, and dose (Dowling & Barry, 2020; Linnan & Steckler, 2002; Rossi et al., 2004; Scheirer, 1981). Fidelity refers to the degree to which the program is implemented with its change methods and practical applications intact; completeness indicates the proportion of intended program activities and components delivered; and dose is the amount of the program that participants receive. For the initial implementation and testing of a new health promotion program, planners usually place greater emphasis on achieving a high level of fidelity and completeness to ensure that the intervention methods and practical applications are applied as intended.

Planners will want to answer the following questions to describe the implementation outcome: "What exactly is the program?" and "What would constitute a level of fidelity and a level of completeness consistent with program effectiveness?" To a greater extent than for adoption, implementation often includes multiple tasks performed by a variety of individual roles. Program implementation outcomes can be stated in this way: The [organization or individual] implements [innovative program] including use of [program components]. For example: *The clinical manager implements the National DPP program, including monitoring the referral system, making referrals to patients, and promoting and educating staff on implementation.*

Another example might be: *The Lay Health Worker Organization delivers the cancer screening program to women in the community, including the use of all three program components.*

The implementation outcome must answer the question: "What constitutes implementation of the essential program components with acceptable completeness, fidelity, and dose?" Once the implementation outcome is clearly stated, the planner can begin to develop the performance objectives for implementation.

Implementation Performance Objectives To create performance objectives, the health promotion planner will think about the steps necessary to deliver the program and about what structural or organizational infrastructure may be required for implementation of the new program. To a greater extent than for adoption, implementation often includes multiple tasks performed by a variety of individual roles. It is important to think about the different implementers and what they have to do to deliver the program or to change the implementation context.

In addition to thinking about the specific actions of implementers, planners should also consider important actions of others who can create needed structural changes or organizational infrastructure required for implementation of the new program. There may be changes in the implementation environment (context) that are necessary to deliver the program, such as hiring new staff or modifying patient flow in clinic settings. These should all be included in the implementation performance objectives specifying who is responsible for what change.

Performance objectives for implementation should be stated as follows: *The [implementer] carries out [specific action] to ensure implementation.*

When writing performance objectives, the planner should refrain from describing how we will go about ensuring that the implementers do these things (that comes later in Tasks 3 and 4), and instead focus here on what successful implementation looks like. Box 9.3 presents the performance objectives for implementation of DPP.

Clearly specifying who has to do what to implement a program ensures that implementation is not treated as a vague or secondary concern, but as a measurable, actionable process that is essential to achieving program impact.

Using Theories, Models, Frameworks, and Empirical Evidence to Inform Performance Objectives for Implementation Using theories, models, and frameworks such as organizational and systems level, those described in Chapter 4, and implementation frameworks such as those mentioned above can help planners identify implementers and the actions they need to take. Frameworks such as the CFIR and the continued use of ISF provide valuable guidance for this process.

For example, the ISF's prevention support and delivery systems help planners determine the capacities and resources—such as personnel, time, and training—needed to support and deliver an intervention. The updated CFIR emphasizes constructs like implementation climate, readiness for implementation, and networks and communication, while also incorporating a stronger focus on equity and recipient-centered implementation. These constructs can guide planners in defining performance objectives. For instance:

- Leaders of the Texas City community health center publicly express their support for the implementation of the intervention and describe their planned involvement.
- Implementation teams engage community representatives to co-design implementation strategies that address local equity concerns.

The CFIR's Process domain continues to be useful for identifying performance objectives related to planning, engaging, executing, and reflecting. For example: The clinic manager monitors phone counseling and provides feedback to counselors on their progress in reaching women in need of mammograms.

Other CFIR domains, such as characteristics of individuals (e.g., self-efficacy, knowledge, and beliefs about the intervention) and characteristics of the innovation, may be more helpful in identifying the determinants of implementers and are discussed below.

BOX 9.3. IMPLEMENTATION PERFORMANCE OBJECTIVES FOR NATIONAL DPP

To determine the performance objectives, the planners of the DPP program asked what clinic administration and staff needed to do to implement the program.

The clinic administration:

1. Educates clinic staff about the National DPP workflow and make changes to improve productivity.
2. Encourages health care providers to make patient referrals.
3. Identifies gaps in data reporting.
4. Conducts monthly reports on patients who meet prediabetes criteria for National DPP referral.
5. Submits referrals data report to National DPP quarterly.

The health care provider:

1. Reviews patient's medical records.
2. Identifies patients with prediabetes.
3. Discusses National DPP referrals with patients with prediabetes.
4. Connects patients to the National DPP providers.
5. Encourages patients to enroll in National DPP.
6. Submits patient referral to National DPP in the EHR.
7. Shares appropriate patient information with National DPP providers.

The program champion:

1. Advocates for the implementation of National DPP.
2. Motivates clinic health care providers to make National DPP referrals.
3. Ensures that the EHR referral process is operational.
4. Communicates with the National DPP provider to ensure referral feedback.
5. Receives confirmation about patients' National DPP referral status.

Source: Adapted from Perkison et al., 2023

Leadership and Performance Objectives for Implementation Leadership is consistently identified across implementation theories and frameworks as a critical driver of successful and sustained implementation. Recent work has expanded this view, emphasizing not only formal authority but also the adaptive, supportive, and equity-driven behaviors of leaders (Aarons & Ehrhart, 2022; Shea, 2021). Frameworks such as the CFIR, EPIS, and the Health Equity Implementation Framework (HEIF) highlight leadership engagement, climate shaping, and modeling of desired behaviors as central to implementation success (Damschroder et al., 2022b; Moullin et al., 2019; Woodward et al., 2021).

Recent studies underscore the importance of adaptive leadership—leaders who adjust to emerging challenges—and the cultivation of psychological safety, where staff feel safe raising concerns and innovating (Aarons & Ehrhart, 2022; Shea, 2021). These insights support performance objectives such as:

- Supervisors create opportunities for open dialogue about implementation progress and challenges.
- Leaders monitor staff well-being and adjust implementation strategies based on feedback.

Implementation leadership also includes proactive and transformational behaviors such as articulating vision, anticipating barriers, coordinating resources, and recognizing staff contributions (Aarons et al., 2017; Bass & Riggio, 2006). These translate into performance objectives like:

- Leaders articulate a shared vision for implementation and celebrate team successes.
- Managers identify and remove structural obstacles to staff participation in the intervention.

Leadership is also essential for advancing equity. Frameworks such as CFIR and HEIF emphasize the leader's role in fostering inclusive processes and addressing structural inequities (Damschroder et al., 2022b; Woodward et al., 2021). For example: Leaders encourage co-design strategies with frontline staff and community stakeholders to promote equity.

By grounding performance objectives in current leadership constructs across implementation frameworks and empirical studies, planners can more effectively specify what leaders need to do to enable successful and equitable implementation.

Stating Outcomes and Performance Objectives for Maintenance

Maintenance (often used interchangeably with sustainment in implementation science) refers to the extent to which an intervention is continued, institutionalized, and integrated into routine practice over time—particularly after initial funding, external support, or key champions are no longer present (Chambers et al., 2013; Shelton, 2020; Shelton et al., 2018). Sustainment can refer to maintaining either the program itself or the outcomes of a program that is no longer needed (Shediac-Rizkallah & Bone, 1998).

Recent frameworks emphasize that sustainment is not a static outcome but a dynamic process shaped by evolving contextual, organizational, and policy environments (Hailemariam et al., 2019; Moullin et al., 2020). Sustainment requires attention to inner setting factors (e.g., leadership, workflow integration, resource allocation), outer setting influences (e.g., reimbursement policies, community partnerships), and ongoing capacity-building efforts. The Dynamic Sustainability Framework (Chambers et al., 2013) highlights the importance of continual adaptation and learning for long-term success. Similarly, the EPIS framework (Aarons et al., 2011; Moullin et al., 2019) includes sustainment as a distinct phase, encouraging planners to define specific performance objectives for maintaining implementation infrastructure, monitoring fidelity, and re-engaging stakeholders.

Many funding agencies now require applicants to demonstrate how an intervention will be maintained after the end of initial funding (Schell et al., 2013; Shelton, 2020). Planning for sustainment—the ongoing integration of a program into routine practice—should begin early and address both facilitators and threats to long-term viability. Recent implementation research views sustainment not as a static endpoint but as a dynamic and adaptive process, responsive to evolving needs, context, and infrastructure (Chambers et al., 2013; Shelton, 2020).

One threat to sustainment is the absence of feedback systems that reinforce an intervention's relevance. Programs that do not continuously demonstrate value often lose priority, even if originally evidence-based. Sustaining value over time requires robust monitoring and continuous quality improvement (CQI) strategies (Quanbeck et al., 2011), along with organizational changes that support institutionalization. For example, updating workflows, job descriptions, or training procedures can ensure that the intervention remains integrated despite turnover or shifting priorities (Zurynski et al., 2023).

Organizational capacity remains a cornerstone of sustainment. While earlier taxonomies described capacity in terms of leadership, resource mobilization, and group processes, recent studies emphasize the importance of aligning inner setting factors (e.g., leadership engagement, implementation climate) with outer system supports, such as policy incentives and financing mechanisms (Lengnick-Hall et al., 2021; Luke et al., 2014).

Planners will consider the contextual factors that may influence long-term sustainment of the intervention and articulate a goal for its maintenance as well as performance objectives delineating who has to do what to ensure the program is maintained. Program maintenance outcomes can be stated in this way: The [organization or individual] maintains [innovative program] as indicated by [the evidence or document to indicate maintenance].

Anticipating the need to adapt over time, planners can write performance objectives such as:

- Administrators will identify funding, staffing, and policy support to ensure continuation of the program.

- Supervisors regularly assess implementation fidelity and identify adaptation needs.
- Teams formalize the intervention into standard operating procedures to ensure continuity during staff turnover.
- Supervisors ensure that key intervention components are embedded into standard operating procedures and staff onboarding materials.

By addressing the dynamic, capacity-driven, and feedback-informed nature of sustainment, these performance objectives can improve the likelihood of long-term implementation success. Box 9.4 presents example maintenance performance objectives for National DPP.

BOX 9.4. MAINTENANCE PERFORMANCE OBJECTIVES FOR NATIONAL DPP

Maintenance outcome: The Federally Qualified Health Center (FQHC) will ensure that the program continues as indicated by established DPP protocols.

The clinic leadership:

1. Ensures that the contract is up to date and renews the data agreement with National DPP as needed.
2. Monitors fidelity of the referral system.

The clinic administration:

1. Updates EHR as needed.
2. Continues to review patient outcomes on a regular basis.
3. Collects referral data and reports to providers.
4. Provides continued guidance and training for current and new staff on completing referrals.

Source: Adapted from Perkison et al., 2023.

Constructing Matrices of Change Objectives for Implementation

This task is similar to Step 2 of IM except that in this case, the planner develops a matrix to guide the design of implementation strategies (rather than intervention components). Now that the performance objectives describing who has to do what to adopt, implement, and maintain the program are complete, the next part of this task is to describe determinants of implementation. Thinking about the specific actions necessary to implement the program and the implementers who will deliver it first will help make sure that determinants are specific to those implementers and actions. The matrix combines performance objectives and determinants in at least three matrices – one for each phase of the process: adoption, implementation, and maintenance.

Determinants of Adoption, Implementation, and Maintenance

During Task 1 of Implementation Mapping (needs and assets assessments) planners likely identified various factors influencing implementation and used TMFs to inform that process. While some of the findings will have informed understanding of who should be involved in implementation and what they have to do to deliver the program (performance objectives), it is likely that some of the barriers and facilitators to implementation identified in Task 1 represent "determinants."

Determinants include both contextual factors influencing implementation as well as personal level factors that influence implementers. These determinants answer the questions: "Why would adopters decide to use the program?" "Why would implementers do what is necessary to implement the program?" and "Why would those responsible for program maintenance carry out actions that ensure the program continues over time?" The answers to these questions are the determinants of adoption, implementation, and maintenance respectively. Examples of determinants are awareness of the program, perceptions about the program's characteristics (e.g., belief that it represents a relative advantage over what is currently done), insight into the program components, perceived benefits of program use, self-efficacy and skills for implementation, and values supportive of program goals.

Program use may also be influenced by social or structural factors that might serve as barriers or facilitators. Indeed, several of the frameworks described above and the many implementation TMFs that have been reviewed and categorized describe contextual factors that exist at the organizational or even community level. Examples are leadership, resources, social support, and reinforcement. Since these factors require changes to the implementation environment, they are best conceptualized as performance objectives by thinking about who has to change what in order to positively influence these contextual factors to support implementation. Here, we will focus on the "personal determinants," that is, those that lie within the implementer and that influence implementation actions.

The Core Processes (Chapter 2) for selecting determinants of program use are the same as those recommended for selecting determinants of health-related behavior and environmental conditions (Chapter 6, Step 2). The team should begin by exploring a list of factors that will facilitate or serve as barriers or facilitators to adoption, implementation, and maintenance (e.g., using brainstorming with the planning group); review evidence from previous research to refine or add to the list; use theories and frameworks to inform determinant identification; and collect new data from potential program adopters and implementers.

Brainstorming Potential Determinants Perkison et al. (2023) identified determinants for why clinics (decision makers and staff) would adopt and implement the National DPP. The planning team held a brainstorming session activity with clinic staff and leaders and identified determinants from the Social Cognitive Theory. Some of the determinants are related to perceptions of the characteristics of the program and align with concepts described in both Diffusion of Innovation Theory as well as CFIR (e.g., compatibility, relative advantage).

On the list of why clinics would *adopt* the National DPP were the following factors:

- Clinic leaders believe that the DPP program is important for diabetes prevention.
- Clinic medical directors have knowledge of the program; they understand the program goals and components.
- Clinic director believes that the program will benefit patients.
- Clinic medical director believes that the program is better than what is currently done (relative advantage).
- Clinic director believes that the program fits with organizational goals (compatibility).

Ideas about the determinants of implementation were more related to capacity, skills, and confidence of the clinic and staff. The answer to the posed question of why implementers would *deliver* the National DPP as planned included:

- Perceived program effectiveness
- Staff capacity and motivation to overcome barriers to implementation
- Skills related to identifying eligible patients and referring them to the DPP
- Expectations that the program would increase referrals and patient enrollment
- Recognize that provider–patient communication increases trust in the patient for the National DPP
- Believe that submitting referrals will facilitate patient enrollment to prevent diabetes
- Skills and self-efficacy of decision makers to garner support for new programs from staff
- Skills and self-efficacy of program champion to garner support for the program
- Skills and self-efficacy of program champion for program coordination
- Skills of champion to communicate with implementers and support their activities.

As the brainstorming group moved to *maintenance*, the determinants became more related to perceptions of the benefits and costs of having adopted and implemented the program. The main agent for maintenance shifted to the decision makers for the clinic (as in adoption) with some consideration for determinants of the ability of the program champion to enact systems changes to ensure survival of the program. On the list of why the clinic would [be able to] maintain the National DPP, the following determinants were brainstormed:

- Expectations that incorporating the National DPP referral process into the clinic's workflow will contribute to the successful implementation of the National DPP referral
- Belief that incorporation of the National DPP into the clinic's workflow will result in increased referrals to National DPP
- Positive attitudes about the importance of continuing education to maintain the referral numbers/processes when new staff are hired
- Perceptions by decision makers that the DPP can fit into normal routines of the clinic with little staff burden

While these issues did not emerge in the DPP example above, factors influencing implementation (determinants) can also be contextual in nature. That is, they can be influenced by the implementation environment. These, also, are often identified in Task 1. For example, consideration of time and space related to where the intervention would be implemented, resources for implementing, opportunities for professional development to train staff on the intervention, are all important considerations that could serve as barriers or facilitators to implementation. Once these are identified, it is important to determine who is responsible for making changes that would benefit implementation and what they would have to do to make that contextual change.

Reviewing Evidence from Previous Research and Using Theory Reviewing theories, frameworks, and empirical evidence to identify the personal determinants that influence adoption, implementation, and maintenance behaviors can help broaden, confirm, or refute the brainstormed list. The goal is to understand the individual-level factors that shape whether key actors—such as adopters, implementers, and sustainers—will engage in the behaviors necessary for successful program delivery and continuation. Drawing from implementation science, organizational science, and social psychology, theoretical constructs and findings from recent studies should inform the selection of relevant determinants. These determinants will later guide the selection of methods and practical applications for the design of implementation strategies.

A review of the theory and evidence from previous research on personal determinants of implementation will help identify individual-level factors that influence whether adopters, implementers, and maintainers engage in and sustain program-related behaviors. These determinants often include skills, self-efficacy, attitudes, values, and perceived social support—factors that are central to many behavior change theories and implementation frameworks. Perceptions of the intervention itself such as its compatibility with organizational values, its relative advantage over other options, and other attitudes and beliefs about the intervention can strongly influence implementation behaviors (Damschroder et al., 2009; Peterson et al., 2007; Rogers, 1983, 1995, 2003).

The planning team must consider characteristics of an innovation as either a facilitator of or a barrier to adoption and implementation, both during IM planning Steps 1–4 during initial program development. During the development phase, the planner should make decisions about program elements while considering such characteristics of diffusible innovations as required time, complexity, compatibility, and ability to be modified. During Step 5, implementation planning, the planner is concerned with the perceptions of the adopters and implementers relative to these characteristics. Determinants related to these constructs then could include attitudes about the intervention's compatibility or value, or perceived benefits of the program in terms of its compatibility; the planner may consider characteristics such as communicability, relative advantage, and required commitment to help identify both performance objectives and determinants.

Theories and frameworks expand upon and provide guidance about personal determinants of implementation actors. For example, CFIR emphasizes the importance of individual characteristics such as motivation, role clarity, and alignment with innovation goals (Damschroder et al., 2022b). These updates reflect a growing recognition that implementers are not passive recipients of interventions but active agents whose beliefs, capabilities, and values shape implementation outcomes.

The Social Cognitive Theory (SCT) continues to be one of the most widely applied social psychology frameworks in implementation science. SCT emphasizes the dynamic interplay between personal factors, behavior, and environmental influences. Among its constructs, self-efficacy—the belief in one's ability to perform a behavior—has consistently emerged as a strong predictor of implementation behavior. A 2024 scoping review of behavior change interventions found that SCT-based strategies such as goal setting, modeling, social reinforcement, and action planning were commonly used to enhance implementers' confidence and motivation (El Kirat et al., 2024).

Other social psychological theories also offer valuable insights. The Reasoned Action Approach (RAA) highlights the roles of attitudes, perceived norms, and perceived behavioral control in shaping intentions and behaviors. These constructs have been widely applied in implementation research to explain why individuals choose to adopt or resist new practices. Similarly, Self-Determination Theory (SDT) emphasizes the importance of autonomy, competence, and relatedness in fostering intrinsic motivation—

factors that are particularly relevant when implementers are expected to sustain behaviors over time.

Recent empirical studies support the relevance of these theories. For example, El Kirat et al. (2024) found that implementers' perceptions of personal relevance, burden, and value alignment significantly influenced their engagement with implementation strategies. Suchland and Carbonaro (2021) demonstrated that SCT-based interventions incorporating reflective practice and self-assessment improved implementers' confidence and persistence in adopting new behaviors.

These findings reinforce that successful implementation depends not only on organizational or structural factors but also on the personal readiness, motivation, and perceived capability of those tasked with delivering and sustaining the intervention. Addressing these personal determinants through targeted methods (modeling, feedback, and reinforcement) and practical applications can significantly enhance implementation outcomes.

Other determinants are characteristics of the implementers, such as perceived needs, values and goals, skills, and perceived social support (Damschroder et al., 2009). It is critical to consider theories of personal behavior because adopters, implementers, and maintainers are all individuals who need to do something for full implementation to occur. Therefore, many of the theories presented in Chapter 3, that predict and explain individual behavior, are also highly relevant when identifying determinants of implementation.

Because program adoption and implementation often involve organizations and community groups making decisions and changing practices to make use of an innovation, the application of organizational change and community development models is critical to identifying performance objectives and determinants of program adoption and implementation (Estabrooks et al., 2018). Several reviews and syntheses of implementation theories and frameworks have identified factors that influence implementation outcomes in various settings at multiple levels of influence (Chaudoir et al., 2013; Nilsen & Bernhardsson, 2019). They include (among others):

- Structural-level factors (including the political and social climate, public policy, economic climate, and infrastructure).
- Organizational-level factors (including leadership effectiveness, culture and climate, organizational values and rewards).
- Implementer-level factors including attitudes toward the program and perceived behavioral control (or self-efficacy) for implementation.
- Innovation-level factors that include characteristics of the program to be implemented, the perceptions of these characteristics by potential adopters and implementers, and the evidence supporting the program's efficacy.

Implementation frameworks and theories of organizational readiness identify concepts, such as change commitment and change efficacy, which even though they are measured at the organizational level represent individual beliefs related to implementation (Wandersman et al., 2024; Weiner et al., 2009).

Environmental influences necessary for program adoption, implementation, and continuation are identified as performance objectives that state *who* will need to do *what* to make the changes or create the conditions necessary to accomplish the program use outcomes. These influences can be anticipated when stating performance objectives in the previous task, or they can be added as determinants of program use. A useful way to determine whether they should be added as a determinant or as another performance objective is as follows: if the answer to the question "Why would the decision maker adopt the program?" is personal or internal (such as knowledge of the goals of the program, perceived benefits of the program, or perceived compatibility with organization values), these are listed as determinants of adoption. If, however, the answers to the "why?" question are external and are characteristics of the adoption context, such as "the patient advisory board requests the program" or the "state primary care association (PCA) recommends the program," then these should be added as additional adoption performance objectives. In this case, the planner may want to think about what additional determinants may be needed to answer the question of why a patient board would request the program and why the PCA would recommend the program.

Collecting Data from Adopters and Implementers Qualitative methods, such as focus groups or interviews, can be helpful in generating new ideas for determinants or in verifying some of the findings from the research literature. Quantitative data collection using questionnaires that measure the determinants and interest or intentions to adopt and implement a program can be especially helpful in judging the strength of the association between determinants and potential adoption and implementation. With both types of data collection, planners can obtain some estimate of the presence or absence of the determinant in the user system.

Integrating mixed-methods approaches can help clearly identify and understand factors influencing implementation to inform implementation strategy design. For example, a study published in BMC Health Services Research used a mixed-methods design to evaluate the implementation of the GUIDED-HF toolkit for heart failure patients in emergency departments. The researchers combined quantitative surveys (ORCA context scale) and qualitative interviews to identify site-specific barriers and facilitators, which informed tailored implementation strategies (Stolldorf et al., 2025).

Organizing and Prioritizing Determinants Eventually, the planning team must refine the list of determinants to create a practical list for implementation planning. Planners should rate each determinant in terms of importance (that is, strength of association with program adoption and implementation) and changeability (that is, how likely it is that an implementation intervention influences a change in the determinant). The planners should focus on determinants (both personal determinants and contextual determinants) that have both high importance and high changeability. However, planners may want to retain some determinants with high importance and low changeability because the determinants are likely to be critical factors in successful program use. For example, the cost of adopting a health promotion program may be a strong determinant, but there may be little that planners can do to lower the cost. Because cost may be a major barrier to adoption, planners should address it in the intervention, for example, by finding sources of compensation or demonstrating that the program costs are worth the benefit.

Constructing Matrices for Program Use

Here, we create detailed change objectives by crossing performance objectives with determinants for adoption, implementation, and maintenance. Planners are now performing the same task as in Step 2, but instead of focusing on change objectives for behavioral and environmental outcomes, they are writing change objectives for adoption, implementation, and maintenance of the health promotion program. To prepare a matrix for program use, planners follow the same process as they did for the matrices developed for planning the intervention. They enter performance objectives in the left column of the table and the determinants in the top row. They then assess the cells to decide whether the determinant is likely to be important to the achievement of the performance objective. Next, they write change objectives for the appropriate cells (see Chapter 5).

Table 9.1 presents a partial matrix for the *Target:BP™*. The planning team used Implementation Mapping to identify determinants of *Target:BP™* use, an intervention developed by the American Heart Association and American Medical Association to assist clinics in improving hypertension management with EBIs (Valerio-Shewmaker et al., 2022). After identifying outcomes for adopters (community health center (CHC) leadership), implementers and maintainers (program champion), the planning team developed performance objectives by asking the question, "Who needs to do what to ensure that the program is adopted, implemented, and maintained?" Following this, determinants of program use were identified based on the theoretical constructs associated with the barriers and facilitators identified in Task 1, including, for example, attitudes, outcome expectations of program use, and normative beliefs concerning adoption and use of *Target:BP™*. Once this was determined, the matrices of change (Table 9.1) were developed to ensure the content and messaging for implementation addressed the performance objectives and determinants.

Table 9.1 Examples of Change Objectives from the *Target:BP*™

Performance Objectives	Attitudes	Knowledge	Outcome Expectations	Normative Beliefs
Personal Determinants				
Adoption: CHC Leadership will adopt the *Target:BP*™ program and associated recommendations within their practice.				
PO1. CHC Leadership agree, approve, and support the adoption of the Target:BP program	A.1a. Explain that the Target:BP is easy to adopt and implement A.1b. Describe Target:BP as an improvement over what is done now A.1c. Describe Target:BP as fitting with organizational goals and needs	K.1a. Describe the components of the Target:BP program K.1b. Describe the rates of uncontrolled BP in clinic	OE.1a Explain that adopting the Target:BP program will provide help with program implementation and clinic resources OE.1b Explain that the program will provide effective/ improved patient reach/ outcomes and satisfaction	NB.1a Express belief that other clinics like theirs are agreeing to implement Target:BP NB.1b Express belief that the state supports Target:BP as an EBI
PO2. CHC Leadership designate a program champion and a point of contact to review Target:BP program and lead the implementation	A.2a Describe that the program champion is an important element of the program	K.2a. Explain the role of program champion in Target:BP	OE.2a Explain that a program champion will enable the Target:BP program to be implemented and maintained	NB.2a List other clinics like theirs that use champions to assist in practice change or program implementation
PO3. CHC Leadership establish and sign MOU with AHA and UTHealth	A.3a. Describe that the MOU will establish guidelines and scope of work for the relationship with AHA and UTHealth	K.3a. Lists terms of the agreement K.3b. Describe what the partnership will entail in detail	OE.3a. Explain that reviewing and approving the MOU will enable the implementation of Target:BP in their practice	
Implementation: The provider and program champion will implement the *Target:BP*™ program into their hypertension management protocol.				
PO1. Program champion enrolls and works with AHA representative in selected public health region to complete online registration and begin implementation of Target:BP program	A.1a. Express positive attitude towards the implementation of Target:BP	K.1a. Describe the components of the Target:BP program K.1b. Describe the rates of uncontrolled BP in CHC K.1c. Describe requirements of the Target:BP program	OE.1a. Explain that by attending the training he/she will be able to successfully implement Target:BP OE.1b. Explain program champion and CHC leadership will reinforce and acknowledge them for completing the training successfully	NB.1a. Express belief that other CHC like theirs are implementing Target:BP NB.1b. Express belief that other coordinators attend training

Table 9.1 (*Continued*)

Personal Determinants				
Performance Objectives	**Attitudes**	**Knowledge**	**Outcome Expectations**	**Normative Beliefs**
PO2. Program champion obtains and distributes program materials focused on hypertension management and protocol recommendations for providers and patients	A.2a. Express that Target:BP program information will help patients with BP management	K.2a. Describe the role of each CHC team member for implementation K.2b. Describe patient education needs K.2c. Describe toolkits and other materials that support program implementation given specific staff role	OE.2a. Explain that by providing staff and patients with information Target:BP uptake will be achieved OE.2b. Explain that patients will use Target:BP information for BP control management	NB.2a. Express belief that other coordinators are identifying Target:BP components for staff and patients
PO3. Program champion develops strategies to identify upcoming appointments for patients with uncontrolled blood pressure daily	A.3a. Describe the importance of identifying upcoming appointments	K.3a. Describe steps to searching schedule to identify upcoming appointments K.3.b. Describe the data system of the CHC K.3c. Describe process of using data systems to identify upcoming appointments	OE.3a. Explain that all scheduled patients will be identified for receiving Target:BP program information	NB.3a. Express belief that other program coordinators are searching schedules for upcoming appointments
PO4. Program champion oversees implementation efforts and provide feedback to CHC staff	A.4a. Express positive feelings about overseeing implementation as important and useful for ensuring fidelity	K.4a. Describe steps needed to oversee implementation K.4b. Describe daily and weekly activities associated with Champion Role	O.E.4a. Explain that through regular oversight and communication, the Target:BP program will be implemented effectively	NB.4a. Describe that other individuals with similar positions in other CHCs act as champions to oversee and provide feedback
Maintenance: Program champions will maintain the *Target:BP*™ program and ensure the successful delivery of program resources and materials to the designated staff.				
PO1. Program champion discusses the integration of the Target:BP program with leadership/decision makers and with implementation team	A.1a. Express that integration of the Target:BP program into the clinic will support patient BP management	K.1a. Describe processes that will help a program survive in an organization (e.g., inclusion in job descriptions, reward structures, budgets)	OE.1a. Describe the program to continue to be value added to patients	NB.1a. Express belief that other coordinators are discussing integration with CHC leadership

(continued)

Table 9.1 (*Continued*)

Personal Determinants				
Performance Objectives	**Attitudes**	**Knowledge**	**Outcome Expectations**	**Normative Beliefs**
PO2. Program champion maintains supply of resources and program materials, as well as any needed changes in any program materials given the CHC setting and patient population (health management action plan review)	A.2a Express positive feelings about maintaining supply of resources and program materials A.2b. Explain in the importance of conducting a health management action plan review to ensure program material changes are made as needed	K.2a. List resources and materials and how to obtain them for Target:BP K.2b. Describe relevant organizational needs for changes in Target:BP implementation for sustainability	OE.2a. Expect Target:BP protocols are stable and will continue to function as specified OE.2b. Expect that decision makers will support Target:BP protocols and steps	NB.2a. Describe that other coordinators are developing a plan for maintaining program resources and materials NB.2b. Describe that other coordinators are engaging in health management action plan review
PO3. Program champion uses EHR to maintain Target:BP patient outcome goals and ensure CHC hypertension evaluation data is submitted in a timely manner to the Target:BP program	A.3a. Explain in the importance of maintaining and submitting EHR data to the Target:BP program	K.3a. Describe how to query EMR for BP data K.3b. Describe how to visualize and share data program data within clinic and patient population	OE.3a. Expect that continued monitoring and evaluation will contribute to likelihood of program continuation	NB.3a. Express belief that other coordinators continue to use the HER to track and maintain patient outcome goals

Source: Adapted from Valerio-Shewmaker et al. (2022).

Task 3: Choosing Theoretical Methods and Selecting or Designing Implementation Strategies

The third task in Step 5 is to choose theoretical methods and operationalize these methods into practical applications that fit with the context and setting. This collection of practical applications of methods will then (in the following task) be organized into comprehensive, and often multilevel, implementation strategies. Much like in Step 3 of IM, here, we consider the theoretical methods (Kok et al., 2016; see also Chapter 7) that will address determinants of implementation, and we operationalize those (create practical applications of the methods) in ways that fit with the setting where implementation will occur and the population that will be reached. Using Implementation Mapping Task 3 provides a systematic process for selecting or designing implementation strategies that logically follow from the determinants and performance objectives identified in earlier tasks.

Selecting Change Methods and Practical Applications for Program Use

In Implementation Mapping, the term "implementation strategy" is consistent with how it is defined by Proctor et al. (2011) in that it refers to both discrete actions (e.g., a training session, a decision aid) and comprehensive packages (e.g., a multicomponent intervention to support clinic adoption). In Implementation Mapping, all strategies, whether they are discrete or multicomponent, will always contain theoretical change methods matched to determinants of implementation and a description of how they are being operationalized.

Theoretical change methods (Kok et al., 2016) are general techniques derived from behavioral and social science theories that are known to influence specific determinants (also called the "function" of implementation strategies), and **practical applications** are the specific ways in which those methods are operationalized (also called the "form" of implementation strategies) (Perez Jolles et al., 2019). For example, a practical application (aka implementation strategy) such as a face-to-face training with a manual and follow-up coaching might operationalize methods such as instruction, rehearsal, and feedback to build implementers' skills and self-efficacy.

Change methods can target individual-level factors (e.g., attitudes, skills, self-efficacy) or organizational-level factors (e.g., leadership, culture, readiness for change). For example, to influence implementers' self-efficacy and outcome expectations, planners might use methods such as modeling, guided practice, and persuasive communication (Kok et al., 2016). There are cases in which multiple methods may need to be used to address a single determinant. Additionally, methods will frequently target more than one determinant. Organizational-level methods may include strategies to foster institutional commitment, build leadership support, or restructure workflows. For example, Ten Hoor and Plasqui (2016) demonstrated how regular engagement with school leadership helped sustain participation in a strength-based physical activity intervention, illustrating the method of "institutional commitment" in action. Simons-Morton et al. (1988) indicate the importance of organizational change for implementation of health promotion interventions, with school health as example. They identify a number of relevant organizational-level methods for change, among others: institutional commitment and strong organizational leadership, primarily from the superintendent, and technical assistance and resources regarding the health promotion intervention.

Recent work in implementation science has emphasized the importance of aligning methods with both the type of determinant and the level of influence (individual, organizational, or system-level). The updated CFIR framework and the SELECT-IT meta-framework provide guidance for selecting appropriate theories and methods based on project goals and contextual fit (Fontaine et al., 2025). Thus, methods should be selected based on their theoretical relevance to the determinant and their empirical support, and they also should be practically feasible and culturally responsive. Once methods are identified, planners can discuss how to operationalize the methods in ways that are most appropriate for the implementers and the setting.

Typically, program planners start with the determinants and the list of change objectives from the matrix and brainstorm change methods and practical applications. Next, they review the relevant theories and research and practice literature to confirm, refute, or modify the provisional list of change methods and their practical applications. As we discussed in Chapter 7, the selection of change methods and practical applications may be an iterative process. For example, when they review performance objectives, planners may find that ideas for practical applications occur to them before their ideas for change methods. They then assess practical applications and link them to theoretical methods considering how to address the parameters for effective use of the methods.

Each method must be applied in a way that respects its parameters for effectiveness—the conditions under which the method is likely to work (see Chapter 7 for discussion about parameters). For instance, for modeling to be effective, the observer must be able to identify with the model and the model must demonstrate overcoming a challenge, not just performing a skill effortlessly. Ignoring these parameters can reduce the impact of the strategy, even if the method is theoretically appropriate.

It is also essential to ensure that strategies are contextually appropriate and feasible. Recent reviews have highlighted the importance of integrating implementation science with quality improvement approaches to enhance strategy design and sustainability (Bierbaum et al., 2025). This includes using tools like logic models to map how strategies are expected to influence determinants and behaviors, ultimately leading to improved implementation outcomes. The Implementation Mapping Logic Model serves this purpose (Walker et al., 2025a).

Next, planners select or design implementation strategies to operationalize methods into practical applications. At this stage, it is essential to ensure that the relevant adopters, implementers, and maintainers are included in planning how the methods are operationalized.

The process outlined here emphasizes the development of implementation strategies that align with the factors influencing implementation behavior; however, this process can also be utilized to identify strategies that have been successfully applied in other contexts. For example, taxonomies such as the ERIC compilation described above (Powell et al., 2015) provides a valuable menu of options to consider during this task. Since there is little consensus on what strategies work best to address specific types of implementation barriers or determinants (Waltz et al., 2019), using Implementation Mapping and the ERIC strategies together can be useful (Kang & Foster, 2022; Lopez et al., 2024; van Nassau et al., 2025; Schroeck et al., 2022, Schol et al., 2025). During Task 3, the planner could explore ERIC strategies for ideas about the types of approaches that may be useful and then tailor them based on the matrices of change objectives created in Task 2 (Powell et al., 2015). Since the list includes strategies that are qualitatively varied (some represent methods, others practical applications, others are processes or general guidelines), planners should use the list to generate ideas about what might work but should still articulate the specific determinants being addressed and the methods and practical applications contained within selected strategies. For example, Kang & Foster (2022) used the CFIR-ERIC Matching tool (Powell et al., 2015) to generate a list of recommended implementation strategies after using CFIR to identify implementation determinants and SCT and the Taxonomy of Behavior Change Methods to develop change objectives and mechanisms of action. The planning team then narrowed down the list of ERIC strategies from 27 to 9 by identifying those that had at least 20% of experts' endorsement from the ERIC selection process. This integration of Implementation Mapping and the ERIC compilation of strategies enabled the planning team to leverage theory-based determinants and change methods in identifying expert recommended implementation strategies that would be appropriate in the context.

Using Task 3 to Develop Implementation Strategies

Implementation Mapping was used to develop and test strategies to incorporate physical movement in the teaching of academic content: Physically Active Breaks (PABs) and Physically Active Lessons (PALS) (Walker et al., 2022b, Walker et al., 2025c). Informed by the question, "What can we do to help schools and teachers implement PABs and PALs?" the research team followed Implementation Mapping Tasks 1–3 to identify who were the, adopters, implementers, and maintainers, what they needed to do to support implementation, and the determinants influencing implementation (the why), enabling them to identify change methods to specify how those determinants would be influenced. Selected change methods included guided practice, persuasive communication, and advanced organizers. Once change methods were identified, the team moved to develop the practical application of those change methods by asking the questions: "How do we engage with school leaders?" and "How do we deliver "intervention" content?" The team decided to utilize a group format for delivering this content in the form of leadership sessions to address attitudes, skills, and self-efficacy. These leadership sessions, over the course of a year, incorporated the selection change methods and practical applications of those methods in the form of slides, a PAB game, and role-play activity. A sample of the change methods and practical applications of the leadership session implementation strategy can be found in Table 9.2.

In another example, the SEMM-DIA planning team selected theoretical methods and designed implementation strategies to address determinants identified in Task 2. These methods were grounded in SCT and informed by prior implementation experiences with SEMM and similar clinic-based interventions. The strategies were operationalized into practical applications that were feasible and contextually appropriate for community health centers (CHCs).

To address determinants such as community health worker (CHW) self-efficacy, skills, and motivation, the team developed testimonial videos

Table 9.2 Magic Leadership Session Implementation Strategy

Change Objectives	Implementation Strategy (Leadership Session)	
	Method	**Practical Application**
K1.1.1 Describe benefits of PABs & PALs	Advance organizers	PowerPoint slides
K1.1.2 Explain importance of PABs & PALs	Persuasive communication	
A1.1.1 Express positive feelings about PABs & PALs		
A1.1.2 Believe that PABs & PALs are beneficial for learning	Direct experience	PAB game
A1.1.3 Describe how PABs & PALs are beneficial for behavior	Persuasive communication	PowerPoint slides
SSE1.1.1 Express confidence in explaining to teachers why they should use PABs & PALs	Guided practice	Role-Play activity

featuring CHWs who had previously implemented SEMM. These videos modeled successful delivery of the intervention, highlighted personal and professional benefits, and illustrated how SEMM contributed to improved patient outcomes (e.g., increased screening and vaccination rates). Testimonials also included patient perspectives to reinforce the value of the program.

The planning team created a train-the-trainer guide for CHW managers, incorporating step-by-step demonstrations and peer-learning facilitation techniques. This guide was designed to build managerial capacity to supervise CHWs and support ongoing implementation through regular team meetings. Additional strategies included adapting existing CHW manager trainings to integrate behavioral change methods such as modeling, verbal persuasion, and guided practice.

To support leadership engagement, the team developed informational videos for clinic managers and champions. These materials communicated the goals, components, and benefits of SEMM, and emphasized alignment with clinic performance measures (e.g., cervical cancer screening targets). Supporting documents included a SEMM implementation guide, a clinic handbook, and a roles and responsibilities SOP manual (see Table 9.3).

All strategies were mapped to specific determinants and change objectives, and organized into a multicomponent implementation plan. This plan included strategies to promote awareness and adoption, build capacity for implementation, and support long-term maintenance. The planning process ensured that each strategy was theoretically grounded, contextually tailored, and aligned with the overall implementation goals of SEMM-DIA.

Task 3 directly addresses the call to articulate mechanisms of implementation strategies (Lewis et al., 2022; Powell et al., 2017). It guides planners in selecting theory- and evidence-based methods that specifically target identified determinants of implementation, ensuring that chosen strategies are systematically linked to the behavioral and contextual factors

Table 9.3 SEMM Program Implementation Strategies

		Implementation Strategies		
Implementer	**Determinants**	**Change Methods**	**Practical Applications**	**Component**
CHW	• Awareness/ perceptions • Outcome Expectations • Skills and Self-Efficacy • Feedback and Reinforcement	• Information • Persuasion • Skill building • Guided practice • Vicarious reinforcement	• Information video on benefits of implementing SEMM • Video testimonials of CHWs discussing implementation benefits and challenges • Computer assisted SEMM training scripts	• SEMM-DIA Online Tool • Program Orientation Session • CHW online training
Program Champion/Manager Clinic Leadership	• Awareness/perceptions • Outcome Expectations • Skills and Self-Efficacy • Perceived positive	• Modeling • Persuasion • Reinforcement • Communication • Mobilization	• Information video describing SEMM goals, components, and benefits • Video tutorial for implementers • Program champion train-the-trainer guide • Technical assistance via tele-monitoring platform • E-newsletter template to engage stakeholders	• Program Orientation Session • Program tracking tools • SEMM manager training • Technical Assistance

they are intended to influence. Task 3 operationalizes the causal logic that connects strategies to outcomes. This rigorous approach enhances the precision of implementation efforts and provides a concrete framework for understanding and testing how and why strategies work.

Task 4: Creating Implementation Protocols and Materials

In the fourth task of Step 5 Implementation Mapping, the planning team takes what was done in Task 3 (selecting methods and creating practical applications) and (1) organizes them in a way that is consistent with the adoption and implementation process (plans the scope and sequence of the multicomponent implementation strategy); and (2) creates the protocols, tools, and materials needed to carry out the implementation strategies. This step translates theoretical methods and practical applications into tangible products that support implementation across different stages—adoption, implementation, and maintenance.

As in Step 4 of IM, this task includes creating a scope and sequence of the implementation strategy, drafting design documents, developing content, pretesting materials with implementers, and refining them based on feedback. Even when planners adopt existing strategies—such as those from the ERIC compilation—it is essential to define the specific content, messages, and delivery mechanisms that will bring those strategies to life in a particular setting. Implementation Mapping provides a structured approach to ensure that each strategy is grounded in theory, tailored to the context, and aligned with the determinants and change objectives identified earlier.

Organizing the Implementation Strategy: Scope, Sequence, and Materials

Implementation strategies that are designed to increase adoption, implementation, and maintenance usually comprise at least three major components: one to stimulate awareness and adoption; a second to provide training, capacity development, and ongoing technical support for implementation; and a final component to help implementers and managers transition an ongoing program to maintenance. Common materials produced in this task are materials to promote awareness, an implementation manual, and materials to support training for implementers. The scope and sequence of the implementation strategy should complement the scope and sequence of the intervention and include the intervention timeline for delivery, details of components and the implementers they target, and materials associated with the components. Figure 9.5 provides a sample scope and sequence of MAGIC (Movement for Academic Growth in Classrooms), an implementation intervention

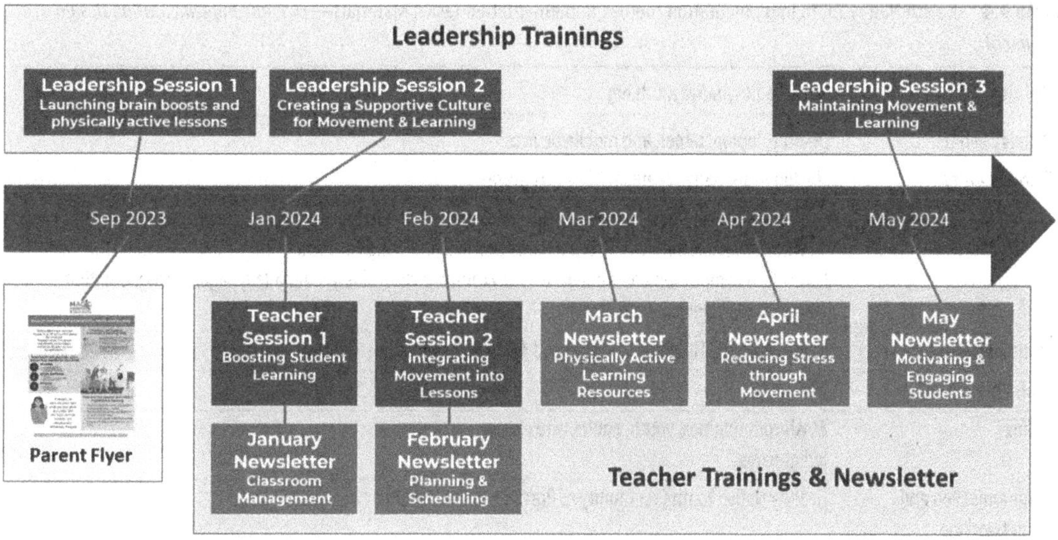

Figure 9.5 MAGIC Scope and Sequence

designed to support classroom-based physical activity approaches in elementary schools.

The implementation strategy included: leadership sessions to support the launch of PABs/PALs and establish a supportive culture at the school, a parent flyer to engage parents to support their children engaging in these activities, monthly newsletters on different tools and resources to support teacher use of PABs/PALs, and teacher trainings to encourage buy-in for using PABs/PALs in the classroom (Walker et al., 2025c).

Design documents for producing materials and procedures for implementation serve as a bridge between planning and production. As in Step 4 of IM, these documents outline the purpose of each material, the intended audience, the targeted determinants and change objectives, the theoretical methods being applied, and any relevant content or imagery. For example, if planners decide to create a testimonial video to encourage program adoption, the design document might specify the video's purpose (e.g., to increase perceived value of the program), the priority audience (e.g., school administrators), the relevant determinants (e.g., outcome expectations, social norms), and the methods (e.g., modeling, persuasive communication). It may also include draft interview questions and visual guidelines for production. These materials are not only essential for implementation but also support evaluation and future adaptation. They provide a clear record of what was delivered, how, and why—facilitating replication and continuous improvement.

For example, to support the implementation of the Healthy Native Youth Implementation Toolbox, an adaptation of iCHAMPSS (CHoosing And Maintaining Effective Programs for Sex Education in Schools) for Native communities (see, Peskin et al., 2017), the planning group

Table 9.4 Health Native Youth Implementation Toolbox Implementation Task 4 Materials—*Example Implementation Design Document*

Website URL	www.healthynativeyouth.org
Delivery vehicle	Desktop, laptop, tablet, and mobile devices
Points of entry	The Big Picture and Where Do I Start? Features
Curriculum selection tools	Curriculum portal provides access to culturally relevant, evidence based sexual health, substance use, suicide prevention, healthy coping, and positive parenting curricula Curriculum Comparison Chart allows users to compare curricula by criteria (e.g., age, setting, duration, cost, and evidence of effectiveness)
Testimonial videos	Stories from the Field from experienced AI/AN sexual health educators
Tools library	20+ tools
Images	AI/AN communities, youth, adults, and elders Indigi-icons
Communication and networking	Healthy Native Youth Community of Practice online sessions
Technical assistance	Request technical assistance feature Recorded Health Native Youth Community of Practice Sessions

developed design documents and drafted content for the production team (Markham et al., 2022). The design documents detailed the content, messages, and tools that the planning group wanted to employ in the Healthy Native Youth Implementation Toolbox. The implementation toolbox can be accessed through the Healthy Native Youth website (www.healthynativeyouth.org). Table 9.4 includes a summary of the design elements including the delivery vehicle and implementation strategies.

Pretesting Implementation Strategy Materials and Protocols

As in Step 4 of IM, in Step 5 Task 4 planners pretest materials and protocols related to the implementation strategy. We distinguish this from formal pilot testing which is often done prior to an evaluation of the intervention and/or implementation strategies (see Task 5 below and Chapter 10). Here we focus on the acceptability and appropriateness of the implementation strategy components and materials.

To ensure that the Health Native Youth Implementation Toolbox proposed tools and design drafts met the needs of those involved in implementation, they were pretested with interested parties. Materials were shared with a community-based workgroup, the Healthy Native Youth AI/AN Adolescent Sexual Health Workgroup, and revised according to feedback prior to final production of the website (Markham et al., 2022). Following the launch of the Health Native Youth Implementation Toolbox, four online Community of Practice sessions were held to gather feedback from AI/AN youth advocates on the tools and content, which is being used to refine the toolbox for version 2.0 (Markham et al., 2022).

Task 5: Evaluate Implementation Outcomes

The final task in Implementation Mapping focuses on evaluating the impact of implementation efforts. This step is essential for understanding whether the strategies developed and applied in the previous tasks have successfully supported the adoption, delivery, and sustainability of the intervention. Implementation outcomes are critical indicators of success because even the most effective interventions cannot achieve their intended impact if they are not implemented—or are implemented inconsistently or incompletely. Evaluating these outcomes helps determine whether implementation strategies are functioning as intended and provides insight into how they can be improved or adapted.

This task aligns with the evaluation planning process evaluation in Step 6 of IM (Chapter 10). It guides planners in developing a plan to assess the extent to which the intervention was implemented and the impact of implementation strategies on program adoption, implementation, and maintenance. While a full discussion of process evaluation is presented in Chapter 10, it is important to briefly distinguish it here from the evaluation of implementation strategies. Both approaches often focus on similar constructs—such as fidelity, reach, and acceptability—and may use overlapping methods. However, their purposes differ. Process evaluation is primarily used as a monitoring tool to assess how well an intervention is delivered, identify gaps in fidelity or reach, and inform interpretation of outcome data. It is often conducted alongside effectiveness evaluations to explain why an intervention did or did not work and to guide improvements in future implementation.

Process evaluation is also used as a continuous quality improvement tool. Chapter 10 stresses the real-time formative function of process evaluation and describes how ongoing monitoring of fidelity, reach, participant engagement, and resource use can identify problems as they emerge and inform mid-course corrections. Methods like process mapping (Kononowech et al., 2020), rapid-cycle improvement (Health Workforce Technical Assistance Center, 2016; Keith et al., 2017), and mixed-methods data collection are used to track and respond to variability in implementation. This dynamic approach allows programs to adapt proactively, improving delivery and effectiveness during the intervention, rather than later.

In contrast, implementation research typically involves formal research questions and hypotheses aimed at understanding the impact of specific implementation strategies on implementation outcomes. For example, an implementation study might test whether a facilitation strategy improves fidelity to a clinical guideline, whereas a process evaluation might simply document whether the guideline was delivered as intended. Implementation science has also introduced hybrid trial designs (discussed earlier in this chapter) that explicitly test both implementation and effectiveness outcomes within the same study, further blurring the lines between these approaches while maintaining distinct goals.

The quality of an assessment of implementation depends on the planning team's ability to: (1) write clear evaluation questions that assess implementation outcomes; (2) identify relevant indicators and measures; (3) select appropriate study designs; and (4) use data to determine the impact of the strategies and refine them if necessary.

Defining Implementation Outcomes

Above we describe various implementation outcomes that refer to the effects of deliberate actions to implement an intervention. Commonly evaluated outcomes include:

1. **Acceptability**: How stakeholders perceive the intervention and its delivery
2. **Adoption**: The initial decision or action to try or employ the intervention
3. **Appropriateness**: The perceived fit or relevance of the intervention
4. **Feasibility**: The extent to which the intervention can be carried out in a given setting
5. **Fidelity**: The degree to which the intervention is delivered as intended
6. **Penetration**: The extent of integration within a service setting
7. **Sustainability**: The extent to which the intervention is maintained over time
8. **Cost**: The financial impact of implementation

Reach. Proportion of women who participate in the SEMM education session among those eligible

Effectiveness. (For screening and HPV vaccination) % of women who complete or initiate screening or vaccination among all clinic patients

Implementation. Extent to which SEMM program components were used

Level of Implementation. Number of implementation steps that have been carried out

Implementation Fidelity. Degree to which SEMM components are implemented by LHWs as prescribed (degree of implementation for each LHW; frequencies and proportion of LHWs performing the required behaviors; proportion of patients recommended for screening and HPV vaccination)

Implementation Dose. Time spent in education sessions; # of navigation calls

Maintenance (intention). Intention to implement the SEMM program in the next 6 months.

Figure 9.6 Implementation Outcomes for SEMM-DIA

These outcomes, as described by Proctor et al. (2011), serve as proximal indicators of whether implementation strategies are working and are often necessary precursors to achieving health or behavioral outcomes.

For example, included below are the implementation outcomes for the SEMM-DIA project (Figure 9.6).

Using Implementation Mapping to Guide Evaluation

The earlier tasks in Implementation Mapping provide a strong foundation for evaluation planning. For example:

- Performance objectives developed in Task 2 can be used to assess fidelity by specifying the exact behaviors expected of implementers.
- Determinants and change objectives help identify potential mediators or moderators of implementation success.
- Matrices of change can inform the development of instruments to measure changes in attitudes, skills, or other relevant constructs.

By linking evaluation measures to these earlier planning elements, the planner ensures that the evaluation is theory-informed and aligned with the logic of the implementation strategy.

Designing the Evaluation

Implementation efforts are often complex and occur in dynamic, real-world settings. As such, mixed-methods approaches are especially valuable for evaluating program implementation. Quantitative methods can test hypotheses about relationships between strategies, determinants, and outcomes, while qualitative methods can explore contextual influences, stakeholder experiences, and reasons for success or failure. For example, quantitative tools might include surveys to assess fidelity or adoption rates, while qualitative methods such as interviews or focus groups can uncover barriers, facilitators, and perceptions of feasibility or acceptability. Palinkas et al. (2015) have emphasized the importance of purposeful sampling and integration of qualitative and quantitative data in implementation research, particularly when evaluating multilevel strategies.

Pilot and Feasibility Studies in Implementation Research

Pilot and feasibility studies are key tools for better understanding the acceptability and potential impact of implementation strategies (Bond et al., 2023). These studies allow researchers to test the feasibility, acceptability, and usability of implementation strategies before launching full-scale trials (Bowen et al., 2009). They can also contribute to the iterative refinement of implementation strategies, helping ensure that subsequent trials are both methodologically sound and contextually appropriate.

Although the terms "pilot" and "feasibility" studies are often used interchangeably, they have distinct meanings. A **feasibility study** broadly investigates whether an intervention or strategy can be done, should be done, and how it might be done. It may explore issues such as recruitment, retention, acceptability, or logistical challenges. A **pilot study**, on the other hand, is a specific type of feasibility study that involves conducting a smaller version of a future study—or a component of it—using the same design, procedures, and measures intended for the full trial. Pilot studies are typically more structured and are often used to test the implementation of trial protocols or to simulate the delivery of an intervention or strategy on a limited scale. A pilot study might test whether a training and coaching strategy improves fidelity to a new clinical guideline, while a feasibility study might explore whether the strategy is acceptable to providers and fits within existing workflows.

In implementation science, both types of studies help researchers assess whether a strategy or approach is practical, acceptable, and appropriate for a given context before committing to a full-scale trial. They are particularly valuable for refining strategies, identifying potential barriers, and exploring mechanisms of action in real-world settings. When there is uncertainty about how a strategy will perform in a specific context or with a particular population, these studies can be extremely useful. A pilot study of the Hoosier Sport program, a program to promote physical activity among school-aged youth, found limited in the reproducibility of the training materials and minimal clarity of the valuation process (Major et al., 2025). This led to the addition of a standardized training module to the onboarding process and a modified evaluation plan (Major et al., 2025). Pearson et al. (2020) provide guidance for conducting feasibility and pilot studies in implementation science, emphasizing the importance of aligning study aims with appropriate designs, selecting relevant implementation outcomes, and using mixed methods to capture both process and outcome data.

Pilot studies can be embedded within hybrid effectiveness-implementation trials (especially Type 1 or Type 2) or conducted as standalone exploratory studies. They help refine implementation strategies, assess research methods, and explore potential mechanisms of action. For example, the SEMM-DIA pilot study tested a multilevel implementation support strategy in community health centers, using mixed methods to evaluate fidelity, reach, and sustainability (Savas et al., 2023). Importantly, pilot and feasibility studies should not be used to estimate effect sizes or test hypotheses about intervention efficacy. Instead, they should focus on implementation outcomes and inform the design of future trials. Guidance from Pearson et al. (2020) and the NCCIH (NCCIH, n.d.) emphasizes the importance of aligning pilot study aims with appropriate methods and avoiding common misuses such as underpowered efficacy testing. Embedding pilot studies within hybrid designs (described below and in

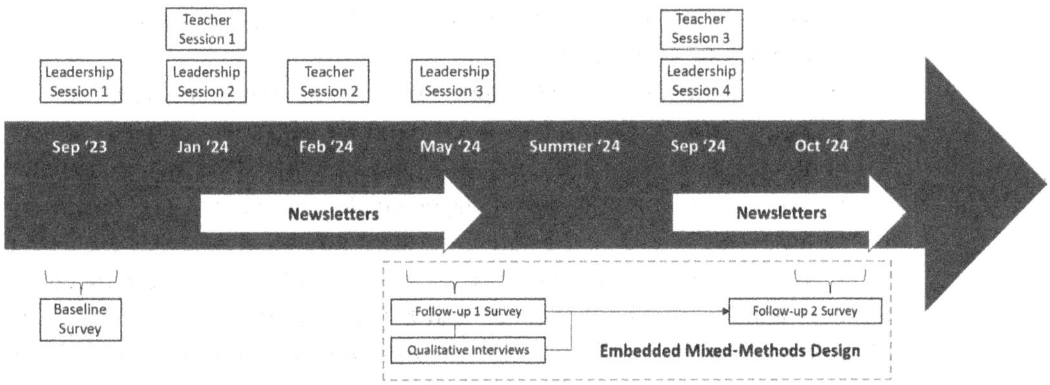

Figure 9.7 MAGIC Study Timeline and Evaluation Plan. Adapted from Walker et al. (2025b)

Chapter 10)—especially Types 1 and 2—can accelerate the development and refinement of implementation strategies.

The MAGIC study, mentioned above, used a mixed-methods design to assess the feasibility and acceptability of MAGIC in one elementary school (Walker et al., 2025b). As shown in Figure 9.7, teachers completed surveys measuring training participation, receipt of newsletters, and perceptions of acceptability. In parallel, researchers conducted interviews with teachers and school leaders to gather qualitative insights into their experiences with the strategy.

Findings showed high levels of engagement with the training sessions and newsletters, and participants reported that the strategy was both feasible and acceptable. Flexible scheduling and integration of training into existing meetings were cited as key facilitators. Teachers also appreciated the practical focus of the training and the simplicity of the newsletters. The results supported further evaluation of MAGIC in additional schools to examine its impact on teacher behavior and student physical activity outcomes.

Hybrid Effectiveness-Implementation Studies

Hybrid effectiveness-implementation studies, described further in Chapter 10, offer an efficient way to evaluate both the effectiveness of an intervention and the strategies used to implement it. Curran et al. (2012, 2022) describe three types of hybrid designs:

1. **Type 1**: Primarily tests intervention effectiveness while gathering information on implementation
2. **Type 2**: Simultaneously tests both intervention effectiveness and implementation strategies
3. **Type 3**: Primarily tests implementation strategies while observing intervention outcomes

These designs allow researchers to explore how strategies function in real-world settings and to gather data on both implementation and clinical outcomes. They are particularly valuable when the goal is to move quickly from research to practice.

Kang and Foster (2022) applied Implementation Mapping to identify implementation determinants, mechanisms of action, implementation strategies, and outcome evaluation plans for "MyGoals," a system designed to support goal setting and management for adults with chronic conditions. To fulfill Task 5, the authors designed a mixed-methods evaluation plan involving occupational therapist–client dyads. Data were gathered on acceptability, feasibility, fidelity, and appropriateness through qualitative interviews and a self-administered survey aligned with previously identified change objectives. The evaluation plan allowed the researchers to assess the degree to which MyGoals was implemented and informed iterative refinements to the strategy. Although the authors noted limitations in relying on self-reported data, the study illustrates how Task 5 can be operationalized in resource-constrained, real-world settings.

FOR OUR CHILDREN EXAMPLE: STEP 5

In Step 5, also referred to as Implementation Mapping (Fernandez et al., 2019), program planners for the ***For Our Children*** or, in Spanish, ***Por Nuestros Hijos (PNH)*** program developed a plan for implementation (adoption, implementation, and maintenance) of the full PNH program (TIMI and fotonovela for parents and HPV Cancer Coach App for providers). They used the Step 5 tasks to develop implementation strategies to enhance the adoption, implementation, and maintenance of the PNH program among Texas primary care practices/clinics (parent and provider component) and community health worker (CHW) organizations (parent component only) that provide health education and facilitate healthcare access, particularly those serving the PNH priority population (Hispanic parents with adolescent children).

Task 1: Conduct a Needs and Assets Assessment and Identify Implementers

In Task 1, program planners conduct (or describe the results of) an implementation-focused needs and assets assessment to determine barriers and facilitators to the program's implementation. They also identify who will decide to adopt the program and who will be responsible for implementing and maintaining the program. For the PNH program, the planners reviewed the theoretical and empirical literature on the dissemination and implementation of clinic-based and CHW-led interventions, conducted key informant interviews and surveys with healthcare providers and community health workers, and consulted with parent and community advisory boards and clinic partners to understand the implementation process. Key decision-makers within healthcare settings and CHW organizations include clinic/agency directors and board members. These individuals were identified as responsible for deciding to adopt as well as to maintain the PNH program components. Regarding individuals responsible for implementation, healthcare providers and CHWs involved in recommending or promoting HPV vaccination would deliver the TIMI and/or fotonovela to parents, while program champions and program coordinators would facilitate training for providers and CHWs and program delivery and maintenance at their respective organizations.

Task 2: Identify Implementation Outcomes, Performance Objectives, and Determinants to Create Matrices of Change

In Task 2, planners first identify program use outcomes for each stage of program delivery (adoption, implementation, and maintenance), the specific tasks (performance objectives) required to achieve these outcomes, and relevant determinants for each performance objective. Then, similar to the procedures in Step 2, they develop a matrix for each adoption, implementation, and maintenance outcome that links performance objectives (row headers) and determinants (column headers) to identified change objectives (cells), or what needs to change in a specific determinant to accomplish associated performance objectives.

First, the PNH program planning group identified outcomes and related performance objectives to facilitate the implementation of all components of the program (see Table 9.5). For adoption of the program, they identified two outcomes (one per type of adopter): *Clinic and agency directors agree to adopt the PNH program to increase HPV vaccination rates in adolescents (11–17 years).* For implementation of the program, four outcomes were identified (one per type of implementer): *Program coordinators (clinic and agency-based), CHWs, and clinic staff will implement the PNH program to increase HPV vaccination rates in adolescents (11–17 years).* For maintenance of the program, two outcomes (one per type of maintainer) were identified: *Clinic/agency directors agree to maintain the PNH program to increase HPV vaccination rates in adolescents (11–17 years), and program coordinators facilitate maintenance of the program.*

The planning group reviewed the literature and conducted qualitative interviews with previous adopters, implementers, and maintainers to identify specific performance objectives or tasks that clinic/agency directors needed to complete to adopt and maintain the program and that program coordinators, CHWs, and clinic staff needed to do to deliver the program with fidelity and/or to maintain it over time. For example, using DOI (Rogers, 2003), they recognized that it was important for potential adopters to assess the relative advantage of PNH compared with current HPV vaccination promotion efforts, and to assess the program's compatibility with existing clinic/agency practices to identify potential barriers to implementation. Guided by the Interactive Systems Framework (Wandersman et al., 2008), they determined that potential implementers would require training, technical assistance, and support to implement the program with fidelity.

Based on their literature review and local research, the planning group identified important and changeable determinants for the adoption, implementation, and maintenance of the PNH program. They found that awareness/knowledge (e.g., awareness of the program's goals and procedural knowledge about how to implement it), outcome expectations or positive attitudes toward program use, and perceived norms were key determinants for program adoption, implementation, and maintenance (Bandura, 1986; Damschroder et al., 2009; Rogers, 2003). Skills and self-efficacy were also critical for program implementation (Bandura, 1986; Damschroder et al., 2009; Peskin et al., 2011; Steckler et al., 1992). The planning group developed a matrix of change objectives for each of the adoption (Tables 9.5 and 9.6), implementation (Tables 9.7–9.10), and maintenance (Tables 9.11 and 9.12) outcomes.

Table 9.5 Partial Matrix for Adoption Outcome: Clinic decision makers will adopt For Our Children, an educational web-based parent and provider Program for FQHCs/clinics to increase HPV vaccination rates in adolescents (11–17 years)

Adoption	**Determinants**				
Performance Objective	**Knowledge/Awareness**	**Skills and Self-efficacy**	**Attitudes**	**Perceived Norms**	**Outcome Expectations**
PO1. The Clinic Director decides to use the **For Our Children** web-based program (parent & provider component).	K.1.a. State the difference between current HPV vaccination rates for Hispanic adolescents and the Healthy People 2030 goals. K.1.b. Describe that the **For Our Children** program, including the provider component **HPV Cancer Coach**, is available at no cost. K.1.c. Recognize that the **For Our Children** program is culturally appropriate for Hispanics. K.1.d. Recognize that **HPV Cancer Coach** is a useful tool for providers. K.1.e. Recognize that the **For Our Children** program will provide resources for the clinic. K.1.f. Describe the program as an evidence-based educational program for parents and providers that was shown to be effective in increasing HPV vaccination rates. K.1.g. Describe the program as a tool for increasing provider's knowledge on HPV vaccination guidelines and recommendation techniques. K.1.h. Describe the program as a tool for increasing HPV vaccination initiation and completion rates among adolescents (11–17 years).	SSE.1.a. Demonstrate the ability to work with the UTHealth research team to start the implementation process. SSE.1.b. Identify a program champion within the clinic to oversee the implementation of the program. SSE.1.c. Demonstrate the ability to identify the necessary resources required to implement the program.	A.1.a. Believe the program will increase HPV vaccination rates among Hispanic adolescents served by the clinic. A.1.b. Believe the program will increase provider knowledge and improve recommendation practices. A.1.c. Believe that the program will improve upon the current HPV vaccination practice. A.1.d. Believe that the program fits with organizational priorities. A.1.e. Believe that the program will be adopted and implemented with minimal risk/changes.	PN.1.a. Recognize that other clinics are prioritizing HPV vaccination for Hispanic adolescents (11–17 years). PN.1.b. Recognize that other clinics are effectively using this program to promote vaccination among Hispanic adolescents. PN.1.c. Recognize that other clinics are following recommended guidelines for HPV vaccination among adolescents aged 11–17.	OE.1.a. Expect that implementing the program will increase HPV vaccination rates among Hispanic adolescents (11–17 years) served by the clinic. OE.1.b. Expect that implementing the program will improve provider recommendations for HPV vaccination.

PO2. Clinic director/medical director obtains administrative approval.	K.2.a Describe the clinic's program approval guidelines. K.2.b. Describe the clinic's management and organizational scheme. K.2.c. Describe health insurance protocols. K.2.d. Explain budget availability. K.2.e. Explain disbursement protocol. K.2.f. Explain budget restrictions. K.2.g. Describe the clinic's need to increase HPV vaccination rates. K.2.h. Describe the clinic's need to improve provider HPV vaccine recommendations.	SSE.2. Demonstrate that approval for the program can be obtained.	A.2.a. Believe that the clinic has the capacity to implement the program. A.2.b. Believe that the program aligns with the clinic's vaccination protocols and goals.	PN.2. Describe other clinics as having successfully implemented the program.	OE.2.a. Recognize that the program is a tool that will help them attain the Healthy People 2030 goals. OE.2.b. Recognize that the program is a tool that will facilitate HPV vaccination goals for Hispanic adolescent patients. OE.2.c. Recognize that the **HPV Cancer Coach** is a tool that will help clinic providers improve HPV vaccination recommendations
PO3. Clinic director/medical director obtains staff buy-in.	K.3.a. Demonstrate the availability of staff capable of implementing the program. K.3.b. Identify the staff, Community group and/or Community Health Worker (CHW) that will be trained to conduct the program **For Our Children**, if the clinic staff is not available. K.3.c. Identify the clinical staff who will receive the **HPV Cancer Coach** training and tool. K.3.d. Describe the support that staff will have for the implementation of the program.	SSE.3.a. Express confidence to promote the program among the staff. SSE.3.b. Express confidence to promote the collaboration between the clinical staff and CHWs implementing the program.	A.3.a. Feel favorable about the clinic staff's capabilities to implement the program. A.3.b. Feel favorable about the community group's capabilities to implement the program. A.3.c. Feel favorable about the CHW's capabilities to implement the program. A.3.d. Feel favorable about the collaboration capabilities between the staff and the Community group or CHW's to implement the program.	PN.3.a. Recognize that the clinic staff sees the need to increase HPV vaccination rates in their clinic. PN.3.b. Recognize that the clinic staff sees the value of having tools to improve HPV vaccine recommendations for clinic patients. PN.3.c. Describe other clinics as using Community/Lay Health Workers to implement programs successfully when clinic staff are unavailable.	OE.3.a. Expect that staff will consider the program as a value add to clinic services. OE.3.b. Expect that staff will accept and take ownership of program implementation. OE.3.c. Expect that collaboration between clinical staff and CHWs will facilitate program implementation. OE.3.d. Expect that greater staff buy-in will lead to successful implementation.

(continued)

Table 9.5 (*Continued*)

Adoption	Determinants				
Performance Objective	**Knowledge/Awareness**	**Skills and Self-efficacy**	**Attitudes**	**Perceived Norms**	**Outcome Expectations**
P04. Clinic director identifies program champion to oversee implementation.	K.4.a. Describe the responsibilities and importance of a program champion. K.4.b. Describe the qualities of an effective program champion. K.4.c. Describe where and how to recruit a program champion.	SSE.4.a. Demonstrate the ability to recruit an effective program champion. SSE.4.b. Express confidence in being able to provide the necessary support to the program champion.	A.4.a. Believe that a program champion is necessary to ensure program implementation. A.4.b. Describe the program champion as a necessary and important part of implementation.	PN.4. Recognize that the program champion has been a necessary and important part of implementation in other clinics.	OE.4.a. Expect that the program champion can effectively implement and maintain the program. OE.4.b. Expect that the program champion can effectively engage staff or Community/Lay Health workers in actively identifying and recruiting participants. OE.4.c. Expect that the program champion can effectively engage clinical staff to use the **HPV Cancer Coach** tool. OE.4.d. Expect that the program champion can effectively manage the resources provided.
P05. Clinic director budgets the program into clinic operations.	K.5.a. Identify current budget. K.5.b. Describe budgetary needs of the program. K.5.c. Describes how to integrate the program's costs to the clinic's budget processes. K.5.d. Identify potential funding sources for the program.	SSE.5.a. Demonstrate the ability to procure necessary funds to implement the program. SSE.5.b. Expresses how program costs can be justified within the clinic's budget. SSE.5.c. Procures necessary funds.	A.5. Feel favorable about allocating necessary funds for the program.	PN.5. Recognize that other clinics have included the program as part of their budget.	OE.5. Recognize that appropriate budget allocation will result in successful program implementation and an increase in HPV vaccination

Table 9.6 Partial Matrix for Adoption Outcome: Agency decision makers will adopt For Our Children, an educational web-based parent and provider program for community-based agencies, to increase HPV vaccination rates in adolescents (11–17 years)

Adoption	**Determinants**				
Performance Objective	**Knowledge/Awareness**	**Skills and Self-efficacy**	**Attitudes**	**Perceived Norms**	**Outcome Expectations**
P01. Agency director decides to use the parent component of the **For Our Children** program.	K.1.a. State current HPV vaccination rates for Hispanic adolescents aged 11–17 years served by their agency. K.1.b. Recognize that the **For Our Children** program is culturally appropriate. K.1.c. Recognize that this program is available at no cost. K.1.d. Recognize that the program will provide resources to the community that it serves. K.1.e. Describe the program as an evidence-based educational program for Hispanic parents that is effective in increasing HPV vaccination rates among adolescents aged 11–17 years. K.1.f. Describe the program as a tool for increasing HPV vaccination initiation and completion rates among Hispanic adolescents (11–17 years) in the community they serve.	SSE.1.a. Express confidence in the ability to implement the program within the agency. SSE.1.b. Demonstrate the ability to work with the clinic to implement the program. SSE.1.c. Demonstrate the ability to identify the necessary resources required to implement the program.	A.1.a. Believe the program will increase HPV vaccination rates among Hispanic adolescents within the community served by the agency. A.1.b. Believe the program will improve upon current practice. A.1.c. Believe that the program fits with the agency's organizational priorities. A.1.d. Believe the program adds value to current services. A.1.e. Believe that the program will be adopted and implemented with minimal risk/changes.	PN.1.a. Recognize that HPV vaccination is recommended for adolescents aged 11 – 17 years. PN.1.b. Recognize that other agencies as effectively using this program to promote vaccination among Hispanic adolescents. PN.1.c. Recognize that other agencies are effectively collaborating with clinics to promote vaccination among Hispanic adolescents. PN.1.d. Recognize that other agencies are following recommended guidelines for HPV vaccination in adolescents.	OE.1.a. Expect that implementing the program will improve staff's knowledge of HPV vaccination. OE.1.b. Expect that implementing the program will increase HPV vaccination rates among Hispanic adolescents (11–17 years) served by the agency.

(*continued*)

Table 9.6 *(Continued)*

Adoption	Determinants				
Performance Objective	**Knowledge/Awareness**	**Skills and Self-efficacy**	**Attitudes**	**Perceived Norms**	**Outcome Expectations**
PO2. Agency director obtains administrative approval.	K.2.a. Describe the agency's program approval guidelines. K.2.b. Describe the agency's management and organizational scheme. K.2.c. Explain budget availability. K.2.d. Explain disbursement protocol. K.2.e. Explain budget restrictions. K.2.f. Describe the agency's need to improve knowledge of HPV vaccine recommendations to improve vaccination rates. K.2.g. Describe the agency's need to increase HPV vaccination rates.	SSE.2. Demonstrate that approval for the program can be obtained.	A.2.a. Believe that the agency has the capacity to implement the program. A.2.b. Believe that the program aligns with the agency's goals. A.2.c. Believe that the program will solidify the agency's collaboration with the clinic.	PN.2. Describe other community-based organizations as having successfully implemented the program.	OE.2.a. Recognize that the program is a tool that will help them attain the Healthy People 2030 goals. OE.2.b. Recognize that the program is a tool that will facilitate HPV vaccination goals for Hispanic adolescent patients. OE.2.c. Recognize that the program will help agency staff improve HPV vaccination knowledge.
PO3. Agency director obtains staff and community buy-in.	K.3.a. Recognize the availability of Community/Lay Health Workers capable of implementing the program. K.3.b. Identify Community/Lay Health Workers that will be trained to facilitate program delivery. K.3.c. Describe how the agency will support Community/Lay Health Workers in delivering the program. K.3.d. Reflect that involving community leaders in planning will help develop a program that communities will accept.	SSE.3.a. Express confidence in promoting the program to staff who will be involved in implementation. SSE.3.b. Express confidence to work with the community to facilitate program implementation.	A.3.a. Feel favorable about the agency's Community/Lay Health Workers' capabilities to implement the program. A.3.b. Describe Community/Lay Health Workers as a resource to build ties to the community. A.3.c. Describe Community/Lay Health Workers as a credible source of health information.	PN.3.a. Recognize that Community Health Workers see the need to increase HPV vaccination rates in the communities they serve. PN.3.b. Describe other agencies that use Community/Lay Health Workers to implement the program successfully.	OE.3.a. Expect that the Community/Lay Health Worker will consider the program as a value add to the services they provide. OE.3.b. Expect the Community/Lay Health Worker to accept and take ownership of program implementation. OE.3.c. Expect that collaboration between the agency's and the clinic's staff will facilitate program implementation. OE.3.d. Expect that greater Community/Lay Health Worker staff buy-in will lead to successful implementation.

PO4. Agency director identifies a program coordinator to support implementation.	K.4.a. Describe the responsibilities and importance of a program coordinator. K.4.b. Describe the qualities of an effective program coordinator. K.4.c. Describe where and how to recruit a program coordinator.	SSE.4.a. Demonstrate the ability to recruit an effective program coordinator. SSE.4.b. Express confidence in being able to provide the necessary support to the program champion.	A.4.a. Believe that a program coordinator is necessary to ensure program implementation. A.4.b. Describe the program coordinator as a necessary and important part of implementation.	PN.4. Recognize that the program coordinator has been a necessary and important part of implementation in other agencies.	OE.4.a. Expect that the program coordinator can effectively implement and maintain the program. OE.4.b. Expect that the program coordinator can effectively engage staff in actively identifying and recruiting participants. OE.4.c. Expect that the program coordinator can effectively promote collaboration with clinical staff in implementing the program. OE.4.d. Expect that the program coordinator can effectively manage the resources provided.
PO5. Agency director budgets the program into agency operations.	K.5.a. Identify current budget. K.5.b. Describe budgetary needs of the program. K.5.c. Describes how to integrate the program's costs to the agency's budget processes. K.5.d. Identify potential funding sources for the program.	SSE.5.a. Demonstrate the ability to procure necessary funds to implement the program. SSE.5.b. Expresses how program costs can be justified within the agency's budget. SSE.5.c. Procures necessary funds.	A.5. Feel favorable about allocating necessary funds for the program.	PN.5. Recognize that other Community/Lay Health Worker agency directors have included the program in their budgets.	OE.5. Recognize that appropriate budget allocation will result in successful program implementation and an increase in vaccination completion rates.

Table 9.7 Partial Matrix for Implementation Outcome: Program Champion (Health Service) implements For Our Children, an educational web-based parent and provider program for FQHCs/clinics, to increase HPV vaccination rates in adolescents (11–17 years)

Implementation	**Determinants**				
Performance Objective	**Knowledge/Awareness**	**Skills and Self-efficacy**	**Attitudes**	**Perceived Norms**	**Outcome Expectations**
P01. Program Champion identifies resources required to implement the **For Our Children** program (parent and provider component)	K.1.a. List resources required to implement the parent and provider components of the program. K.1.b. Describe the process for allocating resources to the parent and provider components of the program. K.1.c. Describe Organizational Readiness to implement the parent and provider components of the program.	SSE.1.a. Demonstrate ability to identify resources required to implement the parent and provider components of the program. SSE.1.b. Demonstrate skills to allocate resources required for the implementation of the parent and provider components of the program. SSE.1.c. Demonstrate the ability to assess Organizational Readiness using the checklist provided.	A.1.a. Express confidence in obtaining the resources needed to implement the parent and provider components of the program. A.1.b. Express confidence in the clinic's organizational capacity to implement the parent and provider components of the program.	PN.1. Recognize that other clinics have allocated resources to implement the parent and provider components of the program.	OE.1.a. Expect that allocating resources will enable the clinic to implement the parent and provider components of the program effectively. OE.1.b. Expect that allocating resources will improve providers' HPV vaccination recommendations. OE.1.c. Expect that allocating resources will contribute to increasing HPV vaccination rates among Hispanic adolescents.
P2. Program Champion identifies staff to implement the **For Our Children** program.	K.2.a. Describe the capabilities that CHWs and/or clinical staff (e.g., RNs, MAs) require to implement the program K.2.b. Identify existing CHWs and clinical staff (e.g., RNs, MAs) to implement FOC K.2.c. Describe the process for recruiting additional CHWs or staff to implement the program (if required).	SSE.2.a. Demonstrate the ability to identify existing staff to implement the program SSE.2.b. Demonstrate the ability to recruit additional staff to implement the program (if required).	A.2.a. Express confidence in identifying existing and staff A.2.b. Express confidence in recruiting staff to implement the program.	PN.2. Recognize that other program champions are involved in identifying and recruiting staff to deliver health education programs.	OE.2. Expect that identifying and recruiting staff to deliver the program will facilitate the successful implementation of the program.

P03. Program Champion designates time for staff to complete program training.	K.3.a. List dates and times when training will be conducted and the staff K.3.b. Lists resources required to conduct training. K.3.c. Describe the importance of delivering training before program implementation.	SSE.3.a. Demonstrates the ability to schedule training times within the clinic's schedule and workflow. SSE.3.b. Demonstrates the ability to identify and allocate resources required for the program training. SSE.3.c. Demonstrates the capacity for the staff to attend training.	A.3. Express confidence that the training session will help staff to implement the program effectively.	PN.3. Recognize that other program champions support staff to participate in training programs.	OE.3.a. Expect that by attending training, staff will be able to increase their knowledge of HPV vaccination guidelines and provider recommendations. OE.3.b. Expect that by attending training, staff will be able to successfully implement the program and increase HPV vaccination rates among Hispanic adolescents.
P04. Program Champion participates in program training.	K.4.a. List dates and times when the training session will be implemented. K.4.b. Describe the importance of participating in the training before program implementation.	SSE.4. Express confidence in attending the training session.	A.4.a. Believe the training session will assist them to implement and coordinate the program. A.4.b. Believe the training session will provide them with the tools to improve HPV vaccination rates among the adolescent population they serve.	PN.4. Recognize that other program champions are participating in the training session.	OE.4. Expect that by completing the training, they will be able to successfully coordinate the program and increase HPV vaccination rates in Hispanic adolescents.
P05. Program Champion supports the identification and recruitment of eligible patients to participate in the program.	K.5.a. Describe the target audience for the program. K.5.b. Describe protocols for identifying, contacting, and recruiting eligible patients using patient records.	SSE.5.a. Demonstrates ability to describe the target audience. SSE.5.b. Demonstrates skills to identify, contact, and recruit eligible clients using patient records. SSE.5.c. Demonstrates ability to support staff in implementing effective recruiting strategies	A.5. Expresses confidence in identifying and recruiting eligible patients to participate.	PN.5. Recognizes that other clinics use patient records to identify patients who will benefit from health education initiatives.	OE.5. Expect that identifying and recruiting eligible patients will increase participation in the program, thereby increasing HPV vaccination rates.

(continued)

Table 9.7 (*Continued*)

Implementation	Determinants				
Performance Objective	**Knowledge/Awareness**	**Skills and Self-efficacy**	**Attitudes**	**Perceived Norms**	**Outcome Expectations**
PO6. Program Champion supports CHWs and clinical staff (e.g., RNs, MAs) to implement the program.	K.6.a. Describes proper protocols for program implementation. K.6.b. Describes role in coordinating the program and supporting staff to implement the program.	SSE.6.a. Demonstrates skills to implement the program according to protocols. SSE.6.b. Demonstrate skills in managing staff who are implementing the program. SSE.6.c. Demonstrate the ability to support staff in implementing the program. SSE.6.d. Demonstrate the ability to problem-solve issues faced by staff when implementing the program	A.6.a. Feels confident in their ability to support staff in implementing the program as per protocols. A.6.b. Feels confident in their ability to manage staff in implementing the program. A.6.c. Feels confident in their problem-solving abilities.	PSN.6. Recognizes that other clinics provide constant support to staff during program implementation.	OE.6. Expect that supporting staff to deliver the program will ensure the program is delivered effectively and with fidelity.
PO7. Program Champion monitors program implementation and reports findings to UTHealth.	K.7.a. Describes the process for monitoring program implementation. K.7.b. Describe the process for collating program data. K.7.c. Describes the process for reporting data to UTHealth.	SSE.7.a. Demonstrates ability to utilize tracking templates to monitor program implementation SSE.7.b. Demonstrates ability to collate data. SSE.7.c. Demonstrates the ability to timely report data on program reach and effectiveness to UTHealth.	A.7.a. Feels confident in their ability to use tracking templates to monitor program implementation. A.7.b. Feels confident in their ability to collate data required for program evaluation. A.7.c. Feels confident in their ability to report data to UTHealth	PSN.7.a. Recognizes the importance of evaluating programs to monitor program reach and effectiveness. PSN.7.b. Recognizes the importance of program monitoring to identify areas for improvement. PSN.7.c. Recognizes the importance of reporting to UTHealth to facilitate program implementation, quality, and support.	OE.7.a. Expects that program evaluation can be used to monitor the reach and effectiveness of the program OE.7.b. Expects that program evaluation facilitates the identification of opportunities to improve program delivery. OE.7.c. Expects that reporting program findings to UTHealth facilitates program implementation quality and support.

Table 9.8 Partial Matrix for Implementation Outcome: Program Coordinator (agency/CHW organization) will implement For Our Children, an educational web-based parent and provider program for community-based agencies, to increase HPV vaccination rates in adolescents (11–17 years)

Implementation	Determinants				
Performance Objective	**Knowledge/Awareness**	**Skills and Self-efficacy**	**Attitudes**	**Perceived Norms**	**Outcome Expectations**
PO1. Program coordinator identifies resources required to implement the **For Our Children** parent component.	K.1.a. Lists resources required to implement the parent component of the program K.1.b. Describes the process of allocating resources. K.1.c. Describes organizational Readiness to implement the parent component.	SSE.1.a. Demonstrates ability to identify and allocate resources required to implement the parent component of the program. SSE.1.b. Demonstrates ability to assess Organizational Readiness using the checklist provided.	A.1.a. Express confidence in obtaining and allocating the resources needed to implement the parent component. A.1.b. Express confidence in the organization's ability to implement the parent component.	PN.1. Recognize that other agencies have allocated resources to implement the parent component.	OE.1.a. Expect that allocating resources will enable the agency to implement the parent component effectively. OE.1.b. Expect that allocating resources will contribute to increasing HPV vaccination rates among Hispanic adolescents.
PO2. Program coordinator identifies staff members to implement the parent component.	K.2.a. Describes the capabilities CHWs require to implement the parent component. K.2.b. Describe the role of CHWs in implementing the parent component. K.2.c. Identify existing CHWs to implement the program. K.2.d. Describes process for recruiting additional CHWs (if required).	SSE.2.a. Demonstrates skills to identify existing CHWs to implement the parent component. SSE.2.b. Demonstrates skills to recruit additional CHWs to implement the parent component (if required).	A.2.a. Express confidence in identifying existing CHWs to implement the parent component. A.2.b. Express confidence in recruiting CHWs to implement the parent component.	PN.2. Recognize that other program coordinators are involved in identifying and recruiting CHWs to deliver health education programs.	OE.2. Expect that identifying and recruiting CHWs to implement the program will facilitate successful implementation.

(*continued*)

Table 9.8 *(Continued)*

Implementation	Determinants				
Performance Objective	**Knowledge/Awareness**	**Skills and Self-efficacy**	**Attitudes**	**Perceived Norms**	**Outcome Expectations**
P03. Program Coordinator designates time for CHWs to complete program training.	K.3.a. List dates and times when training will be conducted for CHWs K.3.b. Lists resources required to conduct training. K.3.c. List ways to support CHWs to participate in training. K.3.d. Describe the importance of delivering training before program implementation.	SSE.3.a. Demonstrates the ability to schedule training times within the agency's schedule and workflow. SSE.3.b. Demonstrates ability to identify and allocate resources required for the program training. SSE.3.c. Demonstrates ability to support CHWs and staff to attend training.	A.3.a. Express confidence that the training session will help CHWs to implement the parent component effectively.	PN.3. Recognize that other program coordinators support CHWs to participate in training programs.	OE.3. Expect that by attending training, CHWs will be able to successfully implement the parent component of the program and increase HPV vaccination rates among the Hispanic adolescents they serve.
P04. Program Coordinator participates in program training.	K.4.a. List dates and times when the training session will be implemented. K.4.b. Describe the importance of participating in the training before program implementation.	SSE.4. Express confidence in attending the training session.	A.4.a. Believe the training session will assist them to implement and coordinate the program. A.4.b. Believe the training session will provide them with the tools to improve HPV vaccination rates among the adolescent population they serve.	PN.4. Recognize that other program coordinators are participating in the training session.	OE.4. Expect that by completing the training, they will be able to successfully coordinate the program and increase HPV vaccination rates in Hispanic adolescents.
P05. Program Coordinator identifies local FQHCs/ health clinics that provide HPV vaccination services.	K.5.a. Identify clinics that provide HPV vaccination services for the target population. K.5.b. Describe the process for establishing referral pathways to local health services that provide HPV vaccination.	SSE.5.a. Demonstrate ability to identify local health services that provide HPV vaccination services. SSE.5.b. Express confidence in documenting referral pathways to local health services that provide HPV vaccination services.	A.5. Believe that locating local health services that provide the HPV vaccine and establishing referral pathways is important to the success of the program.	PN.5. Recognizes that other agencies have established referral pathways to local health services that provide the HPV vaccine.	OE.5. Expect that identifying local HPV vaccination services and establishing referral pathways will support the agency to deliver the program and increase HPV vaccination rates.

PO6. Program Coordinator supports program implementation.	K.6.a. Describes proper protocols for program implementation. K.6.b. Describes role in coordinating the program and supporting CHWs to implement the program.	SSE.6.a. Demonstrate ability to implement the program according to protocols. SSE.6.b. Demonstrate skills in managing CHWs implementing the program. SSE.6.c. Demonstrate the ability to support CHWs to implement the program. SSE.6.d. Demonstrate the ability to problem-solve issues faced by CHWs when implementing the program	A.6.a. Express confidence in the ability to support CHWs to implement the program as per protocols. A.6.b. Demonstrate ability to manage and support CHWs implementing the program. A.6.c. Feels confident in their problem-solving abilities.	PN.6. Recognizes that other program coordinators provide constant support to staff during program implementation.	OE.6. Expect that supporting the CHWs to implement the program will result in increased HPV vaccination rates.
PO7. Program Coordinator monitors the program implementation and reports findings to UTHealth.	K.7.a. Describe the process for monitoring program implementation K.7.b. Describe the process for collating program data. K.7.c. Describe the process for reporting data to UTHealth.	SSE.7.a. Demonstrates ability to monitor program implementation using tracking templates. SSE.7.b. Demonstrates ability to collate data. SSE.7.c. Demonstrates ability to report data on program reach and effectiveness to UTHealth.	A.7.a. Expresses confidence in their ability to monitor program implementation. A.7.b. Expresses confidence to collate data required for program evaluation. A.7.c. Expresses confidence in their ability to report data to UTHealth using templates provided.	PN.7.a. Recognizes the importance of evaluating programs to monitor program reach and effectiveness. PN.7.b. Recognizes the importance of program monitoring to identify areas for improvement. PN.7.c. Recognizes the importance of reporting to UTHealth to facilitate program implementation, quality, and support.	OE.7.a. Expects that program evaluation can be used to monitor the reach and effectiveness of the program OE.7.b. Expects that program evaluation facilitates the identification of opportunities to improve program delivery. OE.7.c. Expects that reporting program findings to UTHealth facilitates program implementation quality and support.

Table 9.9 Partial Matrix for Implementation Outcome: Community Health Workers in FQHCs/clinics will implement For Our Children, an educational web-based parent and provider program for FQHCs/clinics, to increase HPV vaccination rates in adolescents (11–17 years)

Implementation	**Determinants**				
Performance Objectives	**Knowledge**	**Skills and Self-efficacy**	**Attitudes/Beliefs**	**Perceived Social Norms**	**Outcome Expectations**
P01. Community Health Workers (CHWs) participate in the **For Our Children** parent component program training.	K.1.a. List dates and times when the training sessions will be implemented. K.1.b. Describe the importance of participating in the training before program implementation.	SSE.1. Express confidence in attending the training session.	A.1.a. Believe the training session will assist them in using the educational materials for parents (TIMI app, fotonovela, and other educational resources) to improve HPV vaccination rates. A.1.b. Believe the training session will assist them in implementing the program effectively.	PSN.1. Recognize that other community health workers are participating in the training session.	OE.1. Expect that by completing the training, they will be able to successfully implement the program and increase HPV vaccination rates in Hispanic adolescents.
P01. CHWs identify eligible parents and recruit them to participate in the program.	K.2.a. Describe how to identify Hispanic parents with adolescent children who are due for or haven't completed their HPV vaccination series, either by using the clinic's EMR system or by clinician referral. K.2.b. Describe strategies to promote the program to parents with adolescent children who are due for or haven't completed their HPV vaccination series. K.2.c. Describe strategies for recruiting parents to participate in the program. K.2.d. List eligibility requirements such as the child's age and vaccination status.	SSE.2.a. Demonstrate ability to identify and locate Hispanic parents with adolescents in the clinic. SSE.2.b. Demonstrate the ability to use the clinic's EMR and/or communicate effectively with clinicians. SSE.2.c. Demonstrate the ability to promote the program to Hispanic parents. SSE.2.d. Demonstrates the ability to recruit Hispanic parents to participate in the program. SSE.2.e. Demonstrate the ability to identify eligible participants within the recruited parents.	A.2.a. Express confidence in identifying and recruiting parents to participate in the program. A.2.b. Express confidence in their ability to use the clinic's EMR and/or to effectively communicate with clinicians. A.2.c. Believe that parents will benefit from participating in the program.	PSN.2. Recognize that other community health workers are recruiting parents to participate in the program to increase HPV vaccination rates.	OE.2. Expect that identifying and recruiting parents using CHWs to implement the program will facilitate successful implementation.

PO3. CHWs collaborate with clinicians to promote the program and recruit parents to participate (when CHWs don't have access to the clinic's EMR)	K.3.1.a. Describe the clinic workflow and how CHWs can engage with clinicians for parent referrals. K.3.1.b. Describe how clinicians can assist CHWs in identifying parents with adolescent children who are due for or haven't completed their HPV vaccination series. K.3.1.c. Describe how parents with adolescent children who are due for or haven't completed their HPV vaccination series will be contacted and recruited by CHWs.	SSE.3.a. Demonstrate the ability to engage and collaborate with clinicians. SSE.3.b. Demonstrate the ability to contact and promote the program. SSE.3.c. Demonstrate skills to recruit referred parents.	A.3. Believe that collaborating with clinicians is an effective way of promoting the program and recruiting parents to participate.	PSN.3. Recognize that other community/lay health workers collaborate with clinicians to promote health education programs.	OE.3. Expect that collaborating with clinicians will increase participation in the program.
PO4. Deliver education sessions to parents using program materials.	K.4.a. Describe the protocol for delivering education sessions effectively and with fidelity. K.4.b. Describes how to use program materials (TIMI and fotonovela) to educate parents about HPV and motivate them to vaccinate their adolescent children. K.4.c. Describe communication strategies to address common parental concerns and barriers.	SSE.4.a. Demonstrate skills to deliver the intervention with fidelity. SSE.4.b. Demonstrate skills to educate parents about HPV and HPV vaccination using program resources. SSE.4.c. Demonstrate the ability to address parental barriers regarding HPV vaccination using communication strategies and program resources.	A.4. Express confidence in the ability to educate parents about HPV using program materials and motivate them to vaccinate their adolescent children.	PSN.4. Recognize that other community health workers are implementing the program to educate parents about HPV using program materials and to increase HPV vaccination rates at their clinics.	OE.4. Expect that delivering the program with fidelity will motivate parents to vaccinate their adolescent children against HPV.

(*continued*)

Table 9.9 (*Continued*)

Implementation	Determinants				
Performance Objectives	**Knowledge**	**Skills and Self-efficacy**	**Attitudes/Beliefs**	**Perceived Social Norms**	**Outcome Expectations**
PO5. CHWs assist parents in scheduling HPV vaccination services at the clinic.	K.5.a. Describe the process for assisting parents in scheduling HPV vaccination services at the clinic. K.5.b. Describe the financial support available to parents to pay for the HPV vaccine at the clinic.	SSE.5.a. Demonstrate ability to locate the staff or system needed to coordinate HPV vaccination scheduling at the clinic. SSE.5.b. Demonstrate skills required to refer parents or navigate parents to HPV vaccination scheduling services. SSE.5.c. Demonstrate ability to provide parents with information about financial support services to pay for the HPV vaccine.	A.5. Express confidence in referring and/or navigating parents to HPV vaccination scheduling services located within their clinic.	PSN.5. Recognize that other community health workers refer and/or navigate parents to HPV vaccination scheduling services and provide information on financial support for vaccines.	OE.5. Expect that referring or navigating parents to HPV vaccination scheduling services and providing them with information about financial support will increase HPV vaccination rates.
PO6. CHWs follow up with parents to ensure initiation and completion of the vaccine series.	K.6.a. Describe the HPV vaccination guidelines for each age group. K.6.b. Describe communication strategies to address parental concerns and barriers to HPV vaccination. K.6.c. Describe the process for following up with parents to ensure initiation and completion of the HPV vaccine series.	SSE.6.a. Express the methods (phone calls, emails, texts, and/or reminder cards) used by the clinic to follow up with parents. SSE.6.b. Demonstrate the ability to address common parental concerns or barriers that may impede HPV vaccination. SSE.6.c. Demonstrate skills to facilitate HPV vaccination appointments. SSE.6.d. Demonstrate skills to follow-up with parents to ensure initiation and completion of the vaccine series	A.6. Express confidence in following up with patients to ensure initiation and completion of the vaccine series.	PSN.6. Recognize that other CHWs follow up with parents to increase HPV vaccination initiation and completion.	OE.6. Expect that following up with parents will increase HPV vaccination initiation and completion rates.

P07. CHWs record and report interactions with Hispanic parents to monitor program reach and effectiveness.	K.7.a. Lists the type of interactions that need to be recorded, such as education sessions, referrals, vaccination appointments, and parent follow-up. K.7.b. Describe how to monitor program implementation using the tracking template provided. K.7.c. Describe how to address data recording and reporting issues to the Program Champion. K.7.d. Describe how to report data collected to the Program Champion.	SSE.7.a. Demonstrate the ability to use a tracking template to keep records. SSE.7.b. Demonstrates ability to address data recording and reporting issues. SSE.7.c. Demonstrate the ability to report data to the program champion.	A.7.a. Express confidence in monitoring program implementation using tracking templates. A.7.b. Believe that documenting interactions is important for monitoring program reach and effectiveness.	PSN.7. Recognize that other community/lay health workers keep records and report activity to program coordinators.	OE.7.a. Expect that recording interactions contributes to the identification of gaps in program implementation. OE.7.b. Expect that continued monitoring and evaluation will contribute to improved program implementation.

Table 9.10 Partial Matrix for Implementation Outcome: Clinic staff (Physicians, Physician Assistants, RNs, MAs) will implement For Our Children, an educational web-based parent and provider program for FQHCs/clinics, to increase HPV vaccination rates in adolescents (11–17 Years)

Implementation	**Determinants**				
Performance Objectives	**Knowledge**	**Skills and Self-efficacy**	**Attitudes/Beliefs**	**Perceived Social Norms**	**Outcome Expectations**
PO1. Clinic staff participate in the **For Our Children** program training (provider and parent component).	K.1.a. List dates and times when the training sessions will be implemented. K.1.b. Describe the importance of participating in the training before program implementation.	SSE.1.a. Express confidence in attending the training session.	A.1.a. Believe the training session will assist them in using the educational materials for parents (TIMI app, fotonovela, and other educational resources) to improve HPV vaccination rates. A.1.b. Believe the training session will guide them to use provider education resources, including the **HPV Cancer Coach** app, and other clinic resources to improve HPV vaccination rates. A.1.c. Believe the training session will assist them in implementing the program effectively.	PSN.1. Recognize that other staff members are participating in the training session.	OE.1.a. Expect that by completing the training, they will be able to successfully implement the parent component of the program and increase HPV vaccination rates in Hispanic adolescents. OE.1.b. Expect that by completing the training, they will be able to successfully use the **HPV Cancer Coach** app and other clinic resources to increase HPV knowledge and skills needed to effectively recommend HPV vaccination and increase vaccination rates in Hispanic adolescents.
PO2. Clinic staff identify eligible parents using EMR data and recruit them to participate in the program.	K.2.a. Describe how to identify Hispanic parents with adolescent children in the clinic they serve who are due for or haven't completed their HPV vaccination series. K.2.b. Describe strategies to promote the program to parents with adolescent children who are due for or haven't completed their HPV vaccination series. K.2.c. Describe strategies for recruiting parents of children who are due for or haven't completed their HPV vaccination series to participate in the program.	SSE.2.a. Demonstrate ability to identify and locate Hispanic parents with adolescent children who are due for or haven't completed their HPV vaccination series in the clinic served. SSE.2.b. Demonstrate the ability to promote the program to eligible Hispanic parents. SSE.2.c. Demonstrate the ability to recruit eligible Hispanic parents to participate in the program.	A.2.a. Express confidence in identifying and recruiting parents to participate in the program. A.2.b. Believe that parents will benefit from participating in the program.	PSN.2. Recognize that other clinic staff are recruiting parents to participate in the program to increase HPV vaccination rates.	OE.2. Expect that identifying and recruiting parents using the EMR data will facilitate successful implementation.

PO3. Clinic staff deliver education sessions to parents using program materials.	K.3.a. Describe the protocol for delivering a parent education session effectively and with fidelity. K.3.b. Describe how to use program materials (HPV Cancer Coach app, TIMI, and fotonovela) to educate parents about HPV and motivate them to vaccinate their adolescent children. K.3.c. List the communication strategies to address common parental concerns and barriers.	SSE.3.a. Demonstrate skills to deliver the intervention with fidelity. SSE.3.b. Demonstrate skills to educate parents about HPV and HPV vaccination using program resources. SSE.3.c. Demonstrate the ability to address parental barriers regarding HPV vaccination using communication strategies and program resources.	A.3.a. Express confidence in the ability to educate parents about HPV using program materials. A.3.b. Express confidence in the ability to motivate parents of children who are due for or haven't completed their HPV vaccination series to vaccinate their adolescent children.	PSN.3. Recognize that other clinic staff are implementing the program to educate parents about HPV using program materials and to increase HPV vaccination rates.	OE.3.a. Expect that delivering the program with fidelity will motivate parents to vaccinate their adolescent children against HPV. OE.3.b. Expect that educating parents of children who are due for or haven't completed their HPV vaccination series will increase HPV vaccination rates.
PO4. Clinic staff refer and navigate patients for HPV vaccination.	K.4.a. Describe the process for referring or navigating parents to HPV vaccination services. K.4.b. Describe the financial support available to parents to pay for the HPV vaccine.	SSE.4.a. Demonstrate ability to locate HPV vaccination services in the clinic. SSE.4.b. Demonstrate skills required to refer parents or navigate parents to HPV vaccination services. SSE.4.c. Demonstrate the ability to facilitate appointments for HPV vaccinations. SSE.4.d. Demonstrate ability to provide parents with information about financial support services to pay for the HPV vaccine.	A.4.a. Express confidence in referring and/or navigating parents to HPV vaccination services in their clinic A.4.b. Express confidence in the availability of resources to pay for the HPV vaccine.	PSN.4. Recognize that other clinic staff refer and/or navigate parents to HPV vaccination services and provide information on financial support for vaccines.	OE.4. Expect that referring and navigating parents to HPV vaccination services and providing them with information about financial support will increase HPV vaccination rates.

(continued)

Table 9.10 (*Continued*)

Implementation	Determinants				
Performance Objectives	**Knowledge**	**Skills and Self-efficacy**	**Attitudes/Beliefs**	**Perceived Social Norms**	**Outcome Expectations**
P05. Clinic staff follow up with parents to ensure initiation and completion of the vaccine series.	K.5. Describe the process for following up with parents to ensure initiation and completion of the HPV vaccine series.	SSE.5.a. Demonstrate skills to navigate parents to the clinic's HPV vaccination services. SSE.5.b. Demonstrate skills to follow up with parents to ensure initiation and completion of the vaccine series.	A.5. Express confidence in following up with patients to ensure initiation and completion of the vaccine series.	PSN.5. Recognize that other clinic staff follow up with parents to increase HPV vaccination initiation and completion.	OE.5. Expect that following up with parents will increase HPV vaccination initiation and completion rates.
P06. Clinic staff record and report interactions with parents to monitor program reach and effectiveness.	K.6.a. Lists the type of interactions that need to be recorded, such as education sessions, referrals, vaccination appointments, and parent follow-up. K.6.b. Describe how to monitor program implementation using the tracking template provided. K.6.c. Describe how to address data recording and reporting issues to the Program Champion. K.6.d. Describe how to report data collected to the Program Champion.	SSE.6.a. Demonstrate ability to use tracking template to keep records. SSE.6.b. Demonstrates ability to address data recording and reporting issues. SSE.6.c. Demonstrate the ability to report data to the program champion.	A.6.a. Express confidence in monitoring program implementation using tracking templates. A.6.b. Believe that documenting interactions is an important for monitoring program reach and effectiveness.	PSN.6. Recognize that other clinic staff keep records and report activity to program coordinators.	OE.6.a. Expect that recording interactions contributes to the identification of gaps in program implementation. OE.6.b. Expect that continued monitoring and evaluation will contribute to improved program implementation.

Table 9.11 Partial Matrix for Maintenance Outcome: Clinic/Agency Director (Health Services/Community Organization) maintains For Our Children, an educational web-based parent and provider program for FQHCs/Clinics and community-based agencies, to increase HPV vaccination rates in Adolescents (11–17 Years)

Maintenance	**Determinants**			
Performance Objectives	**Knowledge**	**Skills and Self-efficacy**	**Attitudes/Beliefs**	**Outcome Expectations**
P01. Discuss with the senior leadership (e.g., Board of Directors/CEO/Chairman, etc.) about the continuation of the **For Our Children** program training (provider and parent component) after initial funding.	K.1.a. Describe processes that will ensure the program can be continued in the clinic/agency.	SSE.1.a. Demonstrate skills for addressing management issues with senior leadership. SSE.1.b. Express self-efficacy for addressing any management issues/obstacles.	A.1.a. Describe early successes with the program as evidence of its usefulness and reason to continue implementation. A.1.b. Believe that it is important to maintain the program. A.1.c. Express continued satisfaction with enhanced HPV vaccination services and improved vaccination rates.	OE.1. Expect the program to continue to be value add to patients and the community.
P02. Assure the senior leadership that HPV vaccination rates continue to be reported (and remain stable or on an upward trend).	K.2.a. List ways how the vaccination reports will be presented, visualized, and shared from EMR to senior leadership. K.2.b. Describes how HPV vaccination data is interpreted and utilized to support program maintenance.	SSE.2.a. Demonstrate current team capacity, administrative skills to monitor data. SSE.2.b. Express confidence in the ability to monitor, track, visualize, and present data. SSE.2.c. Express confidence in the ability to use data to support program maintenance.	A.2. Describes how data and feedback on HPV vaccination are important to maintain or improve vaccination rates.	OE.2. Expect that continued monitoring and evaluation will contribute to the likelihood of program continuation.
P03. Discuss with Program Champion/Coordinator and clinic/agency staff regarding the continuation of the **For Our Children** program training (provider and parent component) after initial funding.	K.3.a. Describe the importance of continued training to maintain program fidelity and quality. K.3.b. Describe processes that will ensure the program can be continued in the clinic/agency (e.g., inclusion in job descriptions, reward structures, budgets)	SSE.3.a. Express confidence in identifying solutions to sustain training delivery. SSE.3.b. Demonstrate skills for addressing management issues with decision makers. SSE.3.c. Express self-efficacy for addressing any management issues/obstacles.	A.3.a. Describes early successes with the program as evidence of its usefulness and reason to continue it. A.3.b. Believes that it is important to maintain the program. A.3.c. Expresses continued satisfaction with enhanced HPV vaccination services and improved vaccination rates.	OE.3. Expect the program to continue to be a value add to patients and the community.
P04. The senior leadership approves steps to assure the integration of the **For Our Children** program into the clinic/community agency routine.	K.4.a. Describe the program components and the feasibility of integrating them into the workflow. K.4.b. Describe the steps decision makers plan to take to support the continued use of the **For Our Children** program website.	SSE.4.a. Demonstrate the ability to maintain a workforce that is skilled in utilizing the program components. SSE.4.b. Express confidence in the ability to maintain the program website as a part of clinic/agency routine practices.	A.4. Believe that approving the integration of the program into normal clinic/agency routines is an important part of their role in improving clinic/agency practices and meeting patient and community needs.	OE.4.a. Expects that continued monitoring and evaluation will contribute to the likelihood of program continuation. OE.4.b. Expect that integration of the program website into clinic/agency practices will lead to a sustained increase in HPV vaccinations.

Table 9.12 Partial Matrix for Maintenance Outcome: Program Champion/Coordinator (Health Services/Community Organization) maintains For Our Children, an educational web-based parent and provider program for FQHCs/clinics and community-based agencies, to increase HPV vaccination rates in adolescents (11–17 Years)

Maintenance	**Determinants**			
Performance Objectives	**Knowledge**	**Skills and Self-efficacy**	**Attitudes/Beliefs**	**Outcome Expectations**
PO1. Discuss with clinic/agency decision-makers the continuation of the **For Our Children** program training (provider and parent component) after initial funding.	K.1.a. Describe the importance of continued training to maintain program fidelity and quality. K.1.b. List available options to sustain training (internal trainers, integration to orientation requirements, e-learning). K.1.c. Describe processes that will ensure the program can be continued in the clinic/agency (e.g., inclusion in job descriptions, reward structures, budgets)	SSE.1.a. Demonstrate skills for addressing management issues with decision makers. SSE.1.b. Expresses self-efficacy for addressing any management issues/obstacles with decision makers	A.1.a. Describe early successes with the program as evidence of usefulness and reason to continue it. A.1.b. Believe that it is important to maintain the program. A.1.c. Express continued satisfaction with enhanced HPV vaccination services and improved no-show rates.	OE.1. Expect the program to continue to be value add to patients and the community.
PO2. Assure that HPV vaccination rates continue to be reported (and remain stable or on an upward trend).	K.2.a. Describe how to visualize and share data from EMR to the appropriate clinic staff and CHWs. K.2.b. Describes how HPV vaccination data is interpreted and utilized to support program maintenance.	SSE.2.a. Demonstrate administrative skills to monitor data. SSE.2.b. Express confidence in the ability to monitor, track, visualize and present data. SSE.2.c. Express confidence in the ability to use data to support program maintenance.	A.2. Describes how data and feedback on HPV vaccination are important to maintain or improve vaccination rates.	OE.2. Expect that continued monitoring and evaluation will contribute to the likelihood of program continuation.
PO3. Discuss strategies/steps that may be needed to maintain the website and other educational resources/program materials.	K.3.a. Describe the importance of updating and maintaining the program materials. K.3.b. Lists components that require upkeep (fotonovela/TIMI/Website content regarding guidelines and website links to resources). K.3.c. List strategies/steps that will be taken to ensure the FOC website and other resources can be continued in the clinic/agency.	SSE.3.a. Express confidence in the ability to apply practical approaches to maintain program materials. SSE.3.b. Demonstrate skills for addressing potential program website-related issues for continuation with decision makers. SSE.3.c. Expresses self-efficacy for addressing any potential program website-related issues with decision-makers	A.3. Believes that it is important to prepare action steps to ensure the continuation of the program website and other resources.	OE.3. Expect the strategies/steps will allow for the program website and materials to continue and to be a value add to patients.

Task 3: Choose Change Methods and Design Implementation Strategies

Task 3 in Step 5 is analogous to the tasks in Intervention Mapping Step 3. In this case, for program implementation, the PNH planning group selected theoretical and evidence-based methods (e.g., persuasion, guided practice, facilitation) expected to address adoption, implementation, and maintenance determinants and change objectives they identified in the previous task. They then operationalized the methods by selecting and designing implementation strategies (e.g., PNH program website, training for implementers, organizational consultation) to facilitate the adoption, implementation, and maintenance of the PNH program in primary care clinics and CHW organizations across Texas. The final product after completing this task was the PNH program implementation plan (Table 9.13).

Task 4: Produce Implementation Protocols and Materials

In Task 4, program planners develop implementation protocols and other program materials and products in line with selected implementation strategies. For the PNH program, the planning group held brainstorming sessions to discuss how the methods and strategies selected in Task 3 would be put in place and the materials needed to support implementation. This involved designing a PNH program website, promotional resources, parent informational resources, health professional/CHW informational resources, a program manual and corresponding training materials, and other program materials and resources, described in detail below.

To promote the adoption of the PNH program, they developed a program website designed to share information about the program (and how to deliver it) with primary care practices and CHW organizations. The **For Our Children/Por Nuestros Hijos program website**, available in English and Spanish, provides:

- A brief overview of the **PNH program** goals, components, and developers;
- Information about HPV, the HPV vaccine, and why HPV vaccination is important;
- An overview of the parent education component of the PNH program and a link to the **Parent Education program** website, which houses more detailed information about the parent education component and training and program materials to facilitate implementation;
- An overview of the healthcare provider component of the PNH program and a link to the **HPVCancerCoach program** website, which houses more detailed information about the provider component of the PNH program and training and program materials to facilitate implementation; and
- Brief testimonials from organizations who have implemented the program.

The PNH website was designed not only to support adoption but also to facilitate implementation and sustainability of the program beyond the initial funding period.

Additional program promotion materials included promotional flyers (in English & Spanish), which included previous adopters' testimonials and newsletters to be distributed through their

Table 9.13 Partial Implementation Plan for the For Our Children (Por Nuestros Hijos) Program: Table of Methods, Strategies, and Materials to Enhance Adoption, Implementation, and Maintenance

Responsible Person	Sample Performance Objectives	Determinants	Methods and Implementation Strategy	Implementation Materials
Adoption				
Agency/Clinic/Medical Director	Obtains staff and community buy-in (PO3)	• Knowledge • Skills and Self-efficacy • Attitudes • Perceived Norms • Outcome Expectations	Persuasive communication.	Presentations with vaccination rates, HPV-cancer incidence data, key program information, program benefits, and testimonials of previous adopters.
	Obtains administrative approval (PO2) Identifies Program Champion/Coordinator to oversee implementation (PO4) Budgets program into agency operations (PO5)	• Knowledge • Skills and Self-efficacy • Attitudes • Perceived Norms • Outcome Expectations	Persuasive communication through providing evidence. Modeling through testimonials from previous adopters Organizational Consultation and Planning.	Promotion via Partner networks (email and teleconferences). Presentations via webinars, conferences, workshops, and meetings. Promotional flyers (English & Spanish). Introductory package for agencies outlining goals & objectives, program benefits, required resources, materials, and available support.
Implementation				
Program Champion/Coordinator	Identifies resources and staff required to implement PNH. (PO1) Designates time for CHWs to complete program training. (PO2) Identifies local clinics providing HPV vaccination services. (PO2) Supports and monitors PNH implementation. (PO6)	• Knowledge • Skills and Self-efficacy • Attitudes • Perceived Norms • Outcome Expectations	Persuasive communication: During training session Program Champion/Coordinator provides staff with the latest research on HPV, associated cancers, and HPV vaccination. Modeling using testimonials of UTHealth master trainers on how to monitor, track and evaluate program activities. Modeling through trainings provided by UTHealth master trainers demonstrate using program materials on how to monitor, track and evaluate program activities. Guided practice through education sessions in which CHWs receive feedback on using PNH materials to educate parents.	Training materials: PowerPoint presentation and script, case studies, discussion questions, HPV quiz, mini-course on communication strategies, course evaluation, and HPV information/resources. Manual: Step-by-step guide on implementing PNH. PNH website: program materials, training materials, templates, promotional flyers, vaccination reminder cards, and other HPV resources. Referral information: list of local health clinics and county health programs providing HPV vaccination services

Community Health Worker	Participate in PNH program training (P01) Collaborate with community partners to promote program participation. (P03) Identifies and recruits eligible parents to participate. (P02) Delivers educational sessions using program materials. (P04) Refers and/or navigates parents to local clinics providing HPV vaccination. (P05) Follow up with parents to ensure initiation and completion of the vaccine series. (P06) Keeps record and reports interactions with parents to monitor program reach and effectiveness. (P07)	• Knowledge • Skills and Self-efficacy • Attitudes • Perceived Norms • Outcome Expectations	Persuasive communication: During one-on-one education sessions with the parents, providing information on HPV vaccination as cancer prevention. Guided practice through education sessions demonstrates how to use program materials to educate parents. Role-play: CHWs practice using program materials to educate and motivate parents. Case studies demonstrating how to address parental concerns and questions about HPV vaccination. Modeling through training provided by the Program coordinator demonstrates how to complete project-tracking templates.	Training materials: PowerPoint presentation and scripts, case studies, discussion questions, HPV quiz, course evaluation, and HPV information/ resources. PNH manual: a step-by-step guide on program implementation, protocols, and templates. Program website: program materials, training materials, templates, promotional flyer, and other resources.
Maintenance				
Agency/Clinic director Program Champion/Coordinator	Budget for PNH (P01) Report outcomes (P02)	• Knowledge • Skills and Self-efficacy • Attitudes • Perceived Norms • Outcome Expectations	Facilitation through the use of templates to develop the next phase of program goals, implementation plans, and budget.	Sample budget.Template for outcomes report.

partner networks, email distribution lists, and social media channels such as Facebook, Instagram, and X (formerly Twitter). The planning group also developed presentations to disseminate information about the program and study results at academic conferences/professional meetings, and workshops. To prepare program champions/coordinators, CHWs, and clinical staff to implement the program in primary care clinics and CHW organizations, the planning group developed training materials certified by the Texas Department of State Health Services (DSHS), including a standardized training presentation and script (in-person and virtual training versions), a pre-recorded training webinar delivered by the program developers, a training guide for training instructors, quizzes, case studies, and training evaluation templates (Figure 9.8).

Additionally, the program planners developed a compilation of HPV resources for parents and health professionals; a step-by-step guide for how to approach parent education; a program manual to guide planning, implementation, and evaluation of the program; and program

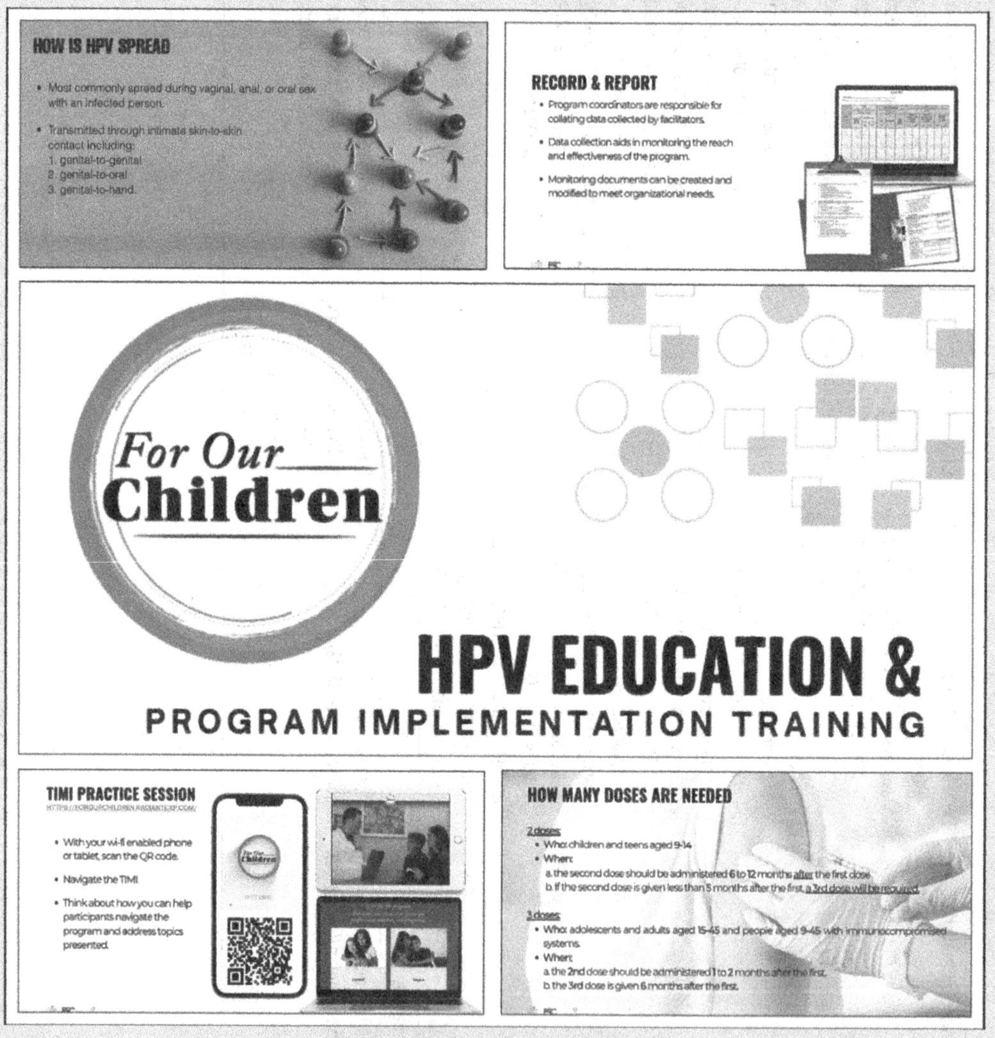

Figure 9.8 PNH Training Presentation for CHWs. Source: vetre / Adobe Stock Photos

websites (noted above) that house all training and program materials including access to the Tailored Interactive Multimedia Intervention (TIMI), fotonovela, and HPVCancerCoach App (Figure 9.9).

Initial training was provided by the PNH staff. These trainings were conducted in-person or virtual to accommodate the adopters' needs. These sessions lasted between 2 and 6 hours depending if it was a full program training or training for a specific component (parental or provider). During the training sessions, the PNH staff provided an overview of the program's content (information transfer) and modeled implementation of program components using the fotonovela, TIMI, and the HPVCancerCoach provider app (modeling). Program champions/coordinators, CHWs, and clinical staff engaged in interactive lesson practice, receiving feedback from the trainers and their peers (guided practice with feedback). They also practiced communication strategies for dealing and addressing parental concerns. To facilitate additional training sessions for new employees, pre-recorded sessions were made available to adopters after the in-person or virtual sessions.

To facilitate maintenance of the PNH program, the program developers created outcome report templates so that implementers could keep track of program reach (number of educated parents and vaccinated children), monthly activities (staff training and outreach

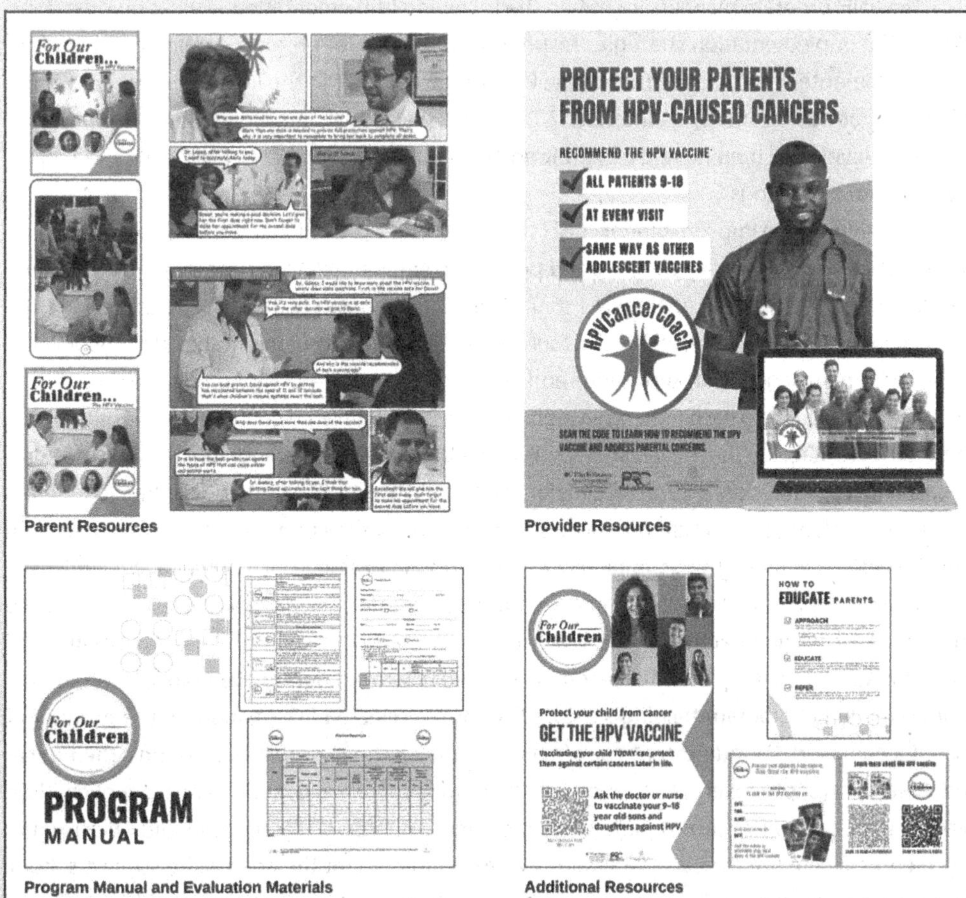

Figure 9.9 PNH Additional Resources

activities) and audit and feedback. Additionally, to ensure healthcare professionals and community organizations have ongoing access to the program and training resources required to implement the program effectively and with fidelity, a PNH staff was assigned to continuously monitor and to maintain the program website indefinitely. To secure and facilitate PNH staff access, content updates, continued monitoring for broken links, and compliance with WCAG 2.0 AA accessibility standards and the State Website Linking and Privacy Policy, the website is hosted at no cost within the institution's (UTHealth) website. The PNH staff also continued to promote the program through its partner networks and social media. Additionally, PNH staff maintains communication with adopters to assess emerging needs, provide technical support, newly developed resources, and retraining (if necessary), and assess if the program would be a good fit for additional clinics/agencies within the implementing organization

Task 5: Evaluate Implementation Outcomes

The final task for step 5 involves developing a plan to evaluate implementation of the program, including adoption, implementation, and maintenance outcomes, and determining the impact of the implementation strategies developed. To accomplish this, the PNH program planners identified implementation evaluation questions, developed indicators and measures for assessment, and specified the implementation evaluation design.

The PNH program planners identified the following implementation evaluation questions: (1) Did the implementation strategies respond to the needs of program implementers (adopters, implementers, and maintainers of the PNH program)? (2) Did the implementers deliver the PNH program components as intended? To assess these evaluation questions, the program planners developed training records, clinic and CHW surveys, interviews, PNH evaluation materials, and follow-up logs.

Prior to program implementation, PNH staff assessed organizational readiness by conducting interviews with clinic/agency directors and program coordinators/champions at adopting organizations. Based on this assessment, PNH staff tailored training and technical support to meet the specific needs of each organization. Factors considered in the assessment included the level of support from managers, staff knowledge and skills, and access to resources required to implement the program. Following each training session, trained staff completed course evaluations to assess program acceptability. These evaluations collected data on trainee demographics, workplace protocols on HPV education and/or vaccination, HPV and HPV-vaccination knowledge acquisition, perceived usefulness of program materials, and training satisfaction. Clinicians participating in HPVCancerCoach training also completed usability surveys to assess app content and usefulness.

To evaluate the fidelity of the implementation, adopting clinics and agencies were asked to keep track of program activities and reach by using the PNH Activities Report Form and the Program Reach Log templates. These forms were provided to program champions/coordinators during the initial program training session. The forms collected information on the number of parents educated, the adolescent's sex (male or female), the materials used during the educational session (photonovella, TIMI, or other), the number of referrals, and the number of children vaccinated as a result of the program. Nonclinical implementers (CHW agencies and CBOs) would also report where the educational sessions were conducted (at the agency, health fair, school, participant's house, etc.). These reports were submitted quarterly. Additionally, PNH staff conducted focus groups and individual interviews with the implementers to assess the fidelity of program implementation. During the interviews, implementers were asked to describe the protocols and processes used to deliver and monitor the program, as well as any barriers or facilitators to implementation. Specifically, they were asked about which materials were used during the educational sessions and how they were used, the usefulness of the TIMI and the fotonovela, and if they adapted any of the materials or the ways in which they were used.

In most cases, implementers indicated that they did adapt PNH to meet organizational and community needs. For example, the parent-educational materials were designed to be used as a bundle; parents would watch the TIMI and then would read the fotonovela, which captured the main points presented in the TIMI. However, implementers reported using the fotonovela more frequently than the TIMI, as parents did not have enough time to complete the TIMI during their clinic visits or educational sessions conducted in community settings. Implementers in rural locations also indicated that limited internet access was another factor that promoted the use of the fotonovela over the TIMI. Following feedback from early adopters and implementers, PNH staff adapted the training curriculum to include additional information about HPV-related topics and developed a communication strategy to address the concerns of hesitant parents. To support continued delivery of high-quality training, a standardized training script and presentation, along with other supporting material, were developed and made available on the PNH webpage.

PNH staff trained clinicians and CHWs from 5 metropolitan areas across Texas (Austin, Brownsville, Dallas-Fort Worth, El Paso, Houston, and San Antonio). Based on course evaluations, participants strongly agreed that the training increased their knowledge of HPV, HPV-related cancers, and the vaccine. Having completed the training, they were confident in their ability to use PNH to educate parents about HPV vaccination. Over the course of the project, implementers used program materials to educate 8,114 Hispanic parents about HPV vaccination, reaching 7,489 adolescents.

Summary

Because the success of any health promotion program depends not only on its effectiveness but also on its adoption, implementation, and maintenance, systematic processes are needed to ensure program use and sustainment. Step 5 of IM—Implementation Mapping—provides a step-by-step process for planning strategies that will increase adoption, implementation, and maintenance. Planning implementation is an essential part of health promotion planning and should be done before the new intervention is delivered. Implementation Mapping can also be used for planning implementation of existing effective interventions. Without deliberate planning, even health promotion programs that have strong evidence of effectiveness risk remaining unused or being delivered inconsistently, limiting their impact. Implementation Mapping integrates concepts from implementation science and health promotion to guide planners in designing strategies that address multilevel determinants of program use and ensure contextual fit. These strategies, previously called "implementation interventions" have clearly defined mechanisms of action, linking determinants of implementation action to implementation outcomes.

The chapter outlines five core Implementation Mapping tasks: conducting an implementation needs and assets assessment; identifying outcomes, performance objectives, and determinants; selecting theoretical methods and designing implementation strategies; producing protocols and materials; and evaluating implementation outcomes. It emphasizes the importance of participatory and co-creation approaches that engage adopters, implementers, and maintainers throughout the process to ensure strategies are feasible and acceptable. Implementation science frameworks such as CFIR (Damschroder et al., 2009), EPIS (Aarons et al., 2011), and ISF (Wandersman et al., 2008), along with theories like Social Cognitive Theory (Bandura, 2001) and Diffusion of Innovations (Rogers, 1983), inform the identification of determinants and the design of strategies. This chapter also includes real-world examples illustrating how matrices of change objectives, logic models, and tailored strategies can be used to operationalize theory-driven methods into actionable plans for adoption, implementation, and sustainment.

Using Step 5 can help bridge the gap between research and practice by ensuring that programs are not only developed using theory, evidence, new data, and community engaged co-creation approaches, but that their delivery also draws upon these processes to ensure use and sustainment. By systematically linking determinants to strategies and grounding decisions in theory and evidence, Implementation Mapping helps planners create robust, contextually appropriate plans that support program uptake and long-term integration into routine practice. This approach enhances the likelihood that health-promotion programs will achieve meaningful population-level impact.

Implementation Mapping is now being applied globally to plan implementation strategies across diverse health systems and community settings. A scoping review of Implementation Mapping studies found that it had been applied to implement health practices and programs in five different countries across diverse settings, including community and primary care settings, residential care, community pharmacy, specialty outpatient clinics, and hospital settings (Warhurst et al., 2025). Its structured, theory-informed approach has advanced the field of implementation science by providing a prescriptive process for linking determinants to strategies and clarifying mechanisms of action (Fernandez et al., 2023; Warhurst et al., 2025).

Discussion Questions and Learning Activities

1. Compare and contrast the tasks in IM Step 5 with Steps 2, 3, and 4. What do they have in common? How are they different?
2. Explain why it is important to plan for program use as part of health promotion program planning.
3. What is meant by a linkage system for program adoption and implementation? Give examples of different ways in which a linkage system can be established.
4. Refer back to Chapter 5, question 2, where you have described your planning group. Do you need to bring any new people to the planning

group to begin planning for program adoption and implementation? Who are they and what will they contribute to planning for program adoption and implementation?

5. What theories can be used to identify determinants of program adoption, implementation, and sustainability? Give an example of determinants that research and theory have shown to be important determinants of program adoption, implementation, and sustainability.
6. Describe how the matrices created in Step 5 can be used to help guide process evaluation of the health promotion program.
7. Continuing with the health promotion program you are proposing, state adoption, implementation, and sustainability outcomes and write performance objectives for each outcome.
8. Create a matrix for adoption and implementation of the program by linking performance objectives with determinants.
9. Describe methods and practical applications you propose to affect the change and performance objectives in the matrices to achieve program adoption and implementation.

References

Aarons, G. A., & Ehrhart, M. G. (2022). Leading implementation by focusing on strategic implementation leadership. In R. C.-W. Frances Rapport & J. Braithwaite (Eds.), *Implementation science: The key concepts.* Routledge. doi:10.4324/9781003109945

Aarons, G. A., Ehrhart, M. G., Farahnak, L. R., Sklar, M., & Horowitz, J. (2017). Discrepancies in leader and follower ratings of transformational leadership: Relationship with organizational culture in mental health. *Administration and Policy in Mental Health, 44*(4), 480–491. doi:10.1007/s10488-015-0672-7

Aarons, G. A., Hurlburt, M., & Horwitz, S. M. (2011). Advancing a conceptual model of evidence-based practice implementation in public service sectors. *Administration and Policy in Mental Health and Mental Health Services Research, 38*(1), 4–23.

Adsul, P., Shelton, R. C., Oh, A., Moise, N., Iwelunmor, J., & Griffith, D. M. (2024). Challenges and opportunities for paving the road to global health equity through implementation science. *Annual Review of Public Health, 45*(Volume 45, 2024), 27–45. doi:10.1146/annurev-publhealth-060922-034822

Ammerman, A. S., Lindquist, C. H., Lohr, K. N., & Hersey, J. (2002). The efficacy of behavioral interventions to modify dietary fat and fruit and vegetable intake: A review of the evidence. *Preventive Medicine, 35*(1), 25–41.

Ashcraft, L. E., Goodrich, D. E., Hero, J., Phares, A., Bachrach, R. L., Quinn, D. A., Qureshi, N., Ernecoff, N. C., Lederer, L. G., Scheunemann, L. P., Rogal, S. S., & Chinman, M. J. (2024). A systematic review of experimentally tested implementation strategies across health and human service settings: Evidence from 2010-2022. *Implementation Science, 19*(1), 43. doi:10.1186/s13012-024-01369-5

Bamford, C., Poole, M., Brittain, K., Chew-Graham, C., Fox, C., Iliffe, S., Manthorpe, J., & Robinson, L. (2014). Understanding the challenges to implementing case management for people with dementia in primary care in England: A qualitative study using Normalization process theory. *BMC Health Services Research, 14*, 549. doi:10.1186/s12913-014-0549-6

Bandura, A. (1986). *Social foundations of thought and action: A social cognitive theory*. Prentice-Hall.

Bandura, A. (2001). Social cognitive theory: An agentic perspective. *Annual Review of Psychology, 52*, 1–26.

Basch, C. E., Sliepcevich, E. M., Gold, R. S., Duncan, D. F., & Kolbe, L. J. (1985). Avoiding type III errors in health education program evaluations: A case study. *Health Education Quarterly, 12*(3), 315–331.

Bass, B. M., & Riggio, R. E. (2006). *Transformational leadership* (2nd ed.). Psychology Press. doi:10.4324/9781410617095

Baumann, A. A., Hooley, C., Kryzer, E., Morshed, A. B., Gutner, C. A., Malone, S., Walsh-Bailey, C., Pilar, M., Sandler, B., Tabak, R. G., & Mazzucca, S. (2022). A scoping review of frameworks in empirical studies and a review of dissemination frameworks. *Implementation Science, 17*(1), 53. doi:10.1186/s13012-022-01225-4

Berkel, C., Mauricio, A. M., Sandler, I. N., Wolchik, S. A., Gallo, C. G., & Brown, C. H. (2018). The cascading effects of multiple dimensions of implementation on program outcomes: A test of a theoretical model. *Prevention Science, 19*(6), 782–794. doi:10.1007/s11121-017-0855-4

Bero, L. A., Grilli, R., Grimshaw, J. M., Harvey, E., Oxman, A. D., & Thomson, M. A. (1998). Closing the gap between research and practice: An overview of systematic reviews of interventions to promote the implementation of research findings. The Cochrane Effective Practice and Organization of Care Review Group. *British Medical Journal (Clinical Research Edition), 317*(7156), 465–468.

Bierbaum, M., Best, S., Williams, S., Fehlberg, Z., Hillier, S., Ellis, L. A., Goodrich, A., Padbury, R., & Hibbert, P. (2025). The integration of quality improvement and implementation science methods and frameworks in healthcare: A systematic review. *BMC Health Services Research, 25*(1), 558. doi:10.1186/s12913-025-12730-9

Bodkin, A., & Hakimi, S. (2020). Sustainable by design: A systematic review of factors for health promotion program sustainability. *BMC Public Health, 20*(1), 964. doi:10.1186/s12889-020-09091-9

Bonawitz, K., Wetmore, M., Heisler, M., Dalton, V. K., Damschroder, L. J., Forman, J., Allan, K. R., & Moniz, M. H. (2020). Champions in context: Which attributes matter for change efforts in healthcare? *Implementation Science, 15*(1), 1–10.

Bond, C., Lancaster, G. A., Campbell, M., Chan, C., Eddy, S., Hopewell, S., Mellor, K., Thabane, L., & Eldridge, S. (2023). Pilot and feasibility studies: Extending the conceptual framework. *Pilot and Feasibility Studies, 9*(1), 24. doi:10.1186/s40814-023-01233-1

Bowen, D. J., Kreuter, M., Spring, B., Cofta-Woerpel, L., Linnan, L., Weiner, D., Bakken, S., Kaplan, C. P., Squiers, L., & Fabrizio, C. (2009). How we design feasibility studies. *American Journal of Preventive Medicine, 36*(5), 452–457.

Breslau, E. S., Weiss, E. S., Williams, A., Burness, A., & Kepka, D. (2015). The implementation road: Engaging community partnerships in evidence-based cancer control interventions. *Health Promotion Practice, 16*(1), 46–54. doi:10.1177/1524839914528705

Brownson, R. C., Ballew, P., Dieffenderfer, B., Haire-Joshu, D., Heath, G. W., Kreuter, M. W., & Myers, B. A. (2007). Evidence-based interventions to promote physical activity: What contributes to dissemination by state health departments. *American Journal of Preventive Medicine, 33*(1), S66–S78.

Brownson, R. C., Fielding, J. E., & Green, L. W. (2018). Building capacity for evidence-based public health: Reconciling the pulls of practice and the push of research. *Annual Review of Public Health, 39*, 27–53.

Brownson, R. C., Jacobs, J. A., Tabak, R. G., Hoehner, C. M., & Stamatakis, K. A. (2013). Designing for dissemination among public health researchers: Findings from a national survey in the United States. *American Journal of Public Health, 103*(9), 1693–1699.

Cabassa, L. J., & Baumann, A. A. (2013). A two-way street: Bridging implementation science and cultural adaptations of mental health treatments. *Implementation Science, 8*(1), 1–14.

Cawley, J. (2010). The economics of childhood obesity. *Health Affairs (Project Hope), 29*(3), 364–371. doi:10.1377/hlthaff.2009.0721

Chambers, D. A., Glasgow, R. E., & Stange, K. C. (2013). The dynamic sustainability framework: Addressing the paradox of sustainment amid ongoing change. *Implementation Science, 8*(1), 117.

Chapman, A., Buccheri, A., Mohotti, D., Wong Shee, A., Huggins, C. E., Alston, L., Hutchinson, A. M., Yoong, S. L., Beks, H., Mc Namara, K., Peeters, A., & Ugalde, A. (2025). Staff-reported barriers and facilitators to the implementation of healthcare interventions within regional and rural areas: A rapid review. *BMC Health Services Research, 25*(1), 331. doi:10.1186/s12913-025-12480-8

Chaudoir, S. R., Dugan, A. G., & Barr, C. H. I. (2013). Measuring factors affecting implementation of health innovations: A systematic review of structural, organizational, provider, patient, and innovation level measures. *Implementation Science, 8*(1), 22.

Chin, M. H., Goddu, A. P., Ferguson, M. J., & Peek, M. E. (2014). Expanding and sustaining integrated health care-community efforts to reduce diabetes disparities. *Health Promotion Practice, 15*(2 Suppl), 29s–39s. doi:10.1177/1524839914532649

Collaborative for Implementation Practice (CIP) & National Implementation Research Network (NIRN) (2021). Fit and feasibility: Best practices and tools to assess programs or practices' contextual fit and feasibility. https://www.implementationpractice.org/wp-content/uploads/2021/05/NIRN-CIP-Practice-Guide-Fit-and-Feasibility_7.29.21.pdf

Craig, D. W., Walker, T. J., Cuccaro, P., Sharma, S. V., Heredia, N. I., Robertson, M. C., & Fernandez, M. E. (2024). Using the R = MC2 heuristic to understand barriers to and facilitators of implementing school-based physical activity opportunities: A qualitative study. *BMC Public Health, 24*(1), 207. doi:10.1186/s12889-024-17744-2

Curran, G. M. (2020). Implementation science made too simple: A teaching tool. *Implementation Science Communications, 1*(1), 27. doi:10.1186/s43058-020-00001-z

Curran, G. M., Bauer, M., Mittman, B., Pyne, J. M., & Stetler, C. (2012). Effectiveness-implementation hybrid designs: Combining elements of clinical effectiveness and implementation research to enhance public health impact. *Medical Care, 50*(3), 217–226.

Curran, G. M., Landes, S. J., McBain, S. A., Pyne, J. M., Smith, J. D., Fernandez, M. E., Chambers, D. A., & Mittman, B. S. (2022). Reflections on 10 years of effectiveness-implementation hybrid studies. *Frontiers in Health Services*, *2*, 125.

Damschroder, L. J., Aron, D. C., Keith, R. E., Kirsh, S. R., Alexander, J. A., & Lowery, J. C. (2009). Fostering implementation of health services research findings into practice: A consolidated framework for advancing implementation science. *Implementation Science*, *4*(1), 50. doi:10.1186/1748-5908-4-50

Damschroder, L. J., Reardon, C. M., Opra Widerquist, M. A., & Lowery, J. (2022a). Conceptualizing outcomes for use with the Consolidated Framework for Implementation Research (CFIR): The CFIR Outcomes Addendum. *Implementation Science*, *17*(1), 7. doi:10.1186/s13012-021-01181-5

Damschroder, L. J., Reardon, C. M., Widerquist, M. A. O., & Lowery, J. (2022b). The updated Consolidated Framework for Implementation Research based on user feedback. *Implementation Science*, *17*(1), 1–16.

de Jong, J. P. J., Rigtering, C., & Spaans, L. (2023). Heroes of diffusion: Making user innovations widely available. *Research Policy*, *52*(8), 104840. doi:10.1016/j.respol.2023.104840

Dearing, J. W. (2009). Applying diffusion of innovation theory to intervention development. *Research on Social Work Practice*, *19*(5), 503–518.

Dias, E. M., Walker, T. J., Balasubramanian, B. A., Cuccaro, P. M., Workman, L., Wandersman, A., & Fernandez, M. E. (2025). Organizational readiness and implementation of colorectal cancer screening evidence-based interventions in federally qualified health centers: A cross-sectional study. *Journal of Clinical and Translational Science*, *9*(1), e26. doi:10.1017/cts.2024.689

Dickson, K. S., Holt, T., & Arredondo, E. (2022). Applying implementation mapping to expand a care coordination program at a federally qualified health center. *Frontiers in Public Health*, *10*, 844898. doi:10.3389/fpubh.2022.844898

Domlyn, A. M., Scott, V., Livet, M., Lamont, A., Watson, A., Kenworthy, T., Talford, M., Yannayon, M., & Wandersman, A. (2021). R = MC(2) readiness building process: A practical approach to support implementation in local, state, and national settings. *Journal of Community Psychology*, *49*(5), 1228–1248. doi:10.1002/jcop.22531

Donaldson, A., & Poulos, R. G. (2014). Planning the diffusion of a neck-injury prevention programme among community rugby union coaches. *British Journal of Sports Medicine*, *48*(2), 151–158. doi:10.1136/bjsports-2012-091551

Dowling, K., & Barry, M. M. (2020). Evaluating the implementation quality of a social and emotional learning program: A mixed methods approach. *International Journal of Environmental Research and Public Health*, *17*(9). doi:10.3390/ijerph17093249

Durlak, J. A., & DuPre, E. P. (2008). Implementation matters: A review of research on the influence of implementation on program outcomes and the factors affecting implementation. *American Journal of Community Psychology*, *41*(3-4), 327–350.

Eccles, M. P., & Mittman, B. S. (2006). Welcome to implementation science. *Implementation Science*, *1*(1), 1. doi:10.1186/1748-5908-1-1

El Kirat, H., van Belle, S., Khattabi, A., & Belrhiti, Z. (2024). Behavioral change interventions, theories, and techniques to reduce physical inactivity and sedentary behavior in the general population: A scoping review. *BMC Public Health, 24*(1), 2099. doi:10.1186/s12889-024-19600-9

Elder, J. P., Lytle, L., Sallis, J. F., Young, D. R., Steckler, A., Simons-Morton, D., Stone, E., Jobe, J. B., Stevens, J., Lohman, T., Webber, L., Pate, R., Saksvig, B. I., & Ribisl, K. (2007). A description of the social-ecological framework used in the trial of activity for adolescent girls (TAAG). *Health Education Research, 22*(2), 155–165. doi:10.1093/her/cyl059

Escoffery, C., Sekar, S., Allen, C. G., Madrigal, L., Haardoerfer, R., & Mertens, A. (2023). A scoping review of outer context constructs in dissemination and implementation science theories, models, and frameworks. *Translational Behavioral Medicine, 13*(5), 327–337. doi:10.1093/tbm/ibac115

Estabrooks, P. A., Brownson, R. C., & Pronk, N. P. (2018). Dissemination and Implementation Science for Public Health Professionals: An Overview and Call to Action. *Preventing Chronic Disease, 15,* E162. doi:10.5888/pcd15.180525

Fernandez, M. E., Melvin, C., Leeman, J., Ribisl, K., Allen, J., Kegler, M., Bastani, R., Ory, M., Risendal, B., Hannon, P., Kreuter, M., & Hebert, J. (2014). The cancer prevention and control research network: An interactive systems approach to advancing cancer control implementation research and practice. *Cancer Epidemiology, Biomarkers & Prevention, 23*(11), 2512–2521.

Fernandez, M. E., ten Hoor, G., van Lieshout, S., Rodriguez, S., Beidas, R., Parcel, G., Ruiter, R., Markham, C., & Kok, G. (2019). Implementation mapping: Using intervention mapping to develop implementation strategies. *Frontiers in Public Health, 7,* 158. doi:10.3389/fpubh.2019.00158

Fernandez, M. E., Damschroder, L., & Balasubramanian, B. (2022). Understanding barriers and facilitators for implementation across settings. In B. J. Weiner, K. Sherr, & C. C. Lewis (Eds.), *Practical implementation science: Moving evidence into action.* Springer Publishing.

Fernandez, M. E., Kang, E., Balasubramanian, B., Walker, T., Unger, K. (2024, December 8–11, 2024). *Optimizing the pace of implementation mapping logic model* [Workshop]. 17th Annual Conference on the Science of Dissemination and Implementation in Health, Arlington, VA.

Fernandez, M. E., Powell, B. J., Ten Hoor, G.A. (2023). *Implementation mapping for selecting, adapting, and developing implementation strategies. Frontiers in Public Health 11,* 12887

Fox, K., Passey, D., Kang, E., Zeigen, L., Kenzie, E., Austin, J. D., Meadows, R. J., Fernandez, M. E., & Perez Jolles, M. (2025). Application of core functions and forms in complex health intervention research: a scoping review protocol. BMJ open, 15(1), e091088. doi: 10.1136/bmjopen-2024-091088

Fontaine, G., Mooney, M., Porat-Dahlerbruch, J., Cahir, K., Ellen, M., Spinewine, A., Taylor, N., Laritz, R., Bourbeau-Allard, È., & Grimshaw, J. M. (2025). Advancing the selection of implementation science theories, models, and frameworks: A scoping review and the development of the SELECT-IT meta-framework. *Implementation Science, 20*(1), 24. doi:10.1186/s13012-025-01436-5

Gabbert, K. D., Tompkins, N. O., & Murphy, E. (2023). Addressing the gap between academic research and grassroots public health practice: Supporting policy, systems, and environmental changes in rural communities. *Health Promotion Practice, 24*(1_suppl), 161s–169s. doi:10.1177/15248399221115452

Gaglio, B., Shoup, J., & Glasgow, R. (2013). The RE-AIM framework: A systematic review of use over time. *American Journal of Public Health, 103*(6), e48–e46.

Glasgow, R. E., Estabrooks, P. A., & Ory, M. G. (2020). Characterizing evolving frameworks: Issues from Esmail et al. (2020) review. *Implementation Science, 15*(1), 53. doi:10.1186/s13012-020-01009-8

Glasgow, R. E., Harden, S. M., Gaglio, B., Rabin, B., Smith, M. L., Porter, G. C., Ory, M. G., & Estabrooks, P. A. (2019). RE-AIM planning and evaluation framework: Adapting to new science and practice with a 20-year review. *Frontiers in Public Health, 7*, 64.

Glasgow, R. E., Klesges, L. M., Dzewaltowski, D. A., Estabrooks, P. A., & Vogt, T. M. (2006). Evaluating the impact of health promotion programs: Using the RE-AIM framework to form summary measures for decision making involving complex issues. *Health Education Research, 21*(5), 688–684.

Glasgow, R. E., McKay, H. G., Piette, J. D., & Reynolds, K. D. (2001). The RE–AIM framework for evaluating interventions: What can it tell us about approaches to chronic illness management? *Patient Education and Counseling, 44*(2), 119–127.

Glasgow, R. E., Vogt, T. M., & Boles, S. M. (1999). Evaluating the public health impact of health promotion interventions: The RE-AIM framework. *American Journal of Public Health, 89*, 1322–1327.

Grimshaw, J. M., Shirran, L., Thomas, R., Mowatt, G., Fraser, C., Bero, L., Grilli, R., Harvey, E., Oxman, A., & O'Brien, M. A. (2001). Changing provider behavior: An overview of systematic reviews of interventions. *Medical Care, 8*(Suppl 2), II2–II45.

Guerin, R. J., Glasgow, R. E., Tyler, A., Rabin, B. A., & Huebschmann, A. G. (2022). Methods to improve the translation of evidence-based interventions: A primer on dissemination and implementation science for occupational safety and health researchers and practitioners. *Safety Science, 152*. doi:10.1016/j.ssci.2022.105763

Hailemariam, M., Bustos, T., Montgomery, B., Barajas, R., Evans, L. B., & Drahota, A. (2019). Evidence-based intervention sustainability strategies: A systematic review. *Implementation Science, 14*(1), 57. doi:10.1186/s13012-019-0910-6

Harden, S. M., Strayer, T. E., 3rd, Smith, M. L., Gaglio, B., Ory, M. G., Rabin, B., Estabrooks, P. A., & Glasgow, R. E. (2019). National working group on the RE-AIM planning and evaluation framework: Goals, resources, and future directions. *Frontiers in Public Health, 7*, 390. doi:10.3389/fpubh.2019.00390

Hartveit, M., Hovlid, E., Øvretveit, J., Assmus, J., Bond, G., Joa, I., Heiervang, K., Stensrud, B., Høifødt, T. S., Biringer, E., & Ruud, T. (2022). Can systematic implementation support improve programme fidelity by improving care providers' perceptions of implementation factors? A cluster randomized trial. *BMC Health Services Research, 22*(1), 808. doi:10.1186/s12913-022-08168-y

Havelock, R. G. (1971). The utilisation of educational research and development. *British Journal of Educational Technology, 2*(2), 84–98.

Hawe, P., Shiell, A., & Riley, T. (2004). Complex interventions: how "out of control" can a randomised controlled trial be?. BMJ (Clinical research ed.), 328(7455), 1561–1563. doi: 10.1136/bmj.328.7455.1561

Health Workforce Technical Assistance Center (2016). Rapid cycle quality improvement (RCQI): A resource guide to accelerate improvement efforts for health resources and services administration (HRSA) grantees. CHWS Studies. https://www.healthworkforceta.org/wp-content/uploads/2024/11/RCQI_Resource_Guide.pdf

Henderson, V., Tossas-Milligan, K., Martinez, E., Williams, B., Torres, P., Mannan, N., Green, L., Thompson, B., Winn, R., & Watson, K. S. (2020). Implementation of an integrated framework for a breast cancer screening and navigation program for women from underresourced communities. *Cancer, 126*(Suppl 10), 2481–2493. doi:10.1002/cncr.32843

Hoelscher, D. M., Springer, A., Menendez, T. H., Cribb, P. W., & Kelder, S. H. (2011). From NIH to Texas schools: Policy impact of the Coordinated Approach to Child Health (CATCH) program in Texas. *Journal of Physical Activity & Health, 8*(Suppl 1), S5–S7. doi:10.1123/jpah.8.s1.s5

Holcomb, J., Ferguson, G. M., Sun, J., Walton, G. H., & Highfield, L. (2022). Stakeholder engagement in adoption, implementation, and sustainment of an evidence-based intervention to increase mammography adherence among low-income women. *Journal of Cancer Education, 37*(5), 1486–1495. doi:10.1007/s13187-021-01988-2

Holtrop, J. S., Estabrooks, P. A., Gaglio, B., Harden, S. M., Kessler, R. S., King, D. K., Kwan, B. M., Ory, M. G., Rabin, B. A., Shelton, R. C., & Glasgow, R. E. (2021). Understanding and applying the RE-AIM framework: Clarifications and resources. *Journal of Clinical and Translational Science, 5*(1), e126. doi:10.1017/cts.2021.789

Holtrop, J. S., Rabin, B. A., & Glasgow, R. E. (2018). Dissemination and implementation science in primary care research and practice: Contributions and opportunities. *Journal of American Board of Family Medicine, 31*(3), 466–478. doi:10.3122/jabfm.2018.03.170259

Hoskins, K., Sanchez, A. L., Hoffacker, C., Momplaisir, F., Gross, R., Brady, K. A., Pettit, A. R., Zentgraf, K., Mills, C., Coley, D., & Beidas, R. S. (2022). Implementation mapping to plan for a hybrid trial testing the effectiveness and implementation of a behavioral intervention for HIV medication adherence and care retention. *Frontiers in Public Health, 10*, 872746. doi:10.3389/fpubh.2022.872746

Johnson, K., Hays, C., Center, H., & Daley, C. (2004). Building capacity and sustainable prevention innovations: A sustainability planning model. *Evaluation and Program Planning, 27*(2), 135–149. doi:10.1016/j.evalprogplan.2004.01.002

Kallam, B., Pettitt-Schieber, C., Owen, M., Agyare Asante, R., Darko, E., & Ramaswamy, R. (2018). Implementation science in low-resource settings: Using the interactive systems framework to improve hand hygiene in a tertiary hospital in Ghana. *International Journal for Quality in Health Care, 30*(9), 724–730. doi:10.1093/intqhc/mzy111

Kang, E., & Foster, E. R. (2022). Use of implementation mapping with community-based participatory research: Development of implementation strategies of a new goal setting and goal management intervention system. *Frontiers in Public Health, 10*, 834473. doi:10.3389/fpubh.2022.834473

Keith, R. E., Crosson, J. C., O'Malley, A. S., Cromp, D., & Taylor, E. F. (2017). Using the Consolidated Framework for Implementation Research (CFIR) to produce actionable findings: A rapid-cycle evaluation approach to improving implementation. *Implementation Science, 12*(1), 15. doi:10.1186/s13012-017-0550-7

Kelder, S. H., Mitchell, P. D., McKenzie, T. L., Derby, C., Strikmiller, P. K., Luepker, R. V., & Stone, E. J. (2003). Long-term implementation of the CATCH physical education program. *Health Education & Behavior, 30*(4), 463–475. doi:10.1177/1090198103253538

King, D. K., Shoup, J. A., Raebel, M. A., Anderson, C. B., Wagner, N. M., Ritzwoller, D. P., & Bender, B. G. (2020). Planning for implementation success using RE-AIM and CFIR frameworks: A qualitative study. *Frontiers in Public Health, 8*, 59. doi:10.3389/fpubh.2020.00059

Kok, G., Gottlieb, N. H., Peters, G.-J. Y., Mullen, P. D., Parcel, G. S., Ruiter, R. A. C., Fernández, M. E., Markham, C., & Bartholomew, L. K. (2016). A taxonomy of behavior change methods: An Intervention Mapping approach. *Health Psychology Review, 10,* 297–312. doi: 10.1080/17437199.2015.1077155

Kononowech, J., Landis-Lewis, Z., Carpenter, J., Ersek, M., Hogikyan, R., Levy, C., Phibbs, C., Scott, W., & Sales, A. E. (2020). Visual process maps to support implementation efforts: A case example. *Implementation Science Communications, 1*(1), 105. doi:10.1186/s43058-020-00094-6

Kwan, B. M., Brownson, R. C., Glasgow, R. E., Morrato, E. H., & Luke, D. A. (2022). Designing for dissemination and sustainability to promote equitable impacts on health. *Annual Review of Public Health, 43,* 331–353. doi:10.1146/annurev-publhealth-052220-112457

Kwok, G., Senger, A., Sharma, A., Mandato, I., & Devine, K. A. (2024). Understanding the multilevel factors influencing the implementation of digital health interventions for supportive care in Adolescents and Young Adult (AYA) cancer survivorship: Determinants of adopting mindfulness-based mobile applications. *Implementation Science Communications, 5*(1), 76. doi:10.1186/s43058-024-00612-w

LeClair, A. M., Kotzias, V., Garlick, J., Cole, A. M., Kwon, S. C., Lightfoot, A., & Concannon, T. W. (2020). Facilitating stakeholder engagement in early stage translational research. *PLoS ONE, 15*(7), e0235400. doi:10.1371/journal.pone.0235400

Lengnick-Hall, R., Stadnick, N. A., Dickson, K. S., Moullin, J. C., & Aarons, G. A. (2021). Forms and functions of bridging factors: Specifying the dynamic links between outer and inner contexts during implementation and sustainment. *Implementation Science, 16*(1), 34. doi:10.1186/s13012-021-01099-y

Lewis, C. C., Klasnja, P., Lyon, A. R., Powell, B. J., Lengnick-Hall, R., Buchanan, G., Meza, R. D., Chan, M. C., Boynton, M. H., & Weiner, B. J. (2022). The mechanics of implementation strategies and measures: Advancing the study of implementation mechanisms. *Implementation Science Communications, 3*(1), 114. doi:10.1186/s43058-022-00358-3

Linnan, L., & Steckler, A. (2002). Process evaluation for public health interventions and research: An overview. In L. Linnan & A. Steckler (Eds.), *Process evaluation for public health interventions and research.* Jossey-Bass.

Livingood, W. C., Bilello, L., Lukens-Bull, K., Smotherman, C., & Choe, U. (2020). Implementation research as applied science: Bridging the research to practice gap. *Health Promotion Practice, 21*(1), 49–57. doi:10.1177/1524839919858082

Lloyd, A., Joseph-Williams, N., Edwards, A., Rix, A., & Elwyn, G. (2013). Patchy 'coherence': Using normalization process theory to evaluate a multi-faceted shared decision making implementation program (MAGIC). *Implementation Science, 8,* 102. doi:10.1186/1748-5908-8-102

Lopez, C. J., Neil-Sztramko, S. E., Tanyoas, M., Campbell, K. L., Bender, J. L., Strudwick, G., Langelier, D. M., Reiman, T., Greenland, J., & Jones, J. M. (2024). Use of implementation mapping to develop a multifaceted implementation strategy for an electronic prospective surveillance model for cancer rehabilitation. *Implementation Science Communications, 5*(1), 108. doi:10.1186/s43058-024-00650-4

Luke, D. A., Calhoun, A., Robichaux, C. B., Elliott, M. B., & Moreland-Russell, S. (2014). The Program Sustainability Assessment Tool: A new instrument for public health programs. *Preventing Chronic Disease, 11*, 130184. doi:10.5888/pcd11.130184

Markham, C. M., Rushing, S. C., Manthei, J., Singer, M., Jessen, C., Gorman, G., Peskin, M. F., Hernandez, B. F., Sacca, L., Evans, G. S., Luna-Meza, C., Merritt, Z., & Shegog, R. (2022). The Healthy Native Youth Implementation Toolbox: Using Implementation Mapping to adapt an online decision support system to promote culturally-relevant sexual health education for American Indian and Alaska Native youth. *Frontiers in Public Health, 10*, 889924. doi:10.3389/fpubh.2022.889924

Major, M. G., King, J. F., Taaffe, S. T., Troyer, L. E., Waggoner, Z., Craig, D. W., Holden, R. J., Martinez Kercher, V. M., & Kercher, K. A. (2025). Refining a college student-led implementation strategy using implementation mapping in a rural school. *Health Behavior Research*, 8(4). doi:10.4148/2572-1836.1330

May, C. R., Mair, F., Finch, T., MacFarlane, A., Dowrick, C., Treweek, S., Rapley, T., Ballini, L., Ong, B. N., Rogers, A., Murray, E., Elwyn, G., Légaré, F., Gunn, J., & Montori, V. M. (2009). Development of a theory of implementation and integration: Normalization process theory. *Implementation Science, 4*(1), 29. doi:10.1186/1748-5908-4-29

May, C. R., Mair, F. S., Dowrick, C. F., & Finch, T. L. (2007). Process evaluation for complex interventions in primary care: Understanding trials using the normalization process model. *BMC Family Practice, 8*(1), 42. doi:10.1186/1471-2296-8-42

May, C., & Finch, T. (2009). Implementing, embedding, and integrating practices: An outline of Normalization Process Theory. Sociology, 43(3), 535–554. doi:10.1177/0038038509103208

McEvoy, R., Ballini, L., Maltoni, S., O'Donnell, C. A., Mair, F. S., & Macfarlane, A. (2014). A qualitative systematic review of studies using the normalization process theory to research implementation processes. *Implementation Science*, 9, 2. doi:10.1186/1748-5908-9-2

McGuier, E. A., Kolko, D. J., Aarons, G. A., Schachter, A., Klem, M. L., Diabes, M. A., Weingart, L. R., Salas, E., & Wolk, C. B. (2024). Teamwork and implementation of innovations in healthcare and human service settings: A systematic review. *Implementation Science, 19*(1), 49. doi:10.1186/s13012-024-01381-9

McNett, M. M., Tucker, S. J., Juckett, L. A., & Bunger, A. C. (2024). Advancing implementation practice: Supplemental tools to aid in selection of implementation strategies and outcomes for healthcare practitioners. *Global Implementation Research and Applications, 4*(3), 286–295. doi:10.1007/s43477-024-00122-w

Merrill, K. G., Silva, J., Sedeño, A., Salgado, S., Vargas, S., Cano, J. K., Nabor, V., Merrill, J. C., DeCelles, J., Guastaferro, K., Baumann, A. A., Fuentes, J., Rodriguez, L., Melgoza, V., & Donenberg, G. R. (2025). Preparing to implement Floreciendo with Latina teens and their female caregivers: Integrating implementation science and the multiphase optimization strategy framework. *Translational Behavioral Medicine, 15*(1). doi:10.1093/tbm/ibaf005

Meyers, D. C., Durlak, J. A., & Wandersman, A. (2012). The quality implementation framework: A synthesis of critical steps in the implementation process. *American Journal of Community Psychology, 50*(3–4), 462–480. doi:10.1007/s10464-012-9522-x

Michie, S. (2008). What works and how? Designing more effective interventions needs answers to both questions. *Addiction, 103*, 886–887. doi:10.1111/j.1360-0443.2007.02112.x

Michie, S., Johnston, M., Abraham, C., Lawton, R., Parker, D., Walker, A., & Psychological Theory, G. (2005). Making psychological theory useful for implementing evidence based practice: A consensus approach. *Quality & Safety in Health Care, 14*(1), 26–33.

Miech, E. J., Rattray, N. A., Flanagan, M. E., Damschroder, L., Schmid, A. A., & Damush, T. M. (2018). Inside help: An integrative review of champions in healthcare-related implementation. *SAGE Open Medicine, 6*. doi:10.1177/2050312118773261

Miller, R. L., & Shinn, M. (2005). Learning from communities: Overcoming difficulties in dissemination of prevention and promotion efforts. *American Journal of Community Psychology, 35*(3–4), 169–183.

Mizuno, T., Dong, M., Taylor, Z. L., Ramsey, L. B., & Vinks, A. A. (2020). Clinical implementation of pharmacogenetics and model-informed precision dosing to improve patient care. *British Journal of Clinical Pharmacology, 88*(4), 1218–1426. doi:10.1111/bcp.14426

Moullin, J. C., Dickson, K. S., Stadnick, N. A., Albers, B., Nilsen, P., Broder-Fingert, S., Mukasa, B., & Aarons, G. A. (2020). Ten recommendations for using implementation frameworks in research and practice. *Implementation Science Communications, 1*, 42. doi:10.1186/s43058-020-00023-7

Moullin, J. C., Dickson, K. S., Stadnick, N. A., Rabin, B., & Aarons, G. A. (2019). Systematic review of the Exploration, Preparation, Implementation, Sustainment (EPIS) framework. *Implementation Science, 14*(1), 1. doi:10.1186/s13012-018-0842-6

Moullin, J. C., Ehrhart, M. G., & Aarons, G. A. (2018). The role of leadership in organizational implementation and sustainment in service agencies. *Research on Social Work Practice, 28*(5), 558–567. doi:10.1177/1049731517718361

Munch, P. K., Jørgensen, M. B., Højberg, H., & Rasmussen, C. D. N. (2020). Nationwide dissemination of a digital checklist to improve work environment in the eldercare sector in Denmark. *Frontiers in Public Health, 8*, 502106. doi:10.3389/fpubh.2020.502106

NCCIH. Pilot studies: Common uses and misuses. US Department of Health and Human Services. Retrieved July 3 from https://www.nccih.nih.gov/grants/pilot-studies-common-uses-and-misuses

Nilsen, P. (2015). Making sense of implementation theories, models and frameworks. *Implementation Science, 10*(1), 53. doi:10.1186/s13012-015-0242-0

Nilsen, P. (2025). Evaluation of implementation: A taxonomy of implementation science theories, models, and frameworks. In A. Kaehne & J. Feather (Eds.), *Handbook of health services evaluation: Theories, methods and innovative practices* (pp. 161–172). Springer Nature Switzerland. doi:10.1007/978-3-031-87869-5_9

Nilsen, P., & Bernhardsson, S. (2019). Context matters in implementation science: A scoping review of determinant frameworks that describe contextual determinants for implementation outcomes. *BMC Health Services Research, 19*(1), 189. doi:10.1186/s12913-019-4015-3

Noonan, R. K., Wilson, K. M., & Mercer, S. L. (2012). Navigating the road ahead: Public health challenges and the interactive systems framework for dissemination and implementation. *American Journal of Community Psychology, 50*(3–4), 572–580.

Nordberg, S. S., Jaso-Yim, B. A., Sah, P., Schuler, K., Eyllon, M., Pennine, M., Hoyler, G. H., Barnes, J. B., Murillo, L. H., O'Dea, H., Orth, L., Rogers, E., Welch, G., Peloquin, G., & Youn, S. J. (2024). Evaluating the implementation and clinical effectiveness of an innovative digital first care model for behavioral health using the RE-AIM framework: Quantitative evaluation. *Journal of Medical Internet Research, 26,* e54528. doi:10.2196/54528

Orlandi, M. A. (1986). The diffusion and adoption of worksite health promotion innovations: An analysis of barriers. *Preventive Medicine, 15*(5), 522–536.

Palinkas, L. A., Horwitz, S. M., Green, C. A., Wisdom, J. P., Duan, N., & Hoagwood, K. (2015). Purposeful sampling for qualitative data collection and analysis in mixed method implementation research. *Administration and Policy in Mental Health, 42*(5), 533–544. doi:10.1007/s10488-013-0528-y

Park, S., Bakko, M., & Pinto, R. M. (2025). Improving delivery of research-supported practices in human service organizations: A narrative review of organizational dimensions in dissemination and implementation. *Human Service Organizations: Management, Leadership & Governance, 50,* 1–43. doi:10.1080/23303131.2025.2471533

Pearson, N., Naylor, P.-J., Ashe, M. C., Fernandez, M., Yoong, S. L., & Wolfenden, L. (2020). Guidance for conducting feasibility and pilot studies for implementation trials. *Pilot and Feasibility Studies,* 6(1), 167. doi:10.1186/s40814-020-00634-w

Perez Jolles, M., Lengnick-Hall, R., & Mittman, B. S. (2019). Core functions and forms of complex health interventions: A patient-centered medical home illustration. *Journal of General Internal Medicine, 34*(6), 1032–1038. doi:10.1007/s11606-018-4818-7

Pérez Jolles, M., Fernández, M. E., Jacobs, G., De Leon, J., Myrick, L., & Aarons, G. A. (2022). Using Implementation Mapping to develop protocols supporting the implementation of a state policy on screening children for Adverse Childhood Experiences in a system of health centers in inland Southern California. *Frontiers in Public Health,* 10, 876769. https://doi.org/10.3389/fpubh.2022.876769

Perkison, W. B., Rodriguez, S. A., Velasco-Huerta, F., Mathews, P. D., Pulicken, C., Beg, S. S., Heredia, N. I., Fwelo, P., White, G. E., Reininger, B. M., McWhorter, J. W., Chenier, R., & Fernandez, M. E. (2023). Application of implementation mapping to develop strategies for integrating the National Diabetes Prevention Program into primary care clinics. *Frontiers in Public Health, 11,* 933253. doi:10.3389/fpubh.2023.933253

Peskin, M. F., Hernandez, B. F., Gabay, E. K., Cuccaro, P., Li, D. H., Ratliff, E., Reed-Hirsch, K., Rivera, Y., Johnson-Baker, K., Emery, S. T., & Shegog, R. (2017). Using intervention mapping for program design and production of iCHAMPSS: An online decision support system to increase adoption, implementation, and maintenance of evidence-based sexual health programs. *Frontiers in Public Health, 5,* 203. doi:10.3389/fpubh.2017.00203

Peskin, M. F., Hernandez, B. F., Markham, C., Johnson, K., Tyrrell, S., Addy, R. C., Shegog, R., Cuccaro, P. M., DeRoulet, P. E., & Tortolero, S. R. (2011). Sexual health education from the perspective of school staff: Implications for adoption and implementation of effective programs in middle school. *Journal of Applied Research on Children,* 2(2), 9.

Peterson, J. C., Rogers, E. M., Cunningham-Sabo, L., & Davis, S. M. (2007). A framework for research utilization applied to seven case studies. *American Journal of Preventive Medicine, 33*(1), S21–S34.

Polo, J., Basile, M. J., Zhang, M., Ordonez, K., Rodriguez, D., Boye-Codjoe, E., Williams, M., Tsang, D., Medina, R., Jacome, S., Mir, P., Khanijo, S., Pekmezaris, R., & Hajizadeh, N. (2023). Application of the RE-AIM framework to evaluate the implementation of telehealth pulmonary rehabilitation in a randomized controlled trial among African-American and Hispanic patients with advanced stage Chronic Obstructive Pulmonary Disease. *BMC Health Services Research, 23*(1), 515. doi:10.1186/s12913-023-09492-7

Powell, B. J., Beidas, R. S., Lewis, C. C., Aarons, G. A., McMillen, J. C., Proctor, E. K., & Mandell, D. S. (2017). Methods to improve the selection and tailoring of implementation strategies. *The Journal of Behavioral Health Services & Research, 44*(2), 177–194. doi:10.1007/s11414-015-9475-6

Powell, B. J., McMillen, J. C., Proctor, E. K., Carpenter, C. R., Griffey, R. T., Bunger, A. C., Glass, J. E., & York, J. L. (2012). A compilation of strategies for implementing clinical innovations in health and mental health. *Medical Care Research and Review, 69*(2), 123–157. doi:10.1177/1077558711430690

Powell, B. J., Waltz, T. J., Chinman, M. J., Damschroder, L. J., Smith, J. L., Matthieu, M. M., Proctor, E. K., & Kirchner, J. E. (2015). A refined compilation of implementation strategies: Results from the Expert Recommendations for Implementing Change (ERIC) project. *Implementation Science, 10*(1), 1–14.

Proctor, E., Luke, D., Calhoun, A., McMillen, C., Brownson, R., McCrary, S., & Padek, M. (2015). Sustainability of evidence-based healthcare: Research agenda, methodological advances, and infrastructure support. *Implementation Science, 10*(1), 88. doi:10.1186/s13012-015-0274-5

Proctor, E., Silmere, H., Raghavan, R., Hovmand, P., Aarons, G., Bunger, A., Griffey, R., & Hensley, M. (2011). Outcomes for implementation research: Conceptual distinctions, measurement challenges, and research agenda. *Administration and Policy in Mental Health and Mental Health Services Research, 38*(2), 65–76.

Proctor, E. K., Bunger, A. C., Lengnick-Hall, R., Gerke, D. R., Martin, J. K., Phillips, R. J., & Swanson, J. C. (2023). Ten years of implementation outcomes research: A scoping review. *Implementation Science, 18*(1), 31. doi:10.1186/s13012-023-01286-z

Proctor, E. K., Powell, B. J., & McMillen, J. C. (2013). Implementation strategies: Recommendations for specifying and reporting. *Implementation Science, 8*, 139. doi:10.1186/1748-5908-8-139

Quanbeck, A. R., Gustafson, D. H., Ford, J. H., 2nd, Pulvermacher, A., French, M. T., McConnell, K. J., & McCarty, D. (2011). Disseminating quality improvement: Study protocol for a large cluster-randomized trial. *Implementation Science, 6*, 44. doi:10.1186/1748-5908-6-44

Quinn, A. K., Neta, G., Sturke, R., Olopade, C. O., Pollard, S. L., Sherr, K., & Rosenthal, J. P. (2019). Adapting and operationalizing the RE-AIM framework for implementation science in environmental health: Clean fuel cooking programs in low resource countries. *Frontiers in Public Health, 7*, 389. doi:10.3389/fpubh.2019.00389

Reilly, K. L., Kennedy, S., Porter, G., & Estabrooks, P. (2020). Comparing, contrasting, and integrating dissemination and implementation outcomes included in the RE-AIM and implementation outcomes frameworks. *Frontiers in Public Health, 8*, 430. doi:10.3389/fpubh.2020.00430

Reis, R. S., Salvo, D., Ogilvie, D., Lambert, E. V., Goenka, S., & Brownson, R. C. (2016). Scaling up physical activity interventions worldwide: Stepping up to larger and smarter approaches to get people moving. *Lancet, 388*(10051), 1337–1348. doi:10.1016/s0140-6736(16)30728-0

Rhodes, R. E., Grant, S., & de Bruijn, G.-J. (2020). Planning and implementation intention interventions. In M. S. Hagger, L. D. Cameron, K. Hamilton, N. Hankonen, & T. Lintunen (Eds.), *The handbook for behavior change* (pp. 572–585). Cambridge University Press. doi:10.1017/9781108677318

Richards, J. E., Simon, G. E., Boggs, J. M., Beidas, R., Yarborough, B. J. H., Coleman, K. J., Sterling, S. A., Beck, A., Flores, J. P., Bruschke, C., Grumet, J. G., Stewart, C. C., Schoenbaum, M., Westphal, J., & Ahmedani, B. K. (2021). An implementation evaluation of "Zero Suicide" using normalization process theory to support high-quality care for patients at risk of suicide. *Implementation Research and Practice, 2.* doi:10.1177/26334895211011769

Ridde, V., Pérez, D., & Robert, E. (2020). Using implementation science theories and frameworks in global health. *BMJ Global Health, 5*(4), e002269. doi:10.1136/bmjgh-2019-002269

Rimer, B. K., Glanz, K., & Rasband, G. (2001). Searching for evidence about health education and health behavior interventions. *Health Education & Behavior, 28*(2), 231–248.

Robinson, K., Elliott, S. J., Driedger, S. M., Eyles, J., O'Loughlin, J., & Riley, B. (2005). Using linking systems to build capacity and enhance dissemination in heart health promotion: A Canadian multiple-case study. *Health Education Research, 20,* 499–513.

Rogers, E. M. (1983). *Diffusion of innovations* (Vol. 3). Free Press.

Rodriguez, S. A., Velasco-Huerta, F., Sampson-Ansah, M., Garza, E. R., Perkison, W. B., Mathews, P. D., Pulicken, C., & Fernandez, M. E. (2025). Factors influencing implementation of a self-measured blood pressure program in community health centers: an implementation mapping approach. *Frontiers in public health,* 13, 1485343. doi: 10.3389/fpubh.2025.1485343

Rogers, E. M. (1995). *Diffusion of innovations* (Vol. 4). Free Press.

Rogers, E. M. (2003). *Diffusion of innovations* (Vol. 5). Free Press.

Rogers, R. (1983). Cognitive and physiological processes in fear-based attitude change: A revised theory of protection motivation. In J. Cacioppa & R. Petty (Eds.), *Social psychophysiology: A sourcebook* (pp. 153–176). Guilford Press.

Rossi, P. H., Lipsey, M. W., & Freeman, H. E. (2004). *Evaluation: A systematic approach* (Vol. 7). Sage.

Rowbotham, S., Conte, K., & Hawe, P. (2019). Variation in the operationalisation of dose in implementation of health promotion interventions: Insights and recommendations from a scoping review. *Implementation Science, 14*(1), 56. doi:10.1186/s13012-019-0899-x

Sacca, L., Shegog, R., Hernandez, B., Peskin, M., Rushing, S. C., Jessen, C., Lane, T., & Markham, C. (2022). Barriers, frameworks, and mitigating strategies influencing the dissemination and implementation of health promotion interventions in indigenous communities: A scoping review. *Implementation Science, 17*(1), 18. doi:10.1186/s13012-022-01190-y

Sanchez, S. H., Sethi, S. S., Santos, S. L., & Boockvar, K. (2014). Implementing medication reconciliation from the planner's perspective: A qualitative study. *BMC Health Services Research, 14*(1), 290.

Savas, L. S., Loomba, P., Shegog, R., Alaniz, A., Costa, C., Adlparvar, E., Allicock, M. A., Chenier, R., Goetz, M., & Markham, C. M. (2023). Using Implementation

Mapping to increase uptake and use of Salud en Mis Manos: A breast and cervical cancer screening and HPV vaccination intervention for Latinas. *Frontiers in Public Health, 11*, 966553.

Scaccia, J. P., Cook, B. S., Lamont, A., Wandersman, A., Castellow, J., Katz, J., & Beidas, R. S. (2015). A practical implementation science heuristic for organizational readiness: R = MC(2). *Journal of Community Psychology, 43*(4), 484–501. doi:10.1002/jcop.21698

Scheirer, M. A. (1981). *Program implementation: The organizational context.* Sage.

Schell, S. F., Luke, D. A., Schooley, M. W., Elliott, M. B., Herbers, S. H., Mueller, N. B., & Bunger, A. C. (2013). Public health program capacity for sustainability: A new framework. *Implementation Science, 8*(1), 15.

Schol, C. M. A., van Mol, M. M. C., & Ista, E. (2025). Developing implementation strategies for digital ICU diaries targeting ICU professionals: an implementation mapping approach. Implementation science communications, *6*(1), 85. doi: 10.1186/s43058-025-00767-0

Schroeck, F. R., Ould Ismail, A. A., Haggstrom, D. A., Sanchez, S. L., Walker, D. R., & Zubkoff, L. (2022). Data-driven approach to implementation mapping for the selection of implementation strategies: A case example for risk-aligned bladder cancer surveillance. *Implementation Science, 17*(1), 58. doi:10.1186/s13012-022-01231-6

Scott, V. C., LaMarca, T. K., Hamm, D., Tolley, A. J., Rachel, S. A., & Wandersman, A. (2024). The ART of readiness: A practical tool for implementation tailoring at the activity level. *Global Implementation Research and Applications, 4*(2), 139–150. doi:10.1007/s43477-023-00115-1

Shato, T., Kepper, M. M., McLoughlin, G. M., Tabak, R. G., Glasgow, R. E., & Brownson, R. C. (2024). Designing for dissemination among public health and clinical practitioners in the USA. *Journal of Clinical and Translational Science, 8*(1), e8. doi:10.1017/cts.2023.695

Shea, C. M. (2021). A conceptual model to guide research on the activities and effects of Innovation Champions. *Implementation Research and Practice, 2.* doi:10.1177/2633489521990443

Shediac-Rizkallah, M. C., & Bone, L. R. (1998). Planning for the sustainability of community-based health programs: Conceptual frameworks and future directions for research, practice and policy. *Health Education Research, 13*(1), 87–108.

Shelton, R. C., & Brownson, R. C. (2024). Enhancing impact: A call to action for equitable implementation science. *Prevention Science, 25*(Suppl. 1), 174–189. doi:10.1007/s11121-023-01589-z

Shelton, R. C., Chambers, D. A., & Glasgow, R. E. (2020). An extension of RE-AIM to enhance sustainability: Addressing dynamic context and promoting health equity over time. *Frontiers in Public Health, 8.* doi:10.3389/fpubh.2020.00134

Shelton, R. C., Cooper, B. R., & Stirman, S. W. (2018). The sustainability of evidence-based interventions and practices in public health and health care. *Annual Review of Public Health, 39*, 55–76. doi:10.1146/annurev-publhealth-040617-014731

Simons-Morton, D. G., Simons-Morton, B. G., Parcel, G. S., & Bunker, J. F. (1988). Influencing personal and environmental conditions for community health: A multilevel intervention model. *Family & Community Health, 11*(2), 25–35.

Springer, A., Evans, A., Ortuno, J., Salvo, D., & Arevalo, M. (2017). Health by design: Interweaving health promotion into environments and settings. *Frontiers in Public Health, 5*, 1–10, Article 268. doi:10.3389/fpubh.2017.00268

Steckler, A., Goodman, R. M., McLeroy, K. R., Davis, S., & Koch, G. (1992). Measuring the diffusion of innovative health promotion programs. *American Journal of Health Promotion, 6*(3), 214–224.

Stensland, K. D., Sales, A. E., Damschroder, L. J., & Skolarus, T. A. (2022). Applying implementation frameworks to the clinical trial context. *Implementation Science Communications, 3*(1), 109. doi:10.1186/s43058-022-00355-6

Stolldorf, D. P., Storrow, A. B., Liu, D., Jenkins, C. A., Hilton, R. A., Miller, K. F., Kim, J., Boopathy, D., Gunaga, S., Kea, B., Miller, J., & Collins, S. P. (2025). A mixed-methods observational study of strategies for success in implementation science: Overcoming emergency departments hurdles. *BMC Health Services Research, 25*(1), 147. doi:10.1186/s12913-024-12102-9

Suchland, C. E., & Carbonaro, S. (2021). Connecting high-impact practices and student self-efficacy: Social cognitive theory as a window into student growth. *Intersection: A Journal at the Intersection of Assessment and Learning, 2*(2), 15.

Szeszulski, J., Craig, D. W., Walker, T. J., Foster, M., Mullen, P. D., & Fernandez, M. E. (2022). Applying evidence-based intervention (EBI) mapping to identify the components and logic of colorectal cancer screening interventions. *Translational Behavioral Medicine, 12*(2), 304–323.

Tabak, R. G., Khoong, E. C., Chambers, D. A., & Brownson, R. C. (2012). Bridging research and practice: Models for dissemination and implementation research. *American Journal of Preventive Medicine, 43*(3), 337–350.

Ten Hoor, G. A., Kok, G., Rutten, G. M., Ruiter, R. A. C., Kremers, S. P. J., Schols, A. M. J. W., & Plasqui, G. (2016). The Dutch 'Focus on Strength' intervention study protocol: Programme design and production, implementation, and evaluation plan. *BMC Public Health, 16*(496). doi:10.1186/s12889-016-3150-6

Thackeray, A., Waring, J., Hoogeboom, T. J., Nijhuis-van Der Sanden, M. W. G., Hess, R., Fritz, J. M., Conroy, M. B., & Fernandez, M. E. (2022). Implementing a Dutch physical therapy intervention into a U.S. health system: Selecting strategies using implementation mapping. *Front Public Health, 10*, 908484. doi:10.3389/fpubh.2022.908484

Towfighi, A., Orechwa, A. Z., Aragón, T. J., Atkins, M., Brown, A. F., Brown, J., ... Yee, H. F., Jr. (2020). Bridging the gap between research, policy, and practice: Lessons learned from academic-public partnerships in the CTSA network. *Journal of Clinical and Translational Science, 4*(3), 201–208. 10.1017/cts.2020.23

Trickett, E. J. (2011). Community-based participatory research as worldview or instrumental strategy: Is it lost in translation(al) research? *American Journal of Public Health, 101*(8), 1353–1355. doi:10.2105/AJPH.2011.300124

Trinkley, K. E., Glasgow, R. E., D'Mello, S., Fort, M. P., Ford, B., & Rabin, B. A. (2023). The iPRISM webtool: An interactive tool to pragmatically guide the iterative use of the Practical, Robust Implementation and Sustainability Model in public health and clinical settings. *Implementation Science Communications, 4*(1), 116. doi:10.1186/s43058-023-00494-4

Turin, T. C., Kazi, M., Rumana, N., Lasker, M. A. A., & Chowdhury, N. (2023). Employing diffusion of innovation theory for 'not missing the mass' in community-engaged research. *BMJ Open, 13*(8), e069680. doi:10.1136/bmjopen-2022-069680

Valerio-Shewmaker, M. A., Heredia, N. I., Pulicken, C., Mathews, P. D., Chenier, R., Swoboda, T. L., Garza, E. R., Velasco-Huerta, F., & Fernandez, M. E. (2022). Using implementation mapping for the adoption and implementation of Target: BP in community health centers. *Frontiers in Public Health, 10*, 928148. doi:10.3389/fpubh.2022.928148

Van Citters, A. D., Dieni, O., Scalia, P., Dowd, C., Sabadosa, K. A., Fliege, J. D., Jain, M., Miller, R. W., & Ren, C. L. (2021). Barriers and facilitators to implementing telehealth services during the COVID-19 pandemic: A qualitative analysis of interviews with cystic fibrosis care team members. *Journal of Cystic Fibrosis, 20*(Suppl. 3), 23–28. doi:10.1016/j.jcf.2021.09.004

van Nassau, F., Nauta, J., Bouma, A. J., Krops, L. A., van den Akker-Scheek, I., Diercks, R. L., de Jong, J., Leutscher, H., Stevens, M., van Twillert, S., van Mechelen, W., Zwerver, J., Verhagen, E. A. L. M., van der Woude, L. H. V., van Keeken, H., van der Ploeg, H. P., & Dekker, R. (2025). Stepwise development of an implementation protocol to support the prescription of Exercise = Medicine by clinicians using the Implementation Mapping approach. *Frontiers in health services*, 5, 1645456. doi: 10.3389/frhs.2025.1645456

Vedel, I., Le Berre, M., Sourial, N., Arsenault-Lapierre, G., Bergman, H., & Lapointe, L. (2018). Shedding light on conditions for the successful passive dissemination of recommendations in primary care: A mixed methods study. *Implementation Science, 13*(1), 129. doi:10.1186/s13012-018-0822-x

Walker, T. J., Are, F., Heredia, N. I., Onadeko, K., Saving, E. E., Kang, E., & Fernandez, M. E. (2025a). Identifying mechanisms of action for implementation strategies using a retrospective implementation mapping logic model approach. *Prevention Science, 26*(2), 161–174. doi:10.1007/s11121-025-01790-2

Walker, T. J., Brandt, H. M., Wandersman, A., Scaccia, J., Lamont, A., Workman, L., Dias, E., Diamond, P. M., Craig, D. W., & Fernandez, M. E. (2020). Development of a comprehensive measure of organizational readiness (motivation × capacity) for implementation: A study protocol. *Implementation Science Communications, 1*(1), 103. doi:10.1186/s43058-020-00088-4

Walker, T. J., Craig, D. W., Pfledderer, C. D., Lee, M., Onadeko, K., Saving, E. E., Bartholomew, J. B., & Fernandez, M. E. (2025b). Feasibility and acceptability of an implementation strategy to enhance use of classroom-based physical activity approaches in elementary schools: A mixed methods study. *BMC Public Health, 26*(1), 36.

Walker, T. J., Craig, D. W., Pfledderer, C. D., Onadeko, K., Saving, E. E., Nicksic, H. M., Patlovich, K., Fumero, K., Bartholomew, J. B., & Fernández, M. E. (2025c). Using implementation mapping to design an implementation strategy for classroom-based physical activity approaches in elementary schools. *Translational behavioral medicine, 15*(1), ibaf021. doi: 10.1093/tbm/ibaf021

Walker, T. J., Foster, M., Szeszulski, J., Craig, D. W., Mullen, P. D., & Fernández, M. E. (2022a). Evidence-Based Intervention (EBI) Mapping: a systematic approach to understanding the components and logic of EBIs. *BMC Public Health, 22*(1), 1300. doi:10.1186/s12889-022-13692-x

Walker, T. J., Kang, E., Savas, L., Are, F., Szuszulski, J., Powell, B., Shelley, D., Saldana, L., Kwak, L., Kirchner, J., Smith, J., & Fernandez, M. E. (2026). Identifying and describing implementation strategy mechanisms using an implementation mapping logic model (IMap logic model). *Implementation Science.* under review

Walker, T. J., Kohl, H. W., 3rd, Bartholomew, J. B., Green, C., & Fernández, M. E. (2022b). Using Implementation Mapping to develop and test an implementation strategy for active learning to promote physical activity in children: A feasibility study using a hybrid type 2 design. *Implementation Science Communications, 3*(1), 26. doi:10.1186/s43058-022-00271-9

Wallerstein, N., & Duran, B. (2010). Community-based participatory research contributions to intervention research: The intersection of science and practice to improve health equity. *American Journal of Public Health, 100*(S1), S40–S46. doi:10.2105/ajph.2009.184036

Wallerstein, N. B., & Duran, B. (2006). Using community-based participatory research to address health disparities. *Health Promotion Practice, 7*(3), 312–323. doi:1524839906289376

Waltz, T. J., Powell, B. J., Fernández, M. E., Abadie, B., & Damschroder, L. J. (2019). Choosing implementation strategies to address contextual barriers: Diversity in recommendations and future directions. *Implementation Science, 14*(1), 1–15.

Waltz, T. J., Powell, B. J., Matthieu, M. M., Damschroder, L. J., Chinman, M. J., Smith, J. L., Proctor, E. K., & Kirchner, J. E. (2015). Use of concept mapping to characterize relationships among implementation strategies and assess their feasibility and importance: Results from the Expert Recommendations for Implementing Change (ERIC) study. *Implementation Science, 10*(1), 109. doi:10.1186/s13012-015-0295-0

Wandersman, A. (2017). *Organizational readiness as capacity building: "Readiness Is All"* [Presentation]. Danish Implementation Network

Wandersman, A., Cook, B. S., Clark, K., Flaspohler, P., Watson, A., & Lamont, A. E. (2024). Commentary: Bridging and reducing the gaps between research and practice: Pathways to outcomes and the interactive systems framework for dissemination and implementation 2.0. *Evaluation & the Health Professions, 47*(4), 494–506. doi:10.1177/01632787241299820

Wandersman, A., Duffy, J., Flaspohler, P., Noonan, R., Lubell, K., Stillman, L., Blachman, M., Dunville, R., & Saul, J. (2008). Bridging the gap between prevention research and practice: The interactive systems framework for dissemination and implementation. *American Journal of Community Psychology, 41*(3-4), 171–181.

Wang, Y., Wong, E. L.-Y., Nilsen, P., Chung, V. C.-h., Tian, Y., & Yeoh, E.-K. (2023). A scoping review of implementation science theories, models, and frameworks—an appraisal of purpose, characteristics, usability, applicability, and testability. *Implementation Science, 18*(1), 43. doi:10.1186/s13012-023-01296-x

Wangen, M., Escoffery, C., Fernandez, M. E., Friedman, D. B., Hannon, P., Ko, L. K., Maxwell, A. E., Petagna, C., Risendal, B., Rohweder, C., & Leeman, J. (2023). Twenty years of capacity building across the cancer prevention and control research network. *Cancer Causes & Control, 34*(Suppl. 1), 45–56. doi:10.1007/s10552-023-01690-2

Warhurst, K., Tyack, Z., Beckmann, M., & Abell, B. (2025). The use of implementation mapping in healthcare settings: A scoping review. *Frontiers Public Health, Article 13*, 1603178. doi:10.3389/fpubh.2025.1603178

Watson, A. K., Hernandez, B. F., Kolodny-Goetz, J., Walker, T. J., Lamont, A., Imm, P., Wandersman, A., & Fernandez, M. E. (2022). Using implementation mapping to build organizational readiness. *Frontiers in Public Health, 10*, 904652.

Weiner, B. J., Lewis, M. A., & Linnan, L. A. (2009). Using organization theory to understand the determinants of effective implementation of worksite health promotion programs. *Health Education Research, 24*(2), 292–305. doi:10.1093/her/cyn019

Weir, N. M., Newham, R., Dunlop, E., & Bennie, M. (2019). Factors influencing national implementation of innovations within community pharmacy: A systematic review applying the Consolidated Framework for Implementation Research. *Implementation Science, 14*(1), 21. doi:10.1186/s13012-019-0867-5

Weiner, B. J. (2020). Chapter 8: A theory of organizational readiness for change. In Per Nilsen & Sarah A. Birken (Eds.), *Handbook on implementation science.* Cheltenham, UK: Edward Elgar Publishing, doi:10.4337/9781788975995.00015

Whelan, J., Fraser, P., Bolton, K. A., Love, P., Strugnell, C., Boelsen-Robinson, T., Blake, M. R., Martin, E., Allender, S., & Bell, C. (2023). Combining systems thinking approaches and implementation science constructs within community-based prevention: A systematic review. *Health Research Policy and Systems, 21*(1), 85. doi:10.1186/s12961-023-01023-4

Williams, N. J., Wolk, C. B., Becker-Haimes, E. M., & Beidas, R. S. (2020). Testing a theory of strategic implementation leadership, implementation climate, and clinicians' use of evidence-based practice: A 5-year panel analysis. *Implementation Science, 15*(1), 10. doi:10.1186/s13012-020-0970-7

Wiltsey Stirman, S., Kimberly, J., Cook, N., Calloway, A., Castro, F., & Charns, M. (2012). The sustainability of new programs and innovations: A review of the empirical literature and recommendations for future research. *Implementation Science, 7*(1), 17. doi:10.1186/1748-5908-7-17

Woodward, E. N., Singh, R. S., Ndebele-Ngwenya, P., Melgar Castillo, A., Dickson, K. S., & Kirchner, J. E. (2021). A more practical guide to incorporating health equity domains in implementation determinant frameworks. *Implementation Science Communications, 2*(1), 61. doi:10.1186/s43058-021-00146-5

Wu, S., Tannous, E., Haldane, V., Ellen, M. E., & Wei, X. (2022). Barriers and facilitators of implementing interventions to improve appropriate antibiotic use in low- and middle-income countries: A systematic review based on the Consolidated Framework for Implementation Research. *Implementation Science, 17*(1), 30. doi:10.1186/s13012-022-01209-4

Zamantakis, A., Merle, J. L., Queiroz, A. A., Zapata, J. P., Deskins, J., Pachicano, A. M., Mongrella, M., Li, D., Benbow, N., Gallo, C., Smith, J. D., & Mustanski, B. (2024). Innovation and implementation determinants of HIV testing and linkage-to-care in the U.S.: A systematic review. *Implement. Science Communication, 5*(1), 111. doi:10.1186/s43058-024-00638-0

Zulman, D. M., Damschroder, L. J., Smith, R. G., Resnick, P. J., Sen, A., Krupka, E. L., & Richardson, C. R. (2013). Implementation and evaluation of an incentivized Internet-mediated walking program for obese adults. *Translational Behavioral Medicine, 3*(4), 357–369.

Zurynski, Y., Ludlow, K., Testa, L., Augustsson, H., Herkes-Deane, J., Hutchinson, K., Lamprell, G., McPherson, E., Carrigan, A., Ellis, L. A., Dharmayani, P. N. A., Smith, C. L., Richardson, L., Dammery, G., Singh, N., & Braithwaite, J. (2023). Built to last? Barriers and facilitators of healthcare program sustainability: A systematic integrative review. *Implementation Science, 18*(1), 62. doi:10.1186/s13012-023-01315-x

CHAPTER 10

INTERVENTION MAPPING STEP 6

Evaluation Plan

with Patricia Dolan Mullen, Melissa Peskin, and Casey Durand

INTERVENTION MAPPING STEP 6 TASKS

1. **Review the logic model of change, matrices, and implementation plan to guide process and effect evaluation**
2. **Develop process evaluation questions and identify measures**
3. **Develop effect evaluation questions, select a design, and identify measures**
4. **Pilot test the intervention and finalize the evaluation plan**
5. **Plan when and how to report evaluation findings**

Overview

The product of Intervention Mapping Step 6 is a comprehensive evaluation plan that has been pretested and includes a plan for strategically reporting and disseminating the findings. This chapter helps planners (also called evaluators here) use the previous steps of Intervention Mapping (IM) to plan an evaluation that can produce useful knowledge about the intervention's implementation and effectiveness and provide information for improving it.

Task 1 reviews the previous IM steps to guide process and effect evaluation planning. Tasks 2 and 3 provide specific details about designs for process (also called implementation evaluation) and effect evaluation (also known as impact, outcome, and summative evaluation). Tasks 4 and 5 focus on pilot testing and dissemination. Thus, this chapter completes intervention planning and provides online resources and textbooks that expand on the concepts described in this chapter.

The first three tasks in evaluation rely heavily on the logic model of change and implementation plan that enable the evaluator to develop evaluation questions. Input from those with a vested interest and consideration of ethical issues and what is already known will help decide the reasons for the evaluation (which questions should have the highest priority).

Reasons for Evaluation

Planning an evaluation begins with thinking about its purpose. Informed by the previous steps of IM, we present several of the most important reasons.

1. To monitor whether the intervention is being implemented as planned and is being delivered to the intended audiences.
2. To determine whether the appeal or effectiveness of an intervention needs to be improved.
3. To demonstrate whether an intervention is achieving the intended effects and to determine whether this investment of resources should continue.
4. To determine whether one intervention should be preferred over another based on its greater effectiveness or its lower cost per unit of effect.

Clarity about the reason(s) for an evaluation is crucial when selecting the evaluation questions to be addressed, the indicators, and measures and designs to be used, and the resources that are needed. Negotiating the perspectives of various parties on the reasons for evaluation is considered in the next section.

Identifying and Engaging Groups with a Vested Interest in the Evaluation

A foundational task for developing an evaluation plan, the results of which are used and trusted, is to identify those with a vested interest and gather their perspectives on the questions an evaluation should address. Many of the individuals selected in Step 1 of IM (see Chapter 5, Table 5.1) will be important for the evaluation, although not all these interested parties will be relevant for every evaluation (Preskill & Jones, 2009). The first step is to identify those with a vested interest and decide the degree and kind of involvement each will have, keeping in mind the potential impact of overlooking individuals key to discussions of study designs and data analysis (Eyre et al., 2017; Simmons et al., 2015). A general list of those with a vested interest or "stake" in the evaluation is provided in Table 10.1.

Different groups will have different evaluation interests. For example, managers will be especially interested in the proportion of the intended beneficiaries or environmental change agents who participate, how much of the intervention they receive, whether staff members have the skills and credentials needed for implementation, and the costs of the intervention. Members of the at-risk group or environmental change agents are likely to be interested in barriers and facilitators to participation, opinions of the intervention by their peers, and assurance that evaluation results will improve its quality and accessibility.

Ensuring involvement is a continuing process. Here are suggested steps:

- Identify potentially interested parties, involve them early, and set realistic expectations about the resources that are available (or potentially available) for the evaluation (e.g., money, personnel, time, administrative

Table 10.1 Potential Groups with a Vested Interest

Policymakers and decision makers	Persons responsible for deciding whether the program is to be initiated, continued, discontinued, expanded, modified, restructured, or curtailed
Program sponsors	Individuals with positions of responsibility in public agencies or private organizations that initiate and fund the program (may overlap with policy makers and decision-makers)
Evaluation sponsors	Individuals with positions of responsibility in public agencies or private organizations who initiate and fund the evaluation (sometimes program sponsors and evaluation sponsors are the same)
Intended beneficiaries	Persons, households, or other units that are intended to receive the ultimate benefit of the intervention or services being evaluated
Targeted environmental change agents	Persons who are intended to receive components of the intervention to help change an environmental condition
Program managers	Personnel responsible for overseeing and administering the intervention
Program staff	Personnel responsible for delivering the program services or functioning in supporting roles
Program competitors	Organizations or groups that compete with the program for available resources
Interested parties in the immediate environment	Organizations, groups, and individuals in the environment of a program with interests in what the program is doing or what happens to it
Evaluation and research community	Evaluation professionals who judge evaluations and their technical quality and credibility and researchers who work in areas related to program

Adapted from Rossi et al. (2019).

support) and the safeguards to protect the confidentiality of all evaluation participants and the reputations of organizational partners;

- Plan structures that are sensitive to the power dynamics among groups. A practical guide for dealing with power imbalances is provided by Bryson and Patton (2015);
- Negotiate clear agreement on the intended purpose, users, and uses of the evaluation, as well as the deliverables, timeline, and budget;
- Help those with a vested interest plan how to use, interpret the evaluation data, and provide feedback, including an explanation of the technical terms used in describing the design (e.g., random assignment) and their meaning and value;
- Present evaluation results on time and in multiple forms and build opportunities for feedback and interpretation (see Task 5 below).

Several of the steps listed above come from the Centers for Disease Control and Prevention's Framework for Program Evaluation in Public Health (Kidder et al., 2024). This framework stresses the importance of reaching an explicit agreement that includes all engaged groups. The agreement might take the form of a detailed protocol (such as a grant proposal), a memorandum of understanding, or even a legal contract. The agreement provides a basis for modifying or renegotiating procedures, if necessary. Bryson and Patton (2015) offer a stakeholder engagement planning matrix (Figure 2.2, pp. 56–57) to help the evaluator plan the extent to which each stakeholder will be involved in each step of the evaluation as it progresses from planning to completion and reporting. Some evaluators use an empowerment approach to enhance the knowledge, research and communication skills, and leadership of the at-risk group, environmental change agents, and intervention implementers, with the aim of encouraging ownership and use of the results for advocacy and change (Fetterman et al., 2014).

Conflicts of Interest

Conflicts can arise when defining the questions to be addressed, when designing the evaluation plan, when the results are reported and there is unhappiness over the outcome, when there are multiple outcomes available with different implications, or when there are misunderstandings of the terms used. Findings may lead to discontinuation of the intervention and with it, jobs and popular services. It might be summed up as "human nature" to form attachments and antipathies – intervention implementers afraid to lose their funding, academics interested in advancing their careers, or funders with their own needs. Evaluations can have real consequences.

Suggestions for dealing with conflicts of interest include the steps above in engaging interested parties, but getting to agreement and effective use of evaluation findings is not always easy. Additional actions can help an evaluator steer through rough waters (see Box 10.1):

BOX 10.1. ACTIONS TO GET AGREEMENT AMONG GROUPS WITH VESTED INTERESTS

- Develop facilitation skills. Excellent people skills are needed in addition to technical skills and social science knowledge.
- Find and train users of evaluation information. This is a natural aspect of empowerment approaches.
- Focus on intervention improvement and comparative effectiveness studies to counterbalance the notion that evaluations result in "all or none" findings.
- Find "tipping point connectors." This refers to people who are looked to by others for information that could influence key decision-makers (Gladwell, 2000 cited by Bryson & Patton, 2015).
- Facilitate high-quality interactions, rather than sheer quantity of interaction.
- Nurture interest in the evaluation. Find out the interests of those involved in the evaluation process and be sure to make those issues are taken into account.

- Demonstrate cultural sensitivity and humility. Understand personal biases, get feedback from interested groups, and use it.
- Anticipate turnover of intended users. Identify backups and possible substitutes and stay in touch with users to see whether their circumstances are changing.

Source: Adapted from Bryson and Patton (2015).

Ethical Issues

Ethical issues can arise in the course of planning and carrying out an evaluation, and also in using the results. How to avoid bias? How to assure informed consent of all parties whose privacy (and safety) may be at stake? What standards of comparison are appropriate? What is acceptable treatment for the control group? How large a sample is needed? Which perspective to adopt in calculating costs and benefits? How should the results be reported and interpreted?

Bias

Bias in an evaluation is an ethics problem. Bias is associated with distorting the design of an evaluation or selectively reporting the results to favor particular conclusions. The American Evaluation Association's Evaluator's Ethical Guiding Principles (2025) provides advice on avoiding bias (American Evaluation Association, 2025).

Informed Consent

All evaluation participants have the right to know exactly what information will be collected, how long it will be kept, to whom and how it will be reported, and whether there are mandatory reporting requirements (e.g., child or elder abuse). They also need to know whether they can refuse consent and what effect this will have on their access to the services they may be receiving and other information that demonstrates respect for their privacy and autonomy (National Commission for the Protection of Human Subjects of Biomedical and Behavioural Research, 1979). Approval of the content and delivery method by the appropriate human subjects protection body (known in the United States as an institutional review board or in Europe as an ethical review committee) will be essential in most cases of effect evaluations and for many process evaluations. Determination of whether an evaluation study meets the criteria of "human subjects research" requires board approval and should be made by an appropriate review group or committee rather than the evaluator alone. Even when conducting exempt studies, evaluators should be aware of the principles of protection of the privacy of human participants. For more detailed information about the General Data Protection Regulation that updates the European Union (EU)-wide law, see Crutzen, Peters, and Mondschein (2019).

Language that is understandable to a potential participant and an organization and that facilitates comprehension, and engagement is at the heart of informed consent. And yet, complexity is increased by the Common Rule (the US guidance for ethical research conduct), which mandates up to 18 elements that must be disclosed to potential research participants. Nevertheless, consents should take literacy into account, using suitable templates and measure literacy levels of the participants and reading levels of the consent documents to assure that all participants can make an informed decision (See Chapter 8, Paying Attention to (Health) Literacy). Examples for minimal risk research are available from the World Health Organization (for clinical research and research with children) and the US Agency for Healthcare Research and Quality.

Organizations associated with the evaluation also need to understand the risks and benefits of participating. What resources will be available to compensate staff time that may be required to pull records, screen potential participants, adapt organizational policies, make referrals to the intervention, modify their records, and so on? Are there other unforeseen costs to participation? Will staff receive training that may benefit the organization or their careers? Will the organization be identified in reports, and can they change their minds about how they will be identified after they see the results? Will any members of the organization staff be co-authors of the report? How quickly will members of the organization get to see the results, and will they have the opportunity to review and provide input to the report before it is distributed? And, finally, are the external evaluation staff trained to keep confidential their observations about the organization or its staff or clients? Appropriate procedures and rules should be put in place to assure institutional confidentiality and respect while appropriately bringing forward any problems that are identified.

Interpreting Results

Clarity about the perspective taken and the standards, criteria, and evidence for the conclusions drawn from an evaluation is essential. Evaluators should express the results of process and effect evaluations in terms of their practical significance, not just statistical significance and not just selected findings that happen to be statistically significant. Also needed are easy-to-understand explanations of the evaluation's strengths and weaknesses; discussion of recommendations for action with their advantages, disadvantages, and resource implications; and a presentation of minority opinions or rejoinder if there are other views (see plan for communicating results, Task 5).

Step 6 Tasks

The five primary tasks for conducting Step 6 are presented in Box 10.2 and described below.

BOX 10.2. INTERVENTION MAPPING STEP 6 TASKS

1. Review the logic model of change, matrices and implementation plan to guide process and effect evaluation
2. Develop process evaluation questions and identify measures
3. Develop effect evaluation questions, select a design, and identify measures
4. Pilot test the intervention and finalize the evaluation plan
5. Plan when and how to report evaluation findings

Task 1: Review the Logic Model of Change, Matrices, and Implementation Plan to Guide Process and Effect Evaluation

This most basic view of the intervention and its mechanisms of action can be seen in the logic model of change (Figure 10.1) that lays out the understanding of the causes of the health problem (Chapter 5, Step 1) and also defines how an intervention is supposed to work to produce change (Chapters 6 and 7, Steps 2 and 3).

IM promotes understanding and appraisal of the intervention's conceptualization and design as the first part of evaluation. This is consistent with classic and modern evaluation texts (Bryson & Patton, 2015; Fetterman et al., 2014; Rossi et al., 2019) that underscore the importance of understanding the components and logic of an intervention as an important part of the evaluation process. Evaluators have used the terms "logic model," "theory of action," "program theory," and "causal model" (McLaughlin & Jordan, 2015; Patton, 2008; Scheirer, 1994; Weiss, 1995).

Below we list several classic questions that evaluators ask when planning the evaluation of an intervention.

- Is the intervention based on evidence of a need in this population?
- Is there evidence for the relationship between the targeted behaviors and environmental conditions to the health problem?
- Is there evidence for the selected determinants, change methods, practical applications, and delivery channels?
- Were the perspectives of those with a vested interest in the intervention incorporated in the design of the intervention logic?

Interventions that have been developed using Steps 1–5 of IM are likely to stand up well to this scrutiny and their logic will be transparent. Sometimes, however, evaluators are asked to plan an evaluation for an

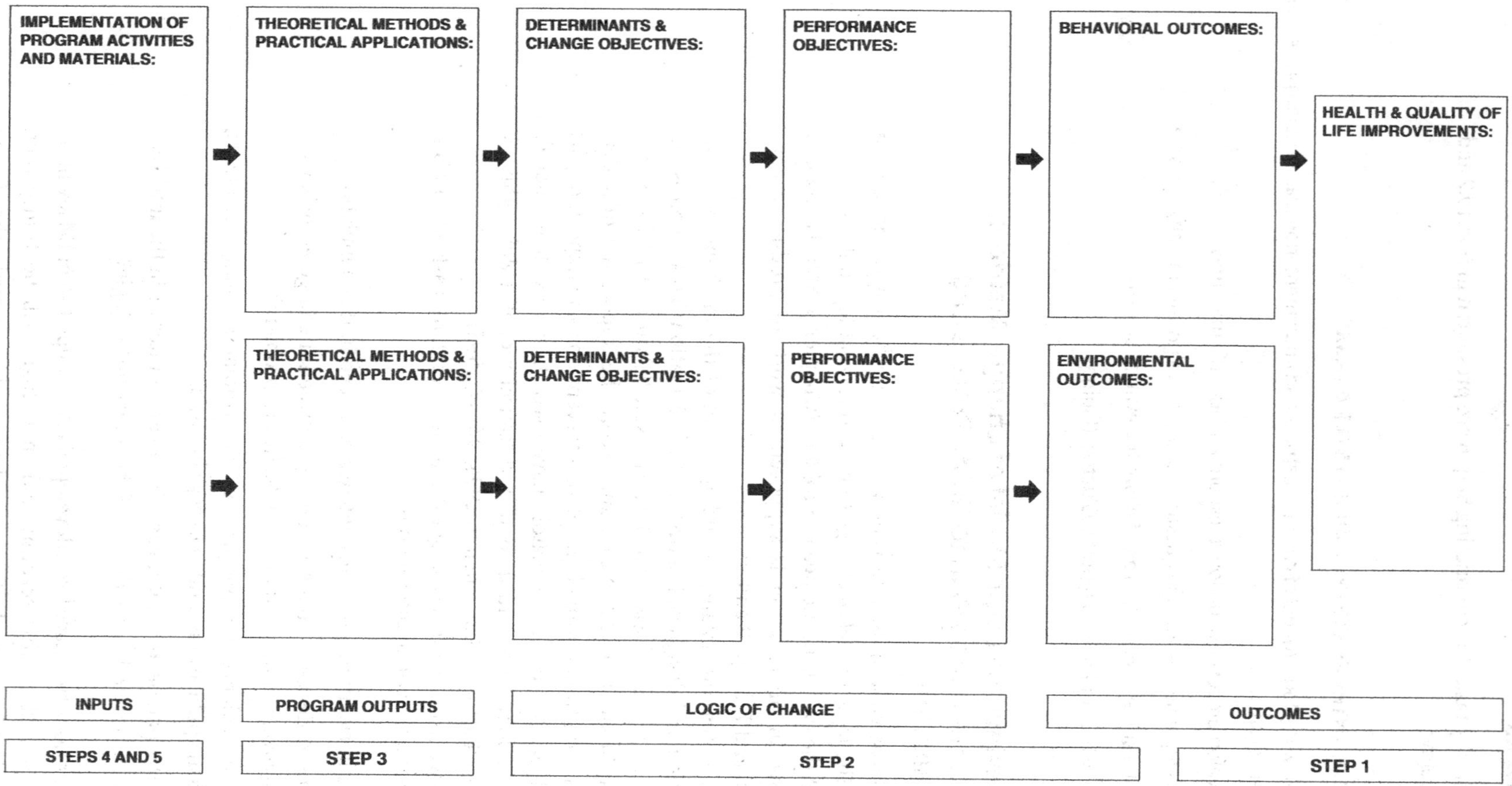

Figure 10.1 Logic Model of the Intervention

intervention without the foundational documents produced in Steps 1–5. In this case, the evaluator must backtrack to reconstruct the logic of the intervention (Chapter 11 on adaptation provides a systematic process, EBI mapping, for deriving the logic of an existing intervention).

The logic model documents can translate directly into evaluation questions. The list of implementers' tasks in **implementation plan**, for example, "police correctly use de-escalation tactics" might become "How often do police correctly use . . .?" (Engel et al., 2022).

Other elements in the implementation plan will bring in the implementation strategy(ies) that have been selected, e.g., training and reinforcement, which will become process evaluation questions. And, the far-left elements of the **logic model**—change methods and their practical applications—provide additional process evaluation questions.

Using the intervention's logic model (Figure 10.1) and matrices developed in Step 2, the evaluator can also readily see that possible effects (or outcomes) of interest (and subsequently effect or outcome evaluation questions) include quality of life, health problems, behaviors, environmental conditions, and intervention objectives (performance objectives, change objectives, and determinants). The notion of identifying effects (and the time frame for expected effects to occur) was also discussed previously in IM Step 1 in relation to SMART objectives. In the needs assessment, the planning team will have set goals for expected changes in these effects. Those goals form the basis for potential effect evaluation questions based on the timeframe selected (discussed below in Task 3). For the effect evaluation, the decision is which constructs should be selected for the final questions. In other words, how far to the right of the logic model of change should the effect evaluation extend? This will depend on how much is known about the health problem and its causes. It is likely that the behavioral or environmental causes of the health problem are well established, as in the case of tobacco cigarette smoking and many forms of cancer and heart disease. In the de-escalation example, only one trial to date has established the positive impact on citizen and officer safety (Engel et al., 2022).

Thus, evaluators will want to consider similarities across interventions and their resources to decide whether to ask about behavior alone or also its impact. To complete the logic of the effect evaluation, questions should include factors further to the left of the selected effects (here, determinants). Next, moving to the left in Figure 10.1, the planner has specified expected changes in objectives from the matrices, that is, performance objectives and change objectives (see Chapter 6). Change objectives combine determinants (supported by theory and/or empirical evidence and expert opinion) with expected performance objectives; both should be well specified and documented from IM Step 2. Planners can easily turnkey change objectives into effect evaluation questions. For example, in an evaluation of It's Your Game. . .Keep it Real, an HIV, STI, and pregnancy prevention intervention for middle-school students, the following effect evaluation questions were derived from the IM work on change objectives: Did the teens who participated in the intervention increase their knowledge of condom use compared to teens who did not receive it? Did participants increase their skills and self-efficacy to use condoms compared to teens who did not receive the intervention (Markham et al., 2012; Tortolero et al., 2010)? These questions form an explicit model that enables an evaluator to analyze their relations with more near-term (distal) effects. This can shed light on how much the determinants were changed and which one(s) were most important in bringing about the outcomes.

Task 2: Develop Process Evaluation Questions and Identify Measures

A well-designed intervention may not be recognizable after it is implemented. Decades ago, a pioneer in evaluation and advocate for the importance of implementation, Carol Weiss, called attention to this problem with the proverb, "There's many a slip between the cup and the lip" (Weiss, 1972). "Process evaluation" is focused on intervention operations and designed to document any "slips" that may have occurred, even including whether the intervention was delivered at all! Process evaluation compares the plan for who is supposed to do what to whom, when, how, where, and with what resources to what actually happens. Subtasks start with defining the purpose of the process evaluation, developing evaluation questions and identifying indicators and measures to complete the plan. (During an effect evaluation, evaluators may also collect process data in a comparison group, to find out whether an unplanned intervention may have contaminated the evaluation.)

Process evaluation is analogous (but not identical) to assessing the impact of implementation strategies (discussed in Chapter 9). Both focus on implementation fidelity and reach and measure similar phenomena. The difference is that the primary purpose of a process evaluation is to help evaluators identify gaps in intervention fidelity and reach that aid interpretation of the findings of the effect evaluation and/or inform improvements in the delivery of the intervention for future implementation (used as a monitoring tool, described below). Process evaluation does not necessarily have formal implementation research questions or hypotheses, whereas implementation studies typically have a research question focused on understanding the impact of one or more specific implementation strategies on fidelity and/or reach. Implementation science has described types of studies that explicitly test both implementation and effectiveness outcomes in the same study (see hybrid studies in Task 3).

A process evaluation may be intended to stand alone as a set of activities focused on monitoring an intervention or as the necessary adjunct to an effect evaluation. To be clear, **a process evaluation is always needed; it is not, however, always necessary to conduct an effect evaluation.**

As a monitoring tool, process evaluation can be seen as part of continuous quality improvement, a concept that originated in business and management science. Its principles have been applied to program evaluation, and in particular, process (and effect) monitoring to ensure that results can be used to continually improve program performance (Linnan & Steckler, 2002; Patton, 2008; Rossi et al., 2019; Scheirer, 1994; Woodhouse et al., 2013). For example, Hawe et al. (2009) suggest that intervention reach for complex interventions can be improved by tracking how interventions impact different social networks. Scott et al. (2020) describe the use of evaluation to conduct rapid-cycle program improvement systems for the evaluation (to monitor intervention dose, quality, and satisfaction) of complex interventions (such as multi-component and multi-level community improvement initiatives). This concept is also referred to "design thinking" or "agile working" which are also discussed in Chapter 8, Step 4 (Dijksterhuis & Silvius, 2017).

Process mapping can be used to demonstrate visually the flow of participants through complex interventions, such as clinical practice activities (Trebble et al., 2010; Zusevics et al., 2021). Ongoing process monitoring can also be used to forecast future program participation (Holzhauser et al., 2018), and in an implementation design, it can be considered the outcome of an implementation strategy.

Develop Process Evaluation Questions

Process evaluation questions could also be called a "learning agenda" (Scheirer, 1994). Evaluators should consider: (1) **reach or coverage**, the extent to which the intervention and its components are reaching the intended audiences and any associated biases in who is served; (2) **delivery**, the extent to which the intervention delivery is faithful to the intervention design and implementation specifications and is received by participants; (3) **participant satisfaction and engagement**, and (4) the **availability of implementation structure and resources**. The answers to these questions are typically followed by a diagnosis of the causes of any gaps that are identified. These four categories of questions are described in more detail below, noting that different authors have used slightly different terms but share similar questions.

We adapt open-ended questions from Rossi et al. (2019) below, noting that it is most helpful if evaluators adopt a **standard of comparison** as part of the question. This is usually a standard of acceptability that may come from the funding agency or other source negotiated among stakeholders. Thus, although intervention developers hope for 100% "fidelity" and 100% "reach" and do not want deficiencies in implementation or for anyone to be left out, standards should not be set unrealistically high. Accountability (e.g., does it meet standards for reach?) tempered with a learning perspective (e.g., why do some priority groups have low rates of participation?) is important to improving the intervention.

1. Intervention Reach

Typical process evaluation questions focus on the extent to which any aspect of the intervention reaches the intended audiences, the ultimate beneficiaries and environmental change agents. Survey researchers use the term "coverage" and some implementation evaluators describe "penetration." (Proctor et al., 2011).

- How many persons are receiving any part of the intervention?
- Are some members of the intended groups not receiving the intervention? (undercoverage)
- Are some participants not members of the intended group(s)? (overcoverage)
- Are subgroups within the intended groups not receiving the intervention? (bias)
- How many of those who start the intervention complete it? (dropout)
- Are expected sources of referral to the intervention referring appropriate participants?
- Are other services available to potential participants and are they using them?

To assess reach, the characteristics of an eligible group member need to be "spelled out," e.g., Is a tobacco smoker someone who smokes occasionally or someone who smokes at least five cigarettes a day? Must environmental change agents be parents or can grandparents and guardians be included? Realistic targets should be set (see standards of comparison above), and evaluators should focus on subgroups less likely to participate (i.e., bias in coverage). Comparing those who were served with nonparticipants and dropouts can reveal systematic differences across subgroups in which more advantaged subgroups have fewer barriers to accessing the intervention, e.g., those with better transportation, less worried about their legal immigration status.

Follow-up questions to understand the reasons for poor reach overall or in particular subgroups could include, "What are organizational and other barriers to participation?" "What is their level of awareness of the intervention?" "What are their perceptions of the intervention or referral sources?" "What factors explain lack of initial contact with the intervention versus dropout (i.e., those who initially decide not to participate in the intervention versus those who initially decide to participate in the intervention but then drop out)?" "Are participation rates changing over time?" "Are language and cultural barriers involved?" and "Who drops out, when, and why?"

Some authors who have written about process evaluation (Steckler & Linnan, 2002) separate recruitment from reach to emphasize the importance of procedures to attract participants to participate initially in the intervention and maintain engagement in intervention activities (i.e., preventing dropout).

2. Intervention Delivery

Questions related to delivery typically include fidelity to the original intervention design and distinguish between the amount or intended intervention components **delivered** (dose delivered) and **received** (dose received) by the intended population:

- Is the intervention delivered as designed (e.g., includes indicated content, change methods, and dose at all intervention levels) (fidelity)?
- Are there differences between the intervention dose delivered and the dose received?
- Does intervention delivery vary significantly across sites or locales?
- What contextual factors influence delivery?

To formulate delivery questions, the planner must first fully describe the intervention that is intended to be delivered as described in Task 1. The IM intervention planner will have done this in Steps 4 and 5 or through EBI Mapping (Chapter 11). Thus, a description of the intervention components and intervention support materials and resources for the delivery plan will be available for the evaluator. This description should be updated to include any contextual factors that might impact intervention delivery, e.g., changes in screening guidelines or state education policies that might affect whether and how the intervention can be delivered.

Fidelity questions should be selected and refined through discussions with implementers and other interested parties and those experienced with the delivery of similar interventions and delivery systems. Some aspects of the intervention might be flagged for more attention because they are expected to be more problematic to deliver at all or to deliver with fidelity. For example, a motivational interviewing approach in a patient counseling protocol may need more attention than other components because of the skill level required to deliver it according to accepted standards. Questions to consider are "Is this component of the intervention typically omitted in its delivery?" and "Was there adequate preparation of the environmental change agents or implementers?"

The **dose** or amount of the intervention that is actually delivered and received is considered a basic aspect of fidelity, but it is also important when considering reach (Saunders et al., 2005; Steckler & Linnan, 2002). Thus, the evaluator must define the minimum **dose delivered** to define when the individual has completed the intervention, e.g., What is the minimum number of sessions of a 10-session church-based exercise intervention that a participant must attend to be considered served (or reached)? All 10 sessions would probably be too high a standard. This decision requires input from the planners as well as those experienced with similar interventions. The main idea here is determining a simple indicator of "complete dose" and then assessing the extent to which this dose was delivered.

As defined by Saunders, Evans, and Joshi (2005), the **dose received** is the "extent to which participants ... interact with, are receptive to, and/or use materials and resources; can include 'initial use' and 'continued use.'" An obvious example is the extent to which the intended groups read print material or download/use an app. Additional questions to consider are "What stood in the way of participants receiving those components?" and "Are there components of the intervention that intervention participants routinely skip?"

3. Participant Engagement and Satisfaction

Engagement is more than attendance or simply logging in. Other indicators are related to the intervention's theoretical change methods or practical applications. And satisfaction can include participants' judgments about the value of the intervention. These perceptions are particularly relevant to environmental change agents who will make judgments about whether their actions "mattered."

- Do participants engage in activities suggested as part of the intervention (e.g., setting a quit date in a smoking cessation program, signing a contract in a parent–child screen-time reduction program, or using their training to recommend an HPV vaccination)?
- Do intervention participants consider the information, skills, etc. they gained from the intervention helpful and impactful (e.g., setting a quit date helped them make the break from cigarettes, planning a family meeting to discuss having their home be smoke free)?
- Are participants satisfied with their interactions with intervention implementers and procedures (e.g., were fliers readily available, trainers gave clear instructions and provided support even when they made mistakes)?
- Are participants satisfied with the messages, delivery channels, vehicles, and other aspects of the intervention they receive? Are practical applications credible and appealing (e.g., did participants understand the message of video-based role models who emphasized that most peers their age were not using drugs)?

Questions related to the decisions made in intervention planning, that is, questions about change methods and practical applications and their operationalization, were also addressed in the pretesting and formative evaluation of the intervention (see Chapter 8). The difference is that in pilot testing (Task 4 below), the planner can test the intervention in its final form and its final setting instead of a provisional form and simulated setting.

4. **Implementation Structure and Resources**

Assessment of implementation focuses on staffing, organization, resources, and execution of planned tasks that were delineated in IM Step 5:

- Are necessary intervention functions being performed adequately?
- Is staffing sufficient in numbers and qualifications for the functions that must be performed?
- Is the program well organized? Do staff work well with one another?
- Does the program coordinate effectively with other programs and agencies with which it must interact?
- Are resources, facilities, and funding adequate to support necessary intervention functions?
- Are resources used effectively and efficiently?
- What is the cost of the intervention?

As with other aspects of process evaluation used to monitor intervention reach and fidelity over time, changes in participants, technology, and the context, the findings from these questions will provide important information that could lead to new decisions about needed changes. Findings from all elements of a process evaluation often generate questions and hypotheses about the reasons for deficiencies and shortfalls. Typically, the motive is to understand and correct them, but sometimes the discoveries uncover better procedures, innovative resources, or even new groups in need.

Identify Indicators and Measures for Process Evaluation

Both quantitative and qualitative methods are fundamental measurement tools for process and effect evaluation. Because the indicators and measures section for effect evaluation will emphasize quantitative tools for measurement, here we highlight qualitative tools and the combination of quantitative and qualitative approaches known as "mixed methods," and administrative records as well as the special cases of Web and "app" analytics and measurement of intervention costs. Process evaluation measures are closely aligned with the outcomes of implementation strategies, the concepts discussed above, and more sources of process evaluation measures can be found in the implementation science literature (Khadjesari et al., 2020; Lengnick-Hall et al., 2021; Lewis et al., 2015; Mettert et al., 2020; Proctor et al., 2011, 2023).

Qualitative Methods Qualitative methods that are often used for process evaluation include focus group discussions, individual interviews, observations, document review, case studies, and open-ended questions on surveys. Qualitative methods are particularly useful in process evaluation because of their ability to help evaluators understand what is happening and why (Hamilton & Finley, 2019). They include many research genres that have in common the intense or prolonged contact with participants to gain a holistic overview of the context under study. Users of qualitative methods analyze most data with words, and the findings are emergent (inductive) rather than having been structured in advance (deductive) (Miles et al., 2013). Traditional pillars of rigor in quantitative research, reliability and validity, also apply to qualitative research, although as described in Chapter 2, the means for addressing them differ somewhat and come from other scientific perspectives (Long & Johnson, 2000; Malterud, 2001; Mays & Pope, 2000; Tobin & Begley, 2004).

Evaluators conducted a qualitative process evaluation using student focus groups and teacher interviews to assess perceived satisfaction and challenges to implementation fidelity for *Fourth R* (Peskin et al., 2019b), an effective school-based teen dating violence intervention (Wolfe et al., 2009). Students and teachers reported that the intervention was engaging, interactive, and helpful. Teachers also said that the intervention included examples that were relevant and realistic for their students, but they also reported disappointment that the lessons were only available in English and that this intervention competed for limited time with existing curricula. Importantly, these findings led to translation of the lessons into Spanish and more attention to coordination with existing programs.

Mixed Methods As introduced in Chapter 5, IM Step 1, the value of a strategic mix of the two sets of methods is now widely recognized (Bamberger, 2012; Creswell et al., 2011; Green et al., 2015), particularly when answering questions about the factors that influence intervention implementation (Green et al., 2015). We have already suggested that qualitative methods are often used for process evaluation. Newer applications in conjunction with quantitative methods, for example, key informant interviews, are a response to the special problem that arises when an effect evaluation is initiated after the intervention begins and qualitative data help reconstruct characteristics of intervention participants and nonparticipants at the time the intervention began. A way in which quantitative methods can strengthen qualitative is by use of the quantitative sampling frame, to help ensure that the individuals providing qualitative data are representative of the population that is being evaluated (Bamberger, 2012).

Quantitative methods are less time consuming; cost less per unit collected; permit evaluator control; are regarded as unbiased, with standard parameters for reliability and validity; and are easily analyzed (Chapel, 2024). Qualitative methods usually require more time for analysis, and they can be costlier per unit collected, although fewer units are collected. A mixed-methods approach balances concerns about the reliability and validity of a single method with a combination of methods that have complementary strengths and nonoverlapping weaknesses (Chapel, 2024). Mixed methods provide corroboration, that is, better understanding, more credibility, and "triangulation" through multiple perspectives on the same event or phenomenon. Mixed methods help the evaluator see patterns and explore new insights (Chapel, 2024).

Two basic categories of mixed methods design (concurrent and sequential) are discussed in Chapter 5. An example of a sequential explanation design, where qualitative data are collected to explain in greater depth the mechanisms underlying quantitative results, can be found in a mixed methods process evaluation of an exercise program for ethnic minority mothers in the Netherlands (Hartman et al., 2013). The evaluators used reply cards and the attendance records to measure reach and participation as well as observations of the recruitment process, interviews with 14 key figures and 32 mothers who responded to the recruitment channel. The qualitative component found that the recruiters were familiar and trusted and could serve as a translator and motivator. Enthusiasm and cultural relevance (for the priority population) and tailoring to the individual appeared to enhance receptivity to the intervention.

Mixed methods also aid cost assessments (discussed below) by capturing the remaining "qualitative residual" of contextual information from both participants' and implementers' perspectives, which cannot be captured by monetary values alone and is particularly prevalent in implementation science research (Dopp et al., 2019).

Administrative Records Evaluators will want to use information collected on a regular basis from records kept by intervention staff or added for the purpose of the evaluation. Typical data for interventions delivered in-person, by telephone or mail capture recruitment, initial and on-going participation. With sociodemographic and other relevant characteristics, evaluators capture the numerator– those who are "reached" (i.e., recruited, percentage of contacts attended, and completed) that can be compared against a denominator–those whom the intervention is intended to reach (i.e., environmental change agents, priority population). The latter are usually drawn from other sources, e.g., pregnant clients of a Women, Infants, and Children feeding program (WIC) or children under the age of two years at a safety net clinic. Delivery data could include records of mailings, appointment logs, checklists provided by implementers, and other reports. For example, program attendance records were completed by process evaluators to monitor student attendance in a school-based program designed to increase physical activity (Wilson et al., 2009). These attendance records were monitored and evaluated on an ongoing basis, and in response to lower attendance in some schools, evaluators instituted a new parent tracking system to increase student attendance and reach during future implementations of the intervention.

The logic of time-series designs discussed in Task 3 can be applied to process evaluations using administrative records. Sometimes, administrative records can be collected periodically, e.g., for one month in every quarter rather than continuously if they are burdensome. Note that all records whether kept by the intervention, evaluator, or another source should be examined closely for completeness and accuracy prior to using them for an evaluation.

Web Analytics Electronic health (eHealth) and mobile health (mHealth) interventions are increasingly important tools for public health, and they present specific challenges for process evaluation (Korda & Itani, 2013; Short et al., 2018; Webb et al., 2010). The editor of the *Journal of Medical Internet Research* and a working group that developed a reporting guideline for Internet, m/eHealth interventions identified "defining and measuring use," "engagement," and "attrition" (nonuse and loss to follow-up) as especially important issues for these interventions (Eysenbach & CONSORT-EHEALTH Group, 2011). Use or engagement is assessed along four dimensions: **frequency** (e.g., number of visits to site, number of log-ins); **intensity** (e.g., number of posts, lessons, or modules viewed); **time or duration** (e.g., amount of time spent at each log-in visit); and **type** (e.g., purpose of engagement) (Barisic et al., 2011; Short et al., 2018).

Google Analytics is commonly used to assess usage and engagement (Crutzen et al., 2013; Song et al., 2018). As an example, Song et al. (2018) used Google Analytics to assess user engagement in the WalkAlong mental health web-based portal and used the data to better understand who was using the website, how they heard about and accessed (e.g., desktop, mobile phone) the website, what tools were most frequently used, and how much time users spent on each tool (Song et al., 2018). Evaluators should also track attrition carefully, using analyses similar to a survival curve or other figures or tables that document use/dose/engagement to assess the proportion of users who are still logging in over time (Eysenbach & CONSORT-EHEALTH Group, 2011). Other advice includes the importance of reporting demographics associated with digital divide issues, such as age, education, gender, socioeconomic status, and computer/Internet literacy. Also, as related to dose, the average session time (a standard Google Analytics) should be accompanied by a description of the timeout policy (e.g., automatic logout after 15 minutes). Other measurement methods, such as qualitative data, self-report data, and sensor data (e.g., global positioning systems [GPS], cameras), may be used to complement usage data obtained from web-based analytics (Short et al., 2018).

Additional discussion of human support to enhance adherence to eHealth interventions in the clinical context provides evaluators with a model for evaluating program reach and use (Mohr et al., 2011). These authors introduce concepts, such as expectations (e.g., by health care providers), social presence (e.g., e-mail reminders from a peer), and bond (e.g., building a therapeutic alliance with the patient). An example of an evaluation of the reach of a Web-assisted tobacco intervention tested the effect of personal referrals by medical and dental providers over and above typical Google advertisements (Sadasivam et al., 2013). They found that recruitment from clinical practices complemented Google recruitment by attracting those who are less motivated to quit and less experienced with this type of delivery channel.

Cost Assessment Analyses of an intervention's costs can provide insight for decisions about maintenance after the evaluation is completed or for potential adopters who need to know the overall cost of implementing and sustaining the intervention, the costs of specific activities, and cost per participant. Cost analyses are needed to build the evidence base for health promotion interventions and are often missing from evaluation reports. And, although cost analyses can be important on their own, they also establish a foundation for other types of economic analysis, such as comparisons of program costs and benefits derived from an effect evaluation, i.e., cost-effectiveness or cost–benefit analyses (Task 3). The precision of these analyses depends, in part, on accurate analysis of intervention costs, which in turn depends on information about the intervention's implementation from the process evaluation. As summed up in one cost analysis guide, a process evaluation defines program inputs and outputs and answers the questions of "what is done," "when," "by whom," and "to whom" (Baldwin et al., 2013).

Specific costs to be included in a cost assessment depend on the perspective that is selected. Another way to put this is cost to whom? Cost analyses commonly consider the perspective of the funding agency or government, the service provider/payer. Other perspectives are the implementing agency, the client or recipient of services, and/or society as a whole. To illustrate, the beneficiary perspective for an HPV vaccination program would include waiting time, time to receive the vaccination, and any co-pays or costs associated with the service. The perspective of the service provider or other payer would not include these costs, but they would include their personnel and material costs of delivering the vaccine. The societal perspective reflects a combination of unduplicated costs to the payer/service provider government (federal, state, or local) or funding agency, the service provider, and the beneficiary of services.

Thus, the perspective is a filter for which costs to include in the cost calculation. For example, waiting time and time spent having a vaccination is a cost from the perspective of the patient and society, but not from the screening provider. (The benefits side of an economic analysis will be discussed in Task 3, and it also depends on the perspective taken.) Thus, it is of utmost importance that evaluators acknowledge their perspective and suggest how other perspectives might affect their conclusions.

Other key concepts in calculating costs are **opportunity costs** (the cost of forgoing the next best alternative use of a resource) and **intervention costs,** which include both fixed and variable costs. Fixed costs are not dependent on the number of services provided, e.g., rent and utilities paid for a clinic or community building; variable costs include items such as screening supplies or vaccine and staff wages. Intervention costs can also be divided into start-up costs, e.g., staff training, materials development, and operational costs, e.g., supplies and staff wages. Start-up costs are sometimes overlooked in calculating costs, but they are very important for others to be aware of to ensure adequate implementation in new settings. **Adjusting costs for the passage of time** refers to inflating costs to allow for comparisons of intervention costs at different times or discounting future costs (and savings) to reflect the assumption that dollars spent or saved in the future are not worth as much as dollars saved today. In addition to costs that appear on an agency's expenditure records and budgets (financial costs), volunteer time and items that an agency receives free of charge (economic costs) are included. Resources to assist an evaluator in determining the cost of an intervention can be found on https://www.cdc.gov/policy/polaris/economics/program-cost/ (CDC, 2024). Table 10.2 provides an example process evaluation plan for a colorectal cancer screening intervention.

Table 10.2 Initial Process Evaluation Plan for a Colorectal Cancer Screening (CRCS) Intervention for Veterans Visiting Veterans Affairs (VA) Healthcare Facilities

Components	Questions	Indicators	Method
(1) Reach (Coverage)	To what extent is the intervention reaching intended participants? Are unintended groups taking part? (overcoverage) Are any subgroups being missed? (undercoverage) How many participants dropped out of the intervention? What are the characteristics of participants who dropped out?	Percentage of the intended participants who used the intervention out of the number who were eligible; distributed by subgroup Percentage and characteristics of users not part of the intended group (e.g., under or over age without family history) Percentage and characteristics of participants who dropped out of the intervention	Project records during the delivery period
(2) Intervention delivery	What message is being delivered? (Fidelity) Are participants segmented according to their stage of change for CRCS? (Fidelity)	Match of message to stage of change	Narrative analysis of message concept booklets against IM matrices, intervention scripts, flow charts, checklists, and transcripts of conversations
	How much of the intervention is being delivered? (Dose delivered) What, if anything, is being omitted/delivered inconsistently? Why? (Dose delivered)	Tailored phone number and length of completed calls and booster sessions	Project records, including phone counselor checklists and reports generated by the telephone counseling system
	What is the average dose received by intervention participants? (Dose received) What parts of the intervention, if any, are not received consistently? Why? (Dose received)	Percentage of intended group calling to request educational materials Attention, recall, understanding, and credibility of messages	Toll-free phone records Participant recall and reaction to intervention Interviews with random sample of those getting CRCS and those not getting CRCS

Table 10.2 (*Continued*)

Components	Questions	Indicators	Method
	During intervention implementation, has the context changed for CRCS? (Context) What changes have been made in screening guidelines, if any? (Context) What changes, if any have been made in organizational capacity for CRCS? (Context) What CRCS interventions or messages have patients been exposed to? (Context)	VA CRCS guidelines VA eligibility for and access to CRCS and follow-up VA CRCS capacity VA capacity to integrate new interventions Participant exposure to non-VA CRCS health promotion efforts	Tracking CRCS guidelines and access policies Interviews with patients Communication with VA staff
(3) Participant engagement and satisfaction with the intervention	Are participants satisfied with the intervention activities? Are participants satisfied with intervention personnel?	Percentage of participants who are satisfied with the intervention activities Percentage of participants who are satisfied with intervention personnel Participants' perceptions of the overall intervention's usefulness and relevance?	Participant reaction survey Participant focus group Survey of periodic samples of participants
(4) Implementation structure and resources	Is there sufficient staffing for the intervention? Does the intervention coordinate effectively with other veteran groups who are necessary for program implementation? Are there appropriate hospital space and resources necessary to support program implementation? What resources (personnel, equipment, supplies, etc.) are required to initiate the intervention and to maintain it	Number of staff needed to operate the intervention List of interested parties List of needed resources and facilities Cost of specific activities Cost per person	Project records, receipts, and personnel timesheets

Source: Eldredge et al. (2016) / with permission of John Wiley & Sons.

Task 3: Develop Effect Evaluation Questions, Select a Design, and Identify Measures

Effect evaluations are highly valued in building the evidence base for health promotion practice. They can answer important questions about an intervention's impact, and they have the potential for influencing decisions about adoption, maintenance, and scale-up/scale-out (dissemination) of the intervention. Because effect evaluations are often costly, however, careful thought should be given to the readiness of the intervention for an effect evaluation (i.e., evaluability assessment) (Trevisan & Walser, 2014), the perceived need for this information, and the feasibility of conducting an evaluation that will yield findings that are likely to be used. Issues to consider include: Is the intervention potentially important enough to merit this investment of resources? Is there a clear description of the intervention? Is there a need for information about the intervention's effect in this population and setting? Have pilot tests of the intervention, measures, and intervention plan been conducted (see Task 4)? Are resources required for a credible evaluation available? Will the results be available within a likely window of time for decision-making? Clarity about the answers to these questions as well as agreement about the questions to be addressed by the evaluation will help the evaluators and others decide whether and how to proceed.

Define the Questions for an Effect Evaluation

An effect evaluation can answer several types of questions. Basic effect evaluation questions, along with their associated design or analytic approach, include the following:

- What is the average effect on the outcomes of interest that can be attributed to the intervention? In other words, what happened to those exposed to the intervention as compared to what would have happened without the intervention? (comparison group designs)
    - What is the effect on the outcomes of interest of an established intervention, compared to the new intervention? (comparative effectiveness evaluation)
    - Does a larger dose of the intervention or added quality produce larger effects? Conversely, can similar outcomes be produced with a smaller dose or with lesser quality? (dose–response evaluation)
- What is the mechanism through which an intervention functions? (mediation analysis)
- What is the differential effect on the outcomes of interest that can be attributed to the intervention by an important characteristic of a subpopulation? (moderation analysis)
- What are the effects of an intervention that offer the opportunity to test the impact of a naturally occurring change? (natural experiment)
- What is the impact of implementation strategies on process (or implementation) evaluation outcomes? (hybrid studies)
- What are the effects or benefits of the intervention compared to its costs? (economic evaluation)

Select the Design for an Effect Evaluation

The essential question in an effect evaluation is the comparison of the magnitude of effect on outcomes with and without the intervention. Thus, the **comparison group design** forms the foundation of our discussion. Other design features and effect evaluation questions described above will build on this.

Comparison Group Designs Conclusions based on this design family are typically expressed as based on the probability or likelihood that an intervention improves the average outcome for the group exposed to the intervention compared to those not exposed. Note that not every member of the exposed group will have a positive outcome; further, some members of the unexposed group will improve. The overall intervention effect is an increased probability or likelihood that those exposed to the intervention will have a desired outcome compared to those not exposed. Certainty about this probability is called **internal validity**, or the accuracy of an effect estimate for the specific sample included in the evaluation. In other words, to what extent can the changes in the desired outcomes be attributed to the intervention? This depends on the comparability of the group that was not exposed to the intervention. And although high internal validity is a critical element in an effect evaluation, generalizability of the effect estimates to the larger population and to other settings, outcomes, and times–**external validity**–is also important to health promotion practice. Here, we focus on internal validity and return to a framework for improving external validity below.

Experimental and "Quasi-experimental" Designs These designs involve some control over the assignment of individual or collections of individual participants to intervention and comparison groups. The distinguishing feature between these two types of design is whether assignment to the intervention to groups is at random (experimental, also called a randomized control trial (RCT) or by some other means (quasi-experimental). Both types of design usually measure the groups before and after exposure to the intervention. See Figure 10.2 for distinguishing features of experimental designs.

We point out that a one-group design in which the intervention group is compared to itself before and after exposure to the intervention is not considered an experimental design (nonexperimental design). It is generally considered a weak design because it is prone to most alternative explanations for the observed outcome (threats to internal validity) (Shadish et al., 2002; Trochim et al., 2016). The addition of multiple measures before and after an intervention can help rule out some of these threats (see time-series designs below).

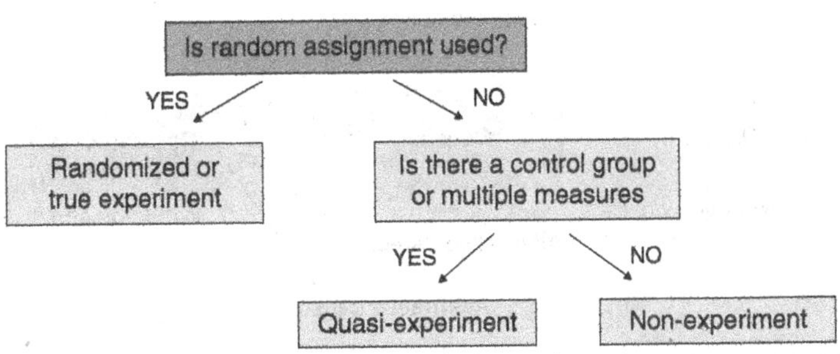

Figure 10.2 Distinguishing Features of Experimental, Quasi-Experimental, and Nonexperimental Designs

In an experimental or quasi-experimental design, defense against many (but not all) threats to internal validity focuses on ensuring the comparability of intervention and control groups on as many factors as possible that may influence the outcomes of interest. Threats to internal validity can be classified in three ways: (1) changes dependent on who was observed (selection, attrition, regression to the mean); (2) changes in participants not caused by the intervention (maturation, secular trends, history), and (3) changes related to how data are collected (testing, instrumentation) (Posavac & Carey, 2002). Definitions and examples of specific threats to internal validity can be found in Shadish et al. and Trochim. See Figure 10.3.

The comparability principle is most easily understood when considering random assignment of participants to the study groups (intervention and comparison) because with random assignment, the threats to internal validity should be distributed randomly across the two groups. Comparability can, however, also be approximated with **"quasi-experimental" designs** in which the intervention group is compared with another similar group by some form of matching (Rossi et al., 2019; Shadish et al., 2002). A group not formed by random assignment is often called a "comparison group"; the term "control group" is often used for a randomized design). The ideal comparison group is as similar as possible to the intervention group but does not receive the intervention at the same time.

Potential sources of comparison groups are drawing its members from within the same population that is eligible to receive the intervention or from an external population. A comparison group that comes from within the same population that is eligible to receive the intervention is more likely to be similar, although it is important that the two groups do not accidentally share the intervention. When matching, it is important to choose variables that the evaluator believes could be related to the intervention outcomes. Of course, the potential flaw in matching is that the evaluator might not know all the potential influencing factors. Two specific methods for creating matched groups are exact matching (where each member of the intervention group is matched to a similar member from the comparison group on the selected matching variables) and propensity score matching (See below) (Rossi et al., 2019). The most common method for assessing

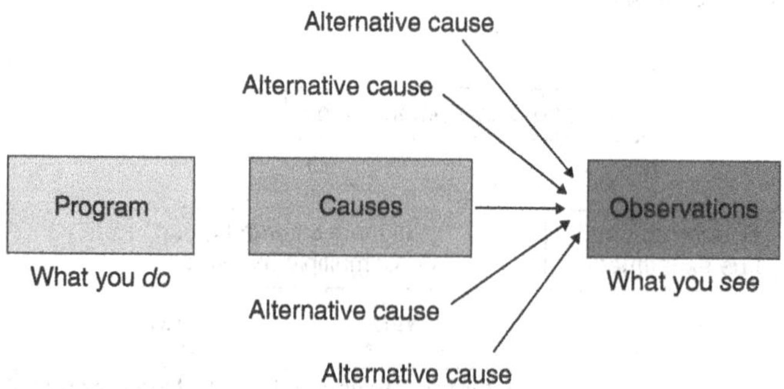

Figure 10.3 Schematic for Understanding Internal Validity

the degree to which the groups are comparable at the beginning of an evaluation is to examine their pretest scores on the matching variables. If the groups differ on these factors, it is often appropriate to make statistical adjustments in the analysis.

Note, however, that ensuring comparability of groups at the start of the evaluation does not guarantee that they are comparable by the end of the study – for example, different rates of dropout between study groups (**differential attrition**) could occur because participants are dissatisfied with either being in the intervention (which they may find too burdensome) or being in the comparison group (see below), or if they are unwilling to complete follow-up measures. Note the importance of paying close attention to potential problems with attrition during pilot testing (Task 4).

Expanding the Number of Measures with a Time-series Design The susceptibility of the one-group nonexperimental design to many threats to internal validity can sometimes be defended against by adding multiple measures at pretest and posttest. This design is best suited to a situation in which data are part of an ongoing monitoring plan for the population potentially affected by the intervention (e.g., law enforcement or health department data kept on motor vehicle crashes, accidental drownings, arrest rates, or fentanyl overdoses in particular geographic areas). The data should be collected from reasonably unbiased sources on an ongoing basis. Time-series designs usually involve a large series of observations on the same variable, consecutively, over time. The **interrupted time-series design** is of particular interest here, where an intervention is introduced at a specific time. The repeated measures allow the evaluator to examine trends before, during, and after the intervention (Shadish et al., 2002). Time-series designs can be with a single group or with a comparison group.

Statistically Constructed Comparison Group Designs Propensity score matching and regression discontinuity designs use statistically constructed comparison groups that can strengthen the internal validity of health promotion evaluations (West et al., 2008). More widespread use of these types of quasi-experimental designs as alternatives to RCTs has grown with greater recognition that RCTs for program evaluation are not always possible in the "real world." These newer designs strengthen internal validity and can solve ethical problems that may accompany the lack of an intervention for a matched comparison group. These designs require statistical expertise to ensure the appropriate choice of analysis and correct interpretation.

Propensity score matching Propensity score matching is a well-developed statistical strategy for reducing "selection bias" (Haviland et al., 2007; Luellen et al., 2005; McCaffrey et al., 2004; Rosenbaum, 2002). Propensity scores are based on baseline measures that must be able to represent participants in the intervention and comparison conditions on all characteristics believed to be potentially related to the treatment election or outcome, or ideally both (West et al., 2008). On the other hand, because the propensity score is a function of covariates and not outcomes, repeated analyses attempting to balance covariate distributions across treatment groups do not bias estimates of the intervention effect on outcomes and enable evaluators to design an observational study, including the analysis in advance, before the outcomes are known (Rubin, 2001).

This design was used to evaluate a mental health treatment diversion program (Special Needs Diversionary Program) to reduce crime among youth in Texas. Evaluators selected the first six counties funded and used administrative data (all juvenile offenses, demographic and education information, and participation in special education programs) together with mental health diagnoses, measured at baseline, before a decision was made to detain the youth or send them home without further processing. Wait-listed youth were an obvious source of a comparison group, but because of the possibility of differences between the two groups (e.g., youth with certain diagnoses or histories are more likely to be assigned to treatment immediately), the evaluators used "propensity scores" based on the administrative data and mental health diagnoses to equate the two groups. Their findings indicated that the diversion program delayed or prevented youth recidivism (Evans Cuellar et al., 2006). For a guide to propensity score analyses, see Guo and Fraser (2014) and Guo et al. (2020).

Regression discontinuity designs In some cases, access to an intervention or treatment is available only to those who have met a defined criterion of need or merit to participate in the intervention. For example, a clinic may offer a behavioral intervention program only to patients with Hgb A1C levels between 5.7 and 6.4 (the range that characterizes pre-diabetes), in an effort to prevent further increases in A1C levels. As a practical matter, however, those just above and just below the cut point of 5.7 are not substantively different from each other. The relatively minor differences between these individuals can be exploited for evaluation purposes using a regression discontinuity design (RDD) (Boon et al., 2021; Bor et al., 2014; Venkataramani et al., 2016). In an RDD, the variable that determines treatment eligibility, called the assignment variable, is used to assign participants to the intervention or comparison group based on their score on a pre-intervention measure. This measure can be the baseline value of the outcome variable, as with the diabetes example, or another characteristic, for example, eligibility for the Women, Infants, and Children's Feeding Program (WIC), which is based on household income. Thus, income could be treated as the assignment variable, even though the question of interest may be the effect of WIC participation on body mass index. Note: the assignment variable must be binary (yes/no).

The RDD offers practical advantages, particularly in cases where it may be considered unethical to withhold treatment from those who otherwise meet established criteria for participation. Consider an evaluation of a health promotion intervention that cannot be implemented in all settings or for all individuals in the initial implementation phase. The intervention could be restricted to those individuals or clinics with the greatest need, and those just below the cutoff could be used as the comparison. In its simplest form, an RDD can be analyzed using a straightforward regression model, where the dependent variable is the post-intervention value of the outcome variable, and the independent variable is the assignment variable indicating whether an individual was above or below the cut point for treatment. Interested readers should see Bor et al. (2014), Venkataramani et al. (2016), Moscoe et al. (2015), and Zuckerman et al. (2006) for more detailed discussion of the particulars of the RDD.

Further Considerations for Experimental and Quasi-Experimental Designs Several additional decisions affect these designs: (1) What will the control/comparison group receive? (2) What is the "unit of assignment" - individuals or a group? (3) What additional analyses about how and for whom the intervention works should be conducted? (4) How should findings be interpreted? and (5) To what extent should aspects of external validity be incorporated?

What Intervention will the Control/Comparison Group Receive? When making this choice, evaluators consider two possibilities: What will provide the most useful contrast with the experimental intervention (a classic evaluator's perspective) and what is acceptable to potential participants (a perspective of many interested parties that may influence participation in the evaluation) Some options include

- Usual care (e.g., an intervention that is in widespread use)
- Delayed intervention (e.g., use of a wait list for the comparison group to receive the intervention in the future if it is effective)
- Minimal intervention (e.g., basic information that ensures the comparison group is aware of a risk factor and resources)
- An attention "placebo" (e.g., the same amount of contact as the experimental intervention but without the content or change methods; could even be a different intervention of benefit to the evaluation participants that is not expected to have an effect similar to the experimental intervention)

Keeping in mind the special circumstances of the statistically constructed designs, the "usual care" option is often ethically and practically desirable. Critics of pharmaceutical trials have pointed out that comparing a new drug against a placebo instead of a drug already established provides misleading data about the magnitude of effect of the new drug (Slutsky & Clancy, 2010). Thus, a fairer contrast is with the current drug, which raises the level of effectiveness the new drug will have to surpass. In health promotion when usual care is an intervention tested previously, the design is known as a "comparative effectiveness" or "noninferiority" trial (Piaggio et al., 2012). "Dose-response" evaluation studies are a variation on this logic. Here, a previously tested intervention might be compared to less intensive versions, e.g., with fewer contacts. This occurred with Project CHOICES, a preconception intervention for women drinking alcohol at excessive levels who are at risk for an unplanned pregnancy. Findings from a second evaluation trial showed that reducing the number of costly one-on-one counseling sessions from four to two did not diminish effectiveness (Velasquez et al., 2017).

In cases when there is little or no usual care in the intervention setting, a minimal intervention should be considered to fulfill the responsibility to provide the comparison group with knowledge about the risk behavior or environmental condition and resources to address it. Placebos are not often used outside of trials of medical devices or drugs or laboratory psychology experiments.

Even though a new intervention has not been shown to be effective, potential participants and sponsors may still view it as more attractive and object to a minimal intervention and even to usual care. The evaluator may have to remind them that the reason for the evaluation is that the new intervention may not "work." Because concealing the group assignment (blinding) is not usually practical in a health promotion evaluation, participants will know that they have been assigned to the comparison group. To prevent comparison group participants from being discouraged (resentful demoralization) and dropping out of the evaluation or having implementers provide the intervention to the comparison group (compensatory equalization of treatment), the evaluator may need to make this assignment as satisfactory as possible, e.g., with the promise that these participants will have access to the intervention–if it is effective–when the evaluation is over. Thus, the prospect of receiving the new intervention in the future may be the most acceptable.

Another view, based on a review of attrition in studies of behavioral interventions, mentioned above, is that more dropout (differential attrition) might occur in the intervention group (Crutzen et al., 2015). And it is possible that the comparison group that is aware of the intervention develops a competitive attitude with the intervention group and improve their outcome scores (compensatory rivalry).

Whatever comparison "treatment" is selected, informed consent based on an understanding of the method of assignment (discussed above) is of critical importance.

What Is the Unit of Assignment? Evaluations of multi-level interventions typically assign clusters of individuals (or groups), e.g., physician practices, classrooms or schools to intervention and comparison groups (Murray et al., 1998). For example, suppose a randomized controlled trial is implemented to test an intervention to improve physician skills to counsel young adult patients about HPV vaccination. In this case, the outcome of interest is change in vaccination rates among the patients whom a physician treats. Because the treatment occurs at the level of the physician practice, however, assignment to intervention and control or comparison group should be by physician practices (at the group level), even though the outcome is measured at the level of the patient. This can be conceptualized as a **clustered design**, where multiple patients are clustered within a smaller number of physicians. The term "unit of assignment" is used to include such collective groups as well as individuals, and it is a signal that the unit needs to be defined.

Clustering may also arise even if the intervention is delivered at the individual level, because the evaluator wants to limit the possibility of diffusion of the intervention to those in the comparison group. If, for example, students in a high school were randomized to receive either a sexual health intervention or a no-treatment control or comparison, it is possible that through close student contact those who received the intervention could intentionally or unintentionally "deliver" the program to control students; thus, contaminating the design. A better design might be to randomize entire schools to treatment or control conditions, such that all students in that school receive whatever condition to which the school was randomized. While possibly more resource intensive, this design would minimize the possibility of contamination. Both the above examples would be considered **cluster-randomized trials**. The cluster (e.g., physicians or schools), not the individual on whom we are measuring outcome (e.g., patients or students), is the unit of assignment (randomization). Ignoring clustering and analyzing individuals as if they were not clustered can result in inflated estimates of program effect (false positives), in part because it appears that we have much more data than we actually do. Effectively, the sample size is reduced to the number of clusters rather than individuals (Campbell et al., 2012). Fortunately, several well-established techniques account for this clustering (Bosker & Snijders, 2011; Murray, 1998).

What Additional Analyses about How and for Whom the Intervention Works Should Be Conducted? Mediation and moderation analyses are now often an expected part of the evaluation process as a way of gaining more information about how an intervention achieved an effect, and for whom it achieved that effect. Hayes (2012) points out that as a research area matures, focus eventually shifts away from whether there is an effect, toward understanding the mechanism(s) by which the effect operates ("how") and establishing the populations and contexts in which it occurs ("for whom"). The "how" questions have typically been approached through **mediation analysis**, and the "for whom" questions, through **moderation analysis**.

Mediation and moderation are both valuable for several reasons, especially for the evaluation of interventions developed with IM. Mediation can help identify the paths by which the intervention achieved an effect, or conversely, the pathways that were not involved in an effect. The intervention's logic model of change will illustrate the proposed pathways that can be tested by mediation analysis. Mediation can help future program planners refine programmatic components, stripping away elements that were not affected by the intervention, and thus did not lead to a change in the behavioral or environmental outcome of interest. Alternatively, any important mediators can be targeted more directly by the intervention, possibly boosting the ultimate effect of the intervention on the outcome. Moderation analyses can help us better target an intervention in the future. For example, a moderation analysis might find that an intervention was effective for middle-school students, but not high-school-age students. This helps guide future implementation and dissemination work by demonstrating where the program should be directed.

As an example of both mediation and moderation, in an evaluation of the Incredible Years BASIC Parent intervention, a parenting program for preschoolers at risk for conduct problems, a mediation analysis found that change in a positive parenting skill (but not a negative parenting skill) predicted change in conduct problems (Gardner et al., 2010). Figure 10.4 depicts the causal chain implied by this mediation analysis.

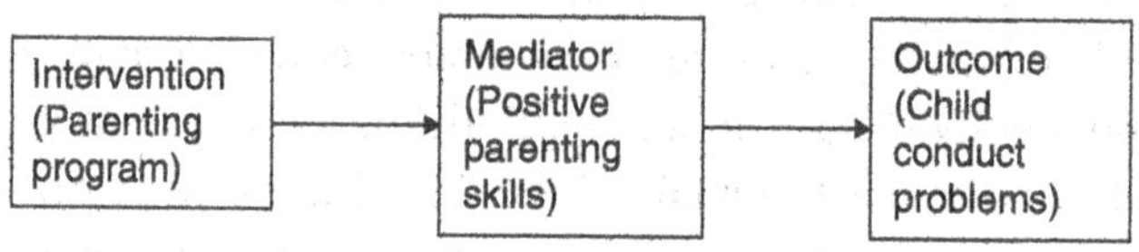

Figure 10.4 Example of Mediation Analysis

Moderation analysis in the same evaluation found that boys and younger children and those with more depressed mothers showed more improvement in conduct problems on posttest. In other words, the relation between the intervention and the outcome depended on other factors. Figure 10.5 depicts how these factors moderate, or alter, the relation between the parenting program and child conduct problems.

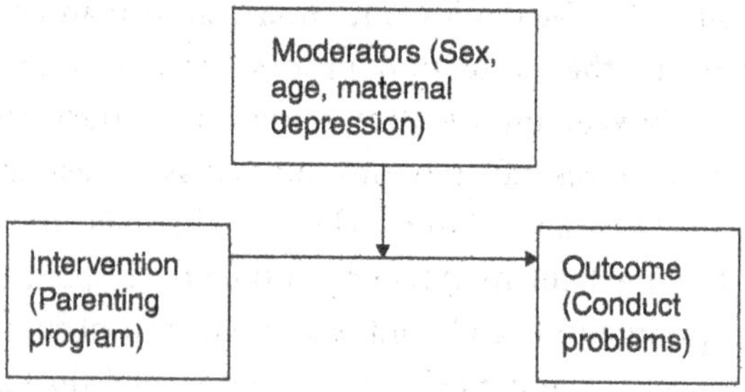

Figure 10.5 Example of Moderation Analysis

Mediation and moderation ultimately are about better understanding an intervention and its components in a more detailed and nuanced way so future work can be more effective.

Another approach to uncover the active ingredients of an intervention is to use a **factorial design** (Baker et al., 2017; Collins et al., 2009). Suppose the intervention planners are designing a program that will consist of two major components A and B, and they wish to know whether the combined

Table 10.3 Logic of a 2 x 2 Factorial Design

		Intervention Component B (Immediate Reinforcement)	
		Present	**Absent**
Intervention component A (Adaptive goal setting)	Present	AB	A alone
	Absent	B alone	Neither (i.e., the no-treatment group)

effects of A and B on the outcome are stronger than receiving just A (or just B). This is known as a 2x2 factorial design and is depicted in the Table 10.3. For example, an evaluation of an intervention for healthy, insufficiently active adults to initiate daily walking tested the independent and combined effects of a mobile health system that automated adaptive goal setting which could adjust up or down for each participant based on an algorithm that approximates an experienced coach (versus goals that did not change) and immediate (versus long-term) reinforcement. The evaluators found independent effects for adaptive goal setting and immediate reinforcement and a significant joint effect (Adams et al., 2022). Factorial designs can be expanded to 2x3 and beyond (Table 10.3).

How Should the Findings Be Interpreted? Exclusive reliance on statistical tests to determine whether the observed differences between groups that are being evaluated (e.g., intervention versus control/comparison) is not always the same as "clinical significance" or population impact. Statistical significance (p-value) simply indicates the likelihood of a finding being caused by chance alone. It does not yield very much practical information. Greater emphasis is now placed on reporting the magnitude of the effect and the confidence intervals around the effect estimate. Thus, how large is the effect and how precise is the estimate? For binary outcome measures, the magnitude is often reported as a risk ratio, or relative risk, or odds ratio. For effects measured as continuous variables, mean difference effect estimates are expressed as standardized effect sizes, such as Cohen's d or its variations. Several nontechnical primers on effect sizes are available (Lakens, 2013).

Although having an effect size and confidence interval is a step forward, the issue of the importance of an effect is still not answered completely. How big does an effect have to be for it to be "important," "useful," or "meaningful"? Practical importance of an effect will of course be specific to both measures and fields. An effect that is considered large in one field may be considered unremarkable in another. Interpretation of blood pressure or other measures provides a clearer interpretation than an intervention's effect on a self-efficacy scale. In the latter case, several options might be considered to communicate the importance of the finding to the reader: Compare your finding with those of other comparable studies using the same self-efficacy scale and consider the potential impact of the observed effects on behavior across a large population.

One last point to consider when interpreting the findings from an evaluation is whether the sample size was planned to be able to detect the hypothesized effect (Sozu et al., 2015). In general, detecting larger effects requires fewer individuals, while detecting smaller effects requires more individuals. This presents ethical concerns because it is not typically considered ethical to expose individuals to an experimental intervention unless this is necessary to answer an important scientific question. Sample size determination is a topic beyond the scope of this chapter, but evaluators are encouraged to consult with an experienced evaluation methodologist in determining sample size since there are various considerations for determining the appropriate number of individuals (and/or units such as schools, clinics, etc.) when conducting an evaluation.

To What Extent Should Elements of External Validity Be Added? External validity is another major concern of effect evaluation (Cook & Campbell, 1979; Shadish et al., 2002), and it can be viewed as a matter of degree, involving a set of design features, not as a "yes" or "no". Before discussing these features, two terms should be introduced. An evaluation that places foremost emphasis on internal validity is known as an efficacy study, in which the intervention is evaluated under optimal conditions, e.g., with a highly selected sample such as volunteers who are likely to stick with the intervention no matter how much time and effort are required. In contrast, an effectiveness evaluation emphasizes external validity, "real-world" circumstances, e.g., representatives of the at-risk group who won't necessarily be motivated to take part in all aspects of the intervention and might even drop out. An evaluation design can have elements of each and may not be strictly one or the other (Gartlehner et al., 2006; Singal et al., 2014).

Emphasis on effectiveness over efficacy **evaluations** for medical and public health interventions, has been driven by the need to better understand the impact of an intervention under less-than-ideal circumstances, and therefore add more relevant evidence to practice (Glasgow et al., 2006; Glasgow et al., 2019; Tunis et al., 2003). The term **pragmatic** was coined by Schwartz and Lellouch (Schwartz & Lellouch, 1967) to describe an attitude in trial design, which recognizes that the difference between effectiveness and efficacy studies is a continuum, not simply an either/or. Thorpe et al. (2009) identified ten dimensions on which trials could be pragmatic, under the acronym PRECIS (PRagmatic-Explanatory Continuum Indicator Summary). These include design dimensions, such as participant eligibility criteria, level of practitioner expertise, follow-up intensity, outcomes, and practitioner adherence (Figure 10.6). In the figure, each spoke represents a design dimension. The web lines connect the dots on each spoke, with dots farther from the center representing a more pragmatic approach. Thus, Figure 10.6A is very pragmatic on all dimensions, in contrast with Figure 10.6B, a classic efficacy trial.

Examples of pragmatic approaches can be found in Thorpe et al. (2009) and Glasgow et al. (2012). According to Zwarenstein et al. (2008), trial results are likely to be more widely applicable if the participants, communi-

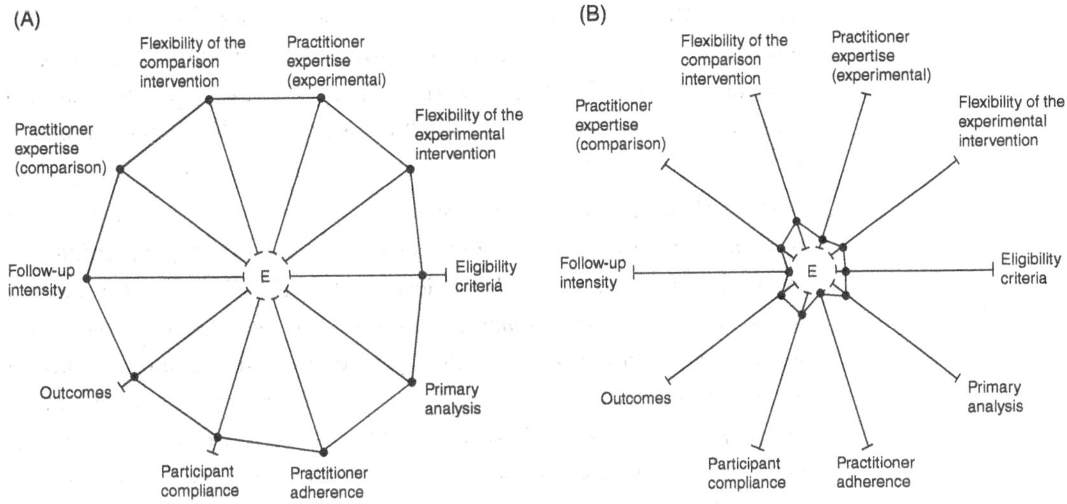

Figure 10.6 Illustration of the PRECIS Criteria to Characterize Research Studies. Source: Reprinted Glasgow and Riley (2013) / with permission of Sage Publications.

ties, practitioners, or institutions resemble the at-risk population, and are not narrowly selected; if the intervention is implemented without strenuous efforts to standardize it; if the comparison group receives care or other interventions widely used; and if outcomes studied are important to relevant decision-makers. Interest in external validity should not stand in the way of demonstrating efficacy, however.

Evaluations of the Smoke-free Homes intervention (three mailings and one coaching call) illustrate a chain of studies that started near (but not completely) the efficacy end of the continuum and proceeded to a full-on pragmatic evaluation. The series began with:

1. An RCT of the intervention was delivered to a "real-world" population of predominantly low-income, female, African American smokers who called a social services help-line in an urban area and who, after their immediate needs were met, told help-line staff there was smoking in their home. Eligibility criteria were minimal, and only eight percent declined to participate. Trained university staff delivered the intervention and conducted follow-up interviews (blinded to the study group), with a sample of those who reported smoking bans validated by home nicotine monitors. A positive effect (40% intervention versus 25% control group at six months) was found with an intent-to-treat analysis (see below) (Kegler et al., 2015).
2. A second RCT moved intervention delivery to trained and monitored help-line staff and was conducted in another state with predominantly low-income, female, current smokers who were urban and rural callers. All other procedures were similar to RCT #1, without mention or implementation of the validation of self-report. The intent-to-treat analyses again found a positive (smaller) increase in home smoking bans (43% versus 33%) (Williams et al., 2016).

3. The third RCT used the same procedures as RCT #2 conducted in a different state with a similar population profile that added English-speaking Hispanic callers. The intent-to-treat analysis found a positive (larger) increase in home smoking bans (63% versus 38%), although the consent rate was lower (Mullen et al., 2016).
4. A dissemination trial selected five call centers (from 31 applicants) and provided a $70,000 grant to cover the staffing costs of implementing and evaluating the intervention for callers meeting the eligibility criteria used in the previous studies. Implementation support included in-person training and two webinars for call center staff, an implementation manual, and a tailored web-based tracking system to guide enrollment, intervention delivery, and evaluation, boosted by monthly calls with implementation coaches. Mixed methods (surveys and in-depth interviews) focused on implementation challenges, with many positive ratings. Challenges included site workflow, recruitment, desire to adapt the intervention, time needed for delivery, and financial sustainability (Thompson et al., 2019).

Thus, some elements of a pragmatic trial were present from the beginning, with more external validity elements added across time. Sequential movement toward broad-scale dissemination was accompanied by safeguards against "drift" that impeded adaptation and concerns about sustainability. The overall findings across the studies provided a strong foundation for scaling up to other social services call-in lines and beyond.

Additional Designs for Effect Evaluations

Natural Experiments Sometimes, health promotion planners and evaluators have a unique opportunity to evaluate the effect of an intervention that does not originate from an IM planner; rather, an initiative could come from a city council, healthcare accrediting body, or other external group that results in the implementation of a program, policy or practice that is of great interest to the field of health promotion and public health. These types of evaluations, known as "natural experiments" are not a design per se, and they are not an experiment in the sense of an experiment with random assignment. In such instances, other comparison group designs, including time series can be employed. The term refers to the intervention when it is not under the control of the evaluator.

Natural experiments are highlighted here because of their importance in adding new interventions to the evidence base, especially for policies. Long advocated by Green and colleagues, such studies can add to "practice-based evidence" (Green & Allegrante, 2020). For example, think back to the time when patient navigation was a new approach without a strong evaluation and a clinic hired laypersons from the community to navigate all patients with positive screening tests for breast, cervical, and colorectal cancer to the next level of assessment and potential treatment. An alert health promotion evaluation specialist could have applied one of the comparison designs described above to assess the impact of the intervention on follow-up rates.

At the outset the evaluator should determine the logic model of the intervention, using EBI mapping techniques described in Chapter 11, and check implementation plans to determine whether the intervention is likely to achieve its objectives. These evaluations pose special challenges, such as having little time to complete the evaluation plan for a feasible design that suits the circumstances. Evaluators should avoid weak designs that provide little useful information. To this point, a review of published examples of natural experiments in obesity found that many used cross-sectional designs, and the authors recommended the use of stronger designs (Bennett et al., 2018). Excellent suggestions for evaluating natural experiments can be found in Leatherdale (2019).

The Houston TRAIN (Travel-related Activity in Neighborhoods) Study presents an example of a natural experiment conducted to understand how macro-level factors can increase population levels of physical activity. The intervention was the expansion of a light-rail transit system designed to influence travel choices and physical activity among residents who live near the new rail lines. The logic behind this connection, supported by prior studies, is that if individuals use public transit in lieu of car travel, then they are more likely to accrue physical activity due to the travel (usually walking) required between the train station and their point of origin or destination.

The regional transit agency exercised sole control over the timing and placement of the rail lines. The evaluators conceptualized the intervention exposure as distance from the new train stations to an individual's home. Thus, those who lived closer to new stations were designated the intervention group, and those living further away were designated the comparison group. *A priori*, the evaluators determined, based on publicly available aggregate data, which sociodemographic and other factors could act as confounders (Durand et al., 2016). The evaluators found that transit users self-reported more physical activity than nonusers. Additionally, most of this activity appeared to be related to transportation specifically, rather than to leisure-time physical activity. This higher physical activity makes transit users seven times more likely to meet physical activity guidelines and consequently achieve the benefits associated with an active lifestyle. These results are substantiated by accelerometer estimates of physical activity that indicate transit users record significantly more moderate-intensity physical activity than nonusers (Knell et al., 2018).

Hybrid Studies "Hybrid studies" (previously, called designs) simultaneously evaluate the impact of interventions (effect evaluation) and implementation (process evaluation) (Bernet et al., 2013; Curran et al., 2022). Looking at effectiveness and implementation together enables the evaluator to identify important interactions, with the idea of scaling up interventions more rapidly (see Chapter 10). The quality-improvement initiative of the largest health care system in the U.S., the Department of Veterans' Affairs, has been an important driver of the hybrid concept (Curran et al., 2012). Interventions most suitable for a hybrid approach are those with at least indirect evidence of effectiveness and strong face validity to support their fit in the new setting or population or to a new delivery method (Bernet et al., 2013). There also should be a solid foundation for the implementation strategy (Curran, 2020; Curran et al., 2012). The degree of certainty for each will dictate how much emphasis to place on implementation versus effectiveness (Curran et al., 2012, 2022). The process evaluation components from Table 10.2 (Reach, Delivery, Participant Engagement and Satisfaction, Implementation Structure and Resources) can also be applied to the evaluation of implementation strategies.

Hybrid studies are classified as Type 1, Type 2, or Type 3, depending on whether intervention effectiveness on substantive outcomes or the utility of proposed implementation strategies are of greater interest. The following classifications are adapted from Curran et al. (2022).

Type 1: Primary aim is intervention effectiveness; secondary aim may be a process evaluation of implementation of the intervention.

Type 2: Two co-primary aims: intervention effectiveness and feasibility/utility of implementation strategies.

Type 3: Primary aim is utility of implementation strategy; secondary aim can examine effect of implementation trial on substantive outcomes.

Further reflection on the hybrid typology and relevance to health promotion and other nonclinical contexts suggests that four questions could be used to decide which type to use (Table 10.4):

Table 10.4 Questions to Guide the Choice of a Hybrid Study

1. What is the nature of the effectiveness data on your intervention of interest?
   - Very-to-moderately strong, especially if not a lot of intervention adaptation needs to take place? Consider type 3 or type 2 depending on how much you expect the intervention will need to be adapted (Question 2).
   - Mixed results? Missing (strong) effectiveness data? Consider types 1 or 2.
2. How much do you expect the intervention will need to be adapted for where you want to study/use it?
   - A little? Consider type 2 or 3, including adaptation process as a step in an implementation-focused project.
   - A lot? Consider focusing on effectiveness in a type 1 or type 2.
3. How much do you already know about implementation determinants for the intervention in your context of interest?
   - Not much? If you also need to focus on effectiveness data, consider type 1.
   - If the effectiveness data are strong, and you know enough already to develop/select a strategy or package of strategies to evaluate? Consider type 2 or 3.
4. How ready are you to evaluate a "real-world" implementation strategy or package of strategies?
   - Not ready? A type 1 is indicated, where you collect information on implementation determinants to help you prepare for developing strategies later.
   - Ready, and you need to focus as well on effectiveness of the intervention (Question 1)? Consider a type 2.
   - Ready, and your effectiveness data are strong (Question 1) and you don't need to adapt a lot (Question 2)? Consider a type 3.

Source: Curran et al. (2022) / Frontiers Media SA / CC BY 4.0.

Examples of hybrid studies are increasingly common in the literature. For example, a Type 1 study focused on testing group versus individual antenatal care on morbidity and mortality of mothers and their infants (intervention effectiveness outcome; primary aim) (Chirwa et al., 2020). The secondary aim was to identify contextual factors associated with successful implementation (continuation of service, reach and fidelity). What is now called a Type 1 study has been standard practice (i.e., conducting effect and process evaluation) in the evaluation literature. A Type 2 study evaluated an intimate partner violence screening instrument for effectiveness (could be disclosure rates and post-screening service utilization), while also assessing the utility of adding implementation facilitation (internal and external) on reach, adoption, fidelity, and maintenance measures (Iverson et al., 2020). A Type 3 study randomized health care providers to use a digital sleep health software platform with their patients exhibiting disordered sleep (with existing evidence to support its effectiveness) either alone, with external facilitation, or with external and internal facilitation (Germain et al., 2021). The primary implementation outcomes were reach, adoption and sustainability. Secondary effectiveness outcomes measured on participating patients included, for example, insomnia, anxiety and pain.

Sequential Multiple Assignment Randomized Trials (SMART Designs) SMART designs are gaining increasing attention in the health promotion literature because they allow practitioners to build and test optimal intervention sequences adapted to initial characteristics and intermediate measures of response by intervention participants (Lei et al., 2012). SMART designs involve multiple decision stages; at the end of each stage, decision rules are used to evaluate participant responsiveness (Almirall et al., 2014). Non-responders are randomized into alternative treatment sequences (i.e., the previous stage treatment is stepped up, augmented or swapped out with another treatment). SMART designs help identify the most effective treatment sequences, rather than individual treatments, as well as sub-groups of individuals that can best benefit from particular treatment sequences. (This chapter's case study uses a SMART design.)

Economic Evaluation Two major types of cost analyses that add intervention outcomes to cost analysis (Task 1) can be differentiated by the way they treat the outcomes. **Cost-effectiveness analysis** compares the costs of an intervention to its key outcomes as specific benefits, e.g., cost per pregnant smoker who refrains from smoking at three months of the pregnancy through delivery or cost per adolescent who reports improved communication with a parent about sexual health or cost per public transport rider who adds a clinically important amount of physical activity. **Cost–benefit analysis** takes that process one step further, attempting to compare costs with the dollar value of all (or most) of an intervention's benefits. This puts the evaluator in search of other studies to estimate the value of smoking cessation during pregnancy or for the additional physical activity. In these cases, estimates are available, but for parent-adolescent communication, while valued as an intermediate outcome likely to lead to less sexual risk, such data are not available. Thus, while cost benefit analysis makes it possible for policy makers to compare different interventions to decide which would yield the most benefit for the investment--a smoking cessation program or a weight gain control program for pregnant women--and incorporate the different prevalence of tobacco and overweight-obesity exposed pregnancies, it may not be feasible. **Budget impact analysis** is a relatively new type of economic analysis focused on the affordability of an intervention to a particular provider in a relatively short time horizon. It has been adopted by national health services, e.g., Canada and Australia, primarily to aid in decisions to adopt a new technology. It differs from most economic analyses in considering the extent to which the new therapy or technology will substitute for an existing therapy or require additional funds and increase or decrease the use of other service delivery resources, the size of the population to be served, and the likely importance of the estimate of affordability in the decision-making process (Trueman et al., 2001). Resources available to assist with cost analyses, include those cited earlier in process evaluation of intervention costs (Mauskopf et al., 2017; Riegg Cellini & Edwin Kee, 2015; Rossi et al., 2019).

Identify Indicators and Measures for the Effect Evaluation Plan

Evaluation in health promotion often concerns multiple effects, and evaluators who have reviewed the logic model of change (Task 1) will have identified the effects of interest. During Step 6, however, it is a good idea to review these identified effects. Before we discuss this further and how to identify indicators and measures of effects and evaluate their reliability and validity for the outcomes of interest, we highlight one other potential effect not part of the logic model of change—unintended effects or side effects.

It is common to think of unintended effects in pharmaceutical trials. Rossi et al. (2019) suggest studying prior research on the topic and keeping in touch with intervention personnel at all levels, including participants and dropouts. For example, teachers charged with implementing a school-based gardening program correctly predicted the positive "side effects" on academic competencies such as science and math, in addition to expected effects on increased fruit and vegetable consumption. Three other ways to capture unintended system-level change include (1) uncovering how the intervention couples with the context, (2) tracking changes in relationships and the distribution and transformation of resources, and (3) assessing the activities that are displaced (Hawe et al., 2009). When reporting unexpected harms and benefits of an intervention, it is important to be clear how these findings were identified.

The worsening of disparities is a negative effect that can occur even when the overall behavior or health status of a disadvantaged group is improved (Mechanic, 2002; Partin & Burgess, 2012). Increased disparity is more likely to occur with interventions that depend on voluntary involvement (because more advantaged individuals have the resources and may be more likely to participate) and with interventions that address prevalent problems when the required behavior is not easy to execute (Mechanic, 2002). An example of mixed effects aside from the hypothesized effect is with interventions to encourage moving out of high-poverty neighborhoods, which in one study were associated with **reduced** rates of depression and conduct disorder among girls and **increased** rates of depression, PTSD, and conduct disorder among boys (Kessler et al., 2014).

Effects to Evaluate Identifying and reviewing intervention effects to evaluate from Task 1 requires thinking about their expected time frame. First, health effects require time to develop. Second, health education, especially for youth, is often directed at future behavior when a risk behavior has not yet emerged. Third, the intervention itself needs time, especially when the goal is long-term change, such as teenage pregnancy for a middle-school population.

Sometimes, changes in behavior may be outside the time frame for an initial evaluation, as in the case of an HIV prevention intervention designed to reach students before they begin having sexual intercourse (Hofstetter et al., 2014). Thus, behavior change may not be an appropriate short-term evaluation goal, although it certainly belongs in the intervention's logic model. In this circumstance, the short-term impacts that program developers expect and seek to measure are changes in determinants such as knowledge, self-efficacy, skills, and/or behavioral intention, personal determinants, which are included in the change objectives.

It is critical to decide in advance the level of effects that can be expected within a given time frame. If health changes are not expected or measured in the evaluation plan, the planner must have strong evidence and logical arguments to justify any assumption of causation. For instance, the evaluator must document the relation between skills improvement now and the use of condoms later and a reduction in HIV infections much later.

Even when there is enough time to achieve a health outcome, as noted in Task 1, there may already be strong evidence that links a behavior or environmental condition with the health outcome, making the latter's measurement unnecessary. At whatever point in the logic model the evaluator begins for assessment of effects, e.g., behavior, all of the effects to the left, e.g., determinants, should also be measured.

Identifying Indicators and Measures for the Effects of Interest The "effect" stated in the logic model of the intervention and incorporated into an evaluation question is often represented as a general idea (measurement construct) and not how the outcome is measured. For example, in an intervention designed to reduce breast cancer by increasing mammography screening, a possible environmental outcome is, "Clinicians recommend mammography screening." This construct is a critical precursor to identifying indicators and measures, but it does not define exactly how we will know whether the recommendation occurred. For the mammography screening example, possible indicators are self-reports by clinicians, notes in the medical record, recordings of patient encounters, and reports by patients. Even then selecting an indicator still does not fully specify how the indicator will be measured. A measure quantifies or categorizes an indicator, usually by applying numbers to the indicator. If the selected indicator is self-report by clinicians, it could be measured on a self-administered questionnaire in several different ways, e.g., Did you recommend mammography to your last eligible patient? (yes/no) or How often do you usually recommend mammography to an eligible patient? (all of the time/most of the time/occasionally/none of the time).

Measurement Considerations Following the discussion of the constructs, evaluators would look for previously established measures in the published literature with evidence for reliability and validity and consider their potential, feasibility and expense.

Reliability is stability or precision in measurement. In choosing a measure to assess the construct we discussed earlier, "clinicians recommend mammography screening," it is important to identify an indicator and measure that have adequate reliability. Barry (2017) assessed this construct using reports by patients as the indicator. The specific measure asked patients to report whether their doctor recommended a mammogram during the past year. For more information on the types of reliability (test-retest, inter-rater, and internal consistency), interested readers can see Bandalos (2018).

Reliability concepts include consideration of sources of random error. For example, clinicians' reports of their mammography recommendation practices for their last patient may not be a reliable method for obtaining their average practice. Further, a child may, for example, understand questions about asthma symptoms or self-confidence differently at two points in time based on the question's complexity, a distraction in the environment, or help they might have received in understanding the question. Reliability can also be diminished through procedural problems, such as asking the question in different ways, or transcribing data inaccurately.

Validity in measurement, means that the evaluators are measuring the construct that they think they are measuring. As with reliability, it is important to identify an indicator and measure that has adequate validity. Note that reliability is the basis for validity. Continuing with the example construct above, "recommend mammography screening," the self-report patient measure of provider mammography screening recommendation (Barry, 2017) can also be examined for validity. In assessing this measure's validity, four types of validity can be considered; more information on these concepts can found in Bandalos (2018).

Established reliable and valid instruments or methods for measurement can be found in the literature for many effects. Furthermore, many entities have developed databases and compendia of measures on health and behavior issues. The National Institute on Alcohol Abuse and Alcoholism, The Child & Adolescent Health Measurement Initative, and Behavioral Measurement

Database Services all have good examples (National Institute on Alcohol Abuse and Alcoholism, 2025; The Child & Adolescent Health Measurement Initiative, n.d.; Behavioral Measurement Database Services, n.d).

Using a reliable and valid measure allows results from one study or program evaluation to be compared with data from other studies. The disadvantage of such measures may be that they are not specific to the effect that the intervention addresses and therefore not sensitive to change even if the effect does improve. Health promotion planners may not be responsible for developing measures and indicators; sometimes, however, it may be necessary as described below. It is important to note that the reliability and/or validity of an existing measure may be altered when it is adapted. The design of reliable and valid instruments to measure the evaluation objectives is beyond the scope of this chapter and requires more advanced methodological expertise (Bandalos, 2018; DeVellis & Thorpe, 2021; Streiner et al., 2015).

Feasibility, burden, and expense also matter. When considering the feasibility of the measure, it is important to consider the way the measure is administered. For example, self-administered surveys are often more feasible for collecting effect evaluation data because they are inexpensive and often require less time and resources to implement than an in-depth interview. Even if a self-administered survey is chosen, however, it is important to consider factors such as survey length and expense. Many measures can be obtained freely from the published literature, but some measures must be purchased.

Measures of Quality of Life and Health Effects Many measures of quality of life and health are readily available from national, state, and local data or from data maintained by health facilities and payers as described in Chapter 5. Careful attention should be paid regarding indicators of health status before measures are sought. In the needs assessment, program planners also identified specific outcomes that they considered to be the consequences of the health problem or the behavioral factors and environmental conditions (Green et al., 2022). The indicators may be stated at the individual level, such as days lost from work, happiness, self-esteem, and alienation; or at a societal level, such as crime, crowding, discrimination, and unemployment. Thus, measurement can be made by collecting data from the population to evaluate the program outcomes for individuals as well as by collecting data from organizations or governmental agencies that track potential social indicators of quality of life. Measurement of quality of life also has important time-related factors that need to be considered when developing a program evaluation model.

Measures of Behavior and Environment Effects For many behaviors and environmental conditions (or behaviors of environmental agents), there is extensive scientific literature on measurement. The best indicator for behavior is the list of performance objectives for behavior changes in IM Step 2, and for environmental conditions it is the list of performance objectives for environmental changes, also in Step 2. The evaluators will need to review the scientific literature to decide whether existing measurement tools match well with the stated performance objectives. If several options are available, then the decision will be to choose the one that best fits the performance objectives and program participants (and has adequate reliability and validity). If there is not a good fit with the performance objectives, then the evaluators may find it necessary to adapt existing reliable and valid measures or develop new questions or instruments to measure the behaviors, though we have noted earlier the limitations of this approach and the required methodological expertise. Measurement of behaviors can also be conducted by observation. However, they are more often measured - for reasons of feasibility - by self-report. Although used less frequently, qualitative methods can also be used to assess behaviors, particularly for interventions that already have demonstrated effectiveness.

Measures of Determinants and Change Objectives Like measures of behavior of the at-risk group and behaviors of environmental agents, measures of determinants can also be found in the published literature or online databases. Change objectives from IM Step 2 matrices are the most specific objectives for program development and for effect evaluation. The evaluator can organize the change objectives by determinant (essentially looking down the determinant columns in the matrix) to create a blueprint for each measure related to effect evaluation questions concerning change in determinants. For example, if change objectives for adolescents in a program to prevent sexually transmitted infections (STIs) included self-efficacy for performance objectives related to condom acquisition, use, negotiation, disposal, refusal, and so on, then the blueprint includes self-efficacy change objectives for all these behaviors. The evaluator would then go to the literature on self-efficacy to determine how the construct is typically measured (Bandura, 1986; Dennis, 2003; Fernandez et al., 2009; Hsu & Chiu, 2004; Maurer & Andrews, 2000; Resnick & Jenkins, 2000). If it is not possible to identify established measures from the literature for specific determinants, the change objectives can be used as the basis for developing the measures.

Table 10.5 provides a summary example of constructs, effect evaluation questions, indicators, measures, and timing for the It's Your Game... Keep it Real intervention (Markham et al., 2012; Tortolero et al., 2010). Measures were adapted from reliable and valid measures that had been used previously with the priority population (Basen-Engquist et al., 1999, 2001; Coyle et al., 2001, 2004; Prinstein et al., 2000, 2001; Vernberg et al., 1999).

Task 4: Pilot Test the Intervention and Finalize the Evaluation Plan

Pilot studies are a critical step before expending the fiscal resources and good will required for a full evaluation. However, reports of completed evaluations are rife with statements such as "recruitment was much slower than expected," "the desired sample size was not achieved," "components of the intervention were not delivered," "some measures had little variability," "follow-up rates were low, especially in the intervention group," and so

Table 10.5 It's Your Game... Keep it Real: Constructs, Effect Evaluation Questions, Indicators, Measures, and Timing (Markham et al., 2012; Tortolero et al., 2010)

Construct	Effect Evaluation Question	Indicator	Measure	Timing
Effect Evaluation: Sample Student Behaviors and Survey Items				
Sexual initiation	Did the intervention decrease the number of students who initiated sexual activity by the 9th grade?	Initiation of vaginal, oral, or anal sex by the 9th grade (among students who reported no sexual activity at baseline)	Student survey item Have you ever had vaginal sex? (item repeated for oral and anal sex) (Yes, No)	Baseline 9th grade Follow-up
Frequency of sex in the past three months	Did the intervention decrease the number of times that students had sex in the past three months?	Frequency of engaging in vaginal, oral, and anal sex in the past three months	Student survey item During the last three months, how many times have you had vaginal sex? (item repeated for oral and anal sex) (Number of times)	Baseline 9th grade Follow-up
Frequency of sex without a condom in the past three months	Did the intervention decrease the number of times that students had sex without a condom in the past three months?	Frequency of engaging in vaginal and anal sex without a condom in the past three months	Student survey item During the last three months, how many times have you had vaginal sex without using a condom? (item repeated for anal sex) (Number of times)	Baseline 9th grade Follow-up
Lifetime sexual partners	Did the intervention decrease the lifetime number of partners with whom the student had vaginal, oral, or anal sex?	Number of partners with whom the student had ever had vaginal, oral, or anal sex	Student survey item How many different boys or girls have you had vaginal sex with? (item repeated for oral and anal sex) (Number of partners)	Baseline 9th grade Follow-up
Physical dating violence victimization	Did the intervention decrease the number of students who reported physical dating violence victimization in the past year?	Experience of physical dating violence victimization (e.g., hitting, kicking, or pushing) by a boyfriend or girlfriend in the past year	Student survey item How often has a boyfriend or girlfriend hit, kicked or pushed you in a mean way in the past year? (Never, Once or Twice, A Few Times, About Once a Week, A Few Times a Week)	Baseline 9th grade Follow-up
Effect Evaluation: Sample Determinants and Items				
Knowledge about HIV/STI transmission	Did the intervention increase the students' knowledge about HIV/STI transmission?	Knowledge about how HIV/STIs are/are not transmitted	4-item HIV/STI knowledge scale on student survey You cannot get an STD from having oral sex. (True, False, Not Sure)	Baseline 8th & 9th grade Follow-ups
Self-efficacy to refuse sex	Did the intervention increase the students' self-efficacy to refuse sex?	Self-efficacy to refuse sex in different scenario	7-item self-efficacy scale on student survey Imagine you are alone with someone you like very much. Could you stop them if they wanted to kiss you on the lips? (I definitely could not, I probably could not, I probably could, I definitely could)	Baseline 8th & 9th grade Follow-ups

forth. And yet, dry runs are not often conducted for local evaluations, and surprisingly, the definition and purpose of pilot studies are not well described (Kegler et al., 2012).

Tasks 1, 2, and 3 have guided the evaluator through important steps in designing the process and effect evaluation plans–crafting specific questions, choosing designs and measures, including standards of comparison and other features that promote more or less external validity. Task 4 begins by filling in the numerous practical details required to make an "operational" plan or protocol and plans the pilot test of the intervention and its implementation and all aspects of the evaluation. The findings help intervention planners and evaluators to make any needed adjustments and finalize the overall evaluation plan.

Develop the Full Evaluation Plan

A full evaluation plan should address questions about how the evaluation operations will be carried out.

- Have the needed resources for the evaluation been described and arrangements made for them to be in place?
- How will study participants be identified, recruited, and screened? Who will get their informed consent, and if needed, who and how will follow-up be conducted? How will loss to follow-up be minimized?
- How will data be collected and from what sources?
- When will data be collected?
- Who will collect the data, who will train and supervise data collectors, and who will calibrate any devices? Have the planned data sources from administrative or other records been checked for permission to use them and for privacy concerns? Are these data sources complete, reliable, and valid?
- If sampling is involved (i.e., individuals or units selected from a population or assignment to an intervention and control group), what methods will be used, and have concerns about equity and acceptability been considered?
- Who will have access to the data and how will privacy be protected? Who will conduct the analyses?
- When and how will reports to stakeholder groups be made?

The plans to answer these and other practical questions should be pretested so that adjustments can be made to improve the successful conduct of the evaluation.

As an example of operationalizing a measurement choice and completing the protocol for an evaluation of It's Your Game. . . Keep It Real, intervention developers had targeted delayed sexual initiation at the ninth-grade follow-up for those students who reported no lifetime sexual activity at baseline. Sexual activity was defined as participation in vaginal, oral, or anal sex (Tortolero et al., 2010). Secondary outcomes included the frequency of sex, frequency of sex without a condom, number of sexual partners, dating violence victimization and perpetration, and the determinants related to these behaviors (Peskin et al., 2014; Tortolero et al., 2010).

To complete the protocol for measurement, however, the evaluators had to decide how these sensitive data would be collected from the students. Thus, they specified that data collectors would be graduate students or other hired employees who were trained to conduct student surveys on laptop computers using an audio-computer-assisted self-interview (ACASI). They noted that ACASI systems are reliable for obtaining sensitive information on sexual risk-taking (Booth-Kewley et al., 2007; Morrison-Beedy et al., 2006). Further, surveys were conducted in a quiet location (e.g., school library) without a teacher present. To protect student confidentiality, headphones were provided and laptops were positioned so screens were not visible to others.

Reporting Guidelines Can Contribute to Writing the Protocol

Reporting guidelines for many types of designs now provide templates for writing evaluation plans (Popham et al., 2012). Although reporting guidelines were designed to increase the transparency of **reporting when writing the evaluation** report or journal article, consulting the appropriate guideline in advance will keep the evaluator from being surprised by the expectation of having to report something that was not anticipated. Guidelines differ in the degree of research and expertise on which they are founded. Literally, hundreds of guidelines are now posted on the EQUATOR (Enhancing the QUAlity and Transparency Of health Research) website at http://www.equator-network.org/. The most helpful (with the strongest foundation) contain checklists of what to report (and plan for), and they are prominently listed, e.g., CONSORT (CONsolidated Standards of Reporting Trials), for randomized trials, StaRI (Standards for Reporting Implementation Studies) for implementation studies, SRQR (Standards for Reporting Qualitative Research for qualitative research), ASSESS for mixed methods focused on implementation, and SQUIRE (Standards for QUality Improvement in Reporting Excellence) for quality improvement studies. Others include recommendations for measuring implementation. Look for "explanation and elaboration" documents that contain examples from published reports of each item on the checklist together with a rationale for including each item. These guidelines also are primers on the particular type of design, including the best practices (and mistakes often made) in analyses. For example, we cited the CONSORT extensions for pragmatic designs, e-interventions, and comparative effectiveness trials in Task 2 and 3 above.

Pilot Test the Intervention, Measures, and Other Protocol Components

Although the terms "feasibility" and "pilot" study are sometimes used interchangeably, a feasibility study has been defined as any type of study that relates to the preparation for a main trial (Bowen et al., 2009). Therefore, "feasibility is a concept encapsulating ideas about whether it is possible to do something and. . .a feasibility study asks whether something can be done, should we proceed with it, and if so, how" (Eldridge et al., 2016). A pilot study can be considered a subset of feasibility studies that looks specifically at design features proposed for the main study, whether full or in part, that is conducted on a small scale (Eldridge et al., 2016). Although a pilot study is also concerned with feasibility study questions, "it has a further dimension; piloting is implementing something, or part of something, in a way you intend to do it in future to see whether it can be done in practice"(Eldridge et al., 2016). Two reporting guidelines that are useful here include the extension of CONSORT (Consolidated Standards of Reporting Trials (CONSORT), 2010) for Pilot and Feasibility Trials, and Guidance for Exploratory Studies of Complex Public Health Interventions. Further guidance for the conduct of feasibility and pilot studies specifically for implementation trials using Hybrid 1 and Hybrid 2 designs is also available (Task 3 above).

Many logistics, especially intervention delivery, participant recruitment and retention, and measurement should be implemented, tested and confirmed in real-life circumstances. An excellent guide to feasibility studies emphasizes pilot studies and suggests designs for addressing acceptability, demand, implementation, practicality, adaptation, integration, and

BOX 10.3. QUESTIONS FOR A PILOT STUDY

- How acceptable is the intervention to the intended beneficiaries?
- How acceptable is the intervention to the implementers?
- Are all levels of implementation procedures realistic?
- Can implementers be recruited and trained to deliver the intervention with acceptable fidelity?
- Are eligibility rates similar to those estimated? If they depend on self-report, are there indications that there is reluctance to endorse a risk factor?
- Can the main subgroups of intended beneficiaries be recruited, and at what rate? Which methods are most productive?
- Do any aspects of the informed consent require additional reassurance or reconsideration of the protocol? How much time does the consent process actually take, and does it fit comfortably into the workflow of the setting (if applicable)?
- Are the indicators and measures available as expected, how much time do they take to collect, and how well do they perform?
- Do follow-up procedures produce the expected completion rates?
- How successful are the planned progress reports and "final" report in helping the various stakeholder groups understand the findings and consider changes to the protocol? Can the reporting be improved to stimulate discussion and suggestions?

Adapted from Bowen et al. (2009).

expansion (Bowen et al., 2009). The questions above (Box 10.3) provide examples of pilot study questions.

For the *Me & You* middle-school healthy relationships intervention described in Chapters 6–8, the developers addressed several of the questions above, particularly those related to intervention acceptability and performance of measures. For example, the program developers pilot tested selected activities and evaluation measures with the priority population which comprised early adolescent ethnic-minority youth (Peskin et al., 2018, 2019). A teen advisory board of 15 ethnically diverse students was recruited. Because few interventions had been conducted with early adolescent youth, it was important to ensure that topics were developmentally appropriate and culturally appropriate for this priority population. For example, based on feedback from the teen advisory board, activities related to active consent (related to dating) were updated to ensure that younger students could relate to the topic (i.e., consent was discussed in general related to borrowing money from someone versus directly teaching about consent in dating and sexual situations). The teen advisory board also pilot-tested the primary behavioral measures which were assessed by the Conflict in Adolescent Dating and Relationship Inventory (CADRI) which was previously only used among high school students (Wolfe et al., 2001). The teens suggested that some words be replaced to ensure comprehension by a younger audience.

A common – and controversial – use of pilot studies is to estimate the findings of an effect evaluation, i.e., the size of the intervention effect (Kistin & Silverstein, 2015). On the one hand, having an accurate estimate helps the evaluator and other interested parties decide whether the intervention is promising enough to be tested in a full trial, and it is a key part of calculating sample size. On the other hand, the small sample size of a pilot study means that the estimate is more likely than not to either overestimate or underestimate the true effect size. If the true effect size is underestimated, a potentially worthwhile intervention may be viewed as not worthwhile to pursue. Worse, even though a promising effect size is shown, it might be mistaken for lack of effect if some interested parties look for a statistically significant difference (when they should not). If the true effect size is overestimated in a pilot study but still used to inform sample size calculations, the sample size for the full evaluation will be too small and may fail to show a statistically significant effect. Thus, it is important to be aware of potential errors and misinterpretation when using small-scale pilot study results to estimate the size of the intervention's effect.

Task 5: Plan When and How to Report to Evaluation Findings

As with other aspects of an evaluation, reporting to relevant audiences the evaluation findings and lessons learned should be discussed in advance with intended users and other interested parties. Reports should be timely, unbiased, and consistent; drafts should be provided so that clarification, alternative interpretations, and other issues can be discussed and resolved. Planning effective communication also requires considering the style, tone, message source, vehicle, and format of information products. *Evaluation Strategies for Communicating and Reporting: Enhancing Learning in Organizations,* by Torres, Preskill and Piontek (2004) and Grob (2015) Chapter 27 (Grob, 2015) and Chapter 28 *(Writing for impact)* in the *Handbook for Practical Program Evaluation* provide excellent guidelines and models. A checklist of items to consider when developing evaluation reports (Box 10.4) includes tailoring the report content for the audience, explaining the focus of the evaluation and its limitations, and listing both the strengths and weaknesses of the evaluation.

BOX 10.4. CHECKLIST FOR ENSURING EFFECTIVE EVALUATION REPORTS

- Provide interim and final reports to intended users in time for comments and questions.
- Tailor the report content, format, and style for the audience(s) by involving audience members.
- Include a summary.
- Summarize the description of the interested groups and how they were engaged.
- Describe essential features of the intervention (e.g., including logic models).
- Explain the focus of the evaluation and its limitations.
- Include an adequate summary of the evaluation plan and procedures.
- Provide all necessary technical information (e.g., in appendices).
- Specify the standards and criteria for evaluative judgments.
- Explain the evaluative judgments and how they are supported by the evidence.
- List both strengths and weaknesses of the evaluation.
- Discuss recommendations for action with their advantages, disadvantages, and resource implications.
- Ensure protections for program clients and other interested groups.
- Anticipate how people or organizations might be affected by the findings.
- Present minority opinions or rejoinders where necessary.
- Verify that the report is accurate and unbiased.
- Organize the report logically and include appropriate details.
- Remove technical jargon.
- Use examples, illustrations, graphics, and illustrative stories.

Adapted from Fitzpatrick et al. (2010).

FOR OUR CHILDREN EXAMPLE: STEP 6

During Step 6 of IM, the planning team described the evaluation of the intervention. This example illustrates some of the key elements of the plan and preliminary findings. The ***For Our Children*** or, in Spanish, ***Por Nuestros Hijos (PNH)*** program was originally designed for parents of girls 11–17 with a focus on vaccine initiation among younger girls (11–12 year olds). It was then adapted because the guidelines for vaccination had changed in the U.S. recommending vaccination for boys (CDC, 2011; Rodriguez et al., 2018).

The parent-focused intervention included two components:

1. **A tailored interactive multimedia intervention (TIMI)** (also available on mobile devices) providing tailored educational content.
2. **A culturally relevant print fotonovela** designed to engage parents with relatable narratives.

Community Health Workers (CHWs) played a critical role in delivering these materials to eligible parents, ensuring accessibility and engagement. Parents also received text message reminders to initiate and complete vaccination for their child.

The provider-focused intervention addressed the most important environmental condition: delivering strong recommendations for HPV vaccination. The **HPVCancerCoach App** (an online/mobile app designed to support providers in delivering strong HPV vaccine recommendations) described in Step 4 was accessible online or via mobile devices and included information, messaging, and videos to target determinants of provider recommendation behavior.

For Step 6, the planning team developed an evaluation plan encompassing a review of the logic model of change and matrices, process evaluation and effect evaluation. The original aim was to assess the effectiveness of this multilevel intervention targeting both parents and providers simultaneously. However, because the provider component was not ready for inclusion in the parent trial, two separate evaluations were conducted. The primary trial focused on the parent component, while the provider intervention was evaluated in a pilot study using a pre–post design to examine changes in self-reported provider recommendations and clinic-level vaccination rates. These evaluations were independent and conducted at different times; therefore, their outcomes were not linked.

Task 1: Review the Logic Model of Change, Matrices and Implementation Plan to Guide Process and Effect Evaluation

Figure 10.7 is a summarized version of the final logic model for **PNH**. Along with the matrices developed in Step 2, it enabled the planning group to develop a plan to assess implementation (process evaluation) and intended outcomes (effect evaluation) of the program and identify outcomes from the work completed in Steps 1–5. The logic model also clearly stipulates the intended mechanisms of change (how the intervention is supposed to lead to desired outcomes) and can guide evaluation questions related to what determinants were impacted and how they mediated change in behaviors.

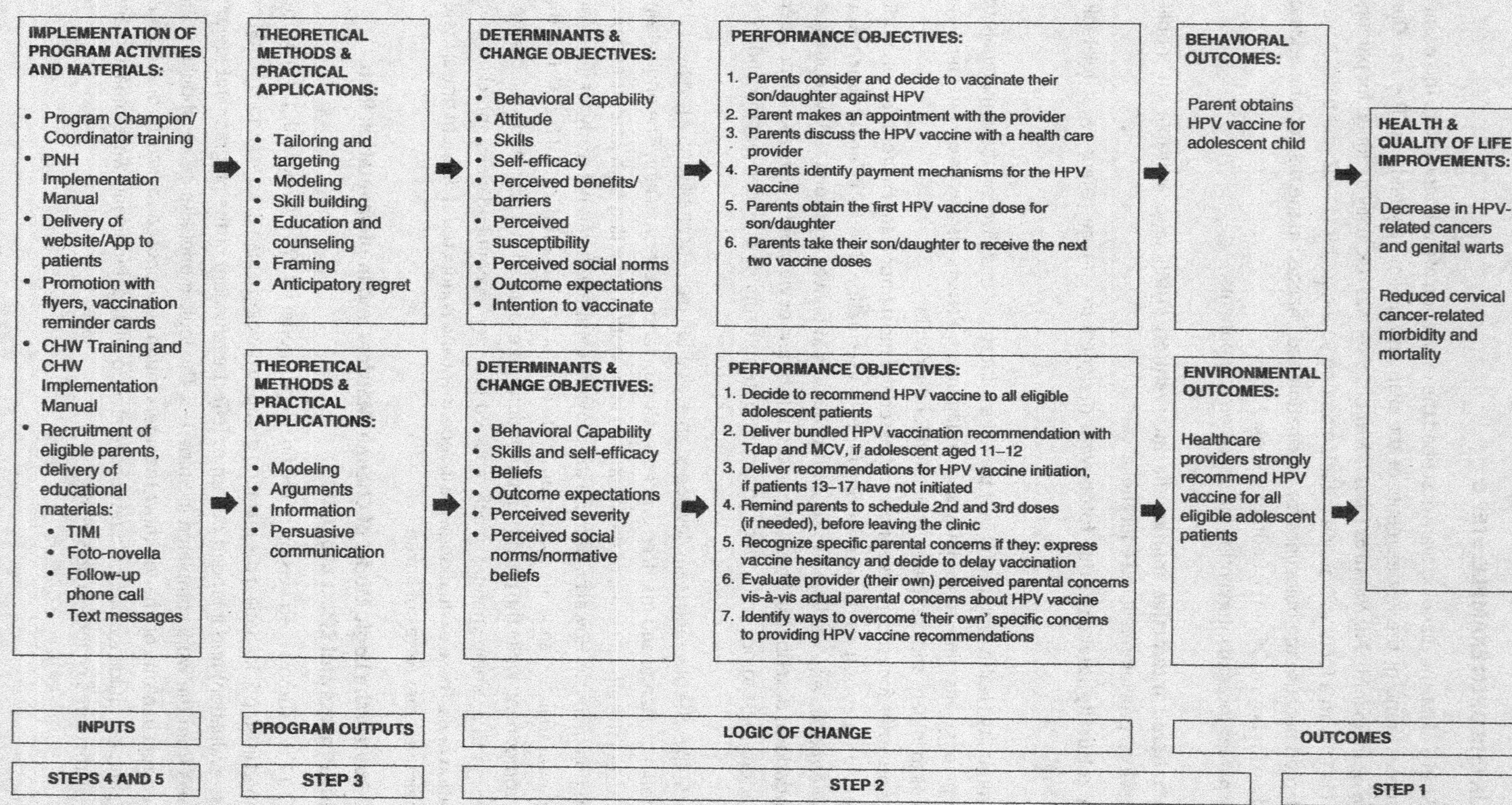

Figure 10.7 PNH Intervention Logic Model of the Intervention

Task 2: Develop Process Evaluation Questions and Identify Measures

For the parent component, the process evaluation focused on key implementation outcomes: reach (number of parents who received the intervention), delivery (which components were delivered and to what extent), participant engagement and satisfaction (completion of intervention activities), and availability of implementation structures and resources.

Examples of process evaluation questions were as follows:

Reach:

- How many eligible parents were contacted and received the intervention materials?
- What proportion of the priority population accessed the web-based app or fotonovela?

Delivery and Fidelity:

- Were all intended components (web app, fotonovela) delivered as planned?
- Did CHWs follow the protocol for introducing and explaining the intervention?

Dose and Engagement:

- How much time did parents spend using the web-based app?
- Did parents read the fotonovela and complete the interactive modules?

Satisfaction:

- How satisfied were parents with the content and delivery of the intervention?

Evaluators measured reach by tracking the number of parents contacted through CHW outreach who received PNH education (TIMI and fotonovella). CHWs used an Intervention Delivery checklist to document the number of potential participants approached, the number eligible, and the number agreeing to participate. Delivery was assessed by documenting the "dose" of each component (e.g., time CHW spent with participants, time on the TIMI, and whether CHWs provided all intended materials). Implementation fidelity was measured by intervention delivery checklists (based on implementation performance objectives, see Table 9. 7–9.10). Indicators and measures are summarized in Table 10.6.

For the provider component, which included the HPVCancerCoach App, the process evaluation aimed to assess reach (number of providers, among all providers offered the tool, who accessed the app), dose delivered (extent of app use and completion of modules), and acceptability/usability (provider satisfaction and perceived usefulness). Process evaluation questions included: (1) to what extent does the provider intervention reach all physicians and nurse practitioners in each clinic recruited to participate?; (2) to what extent is the HPVCancerCoach App accessed?; (3) What is the acceptability of the provider level intervention?

The evaluation team tested the usability and feasibility of the HPVCancerCoach App with a group of 15 healthcare workers, which included physicians, nurses, physician assistants, nurse practitioners, and medical assistants who provide vaccination services to adolescents. After

Table 10.6 Partial Evaluation Plan for the For Our Children/Por Nuestros Hijos (PNH) program

Variable	Evaluation Question	Indicator	Measure	Timing
		Process Evaluation		
Parent Component				
Reach (coverage)	How many eligible parents received PNH (TIMI + fotonovela)?	Number of parents receiving PNH intervention among all screened eligible	Intervention Delivery Checklist completed by CHW	Baseline
Fidelity	To what extent was the parent intervention delivered as planned?	Number of persons marked as "completed intervention" on the REDCap log and the number of components delivered to each participant	Intervention Delivery Checklist completed by CHW	Baseline
Dose and engagement	How many parents received the PNH TIMI?	Percent of parents enrolled in PNH who received a visit from the CHW and received materials	PNH Encounter form that tracked delivery of program components and time of interaction with the CHW	Baseline
	How many received the fotonovela? How much time was the parent exposed to intervention material?	Percent of parents enrolled in PNH who received a visit from the CHW and received materials Number of minutes participating in CHW encounter and using TIMI	PNH Encounter form that tracked delivery of program components and time of interaction with the CHW Encounter logs and TIMI tracking	Baseline
	How much time did the CHW spend with each participant?	Number of minutes CHW spent with each patient Percent of parents enrolled in PNH who received the 2-week phone call Total number of minutes spent on phone call	Encounter forms Phone log tracking parents reached	Baseline 2 weeks following baseline
Provider component				
Reach (providers)	How many eligible providers (and what proportion) accessed the HPVCancerCoach App intervention?	Number of providers in each clinic who accessed the App among all those who see patients of eligible age	Access and registration record captured on App	30 days following training activity (baseline)

Table 10.6 (*Continued*)

Variable	Evaluation Question	Indicator	Measure	Timing
Dose and engagement (providers)	To what extent does the provider intervention reach all physicians and nurse practitioners in each clinic recruited to participate? To what extent is the HPVCancerCoach App accessed?	Number of providers in each clinic who attended training among all those who see patients of eligible age Numbers of minutes each provider used the App	Training sign-in sheets Recorded time in use (captured on the App)	Baseline 30 days following training activity (baseline)
Acceptability and usability	What is the usability and acceptability of the provider level intervention (HPVCancerCoach App)?	The extent to which providers reported usability and acceptability following exposure to the tool	Usability survey and discussions	Following completion of the App, preceding implementation of the trial (baseline)
Effect Evaluation: Sample Participant Behaviors				
Parent component				
HPV vaccine initiation	Did the intervention increase the HPV vaccination in adolescents whose parents received the intervention as compared to those who did not?	Initiation of the HPV vaccine series after program recruitment (among parents who reported adolescents had not been vaccinated at baseline)	Parental report and EMR vaccination record verification	**Intervention participants:** Survey: 2 weeks after the intervention **All participants:** Survey and EMR verification: 3 months after baseline EMR verification: 9 months after baseline
HPV vaccine completion	Did the intervention increase the number of adolescents who completed their HPV vaccination series?	Number of doses of the HPV vaccine series after program recruitment (among all adolescents regardless of vaccination status at baseline)	EMR vaccination record verification	**All participants:** Survey and EMR verification: 3 months after baseline EMR verification 9 months after baseline
Provider component				
HPV vaccination recommendation	Did providers in intervention clinics deliver stronger and more consistent HPV vaccine recommendations compared to providers in control clinics?	Frequency of provider strong recommendation for HPV vaccination	In depth interviews	Follow-up (6 months following baseline)

(*continued*)

Table 10.6 *(Continued)*

Variable	Evaluation Question	Indicator	Measure	Timing
Impact of provider intervention on vaccination rates	Did the provider intervention result in increased HPV vaccination in participating clinics as compared to clinics without the provider intervention?	HPV vaccination rates over time among intervention and comparison clinics	Electronic health record (EHR) data were used to calculate monthly HPV vaccination rates	Monthly; final assessment 6 months following baseline
Effect Evaluation: Sample Determinants				
Parent component				
Behavioral capability about HPV transmission, prevention, and associated diseases	Did the intervention increase the parents' behavioral capability about HPV?	Behavioral capability about how HPV is/is not transmitted, prevented, and which diseases it causes	HPV knowledge true or false questions on the parent survey. (14 items) (NCI, 2005; Savas et al., 2012)	Baseline survey 3-month follow-up survey
Self-efficacy to get their child vaccinated against HPV	Did the intervention increase the parents' self-efficacy to vaccinate their child?	Self-efficacy to make an appointment with their child's healthcare provider and get them vaccinated	Self-efficacy scale on the parent survey. (6 items) (Richman et al., 2012)	Baseline survey 3-month follow-up survey
Normative beliefs about HPV vaccination	Did the intervention increase the parents' belief that other parents endorse HPV vaccination?	Perceived peers' beliefs about HPV vaccination	Normative beliefs scale on the parent survey. (5 items) (Savas et al., 2012)	Baseline survey 3-month follow-up survey
Provider component				
Self efficacy for providing a strong recommendation	Did provider self-efficacy related to HPV vaccine recommendation improve following exposure to the HPVCancerCoach App?	Level of confidence in their ability to deliver a strong recommendation	Provider survey	Baseline and follow-up (6 months later)
Outcome expectation that delivery the recommendation will result in increased HPV vaccination	Did provider outcome expectations related to HPV vaccine recommendation improve following exposure to the HPVCancerCoach App?	Belief that providing a recommendation will lead to increased vaccination	Provider survey	Baseline and follow-up (6 months later)

installing and reviewing the app, providers completed a usability survey addressing key constructs such as perceived usefulness, ease of use, job relevance, and intent to use the system. The survey included questions regarding specific benefits, challenges, facilitators, and barriers to app usage.

Task 3: Develop Effect Evaluation Questions, Select a Design, and Identify Measures

Evaluation of Parent Component

Using the logic model of change and matrices developed in earlier IM steps, the evaluation team identified key determinants, behaviors, and health-related outcomes for the parent component of the PNH intervention. The team formulated effect evaluation questions to assess whether the intervention produced expected changes in theoretically grounded determinants, parental intention to vaccinate their child, and adolescent HPV vaccine uptake.

Effect Evaluation Questions Consistent with Task 3 guidance, the team used the logic model to guide the effect evaluation questions, moving from proximal determinants to behavioral and health outcomes. Example effect evaluation questions included:

Determinant-Level Questions

- Did parents who received the PNH educational intervention demonstrate greater increases in HPV vaccination-related behavioral capability compared to parents receiving usual care?
- Did the intervention increase parents' self-efficacy to obtain HPV vaccination for their adolescent child?
- Did parents exposed to the intervention report more positive outcome expectations regarding HPV vaccination?
- Did perceived social norms supporting HPV vaccination increase among intervention parents relative to controls?

Behavioral Outcome Questions

- Did the PNH intervention increase HPV vaccine initiation among Hispanic girls aged 11–17?
- Did the PNH intervention increase HPV vaccine initiation among Hispanic boys aged 11–17?
- Was the intervention effective for increasing HPV vaccination and vaccine completion in young girls and boys aged 11–12?

These questions reflect both main effects of intervention components and sequencing effects, consistent with the adaptive nature of the intervention.

Measures Measures were selected based on the intervention's change objectives and determinants specified in the logic model and matrices. Some measures were adapted from validated instruments found in the literature or used in previous studies (Allen et al., 2010; Escoffery et al., 2023; Richman et al., 2012; Savas et al., 2021). Parent-reported survey measures assessed HPV vaccination-related behavioral capability, self-efficacy, outcome expectations, and normative beliefs using items adapted from existing validated instruments and tailored to the intervention content. All measures were translated into Spanish using established translation procedures (Cruchinho et al., 2024).

Behavioral outcomes—HPV vaccine initiation and series completion—were assessed using EMR data to minimize self-report bias. Timing of measures was selected to capture both proximal determinant changes and longer-term behavioral outcomes, consistent with the expected causal sequence specified in the logic model.

Design The evaluation team used a Sequential Multiple Assignment Randomized Trial (SMART) design to evaluate the effectiveness of the primary intervention components and their sequencing over time. This design was chosen to align with the intervention's adaptive logic and to inform the development of optimized intervention strategies.

At baseline, eligible parents of Hispanic adolescents aged 11–17 who had not initiated the HPV vaccine series were randomized to receive either the PNH parent educational intervention (TIMI and fotonovella) or usual care. All participants completed a baseline survey at recruitment.

Follow-up surveys were administered at three months post-recruitment (all participants) to assess intermediate outcomes. Participants were re-randomized to receive either tailored HPV vaccination text message reminders or no text messages. The reminder intervention consisted of eight weekly messages tailored by language preference (English or Spanish), adolescent sex, and vaccination status (unvaccinated or initiated). This second-stage randomization allowed examination of the effectiveness of reminder messages and whether their impact differed depending on prior exposure to the educational intervention.

Data collectors contacted participants by phone at baseline, three months, and nine months post-recruitment to obtain self-reported status of the child's HPV vaccination. Electronic medical record (EMR) reviews were conducted to objectively verify adolescent HPV vaccination initiation and completion.

Evaluation of Provider Component

For the provider-focused HPVCancerCoach App intervention, effect evaluation questions targeted providers' role as environmental change agents informing parental vaccination decisions. They included the following:

- Did providers in intervention clinics deliver stronger and more consistent HPV vaccine recommendations compared to providers in control clinics?
- Did provider self-efficacy and outcome expectations related to HPV vaccine recommendation improve following exposure to the HPVCancerCoach App?
- Did the provider intervention result in increased HPV vaccination in participating clinics as compared to clinics without the provider intervention?

Measures Electronic health record (EHR) data were used to calculate monthly HPV vaccination rates, defined as the percentage of eligible adolescents vaccinated during each month.

Pre-intervention rates were calculated for August 2023–January 2024 and post-intervention rates for February–July 2024. The primary outcome was the change in HPV vaccination rates among eligible adolescents, assessed using paired t-tests within intervention clinics and difference-in-differences analyses comparing intervention and comparison clinics over time.

Design The study was a cluster-randomized controlled trial in 13 Federally Qualified Health Center clinics, assigning clinics to intervention or comparison conditions using a covariate-adaptive allocation procedure (minimization) to balance key characteristics such as clinic size, baseline HPV vaccination rates, and patient demographics. Providers in intervention clinics received training on implementing the HPVCancerCoach App.

Task 4: Pilot Test the Intervention and Finalize the Evaluation Plan

Parent Component

Before launching the trial, the team conducted pilot activities focused on usability and feasibility rather than formal impact testing. Study protocols were tested in two Federally Qualified Health Centers (FQHCs) to evaluate recruitment and data collection procedures, including the ability to identify eligible participants through electronic health records (EHR) and verify vaccination status for outcome validation.

To ensure cultural and linguistic appropriateness, community health workers (CHWs) and parents participated in user testing of the PNH program materials. Using in-depth interviews and the "think-aloud" method, the team assessed usability, functionality, and satisfaction with the TIMI and fotonovela. Participants provided feedback on content clarity, navigation, and motivational appeal, as well as suggestions for improvement. Findings from this testing informed refinements to program content and finalization of the trial protocol.

The team also conducted a pilot study to optimize HPV vaccination reminder messages. Eight message variations were tested to examine the effect of linguistic agency assignment—specifically prevention versus threat framing—on parental perceptions and intentions. Results indicated that assigning threat agency to HPV (rather than to humans) increased perceived susceptibility and strengthened intentions to seek vaccination. These insights guided the development of tailored text-message content for the adaptive intervention component (McGlone et al., 2017).

Provider Component

For the healthcare provider assessment, we conducted a usability assessment of the HPVCancerCoach App. Usability testing with 15 providers indicated high acceptability. Usability was measured using validated scales, including the System Usability Scale (SUS) (Brooke, 1996) and Technology Acceptance Model (TAM) (Lewis, 2019), supplemented by open-ended feedback on content, functionality, and barriers to adoption. Providers in participating healthcare centers completed the assessment. Overall, providers found the app provided useful resources, was easy to use, and motivated them to recommend the HPV vaccine. Providers highlighted features such as succinct, up-to-date content and practical communication tips, while recommending shorter videos and improved navigation for easier access to content.

Task 5: Plan When and How to Report Evaluation Findings

Effectiveness of the Parent Component

The study assessed the effectiveness of a multicomponent intervention that included small media materials delivered by CHWs and parental text message reminders. Using a Sequential Multiple Assignment Randomized Trial (SMART) design (Dawson & Lavori, 2012), the PNH was evaluated in a randomized controlled trial conducted in the Houston metropolitan area. In the trial, participants who were recruited at clinics and community events serving a low-income, Hispanic, urban population were randomly assigned to the intervention or control conditioning. The trial comprised a cohort of predominantly Spanish-speaking Hispanic parents of adolescents aged 11–17 followed for nine months. The evaluation demonstrated that the For Our Children (PNH) intervention (TIMI + fotonovela) was effective for girls, particularly younger girls, but not for boys.

Girls whose parents received the PNH educational intervention had significantly higher odds of initiating HPV vaccination compared to those in the control group. At nine-month follow-up, multivariate analysis indicated that exposure to the intervention increased the likelihood of vaccine initiation by 82% (OR = 1.82; 95% CI: 1.03–3.26; $p = 0.041$). Age was a strong predictor: younger girls aged 11–12 were nearly three times more likely to initiate vaccination than older girls aged 13–17 (OR = 2.94; 95% CI: 1.61–5.58; $p < 0.001$).

The adapted intervention did not significantly increase HPV vaccination initiation among boys. Multivariate logistic regression showed no difference between intervention and control groups (OR = 0.86; 95% CI: 0.43–1.68; $p = 0.653$). Parent education level was associated with vaccination initiation among boys: parents with higher education had greater odds of vaccinating their sons (OR = 1.13; 95% CI: 1.02–1.26; $p = 0.021$). These results suggest that additional strategies are needed to address barriers specific to male adolescents.

Tailored text message reminders did not significantly increase HPV vaccination initiation for either girls or boys. Across both sexes, parents who received text messages were only slightly more likely to vaccinate their child, but this difference was not statistically significant (OR = 1.06; 95% CI: 0.75–1.49; $p = 0.73$). Similar null results were observed when analyzing text message effects separately for girls and boys.

These findings highlight the need for sex-specific strategies and more intensive approaches to address barriers to HPV vaccination among boys.

Effectiveness of Provider Component

In the six months following the intervention, five of the six intervention clinics demonstrated higher average HPV vaccination rates post-intervention compared to pre-intervention, with percentage increases ranging from 1.4 to 21.4%. Despite these upward trends, paired t-tests revealed that the increases within intervention clinics were not statistically significant.

Similarly, when comparing the percentage change in vaccination rates between intervention and comparison clinics from the pre- to post-intervention periods, no statistically significant differences were observed.

Although the intervention condition showed a modest positive trend, the limited implementation period and variability across clinics likely constrained the ability to detect significant effects. These findings suggest that while the provider intervention was feasible and acceptable, additional time, reinforcement, and potentially enhanced support may be needed to achieve measurable improvements in HPV vaccination uptake.

Reporting Evaluation Findings

The planning team developed a structured plan for when and how evaluation findings would be reported to ensure timely dissemination, transparency, and meaningful use of the data. Early in Step 6, the team mapped reporting activities onto the evaluation timeline for both the parent and provider components. Interim process evaluation findings (e.g., reach, fidelity, engagement, usability) were scheduled to be shared quarterly with the implementation team and collaborating clinics to support rapid-cycle improvements during implementation. For effect evaluation findings, the team planned to share preliminary results (such as three-month survey outcomes and early EMR updates) with project leadership at mid-point checkpoints, followed by full results after the nine-month parent follow-up and the six-month provider follow-up periods.

The final reporting plan included multiple formats tailored to the needs of different audiences:

1. **Internal technical reports** summarizing all process and effect evaluation metrics for use by the full research team.
2. **Presentations to community partners and participating families**, ensuring that CHWs, parents, and community clinic leaders received accessible summaries of the findings and had the opportunity to provide feedback.
3. **Briefs for interested parties** designed for program funders and health system administrators to support future decision-making, sustainability planning, and resource allocation.
4. **Academic dissemination**, including peer-reviewed manuscripts and conference presentations describing the intervention, evaluation methods, and results.

By planning in advance when, how, and to whom evaluation findings would be communicated, the team ensured that results would not only meet scientific and funder expectations but also be shared with community members who contributed to the project and would benefit from the knowledge gained. This approach supported both accountability and equitable dissemination.

Summary

Chapter 10 describes how to plan an evaluation of a health promotion intervention based on the previous five IM steps. The questions to be answered by the evaluation –out of many possibilities–should be based on consultation with those with a vested interest in the conduct or results, with the highest priority given to questions that have the greatest potential for use. Some evaluations will focus on one or more **process** questions alone, e.g., "To what extent is the intervention reaching the intended population?" "Are any groups missing?" "How well does the intervention that is delivered match what was planned?" "What is its cost?" and "Did those responsible for implementing the intervention follow the implementation plan?" Many times, the process evaluation will stand on its own, especially in cases of already tested, lightly adapted interventions or newly developed interventions that need testing. Process evaluation questions can be incorporated into ongoing or periodic monitoring using administrative records and can be used in short feedback loops for quality improvement.

Evaluators, especially those who have completed IM Steps 1–5, will have enough confidence in the theory and evidence behind the intervention's logic and implementation planning to extend their evaluation to effect evaluation questions, "Does the intervention 'work'?" "How well does it work?" "Is the new intervention more effective (or more cost effective) than another intervention currently in use?" and "Is the intervention more (or less) effective with one subgroup of the intended beneficiaries than others?" To avoid a "black box" evaluation, a process evaluation is *always* needed. Thus, although a process evaluation might stand alone, an effect evaluation cannot deliver the whole picture by itself.

Numerous designs are available for effect evaluations to suit particular circumstances, together with additional considerations such as strong measures with appropriate length and a timeframe for the measures based on what is already known, and the choice of treatment for the comparison group. Development of indicators and measures for the constructs being measured is a major task in the development of all evaluation plans. Clear specification of intervention effects in the logic model and change objectives from the matrices allow the selection and/or development of reliable, valid and feasible measures that can test the effect of the intervention and characteristics of its implementation.

Evaluation plans need a dress rehearsal, a pilot test, and readjustment of key processes such as recruitment, implementation tasks, and intervention components or delivery. Thus, the final product of Step 6 is an evaluation plan, which includes the evaluation protocol (e.g., questions, design, indicators and measures, timing of the measures), resources required, and plan for reporting to interested parties – pilot tested so that weaknesses can be corrected before a more resource-intensive evaluation is initiated.

The chapter has emphasized ethical issues, such as informed consent by potential participants and partner organizations, choosing appropriate and acceptable standards of comparison, and transparency regarding the evaluation perspective. We stress that communication of findings and comments on the findings by affected groups are key actions for a learning organization. As a result of evaluation, some interventions should be discarded; many interventions can be improved or adapted to have a better fit to a new population or setting, or delivered more efficiently. Transparent evaluations can provide the knowledge to inform these important decisions and move health promotion practice forward.

Discussion Questions and Learning Activities

1. Explain how the products from Steps 1 through 5 of IM can be used to help plan for evaluation.
2. Identify the most important organizations and individuals with vested interests in your proposed evaluation and what their interests are.
3. Explain the difference between process and effect evaluation.
4. Use the health promotion intervention you proposed in the preceding chapters and consult the intervention logic, performance measures, and implementation plan to draft process and effect evaluation questions.
5. Explain reliability and validity when considering measures.
6. Briefly describe the measures you will use to answer your process evaluation questions. Provide your rationale for your choice of measures.
7. Briefly describe the measures you will use to answer your effect evaluation questions. Provide your rationale for your choice of measures.
8. Choose an effect-evaluation design to evaluate your health promotion intervention and discuss its strengths and limitations, including consideration of the degree to which it will emphasize internal and external validity.

References

Adams, M. A., Todd, M., Angadi, S. S., Hurley, J. C., Stecher, C., Berardi, V., Phillips, C. B., McEntee, M. L., Hovell, M. F., & Hooker, S. P. (2022). Adaptive goals and reinforcement timing to increase physical activity in adults: A factorial randomized trial. *American Journal of Preventive Medicine, 62*(2), e57–e68. doi:10.1016/j.amepre.2021.09.014

Allen, J. D., Coronado, G. D., Williams, R. S., Glenn, B., Escoffery, C., Fernandez, M., Tuff, R. A., Wilson, K. M., & Mullen, P. D. (2010). A systematic review of measures used in studies of human papillomavirus (HPV) vaccine acceptability. *Vaccine, 28*(24), 4027–4037. doi:10.1016/j.vaccine.2010.03.063

Almirall, D., Nahum-Shani, I., Sherwood, N. E., & Murphy, S. A. (2014). Introduction to SMART designs for the development of adaptive interventions: with application to weight loss research. *Translational behavioral medicine*, 4(3), 260–274. doi: 10.1007/s13142-014-0265-0

American Evaluation Association (2025). American Evaluation Association guiding principles for evaluators. https://www.eval.org/About/Guiding-Principles

Baker, T. B., Smith, S. S., Bolt, D. M., Loh, W.-Y., Mermelstein, R., Fiore, M. C., Piper, M. E., & Collins, L. M. (2017). Implementing clinical research using factorial designs: A primer. *Behavior Therapy, 48*(4), 567–580.

Baldwin, M., Bell, J., Bess, R., Burwick, A., Collins-Camargo, C., Corso, P., & ... Yates, B. (2013). Cost analysis in program evaluation: A guide for child welfare researchers and service providers. Administration for Children and Families, U.S. Department of Health and Human Services.

Bamberger, M. (2012). *Introduction to mixed methods in impact evaluation: Impact evaluation guidance notes No. 3.* InterAction and The Rockefeller Foundation.

Bandalos, D. L. (2018). *Measurement theory and applications for the social sciences.* Guilford Publications.

Bandura, A. (1986). *Social foundations of thought and action: A social cognitive theory.* Prentice-Hall.

Barisic, A., Leatherdale, S. T., & Kreiger, N. (2011). Importance of frequency, intensity, time and type (FITT) in physical activity assessment for epidemiological research. *Canadian Journal of Public Health, 102,* 174–175.

Barry, J. (2017). The relationship between the supply of primary care physicians and measures of breast health service use. *Journal of Women's Health, 26*(5), 511–519.

Bartholomew Eldredge, L. K., Markham, C. M., Ruiter, R. A. C., Fernández, M. E., Kok, G., & Parcel, G. S. (2016). *Planning health promotion programs: An intervention mapping approach* (4th ed.). Jossey-Bass.

Basen-Engquist, K., Coyle, K. K., Parcel, G. S., Kirby, D., Banspach, S. W., Carvajal, S. C., & Baumler, E. (2001). Schoolwide effects of a multicomponent HIV, STD, and pregnancy prevention program for high school students. *Health Education & Behavior, 28*(2), 166–185.

Basen-Engquist, K., Masse, L. C., Coyle, K., Kirby, D., Parcel, G. S., Banspach, S., & Nodora, J. (1999). Validity of scales measuring the psychosocial determinants of HIV/STD-related risk behavior in adolescents. *Health Education Research, 14*(1), 25–38.

Behavioral Measurement Database Services. (n.d.). *HaPI Database.* https://www.bmdshapi.com/hapi-database/.

Bennett, W. L., Wilson, R. F., Zhang, A., Tseng, E., Knapp, E. A., Kharrazi, H., Stuart, E. A., Shogbesan, O., Bass, E. B., & Cheskin, L. J. (2018). Methods for evaluating natural experiments in obesity: A systematic review. *Annals of Internal Medicine, 168*(11), 791–800.

Bernet, A. C., Willens, D. E., & Bauer, M. S. (2013). Effectiveness-implementation hybrid designs: Implications for quality improvement science. *Implementation Science, 8*(S2).

Boon, M. H., Craig, P., Thomson, H., Campbell, M., & Moore, L. (2021). Regression discontinuity designs in health: A systematic review. *Epidemiology (Cambridge, Mass.), 32*(1), 87.

Booth-Kewley, S., Larson, G. E., & Miyoshi, D. K. (2007). Social desirability effects on computerized and paper-and-pencil questionnaires. *Computers in Human Behavior, 23*(1), 463–477.

Bor, J., Moscoe, E., Mutevedzi, P., Newell, M.-L., & Bärnighausen, T. (2014). Regression discontinuity designs in epidemiology: Causal inference without randomized trials. *Epidemiology (Cambridge, Mass.), 25*(5), 729.

Bosker, R., & Snijders, T. A. (2011). Multilevel analysis: An introduction to basic and advanced multilevel modeling. *Multilevel Analysis*, 1–368.

Bowen, D. J., Kreuter, M., Spring, B., Cofta-Woerpel, L., Linnan, L., Weiner, D., Bakken, S., Kaplan, C. P., Squiers, L., & Fabrizio, C. (2009). How we design feasibility studies. *American Journal of Preventive Medicine, 36*(5), 452–457.

Brooke, J. (1996). SUS: A 'Quick and dirty' usability scale. In P. W. Jordan, B. Thomas, I. L. McClelland, & B. Weerdmeester (Eds.), *Usability evaluation in industry* (1st ed.). CRC Press. doi:10.1201/9781498710411

Bryson, J. M., & Patton, M. Q. (2015). Analyzing and engaging stakeholders. In H. P. Hatry, K. E. Newcomer, & J. S. Wholey (Eds.), *Handbook of practical program evaluation* (pp. 36–61). doi:10.1002/9781119171386.ch2

Campbell, M. K., Piaggio, G., Elbourne, D. R., & Altman, D. G. (2012). Consort 2010 statement: Extension to cluster randomised trials. *The BMJ, 345*, e5661.

CDC (2011). Recommendations on the use of quadrivalent human papillomavirus vaccine in males–Advisory Committee on Immunization Practices (ACIP), 2011. *MMWR Morbidity and Mortality Weekly Report, 60*(50), 1705–1708.

CDC (2024). Program cost analysis. Centers for Disease Control and Prevention. Retrieved March 14 from https://www.cdc.gov/polaris/php/economics/cost-analysis.html

Chapel, T. (2024). Mixed methods in program evaluation. https://www.cdc.gov/national-asthma-control-program/php/program_eval/webinars.html#cdc_generic_section_9-tutorial-4b

Chirwa, E., Kapito, E., Jere, D. L., Kafulafula, U., Chodzaza, E., Chorwe-Sungani, G., Gresh, A., Liu, L., Abrams, E. T., & Klima, C. S. (2020). An effectiveness-implementation hybrid type 1 trial assessing the impact of group versus individual antenatal care on maternal and infant outcomes in Malawi. *BMC Public Health, 20*(1), 1–13.

Collins, L. M., Dziak, J. J., & Li, R. (2009). Design of experiments with multiple independent variables: A resource management perspective on complete and reduced factorial designs. *Psychological Methods, 14*(3), 202.

Cook, T. D., & Campbell, D. T. (1979). *Quasi-experimentation: Design and analysis issues for field settings*. Houghton Mifflin.

Coyle, K., Basen-Engquist, K., Kirby, D., Parcel, G., Banspach, S., Collins, J., Baumler, S., Carvajal, S., & Harrist, R. (2001). Safer choices: Reducing teen pregnancy, HIV, and STDs. *Public Health Reports, 116*, 82–93. doi:10.1093/phr/116.S1.82

Coyle, K. K., Kirby, D. B., Marin, B. V., Gomez, C. A., & Gregorich, S. E. (2004). Draw the line/respect the line: A randomized trial of a middle school intervention to reduce sexual risk behaviors. *American Journal of Public Health, 94*(5), 843–851.

Creswell, J. W., Klassen, A. C., Plano Clark, V. L., & Clegg Smith, K. (2011). Best practices for mixed methods research in the health sciences. Report Commissioned by the Office of Behavioral and Social Sciences Research (OBSSR). (Vol. 2014).

Cruchinho, P., López-Franco, M. D., Capelas, M. L., Almeida, S., Bennett, P. M., Miranda da Silva, M., Teixeira, G., Nunes, E., Lucas, P., & Gaspar, F. (2024). Translation, cross-cultural adaptation, and validation of measurement instruments: A practical guideline for novice researchers. *Journal of Multidisciplinary Healthcare, 17*, 2701–2728. doi:10.2147/jmdh.S419714

Crutzen, R., Peters, G.-J. Y., & Mondschein, C. (2019). Why and how we should care about the general data protection regulation. *Psychology & Health, 34,* 1347–1357.

Crutzen, R., Roosjen, J. L., & Poelman, J. (2013). Using google analytics as a process evaluation method for internet-delivered interventions: An example on sexual health. *Health Promotion International, 28*(1). doi:10.1093/heapro/das008

Crutzen, R., Viechtbauer, W., Spigt, M., & Kotz, D. (2015). Differential attrition in health behaviour change trials: A systematic review and meta-analysis. *Psychology and Health, 30*(1). doi:10.1080/08870446.2014.953526

Curran, G. M. (2020). Implementation science made too simple: A teaching tool. *Implementation Science Communications, 1*(1), 27. doi:10.1186/s43058-020-00001-z

Curran, G. M., Bauer, M., Mittman, B., Pyne, J. M., & Stetler, C. (2012). Effectiveness-implementation hybrid designs: Combining elements of clinical effectiveness and implementation research to enhance public health impact. *Medical Care, 50*(3), 217–226.

Curran, G. M., Landes, S. J., McBain, S. A., Pyne, J. M., Smith, J. D., Fernandez, M. E., Chambers, D. A., & Mittman, B. S. (2022). Reflections on 10 years of effectiveness-implementation hybrid studies. *Frontiers in Health Services, 2,* 125.

Dawson, R., & Lavori, P. W. (2012). Efficient design and inference for multistage randomized trials of individualized treatment policies. *Biostatistics, 13*(1), 142–152. doi:10.1093/biostatistics/kxr016

Dennis, C. (2003). The breastfeeding self-efficacy scale: Psychometric assessment of the short form. *Journal of Obstetric, Gynecologic, & Neonatal Nursing, 32*(6), 734–744.

DeVellis, R. F., & Thorpe, C. T. (2021). *Scale development: Theory and applications.* Sage publications.

Dijksterhuis, E., & Silvius, G. (2017). The design thinking approach to projects. *The Journal of Modern Project Management, 4*(3).

Dopp, A. R., Mundey, P., Beasley, L. O., Silovsky, J. F., & Eisenberg, D. (2019). Mixed-method approaches to strengthen economic evaluations in implementation research. *Implementation Science, 14,* 1–9.

Durand, C. P., Oluyomi, A. O., Gabriel, K. P., Salvo, D., Sener, I. N., Hoelscher, D. M., Knell, G., Tang, X., Porter, A. K., & Robertson, M. C. (2016). The effect of light rail transit on physical activity: Design and methods of the travel-related activity in neighborhoods study. *Frontiers in Public Health, 4,* 103.

Eldridge, S. M., Lancaster, G. A., Campbell, M. J., Thabane, L., Hopewell, S., Coleman, C. L., & Bond, C. M. (2016). Defining feasibility and pilot studies in preparation for randomised controlled trials: Development of a conceptual framework. *PLoS ONE, 11*(3), e0150205.

Engel, R. S., Corsaro, N., Isaza, G. T., & McManus, H. D. (2022). Assessing the impact of de-escalation training on police behavior: Reducing police use of force in the Louisville, KY Metro Police Department. *Criminology & Public Policy, 21*(2), 199–233. doi:10.1111/1745-9133.12574

Escoffery, C., Petagna, C., Agnone, C., Perez, S., Saber, L. B., Ryan, G., Dhir, M., Sekar, S., Yeager, K. A., Biddell, C. B., Madhivanan, P., Lee, S., English, A. S., Savas, L., Daly, E., Vu, T., & Fernandez, M. E. (2023). A systematic review of interventions to promote HPV vaccination globally. *BMC Public Health, 23*(1), 1262. doi:10.1186/s12889-023-15876-5

Evans Cuellar, A., McReynolds, L. S., & Wasserman, G. A. (2006). A cure for crime: Can mental health treatment diversion reduce crime among youth? *Journal of Policy Analysis and Management, 25*(1), 197–214.

Eyre, L., Farrelly, M., & Marshall, M. (2017). What can a participatory approach to evaluation contribute to the field of integrated care? *BMJ Quality and Safety, 26*(7), 588–594.

Eysenbach, G., & CONSORT-EHEALTH Group (2011). CONSORT-EHEALTH: Improving and standardizing evaluation reports of Web-based and mobile health interventions. *Journal of Medical Internet Research, 13*(4), e126. doi:10.2196/jmir.1923

Fernandez, M. E., Diamond, P. M., Rakowski, W., Gonzales, A., Tortolero-Luna, G., Williams, J., & Morales-Campos, D. Y. (2009). Development and validation of a cervical cancer screening self-efficacy scale for low-income Mexican American women. *Cancer Epidemiology, Biomarkers & Prevention, 18*(3), 866–875.

Fetterman, D. M., Kaftarian, S. J., & Wandersman, A. (2014). *Empowerment evaluation: Knowledge and tools for self-assessment, evaluation capacity building, and accountability.* Sage.

Fitzpatrick, J. L., Sanders, J. R., & Worthen, B. R. (2010). *Program evaluation: Alternative approaches and practical guidelines* (4th ed.). Pearson

Gardner, F., Hutchings, J., Bywater, T., & Whitaker, C. (2010). Who benefits and how does it work? Moderators and mediators of outcome in an effectiveness trial of a parenting intervention. *Journal of Clinical Child & Adolescent Psychology, 39*(4), 568–580.

Gartlehner, G., Hansen, R. A., Nissman, D., Lohr, K. N., & Carey, T. S. (2006). *Criteria for distinguishing effectiveness from efficacy trials in systematic reviews: Technical review 12 (Prepared by the RTI-International University of North Carolina Evidence-Based Practice Center under contract No. 290-02-0016.).* Agency for Healthcare Research and Quality (US).

Germain, A., Markwald, R. R., King, E., Bramoweth, A. D., Wolfson, M., Seda, G., Han, T., Miggantz, E., O'Reilly, B., & Hungerford, L. (2021). Enhancing behavioral sleep care with digital technology: Study protocol for a hybrid type 3 implementation-effectiveness randomized trial. *Trials, 22*(1), 1–14.

Glasgow, R. E. & Riley, W. T. (2013). What does it mean to be pragmatic? Pragmatic methods, measures, and models to facilitate research translation. *Health Education & Behavior, 40*(3), 257–265.

Glasgow, R. E., Gaglio, B., Bennett, G., Jerome, G. J., Yeh, H., Sarwer, D. B., Appel, L. J., Colditz, G., Wadden, T. A., & Wells, B. (2012). Applying the PRECIS criteria to describe three effectiveness trials of weight loss in obese patients with comorbid conditions. *Health Services Research, 47*(3, Pt. 1), 1051–1067.

Glasgow, R. E., Harden, S. M., Gaglio, B., Rabin, B., Smith, M. L., Porter, G. C., Ory, M. G., & Estabrooks, P. A. (2019). RE-AIM planning and evaluation framework: Adapting to new science and practice with a 20-year review. *Frontiers in Public Health, 7*, 64.

Glasgow, R. E., Klesges, L. M., Dzewaltowski, D. A., Estabrooks, P. A., & Vogt, T. M. (2006). Evaluating the impact of health promotion programs: Using the RE-AIM framework to form summary measures for decision making involving complex issues. *Health Education Research, 21*(5), 688–684.

Green, C. A., Duan, N., Gibbons, R. D., Hoagwood, K. E., Palinkas, L. A., & Wisdom, J. P. (2015). Approaches to mixed methods dissemination and implementation research: Methods, strengths, caveats, and opportunities. *Administration and Policy in Mental Health and Mental Health Services Research, 42*, 508–523.

Green, L., Gielen, A., Peterson, D., Kreuter, M., & Ottoson, J. (2022). *Health program planning, implementation, and evaluation*. Johns Hopkins University Press.

Green, L. W., & Allegrante, J. P. (2020). Practice-based evidence and the need for more diverse methods and sources in epidemiology, public health and health promotion. *The American Journal of Health Promotion, 34*, 946–948.

Grob, G. F. (2015). Writing for impact. In Newcomer, K.E., Hatry, K.P., & Wholey, J.S. (Eds.). *Handbook of practical program evaluation* (4th ed., pp. 739–764). doi:/10.1002/9781119171386.ch28

Guo, S., Fraser, M., & Chen, Q. (2020). Propensity score analysis: Recent debate and discussion. *Journal of the Society for Social Work and Research, 11*(3), 463–482.

Guo, S., & Fraser, M.W. (2014). Propensity score analysis statistical methods and applications. In *Advanced quantitative techniques in the social sciences* (2nd ed., p. 448). SAGE Publications, Inc. https://us2.sagepub.com/en-us/nam/propensity-score-analysis/book238151

Hamilton, A. B., & Finley, E. P. (2019). Qualitative methods in implementation research: An introduction. *Psychiatry Research, 280*, 112516.

Hartman, M. A., Nierkens, V., Cremer, S. W., Stronks, K., & Verhoeff, A. P. (2013). A process evaluation: Does recruitment for an exercise program through ethnically specific channels and key figures contribute to its reach and receptivity in ethnic minority mothers? *BMC Public Health, 13*, 768.

Haviland, A., Nagin, D. S., & Rosenbaum, P. R. (2007). Combining propensity score matching and group-based trajectory analysis in an observational study. *Psychological Methods, 12*(3), 247.

Hawe, P., Shiell, A., & Riley, T. (2009). Theorising interventions as events in systems. *American Journal of Community Psychology, 43*(3-4), 267–276. doi:10.1007/s10464-009-9229-9

Hayes, A. F. (2012). PROCESS: A versatile computational tool for observed variable mediation, moderation, and conditional process modeling [white paper]. http://www.afhayes.com/public/process2012.pdf

Hofstetter, H., Peters, L., Meijer, S., Van Keulen, H., Schutte, L., & van Empelen, P. (2014). Evaluation of the effectiveness and implementation of the sexual health program Long Live Love IV. *European Health Psychologist, 16*(S), 489.

Holzhauser, C., Da Rosa, P., & Michael, S. (2018). Peer reviewed: Forecasting participants in the all women count! Mammography program. *Preventing Chronic Disease, 15*. doi:10.5888/pcd15.180177

Hsu, M., & Chiu, C. (2004). Internet self-efficacy and electronic service acceptance. *Decision Support Systems, 38*(3), 369–381.

Iverson, K. M., Dichter, M. E., Stolzmann, K., Adjognon, O. L., Lew, R. A., Bruce, L. E., Gerber, M. R., Portnoy, G. A., & Miller, C. J. (2020). Assessing the Veterans Health Administration's response to intimate partner violence among women: Protocol for a randomized hybrid type 2 implementation-effectiveness trial. *Implementation Science, 15*(1), 1–10.

Kegler, M. C., Bundy, L., Haardörfer, R., Escoffery, C., Berg, C., Yembra, D., Kreuter, M., Hovell, M., Williams, R., & Mullen, P. D. (2015). A minimal intervention to promote smoke-free homes among 2-1-1 callers: A randomized controlled trial. *American Journal of Public Health, 105*(3), 530–537.

Kegler, M. C., Escoffery, C., Bundy, L., Berg, C. J., Haardörfer, R., Yembra, D., & Schauer, G. (2012). Pilot study results from a brief intervention to create smoke-free homes. *Journal of Environmental and Public Health, 2012*. doi:10.1155/2012/951426

Kessler, R. C., Duncan, G. J., Gennetian, L. A., Katz, L. F., Kling, J. R., Sampson, N. A., Sanbonmatsu, L., Zaslavsky, A. M., & Ludwig, J. (2014). Associations of housing mobility interventions for children in high-poverty neighborhoods with subsequent mental disorders during adolescence. *JAMA, 311*(9), 937–948.

Khadjesari, Z., Boufkhed, S., Vitoratou, S., Schatte, L., Ziemann, A., Daskalopoulou, C., Uglik-Marucha, E., Sevdalis, N., & Hull, L. (2020). Implementation outcome instruments for use in physical healthcare settings: A systematic review. *Implementation Science, 15*(1), 66. doi:10.1186/s13012-020-01027-6

Kidder, D. P., Fierro, L. A., Luna, E., Salvaggio, H., McWhorter, A., Bowen, S. A., ... Young, K. (2024). CDC program evaluation framework, 2024. *MMWR - Recommendations and Reports, 73*(6), 1–37. doi:10.15585/mmwr.rr7306a1

Kistin, C., & Silverstein, M. (2015). Pilot studies: A critical but potentially misused component of interventional research. *JAMA, 314*(15), 1561–1562.

Knell, G., Durand, C. P., Shuval, K., Kohl, I. I. I. H. W., Salvo, D., Sener, I. N., & Gabriel, K. P. (2018). Transit use and physical activity: Findings from the Houston travel-related activity in neighborhoods (TRAIN) study. *Preventive Medicine Reports, 9*, 55–61. doi:10.1016/j.pmedr.2017.12.012

Korda, H., & Itani, Z. (2013). Harnessing social media for health promotion and behavior change. *Health Promotion Practice, 14*(1), 15–23.

Lakens, D. (2013). Calculating and reporting effect sizes to facilitate cumulative science: A practical primer for *t*-tests and ANOVAs. *Frontiers in Psychology, 4*, 863.

Leatherdale, S. T. (2019). Natural experiment methodology for research: A review of how different methods can support real-world research. *International Journal of Social Research Methodology, 22*(1), 19–35.

Lei, H., Nahum-Shani, I., Lynch, K., Oslin, D., & Murphy, S. A. (2012). A "SMART" design for building individualized treatment sequences. Annual review of clinical psychology, 8, 21–48. doi: 10.1146/annurev-clinpsy-032511-143152.

Lengnick-Hall, R., Proctor, E. K., Bunger, A. C., & Gerke, D. R. (2021). Ten years of implementation outcome research: A scoping review protocol. *BMJ Open, 11*, Article 11, e049339. doi:10.1136/bmjopen-2021-049339

Lewis, C. C., Fischer, S., Weiner, B. J., Stanick, C., Kim, M., & Martinez, R. G. (2015). Outcomes for implementation science: An enhanced systematic review of instruments using evidence-based rating criteria. *Implementation Science, 10*, 155. doi:10.1186/s13012-015-0342-x

Lewis, J. R. (2019). Comparison of four TAM item formats: Effect of response option labels and order. *Journal of Usability Studies, 14*(4), 224–236.

Linnan, L., & Steckler, A. (2002). Process evaluation for public health interventions and research: An overview. In L. Linnan & A. Steckler (Eds.), *Process evaluation for public health interventions and research*. Jossey-Bass.

Long, T., & Johnson, M. (2000). Rigour, reliability and validity in qualitative research. *Clinical Effectiveness in Nursing, 4*(1), 30–37.

Luellen, J. K., Shadish, W. R., & Clark, M. H. (2005). Propensity scores: An introduction and experimental test. *Evaluation Review, 29*(6), 530–558.

Malterud, K. (2001). Qualitative research: Standards, challenges, and guidelines. *The Lancet, 358*(9280), 483–488.

Markham, C. M., Tortolero, S. R., Peskin, M. F., Shegog, R., Thiel, M., Baumler, E. R., Addy, R. C., Escobar-Chaves, S. L., Reininger, B. M., & Robin, L. (2012). Sexual risk avoidance and sexual risk reduction interventions for middle school youth: A randomized controlled trial. *Journal of Adolescent Health, 50*(3), 279–288.

Maurer, T. J., & Andrews, K. D. (2000). Traditional, Likert, and simplified measures of self-efficacy. *Educational and Psychological Measurement, 60*(6), 965–973.

Mauskopf, J., Earnshaw, S. R., Brogan, A., Wolowacz, S., & Brodtkorb, T.-H. (2017). *Budget-impact analysis of health care interventions*. Springer.

Mays, N., & Pope, C. (2000). *Assessing quality in qualitative research. BMJ (Clinical Research ed.), 320*(7226), 50–52. doi:10.1136/bmj.320.7226.50

McCaffrey, D. F., Ridgeway, G., & Morral, A. R. (2004). Propensity score estimation with boosted regression for evaluating causal effects in observational studies. *Psychological Methods, 9*(4), 403.

McGlone, M. S., Stephens, K. K., Rodriguez, S. A., & Fernandez, M. E. (2017). Persuasive texts for prompting action: Agency assignment in HPV vaccination reminders. *Vaccine, 35*(34), 4295–4297.

McLaughlin, J. A., & Jordan, G. B. (2015). Using logic models. *Handbook of practical program evaluation*, 62–87.

Mechanic, D. (2002). Disadvantage, inequality, and social policy. *Health Affairs, 21*(2), 48–59.

Mettert, K., Lewis, C., Dorsey, C., Halko, H., & Weiner, B. (2020). Measuring implementation outcomes: An updated systematic review of measures' psychometric properties. *Implementation Research and Practice, 1*. doi:10.1177/2633489520936644

Miles, M. B., Huberman, A. M., & Saldaña, J. (2013). *Qualitative data analysis: A methods sourcebook*. Sage.

Mohr, D. C., Cuijpers, P., & Lehman, K. (2011). Supportive accountability: A model for providing human support to enhance adherence to eHealth interventions. *Journal of Medical Internet Research, 13*(1), e30.

Morrison-Beedy, D., Carey, M., & Tu, X. (2006). Accuracy of audio computer-assisted self-interviewing (ACASI) and self-administered questionnaires for the assessment of sexual behavior. *AIDS and Behavior, 10*(5), 541–552.

Moscoe, E., Bor, J., & Bärnighausen, T. (2015). Regression discontinuity designs are underutilized in medicine, epidemiology, and public health: A review of current and best practice. *Journal of Clinical Epidemiology, 68*(2), 132–143.

Mullen, P., Savas, L., Bundy, L., Haardörfer, R., Hovell, M., Fernández, M., Monroy, J., Williams, R., Kreuter, M., Jobe, D., & Kegler, M. (2016). Minimal intervention delivered by 2-1-1 information and referral specialists promotes smoke-free homes among 2-1-1 callers: A Texas generalization trial. *Tobacco Control, 25*, i10–i18. doi:10.1136/tobaccocontrol-2016-053045]

Murray, D. M. (1998). *Design and analysis of group-randomized trials* (Vol. 29). Monographs in Epidemiology and Biostatistics. Oxford University Press.

Murray, N., Kelder, S., Parcel, G., & Orpinas, P. (1998). Development of an intervention map for a parent education intervention to prevent violence among. *Journal of School Health, 68*(2), 46.

National Commission for the Protection of Human Subjects of Biomedical and Behavioural Research (1979). The Belmont Report: Ethical principles and guidelines for the protection of human subjects of research. U.S. Department of Health, Education and Welfare. DHEW Publication No: (OS) 78-0014

National Institute on Alcohol Abuse and Alcoholism (2025). *Screen and assess: Use quick, effective methods.* National Institutes of Health. https://www.niaaa.nih.gov/health-professionals-communities/core-resource-on-alcohol/screen-and-assess-use-quick-effective-methods

NCI (2005). Health information national trends survey 2005 (HINTS 2005): Main study interview instrument – English. https://hints.cancer.gov/docs/Instruments/HINTS_2005_Instrument-English.pdf

Partin, M. R., & Burgess, D. J. (2012). Reducing health disparities or improving minority health? The end determines the means. *Journal of General Internal Medicine, 27*(8), 887–889.

Patton, M. Q. (2008). *Utilization-focused evaluation.* Sage.

Peskin, M. F., Markham, C. M., Gabay, E. K., Shegog, R., Cuccaro, P. M., Temple, J. R., Hernandez, B., Thiel, M., & Emery, S. T. (2018). Using intervention mapping to develop "Me & You: Building Healthy Relationships," a healthy relationship intervention for early middle school students. In D. A. Wolfe & J. R. Temple (Eds.), *Adolescent dating violence* (pp. 467–501). Academic Press.

Peskin, M. F., Markham, C. M., Shegog, R., Baumler, E. R., Addy, R. C., Temple, J. R., Hernandez, B., Cuccaro, P. M., Thiel, M. A., Gabay, E. K., & Tortolero-Emery, S. R. (2019a). Adolescent dating violence prevention program for early adolescents: The Me & You Randomized Controlled Trial, 2014-2015. *AJPH Open-Themed Research, 109*(10). doi:10.2105/ajph.2019.305218

Peskin, M. F., Markham, C. M., Shegog, R., Baumler, E. R., Addy, R. C., & Tortolero, S. R. (2014). Effects of the It's Your Game. . .Keep It Real program on dating violence in ethnic-minority middle school youths: A group randomized trial. *American Journal of Public Health, 104*(8), 1471–1477.

Peskin, M. F., Sadruddin, S., Addy, R., & Hernandez, B. (2019b). *City of Houston teen dating violence and youth violence project: Evaluation results from calendar year 2019.* [Unpublished report].

Piaggio, G., Elbourne, D. R., Pocock, S. J., Evans, S. J., Altman, D. G., & CONSORT Group (2012). Reporting of noninferiority and equivalence randomized trials: Extension of the CONSORT 2010 statement. *JAMA, 308*(24), 2594–2604.

Popham, K., Calo, W. A., Carpentier, M. Y., Chen, N. E., Kamrudin, S. A., Le, Y. L., Skala, K. A., Thornton, L. R., & Mullen, P. D. (2012). Reporting guidelines: Optimal use in preventive medicine and public health. *American Journal of Preventive Medicine, 43*(4), e31–e42.

Posavac, E. J., & Carey, R. G. (2002). *Program evaluation: Methods and case studies* (6th ed.). Prentice Hall.

Preskill, H., & Jones, N. (2009). *A practical guide for engaging stakeholders in developing evaluation questions.* Robert Wood Johnson Foundation.

Prinstein, M. J., Boergers, J., Spirito, A., Little, T. D., & Grapentine, W. L. (2000). Peer functioning, family dysfunction, and psychological symptoms in a risk factor model for adolescent inpatients' suicidal ideation severity. *Journal of Clinical Child Psychology, 29*(3), 392–405.

Prinstein, M. J., Boergers, J., & Vernberg, E. M. (2001). Overt and relational aggression in adolescents: Social - psychological adjustment of aggressors and victims. *Journal of Clinical Child Psychology, 30*(4), 479–491.

Proctor, E., Silmere, H., Raghavan, R., Hovmand, P., Aarons, G., Bunger, A., Griffey, R., & Hensley, M. (2011). Outcomes for implementation research: Conceptual distinctions, measurement challenges, and research agenda. *Administration and Policy in Mental Health and Mental Health Services Research, 38*(2), 65–76.

Proctor, E. K., Bunger, A. C., Lengnick-Hall, R., Gerke, D. R., Martin, J. K., Phillips, R. J., & Swanson, J. C. (2023). Ten years of implementation outcomes research: A scoping review. *Implementation Science, 18*(1), 31. doi:10.1186/s13012-023-01286-z

Resnick, B., & Jenkins, L. S. (2000). Testing the reliability and validity of the self-efficacy for exercise scale. *Nursing Research, 49*(3), 154–159.

Richman, A. R., Coronado, G. D., Arnold, L. D., Fernandez, M. E., Glenn, B. A., Allen, J. D., Wilson, K. M., & Brewer, N. T. (2012). Cognitive testing of human papillomavirus vaccine survey items for parents of adolescent girls. *Journal of Lower Genital Tract Disease, 16*(1), 16–23. doi:10.1097/LGT.0b013e3182293a49

Riegg Cellini, S., & Edwin Kee, J. (2015). Cost-effectiveness and cost-benefit analysis. In *Handbook of practical program evaluation* (pp. 636–672). doi: 10.1002/9781119171386.ch24

Rodriguez, S. A., Roncancio, A. M., Savas, L. S., Lopez, D. M., Vernon, S. W., & Fernandez, M. E. (2018). Using intervention mapping to develop and adapt two educational interventions for parents to increase HPV vaccination among Hispanic adolescents. *Frontiers in Public Health, 6*, 164.

Rosenbaum, P. R. (2002). *Observational studies* (2nd ed.). Springer.

Rossi, P. H., Lipsey, M. W., & Henry, G. T. (2019). *Evaluation: A systematic approach.* Sage publications.

Rubin, D. B. (2001). Using propensity scores to help design observational studies: Application to the tobacco litigation. *Health Services and Outcomes Research Methodology, 2*(3–4), 169–188.

Sadasivam, R. S., Kinney, R. L., Delaughter, K., Rao, S. R., Williams, J. H., Coley, H. L., Ray, M. N., Gilbert, G. H., Allison, J. J., Ford, D. E., Houston, T. K., National Dental PBRN Group, & QUIT-PRIMO Collaborative Group (2013). Who participates in web-assisted tobacco interventions? The QUIT-PRIMO and National Dental Practice-Based Research Network Hi-Quit studies. *Journal of Medical Internet Research, 15*(5), e77.

Saunders, R. P., Evans, M. H., & Joshi, P. (2005). Developing a process-evaluation plan for assessing health promotion program implementation: A how-to guide. *Health Promotion Practice, 6*(2), 134–147. doi:10.1177/1524839904273387

Savas, L. S., Atkinson, J. S., Figueroa-Solis, E., Valdes, A., Morales, P., Castle, P. E., & Fernandez, M. E. (2021). A lay health worker intervention to improve breast and cervical cancer screening among Latinas in El Paso, Texas: A randomized control trial. *Preventive Medicine, 145*, 106446.

Savas, L. S., Fernández, M. E., Jobe, D., & Carmack, C. C. (2012). Human papillomavirus vaccine: 2-1-1 helplines and minority parent decision-making.

American Journal of Preventive Medicine, 43(6 Suppl 5), S490–S496. doi:10.1016/j.amepre.2012.09.003

Scheirer, M. A. (1994). Designing and using process evaluation. In J. S. Whole, H. P. Hatry, & K. E. Newcomer (Eds.), *Handbook of practical program evaluation.* Jossey-Bass.

Schwartz, D., & Lellouch, J. (1967). Explanatory and pragmatic attitudes in therapeutical trials. *Journal of Chronic Diseases, 20*(8), 637–648.

Scott, V., Alia, K., Scaccia, J., Ramaswamy, R., Saha, S., Leviton, L., & Wandersman, A. (2020). Formative evaluation and complex health improvement initiatives: A learning system to improve theory, implementation, support, and evaluation. *American Journal of Evaluation, 41*(1), 89–106.

Shadish, W., Cook, T., & Campbell, D. (2002). *Experimental and quasi-experimental designs for generalized causal inference.* Houghton Mifflin.

Short, C. E., DeSmet, A., Woods, C., Williams, S. L., Maher, C., Middelweerd, A., Müller, A. M., Wark, P. A., Vandelanotte, C., Poppe, L., Hingle, M. D., & Crutzen, R. (2018). Measuring engagement in e- & mHealth behaviour change interventions: Viewpoint of methodologies. *Journal of Medical Internet Research, 20,* e292.

Simmons, V. N., Klasko, L. B., Fleming, K., Koskan, A. M., Jackson, N. T., Noel-Thomas, S., Luque, J. S., Vadaparampil, S. T., Lee, J.-H., & Quinn, G. P. (2015). Participatory evaluation of a community—academic partnership to inform capacity-building and sustainability. *Evaluation and Program Planning, 52,* 19–26.

Singal, A. G., Higgins, P. D. R., & Waljee, A. K. (2014). A primer on effectiveness and efficacy trials. *Clinical and Translational Gastroenterology, 5*(1), e45.

Slutsky, J. R., & Clancy, C. M. (2010). Patient-centered comparative effectiveness research: Essential for high-quality care. *Archives of Internal Medicine, 170*(5), 403–404.

Song, M. J., Ward, J., Choi, F., Nikoo, M., Frank, A., Shams, F., Tabi, K., Vigo, D., & Krausz, M. (2018). A process evaluation of a web-based mental health portal (WalkAlong) using google analytics. *JMIR Mental Health, 5*(3), e8594.

Sozu, T., Sugimoto, T., Hamasaki, T., & Evans, S. R. (2015). *Sample size determination in clinical trials with multiple endpoints.* Springer.

Steckler, A., & Linnan, L. A. (Eds.). (2002). *Process evaluation for public health interventions and research.* Jossey-Bass.

Streiner, D. L., Norman, G. R., & Cairney, J. (2015). *Health measurement scales: A practical guide to their development and use.* Oxford University Press.

The Child & Adolescent Health Measurement Initiative. (n.d.). *National Maternal and Child Health Measures Compendium.* https://www.cahmi.org/our-work-in-action/measurement-in-action/compendium.

Thompson, T., Kreuter, M. W., Caito, N., Williams, R. S., Escoffery, C., Fernandez, M. E., & Kegler, M. C. (2019). Implementing an evidence-based tobacco control program at five 2-1-1 call centers: An evaluation using the Consolidated Framework for Implementation Research. *Nicotine and Tobacco Research, 21*(2), 180–187.

Thorpe, K. E., Zwarenstein, M., Oxman, A. D., Treweek, S., Furberg, C. D., Altman, D. G., … Magid, D. J. (2009). A pragmatic–explanatory continuum indicator summary (PRECIS): A tool to help trial designers. *Journal of Clinical Epidemiology, 62*(5), 464–475.

Tobin, G. A., & Begley, C. M. (2004). Methodological rigour within a qualitative framework. *Journal of Advanced Nursing, 48*(4), 388–396.

Torres, R. T., Preskill, H., & Piontek, M. E. (2004). *Evaluation strategies for communicating and reporting: Enhancing learning in organizations* (Vol. 2). Sage.

Tortolero, S. R., Markham, C. M., Peskin, M. F., Shegog, R., Addy, R. C., Escobar-Chaves, S. L., & Baumler, E. R. (2010). It's your game: Keep it real: Delaying sexual behavior with an effective middle school program. *Journal of Adolescent Health, 46*(2), 169–179.

Trebble, T. M., Hansi, N., Hydes, T., Smith, M. A., & Baker, M. (2010). Process mapping the patient journey: An introduction. *The BMJ, 341*, c4078.

Trevisan, M. S., & Walser, T. M. (2014). *Evaluability assessment: Improving evaluation quality and use.* Sage Publications.

Trochim, W. M., Donnelly, J. P., & Arora, K. (2016). *Research methods: The essential knowledge base* (Vol. 2). ProtoView.

Trueman, P., Drummond, M., & Hutton, J. (2001). Developing guidance for budget impact analysis. *PharmacoEconomics, 19*, 609–621.

Tunis, S. R., Stryer, D. B., & Clancy, C. M. (2003). Practical clinical trials: Increasing the value of clinical research for decision making in clinical and health policy. *JAMA, 290*(12), 1624–1632.

Velasquez, M. M., von Sternberg, K. L., Floyd, R. L., Parrish, D., Kowalchuk, A., Stephens, N. S., Ostermeyer, B., Green, C., Seale, J. P., & Mullen, P. D. (2017). Preventing alcohol and tobacco exposed pregnancies: CHOICES Plus in primary care. *American Journal of Preventive Medicine, 53*(1), 85–95.

Venkataramani, A. S., Bor, J., & Jena, A. B. (2016). Regression discontinuity designs in healthcare research. *BMJ, 352*.

Vernberg, E. M., Jacobs, A. K., & Hershberger, S. L. (1999). Peer victimization and attitudes about violence during early adolescence. *Journal of Clinical Child Psychology, 28*(3), 386–395.

Webb, T. L., Joseph, J., Yardley, L., & Michie, S. (2010). Using the Internet to promote health behavior change: A meta-analysis of the impact of theoretical basis, use of behavior change techniques, and mode of delivery on efficacy. *Journal of Medical Internet Research, 12*(1), e4.

Weiss, C. H. (1972). *Evaluation research: Methods for assessing program effectiveness.* Prentice-Hall.

Weiss, C. H. (1995). Nothing as practical as good theory: Exploring theory-based evaluation for comprehensive community initiatives for children and families. In *New approaches to evaluating community initiatives: Concepts, methods, and contexts* (Vol. 1, pp. 65–92). The Aspen Institute.

West, S. G., Duan, N., Pequegnat, W., Gaist, P., Des Jarlais, D. C., Holtgrave, D., Szapocznik, J., Fishbein, M., Rapkin, B., & Clatts, M. (2008). Alternatives to the randomized controlled trial. *American Journal of Public Health, 98*(8), 1359–1366.

Williams, R. S., Stollings, J. H., Bundy, L., Haardörfer, R., Kreuter, M. W., Mullen, P. D., Hovell, H., Morris, M., & Kegler, M. C. (2016). Testing a minimal intervention to promote smoke-free homes among 2-1-1 callers: The North Carolina effectiveness trial. *PLoS ONE, 11*(11), e0165086. doi:10.1371/journal.pone.0165086

Wilson, D. K., Griffin, S., Saunders, R. P., Kitzman-Ulrich, H., Meyers, D. C., & Mansard, L. (2009). Using process evaluation for program improvement in dose, fidelity and reach: The ACT trial experience. *International Journal of Behavioral Nutrition and Physical Activity, 6*, 1–10.

Wolfe, D. A., Crooks, C., Jaffe, P., Chiodo, D., Hughes, R., Ellis, W., Stitt, L., & Donner, A. (2009). A school-based program to prevent adolescent dating violence: A cluster randomized trial. *Archives of Pediatrics & Adolescent Medicine, 163*(8), 692–699. doi:10.1001/archpediatrics.2009.69

Wolfe, D. A., Scott, K., Reitzel-Jaffe, D., Wekerle, C., Grasley, C., & Straatman, A.-L. (2001). Development and validation of the conflict in adolescent dating relationships inventory. *Psychological Assessment, 13*(2), 277.

Woodhouse, L. D., Toal, R., Nguyen, T., Keene, D., Gunn, L., Kellum, A., Nelson, G., Charles, S., Tedders, S., & Williams, N. (2013). A merged model of quality improvement and evaluation: Maximizing return on investment. *Health Promotion Practice, 14*(6), 885–892.

Zuckerman, I. H., Lee, E., Wutoh, A. K., Xue, Z., & Stuart, B. (2006). Application of regression-discontinuity analysis in pharmaceutical health services research. *Health Services Research, 41*(2), 550–563.

Zusevics, K. L., Kaemmerer, N., Lang, J., Link, J., & Bluma, D. (2021). A unique approach to quality improvement within the stroke system of care utilizing developmental evaluation. *Health Promotion Practice, 22*(2), 224–235.

Zwarenstein, M., Treweek, S., Gagnier, J. J., Altman, D. G., Tunis, S., Haynes, B., Oxman, A. D., Moher, D., & the CONSORT and Pragmatic Trials in Healthcare (Practihc) groups (2008). Improving the reporting of pragmatic trials: An extension of the CONSORT statement. *BMJ (Clinical Research ed.), 337*, a2390. doi: 10.1136/bmj.a2390

Wilson, D. K., Griffin, S., Saunders, R. P., Kitzman-Ulrich, H., Meyers, D. C., & Mansard, L. (2009). Using process evaluation for program improvement in dose, fidelity and reach: the ACT trial experience. *International Journal of Behavioral Nutrition and Physical Activity*, 6, 1–10.

Wolfe, D. A., Crooks, C., Jaffe, P., Chiodo, D., Hughes, R., Ellis, W., Stitt, L., & Donner, A. (2009). A school-based program to prevent adolescent dating violence: A cluster randomized trial. *Archives of Pediatrics & Adolescent Medicine*, 163(8), 692–699.

[illegible]

CHAPTER 11

INTERVENTION MAPPING FOR ADAPTATION OF EVIDENCE-BASED INTERVENTIONS: IM ADAPT

with Patricia Dolan Mullen, Eunyoung Kang, Jessica D. Austin, and Lara Staub Savas

Overview

In this chapter, we describe how to use Intervention Mapping (IM) to adapt evidence-based interventions (EBIs) for new populations and settings—using a process called IM ADAPT. EBIs can include policies, strategies, clinical practice guidelines, or health promotion interventions that have been proven to work through evaluation research or evaluation. Adaptations can be additions, deletions, or modifications to an EBI or its implementation strategies (Escoffery et al., 2018). Adaptations to the EBI can include modifying images, messages, language, determinants targeted, or changes related to the population or setting where the intervention is delivered. Adaptations also include changes to implementation strategies and protocols. Implementation-related adaptations may include the type of personnel delivering the EBI, the format or mode of delivery, the frequency of delivery, etc. (Wiltsey Stirman et al., 2013b). Although the process for making adaptations—using IM ADAPT—described in this chapter can be used for various types of EBIs, including evidence-based *approaches* (EBAs) or "strategies" such as those described by the Guide to Community Preventive Services (e.g., mass media, provider reminders, one-on-one education, and policies), this chapter focuses on the adaptation of specific, tangible multilevel health promotion interventions delivered in community or healthcare settings rather than general approaches to address a health problem (Williams, 2006). In this chapter, we provide the background about the science and logic of adaptation, followed by a step-by-step description of IM ADAPT followed by a real-world example. In addition to the written description provided in this chapter, IM ADAPT is also available as an online tool (IMADAPT.org).

IM ADAPT Tasks

1. **Assess the needs and assets of the new population and/or setting and develop a logic model of change**
2. **Discover EBIs that potentially match the targets for change and assess level of evidence and fit OR (if EBI has been selected already) Determine level of evidence and fit for a selected EBI**
3. **Assess fit and plan adaptation**
4. **Adapt intervention components**
5. **Plan for implementation of the adapted EBI**
6. **Test the adapted intervention**

Why Adapt?

Rather than developing an intervention from scratch, it is often more efficient and effective to find an EBI that has already been shown to work and to adapt it to fit a new population or setting. This approach can save time and resources and allow planners to take advantage of already developed protocols and materials, even if the existing EBI is not exactly relevant or appropriate for a new setting or population, which may have a different set of characteristics (e.g., norms, beliefs, culture) and/or different or insufficient resources for implementation. When performed in a systematic way, adaptation allows planners to achieve "fit" in a new context so that the EBI will achieve the desired outcomes. Adapting EBIs can enhance engagement, acceptability, and health outcomes, especially when working with traditionally underserved populations like diverse racial and ethnic groups (Ellis et al., 2022).

Types and Timing of Adaptations

EBI adaptation can be planned or spontaneous. We define *planned* adaptation as a careful consideration of what should be adapted and a deliberate process for doing so. This can occur *prospectively* (before implementation has begun) or in *real time* (during implementation). Typically, prospective adaptation planning occurs when planners have identified an EBI and a need for adaptation. The goal, in this case, is to clearly understand both the EBI and the needs of the new population and setting, and their potential fit, allowing adaptations to be made *before* implementation. For example, a planner may decide that an EBI could be improved by making the content more culturally relevant to the populations or changing the format of delivery (in-person versus online) based on the resources of the new setting. Planners may also add content to an existing EBI to address missing information or messaging designed to influence important factors in the new population. While prospectively planned modifications often occur prior to implementation, planners also have the option to make deliberate/systematic "planned" adaptations in *real time*, even while implementation is ongoing.

IM ADAPT is used mostly for prospective planned adaptation. Reed et al. (2022), for example, used IM ADAPT to modify a patient navigation program for enhancing genetic counseling referral and receipt for indicated colorectal cancer (CRC) patients (Reed et al., 2022). Austin et al. used IM to develop training for clinicians working in a Federally Qualified Health Center (FQHC) to deliver strong and consistent recommendations for the HPV vaccine (Austin et al., 2020). The planning team initially designed the provider training to be delivered during a one-hour, in-person session by a gynecological oncologist. They employed IM ADAPT for prospective adaptation of existing provider-level interventions for increasing HPV vaccination. Shortly after implementation, program planners received feedback from stakeholders and clinicians, prompting them to use IM

ADAPT again to make real-time adaptations that resulted in changes to the EBI content. New information was incorporated into the training that outlined the vaccination recommendations for all eligible age groups as well as the LGBTQ community, transgender people, and people living with HIV. The education and training session for providers were also adapted from in-person to a video webinar using the FQHC's online learning management system in response to clinician input about the difficulty in attending in-person training. These changes increased *relevance* to the specific needs of the patient population and also addressed the *delivery* of the training (to increase provider participation).

In some cases, adaptation can occur spontaneously, without planning. After realizing that adaptation occurred, modifications can (and should) be documented *retrospectively* (Wiltsey Stirman et al., 2019). The schema for describing adaptations known as FRAME is a useful and comprehensive guide for documenting adaptations (Wiltsey Stirman et al., 2019). Recommended reporting elements of FRAME include (1) when and how in the implementation process the modification was made, (2) whether the modification was planned/proactive (e.g., an adaptation) or unplanned/reactive, (3) who determined that the modification should be made, (4) what is modified, (5) at what level of delivery the modification is made, (6) type or nature of context or content-level modifications, (7) the extent to which the modification is fidelity-consistent, and (8) the reasons for the modification, including (a) the intent or goal of the modification (e.g., cultural adaptations, to reduce costs, etc.) and (b) contextual factors that influenced the decision. IM ADAPT can also be useful for documenting the types of, and reasons for, adaptations. This can either be done prior to, during, or after implementation.

In this chapter, the primary focus is to describe how IM ADAPT can be used to make decisions about the adaptation of existing EBIs *before they are implemented* in a new population or setting. This still allows the flexibility to continue to make, document, and pretest adaptations during implementation, if needed.

Adaptation at Multiple Levels

Most health problems have causes at multiple levels and most improvements to health can best be influenced by interventions that are multilevel. Health promotion interventions developed using IM will likely address more than one level: the individual level (e.g., patient, community member, student) and one or more environmental levels (e.g., interpersonal, organizational, community, and societal). After assessing the needs of a new population in a specific setting such as a clinic or school (Task 1 of IM ADAPT described below), a planner may realize that an existing EBI addresses some but not all levels. Thus, during adaptation planning, planners may realize (based on the needs assessment) that they need to add intervention components that address one or more levels that are missing in an existing

EBI. In this case, there may be some adaptation of existing components and levels, and some creation or development of intervention components for levels that were not included in the original EBI. IM can be used for this purpose.

Even when an EBI does address all of the levels that influence the health problem in a new population and setting, changes may be needed in its original implementation protocols and materials. The IM ADAPT process described below helps planners identify and plan for needed adaptations in implementation as well as adaptations to the EBI itself. For some interventions, new implementation strategies must be developed (either because they have been adapted in such a way that the prior strategies are no longer valid, or because there are new challenges to adoption and implementation in the new setting). In this case, planners can use Implementation Mapping (IM Step 5).

It is often necessary, for example, to improve an implementing organization's capacity to better deliver an EBI. Whether or not an adaptation of the EBI is needed, the planners may also want to use IM Step 5, Implementation Mapping, to design implementation strategies that improve capacity for EBI delivery within the implementing organization. For example, initially, a clinic may not have implementers needed to deliver an intervention (e.g., community health workers), but may decide to change their infrastructure by hiring community health workers rather than adapting the intervention so that it can be delivered by other clinic staff. The concept of capacity building for implementation is consistent with Wandersman et al. (2008) Interactive Systems Framework (ISF) in which both intervention-specific capacity and general organizational capacity-building efforts are essential for effective implementation (Wandersman et al., 2008).

Addressing Health Equity through Adaptation of EBIs

Despite the development and availability of EBIs that could reduce health disparities, serious challenges related to their fit, and use in populations and settings that could benefit the most from them, remain. In many cases, appropriate and timely adaptation could help address these challenges (Alvidrez et al., 2019; Baumann & Cabassa 2020). Disadvantaged and underserved populations are often underrepresented in efficacy and effectiveness trials informing EBIs, and implementation of EBIs into new context often overlooks the importance of unique factors, such as economic, social, and historical factors that perpetuate health inequity (Patel et al., 2018; Santiago & Miranda 2014; Yapa & Bärnighausen 2018).

Ideally, an EBI implemented with fidelity will exhibit the same or similar effects across diverse cultural groups and settings, yet this is often not the case. When an EBI is less effective across different populations or settings, this may indicate an erosion in the EBI's social validity (also called external validity) (Burlew et al., 2013). This may occur due to a lack of cultural relevance of the EBI in the new population or setting and may indicate a need for improved cultural adaptation (Fernandez et al., 2025).

Adapting EBIs to better fit the needs of new populations and settings has the potential for reducing or eliminating several health disparities and promoting health equity (Alvidrez et al., 2019; Baumann et al., 2016; Fernandez et al., 2025). Landais et al. (2021) used IM ADAPT to adapt evidence-based smoking cessation programs for individuals from lower socioeconomic groups because the existing program was not relevant or accessible to them (Landais et al., 2021). Willams and Anyimukwu (2020) adapted evidence-based lifestyle interventions for African American individuals with breast cancer using IM ADAPT to improve health equity in utilizing EBIs in this high risk and disadvantaged population (Williams & Anyimukwu, 2020).

Cultural adaptations are "systematic modifications of EBIs or intervention protocols that considers culture, language, context, norms, or other determinants so that the intervention will be more compatible with cultural patterns, beliefs, and values" (Fernandez et al., 2025; Baumann et al., 2015). There is increasing recognition of the need to develop culturally informed and responsive interventions that deliver the best science while also addressing the practical considerations of a local community (Alvidrez et al., 2019; Carvalho et al., 2013; Castro & Yasui, 2017; Escoffery et al., 2019). Cultural adaptations have the potential to improve the implementation of EBIs in underserved communities, reduce disparities, and ultimately promote health equity (Barrera et al., 2017). For instance, a health education program designed to increase CRC screening was adapted to the Puerto Rican culture in Spanish and the health literacy level of the target community while maintaining the core EBA (Serra et al., 2017). Cho et al. (2020) adapted an existing evidence-based lifestyle using IM ADAPT to address the unmet needs of African American individuals with prostate cancer and their partners to make the intervention more culturally appropriate (Cho et al., 2020). When cultural adaptations are made to EBIs they may modify EBI content, activities, or language (among other features) to better fit the needs, preferences, or life context of a priority group, while maintaining fidelity to core elements of those EBIs (Castro & Yasui, 2017; Castro et al., 2004).

Various aspects of culture and whether or not they are reflected in an intervention could affect the extent to which it will be adopted, used, and maintained as well as its level of effectiveness in a new setting (Bernal et al., 2009). Identifying and prioritizing these elements and comparing them to what exists in an EBI is an important part of determining what should change and what can stay the same. For instance, McCarthy et al. (2022) used qualitative approaches (focus groups and in-depth interviews) to determine the potential fit of an existing EBI on contraceptive behavior for Zimbabwean youth (McCarthy et al., 2022). The findings informed the iterative adaptation and refinement of intervention messages. Adaptation is considered an iterative process since understanding which cultural factors could influence EBI use and/or effectiveness may not all be known initially.

Community Engagement for Adaptation

Delivering an intervention that does not align with the needs and values of the community will likely result in poor engagement; thus, reducing intervention effectiveness (Castro & Yasui, 2017; Kumpfer et al., 2017). For example, Pot et al. (2018) found that their priority population perceived the existing component of an HPV vaccine intervention that focused on eliciting anticipatory regret could lead to resistance. Thus, they refined the original intervention component tailored to the priority population's preference through an iterative collaboration process (Pot et al., 2018). IM ADAPT is grounded in the principles of community-based participatory research and participatory action research and incorporates a high level of community participation and collaboration; as such, the use of IM ADAPT leads to a better fit between the EBI and the new context. Engaging communities and key stakeholders is a strength of the IM ADAPT process that may facilitate the acceptability and use of the EBI, address health disparities, and advance health equity (Movsisyan et al., 2021). Community engagement is particularly important during the early stages of the adaptation process when exploring the needs and unique contextual factors of the new setting and population, while encouraging a sense of local ownership (Castro et al., 2004; Chambers & Norton, 2016; Chen et al., 2013). Prioritizing community engagement results in a process that is more inclusive, generates buy-in among the priority population, and ensures that the results of the process (interventions, recommendations, materials, strategies, etc.) more accurately reflect the needs and preferences of the community.

Frameworks such as the *Multiphase Optimization Strategy (MOST)* and the *Method for Program Adaptation through Community Engagement (M-PACE)* provide guidance and examples of how to incorporate community engagement principles throughout the adaptation process (Broder-Fingert et al., 2019). Similar to IM, and IM ADAPT, these frameworks recommend forming a planning committee that include representatives of the community that have an equal opportunity to review, select, and revise the EBI to ensure that it aligns with the local culture and context. These frameworks also emphasize the need for community input throughout the adaptation process to generate reactions and recommendations for change from members of the new population and setting. Community engagement plays a central role throughout the implementation process, particularly if the implementation plan has also been adapted. Community engagement (including the participation of implementers) can inform adaptations necessary to build capacity and address challenges that may arise in program adoption, implementation, and/or maintenance (Broder-Fingert et al., 2019).

Adaptation Challenges

Identifying and Retaining Core Elements of the EBI

A central theme in adaptation is the importance of identifying and retaining core components, elements, or essential ingredients of an EBI that are necessary for achieving desired outcomes. Unfortunately, identifying these core elements is not always a simple exercise, given that intervention elements are rarely tested independently (Peters et al., 2015). Typically, the data available in program evaluation efforts does not elucidate which features of an intervention constitute "core elements" and what can be deleted or modified without compromising the EBI's impact. Nevertheless, when adaptation is necessary to improve an EBI's fit, planners must determine which elements were likely to have been essential in making that intervention effective in the first place. But *what* are those core elements and *how* can they be identified?

Core elements can include different aspects of an EBI, including delivery channels, design features, theoretical change methods or their practical applications, or intervention dose. They are the "active ingredients" of an intervention that make it effective and are sometimes referred to as core functions (Wiltsey Stirman et al., 2019). They are distinguished from peripheral elements which are features of the EBI that are not critical for effectiveness. Some processes have been described to help identify core components (e.g., CORE), however, without understanding to full logic of a program, expert consensus approaches will be limited (Kalver et al., 2021).

Before planners can establish which EBI elements are "core," the underlying *logic* of the EBI must be established. An EBI's logic is derived from the theory informing the development of the original EBI, and by specifying the relation between an intervention and its outcomes. Lee et al. (2008) encouraged intervention developers to provide guidance both by describing the theory of change, including mediators and moderators of effects, and by suggesting which parts of the EBI they believe are essential and cannot be changed without modifying the EBI's effectiveness (Lee et al., 2008). Such guidance can serve as a vital roadmap for planners seeking to use that EBI in a new setting. In some instances, websites or other mediums that catalog EBIs provide this information. More generally, however, EBI developers do not provide such guidance, leaving the planner to describe the logic of an EBI. Thus, Task 3 below, EBI Mapping, can be very helpful (Szeszulski et al., 2022; Walker et al., 2022).

IM ADAPT Task 3 (*EBI Mapping*, described below) provides a process that planners can use to identify the intervention logic and mechanisms of change. This process results in the creation of a *logic model* of an EBI and includes the following items/information: (1) the determinants of behavior of the at-risk group and/or environmental change agents that the EBI is intended to target, (2) theoretical change methods that are intended to influence those determinants, and (3) the practical applications of the change methods in accordance with the method's theoretical parameters of use. Understanding *how* an EBI is supposed to create the desired change is an important step in identifying possible core elements, and reducing the risk of an adaptation that reduces an EBI's effectiveness.

In addition to the core elements noted above (design features, theoretical change methods), which can inform the "logic" of how an EBI is intended to work, other core elements or components could also include intervention delivery channels (especially sensitivity to reaching the intended at-risk group with culturally accessible and credible channels), and dose and intensity (how much of the intervention the participants are getting). Because information about an EBI's core elements is often unavailable, in addition to the suggestions above, the planner should reach out to the original developer of the intervention to gain insight into which elements they consider to be core and consult with other experts. While not foolproof, following the suggestions provided here and utilizing the IM ADAPT process can help planners carefully adapt EBIs to simultaneously increase fit while maintaining sufficient fidelity of core components such that effectiveness is maintained.

Balancing EBI Fit and Fidelity

Resolving tensions between: (1) adapting EBIs to "fit" the new population and setting and (2) implementing the EBI as intended (fidelity) remains one of the most challenging tasks of adaptation. There is an understanding that EBIs must be delivered with some level of fidelity to reduce program drift that could lower the impact of the EBI on intended outcomes (Kendall & Frank 2018; Wiltsey Stirman et al., 2013a). Indeed, research has shown that interventions delivered with high levels of fidelity were associated with better outcomes than those delivered with lower fidelity (Durlak, 2008; Eisman et al., 2020; Ginsburg et al., 2020; Schoenwald et al., 2009). On the other hand, there is growing recognition that adaptations to EBIs are not only common (Aarons et al., 2012; Chambers & Norton 2016; Wiltsey Stirman et al., 2013a) but are also necessary to maximize effectiveness in certain settings and populations (Chambers et al., 2013; Marques et al., 2019; Wiltsey Stirman et al., 2012).

Nevertheless, making too many (unnecessary) changes to an EBI can reduce effectiveness, or worse, introduce unintended and harmful outcomes. Planners must balance adaptations that can improve fit while maintaining fidelity to the core components of the EBI. Planners can think about possible adaptations as if they were considering a green, yellow, or red traffic light (NCI, n.d.): *Green light changes* are usually minor and intended to increase the reach, receptivity, and engagement of the community. They may include changes to the program name, updating information like statistics to match the priority population, and tailoring language, figures, and wording to be culturally relevant. *Yellow light changes* should be approached with caution. They include adding and/or modifying EBI components and content, such as adding activities, changing program sequences, expanding the primary audience, and changing who delivers the EBI and the format of the EBI. Finally, *red light changes* are major adaptations that should be avoided when possible, such as changing the core components of the intervention. Red light adaptations may include changing the underlying health behavior theory, changing the health topic, deleting core components of the program, and/or decreasing the program dose. Any adaptations, whether planned or spontaneous (real-time), should be carefully and extensively described.

Knowing When Not to Adapt

Another challenge with adaptation is knowing when to decide against adaptation (or abandon the process of adaptation) in favor of designing a new intervention. A planner may learn early on in the adaptation process, for example, that too many changes would be needed to accommodate mismatches between the original EBI and the new context. For example, if the EBI far exceeds the capacity of the new setting, or extensive modification of the EBI materials and activities would be required, perhaps adaptation is not a viable option. Or, planners may not learn until the pilot testing phase that the adapted intervention is unlikely to be beneficial or feasible in the new context. For example, a weight-management program designed for primary school-aged children and their fathers in Australia was culturally adapted to a multi-ethnic UK population (Moore et al., 2021). Planners learned during the pilot phase that meeting recruitment targets and identifying skilled program facilitators were challenging. Thus, they decided to not proceed further. The decision to abandon or continue with adaptation should be systematic and involve community partners. If there is consensus to abandon a particular EBI, planners could look for another EBI (IM ADAPT Task 2) or abandon adaptation altogether and instead, design a new intervention using IM (beginning at Step 1 or Step 2 if the needs are clearly understood).

Adaptation Frameworks

Originally adaptation frameworks were developed to: (1) discourage unplanned adaptation which could lead to deletion of core components or (2) encourage cultural adaptation for particular health problems such as HIV (Card et al., 2011; Wingood, 2008) or substance abuse (Kumpfer et al., 2008; Smith, 2007). Several of these frameworks focused exclusively on cultural adaptation (e.g., Kumpfer et al., 2008). Frameworks developed over the past 10 years provide more general guidance for adaptation across topics, and most emphasize adaptation through community engagement (Chen et al., 2013; Fernandez et al., 2025). Van Deale and colleagues (2012) present the concept of "empowerment evaluation" as a framework for implementing the core elements of an intervention with fidelity while allowing for adaptation of the intervention to fit the needs of the new population or setting (van Daele et al., 2012).

Between 2012 and 2020, three reviews of frameworks identified commonalities while contrasting their differences and gaps (Escoffery et al., 2018; Krivitsky et al., 2012). These, along with the more recent ADAPT guidance framework by Moore (2021), collectively reveal several significant insights.

1. Most frameworks outline similar step-by-step processes for adapting EBIs, including assessing priority populations, evaluating candidate EBIs, gauging implementation capacity, deciding on adaptation, material adaptation and pretesting, developing an implementation protocol, pilot testing, and full implementation.

2. Some frameworks are conceptual models, while earlier ones are specific to particular health issues.
3. Certain frameworks highlight specific aspects like community engagement (Chen et al., 2013) or empowerment (van Daele et al., 2012).
4. Most frameworks focus on individual-level EBIs and their application to subgroups or at-risk populations, neglecting organizational or policy-level interventions.
5. Many frameworks lack emphasis on theorization, intervention mechanisms, or broader systems thinking.
6. Frameworks often overlook theoretical change methods and mechanisms of action, as well as the critical examination of underlying mechanisms and contextual interactions for replicating EBI effects.
7. Adaptations need better documentation and reporting (Escoffery et al., 2018).

Thus, while many frameworks for adaptation exist, there are many challenges that limit their usefulness. The IM ADAPT framework, presented and described in detail in this chapter, effectively addresses most of these criticisms and shortcomings.

Intervention Mapping for Adaptation—IM ADAPT

The name (IM ADAPT) of the planning framework described here is short for "Intervention Mapping (IM) for Adaptation." The acronym ADAPT spells out the six tasks that outline the process.

- (Task 1) **Assess** the needs and assets of the new population and/or setting and develop a logic model of change.
  - Subtask 1.1: Conduct a needs and assets assessment and develop a logic model of the problem.
  - Subtask 1.2: Develop a logic model of change.
  - Subtask 1.3: Assess capacity to implement.
  - Subtask 1.4: Write goals for expected outcomes from implementing the EBI at the new site.
- (Task 2) **Discover** EBIs that potentially match the targets for change and assess level of evidence and fit **OR** (if EBI has been selected already) **Determine** level of evidence and fit for a selected EBI.
  - Subtask 2.1: Search for EBIs and evaluate the level of evidence OR determine level of evidence of a previously selected EBI.
  - Subtask 2.2: Judge basic fit.

- (Task 3) **Assess** fit and plan adaptation.
  - Subtask 3.1: Use EBI Mapping to describe and create a logic model of the existing intervention.
  - Subtask 3.2: Compare the logic model of change to the logic model of the EBI; judge fit of behavioral and environmental targets, determinants addressed, methods and practical applications used, delivery fit, and design features including cultural elements.
  - Subtask 3.3: Judge implementation fit and make decisions about what should change considering core elements (core functions) and how to retain them.
- (Task 4) Adapt intervention components.
  - Subtask 4.1: Prepare design documents for the adaptations.
  - Subtask 4.2: Create and pretest adapted materials.
  - Subtask 4.3: Produce final adapted materials and activities.
- (Task 5) **Plan** for implementation of the adapted EBI.
  - Subtask 5.1: Use Implementation Mapping processes to identify implementers, implementation behaviors, and outcomes of the adapted intervention and create/adapt strategies if needed.
  - Subtask 5.2: Develop implementation scope, sequence, and protocols.
  - Subtask 5.3: Plan logistics including budget, staffing, and materials.
- (Task 6) **Test** the Adapted Intervention (see Chapter 10).
  - Subtask 6.1: Review the logic model of change, matrices, and implementation plan to guide process and effect evaluation.
  - Subtask 6.2: Develop process evaluation questions and identify measures.
  - Subtask 6.3: Develop effect evaluation questions, identify measures, and select a design.
  - Subtask 6.4: Pilot test and finalize the evaluation plan.
  - Subtask 6.5: Plan when and how to report evaluation findings.

The IM ADAPT process at **Task 1** begins with the creation of a *logic model of problem and a logic model of change* based on a *needs and assets assessment* of the new population and setting (much like in Steps 1 and 2 of IM). This is typically followed by the selection of an existing EBI and careful analysis of the core logic, including the identification of core components that should be maintained and implemented with fidelity. By following the IM ADAPT process, shown in Figure 11.1, planners can more efficiently and effectively make decisions about the modification of both content (materials, protocols, resource lists, etc.) and/or implementation strategies, and plan the evaluation of the newly adapted EBI. Some users, as we shall see in the case study at the end of the chapter, will begin the process with a preselected EBI and skip most of Task 2. Others will search for EBIs to match the basic fit of the identified logic model of problem and change.

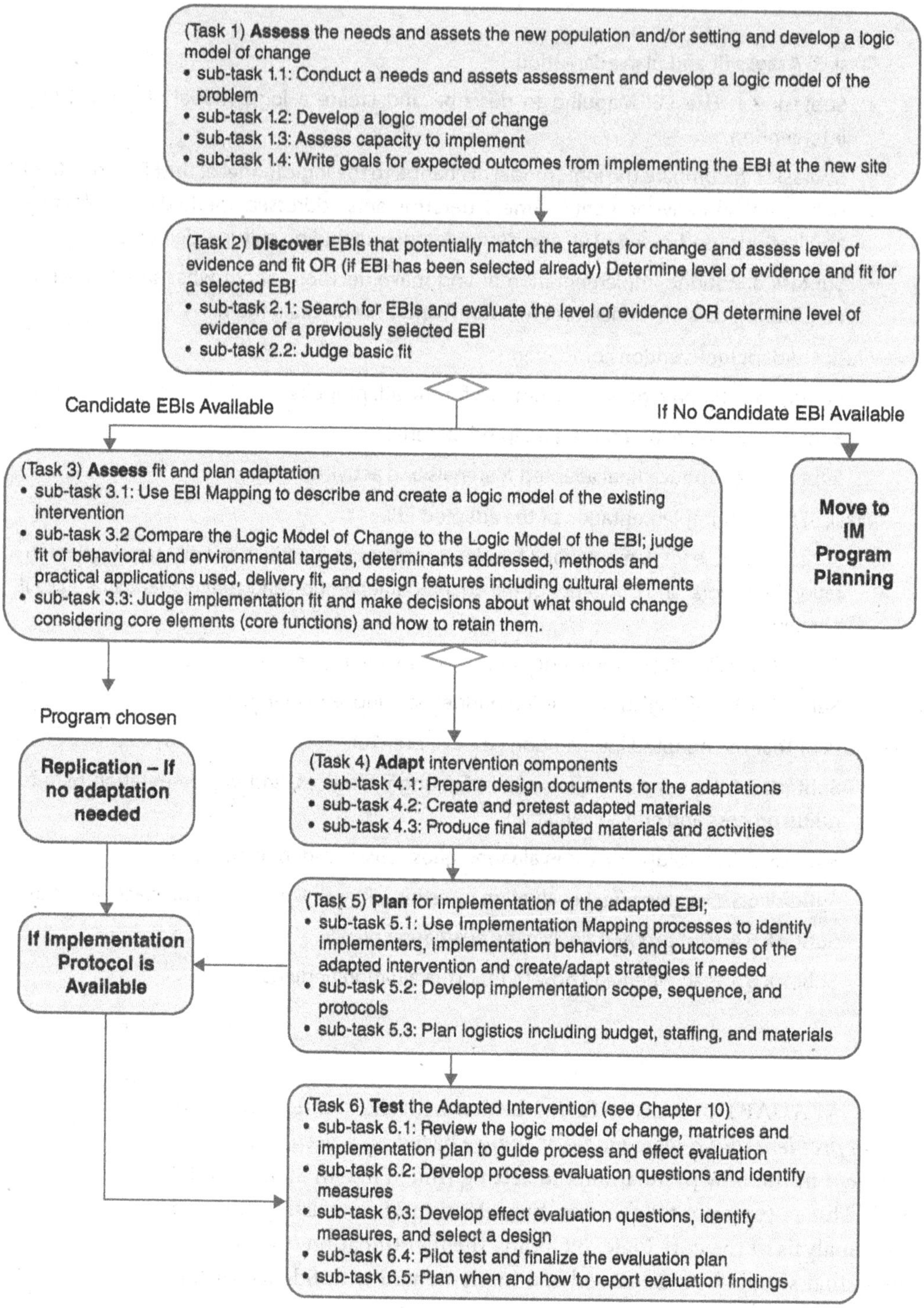

Figure 11.1 Adapting an Evidence-based Health Promotion Intervention (Note: All Steps Include Work with Stakeholders)

Following the description of tasks below, we provide a real-world example that used IM ADAPT to improve the fit of a lay health worker delivered breast and cervical cancer screening intervention. The program was effective in increasing screening in Mexican-American women living in farmworker communities (Fernández, 2005), for Hispanic women in Houston

(*Salud en Mis Manos*—SEMM) (Savas et al., 2023) and El Paso (Savas et al., 2021). We use this case study to provide an example of the application of IM ADAPT for adapting SEMM for a new population and setting.

Task 1: Assess Needs and Assets and Develop a Logic Model of Change

Task 1 of IM ADAPT is divided into four subtasks, which are derived from IM Steps 1 and 2. Subtask 1.1: conduct a needs and assets assessment and develop a logic model of the problem; subtask 1.2: develop a logic model of change; subtask 1.3: assess capacity to implement; and subtask 1.4: write goals for expected outcomes from implementing the EBI at the new site. Task 1 is important for informing the selection of an existing EBI but also plays a key role for planners who already have a preselected EBI. In either case, planners need a good understanding of the needs of the new population and setting conditions that contribute to a health problem, its behavioral and/or environmental causes, the expected changes that need to occur to improve the problem, and the resources and support that are available for implementation. Creating a logic model of the problem and a logic model of change can also serve as a blueprint for tracking adaptations.

Conduct a Needs and Assets Assessment and Develop a Logic Model of the Problem

This iterative process involves formative research and community partner engagement and is essential for understanding the health, behavior, and environmental conditions in the new population and setting (prevalence, incidence, impact), the environmental factors potentially influencing the implementation of an intervention, and the capacity and resources available. See Chapter 5 (IM Step 1) for a thorough description of this process. IM ADAPT Task 1 should be completed regardless of whether the planner has selected an EBI or will be searching for an EBI to adapt.

In Task 1 of IM ADAPT, information about factors contributing to health and quality of life (QOL) concerns in the new population and setting is first organized into a logic model of the problem as in IM Step 1 (see Chapter 5). Information from the needs and assets assessment will inform the logic model of the problem, depicting the relation between the health problem and its causal behaviors and environmental conditions and their determinants (see Figure 11.2). For example, Koutoukidis et al. (2018) aimed to adapt an existing weight-management intervention for endometrial cancer survivors. They began with a needs assessment, which comprised a literature review and a qualitative study. They identified both health problems (i.e., a high risk of cardiovascular diseases, diabetes, and secondary cancers) and health-related QOL issues (i.e., diminished physical function). These health problems were linked to suboptimal diet and limited physical activity behavior factors. Informed by social cognitive theory, they identified personal determinants

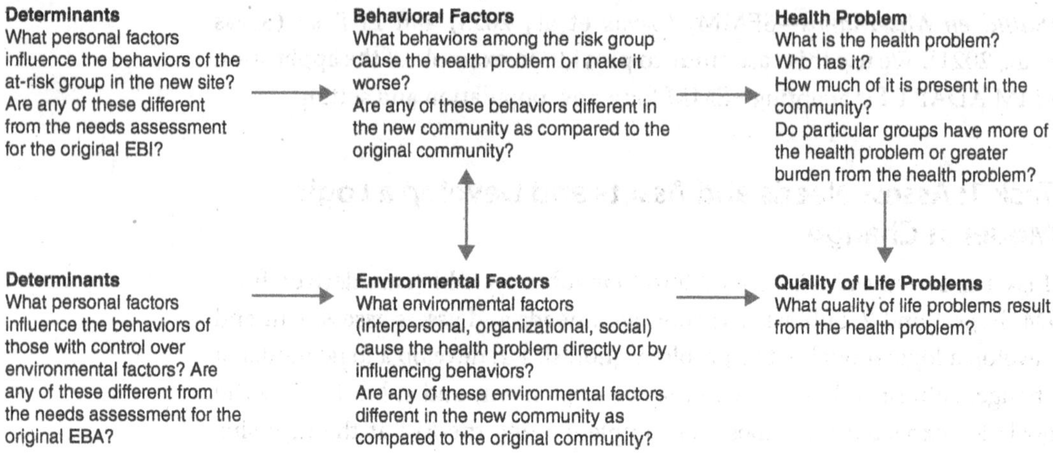

Figure 11.2 Logic Model of the Problem with Guiding Questions

that are thought to be associated with the identified behavioral factors. These determinants included outcome expectations, knowledge, self-efficacy, and goals. Incorporating all findings from the needs assessment, they developed a logic model of the problem. Overall, this understanding laid the foundation for the subsequent subtask of developing a change logic model (Koutoukidis et al., 2018). In some cases, for example, when there is a clear understanding of factors influencing the problem, planners may wish to begin with the logic model of change (describe din the section below).

Develop a Logic Model of Change

As in Step 2 of IM (see Chapter 6), planners create a logic model of the *change* that is informed by the logic model of the problem but which now focuses on the expected changes in determinants, behaviors, and environmental conditions that will lead to the expected outcomes. The logic model of change will provide a guidepost that will be used to compare how well a potential EBI meets the needs and priorities of the new priority population and setting. It can help confirm for planners the appropriateness of the EBI and help identify potential areas of modification. Recall, the logic model of change depicts how determinants (stated positively, e.g., increased knowledge, positive attitudes, perceived social norms) influence health-promoting behaviors and environmental conditions, and how these positively influence health and QOL. When listing behaviors and environmental conditions, planners may choose to be more specific and detail performance objectives (subbehaviors and subtasks to create environmental change). They will then assess the probable determinants of that change (See Figure 11.3).

In IM ADAPT, after describing these components of the logic model of change (which represent expected outcomes), planners also consider what change methods may be used to influence the determinants of behavior and environmental conditions. This thought process can help

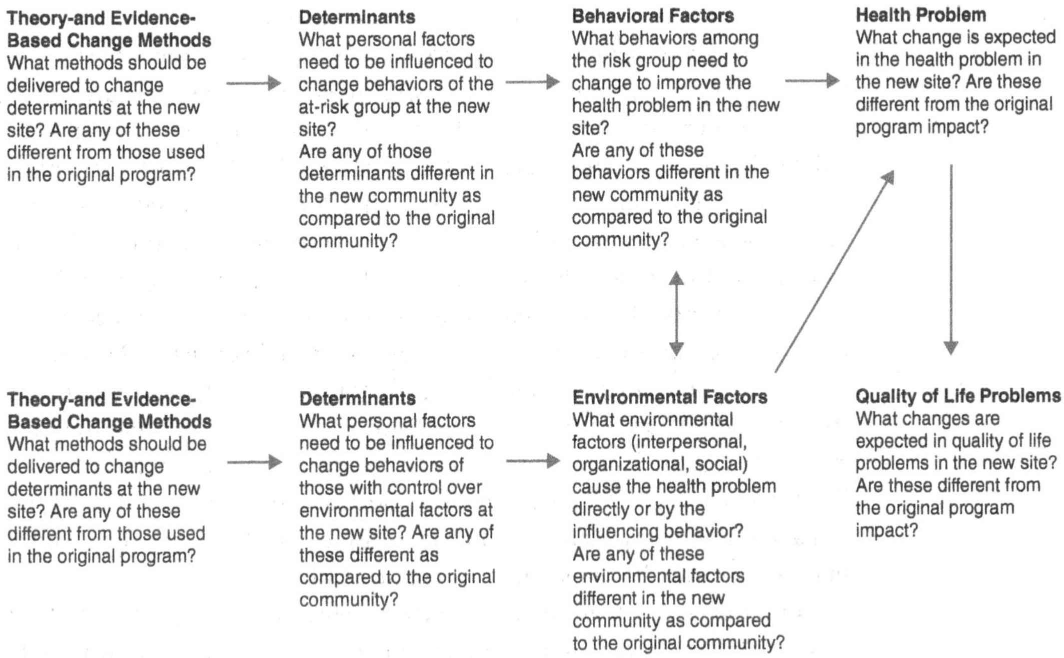

Figure 11.3 Logic Model of Change with Guiding Questions

planners as they search for EBIs (or analyze a preselected EBI) and determine whether the EBI contains relevant methods needed to influence positive change. This may affect whether it is chosen or can inform subsequent adaptation decisions in Task 3.

Assess Capacity to Implement

Implementing existing EBIs among a new population and context requires sufficient capacity (e.g., resources, structures, and workforce) to deliver the EBI (Brownson et al., 2018; Ramanadhan et al., 2022). Public health and other community-based practitioners often lack the time, funding, awareness, knowledge, skills, self-efficacy, and motivation to facilitate the necessary adaptation and implementation process. Resource constraints, insufficient leadership, and turnover also hinder the successful adaptation of EBIs and their subsequent use. Planners need to understand what resources and structures are in place within the new setting that can support the implementation of an existing EBI and what is needed to support implementation efforts. When a planner is using IM ADAPT with a specific EBI in mind, it is easier to assess the potential capacity to implement it. Nevertheless, even if the planner has not yet looked for potential EBIs, it is possible to describe potential resources (personnel, space, technology available, implementers, and other possible resources) that could be used for implementation.

Assessing the potential capacity for implementing a health promotion intervention in healthcare or public health settings in the context of an initial assessment before searching for EBIs to adapt can be informed by recent literature. Brownson et al. (2018) emphasize the importance of considering the availability of resources, structures, and workforce as prerequisites for successful EBI implementation (Brownson et al., 2018). Resource constraints, leadership issues, and workforce turnover are highlighted as potential barriers that planners must typically address. While IM ADAPT offers flexibility in assessing capacity (Vroom et al., 2022), established implementation science frameworks like the Consolidated Framework for Implementation Research 2.0 (CFIR 2.0) (Damschroder et al., 2009, 2022) and the Evidence-Based System for Innovation Support (EBSIS) (Leeman et al., 2015; Wandersman et al., 2008; Wandersman and Scheier, 2024) provide valuable guidance in understanding the factors influencing implementation success and resource requirements. Frameworks related to organizational readiness for implementation can also be helpful (Scaccia et al., 2015; Watson et al., 2022). Planners should explore questions related to organizational alignment, available staff, budget, readiness, and support when assessing capacity even before identifying specific EBIs.

Questions considering capacity even before searching for an EBI (in Task 2) that can guide an initial assessment of potential fit and feasibility include: Does the mission of the organization coincide with the goals of the intervention? What staff are available to work on the adoption and implementation of a new EBI? What is the implementation culture of the organization (from CFIR)? What is the budget available for this project? What is the organization's readiness for implementing this intervention? Who might the potential implementers be (considering sustainability)? What support can be expected from management and staff? What technical assistance might be required to complete implementation and sustainment (Damschroder, 2013; Weiner et al., 2017)? These questions can help determine whether certain EBIs can be feasibly implemented in certain settings and what changes (either to the setting or to the EBI) or strategies may be needed to increase intervention fit and feasibility.

Engagement of leaders and potential implementers is also important to assess capacity. In a study by Vroom (2022), community-based organizations (CBOs) were investigated to assess their capacity for adopting, implementing, and sustaining evidence-based practices (EBPs) (Vroom et al., 2022). The research aimed to understand how staff within these organizations perceive their implementation practice capacity, identify factors necessary for adequate capacity in implementing EBPs, and explore whether perspectives on capacity are consistent across different organizational levels. The study surveyed 97 administrators and practitioners from CBOs using the Implementation Capacity Survey, which evaluated the perceived importance, presence, and organizational capacity of the CBO in nine implementation practice areas. This study is a good example of using assessments and community engagement to assess capacity in community settings and emphasizes the importance of assessing perspectives across organizational levels.

Write Goals for Expected Outcomes from Implementing the EBI at the New Site

The planning team determines goals for the expected outcomes from implementing the EBI at the new site. These outcomes will include changes in QOL, health outcomes, health behavior, and environmental outcomes. They also need to consider the extent to which change is reasonably expected and the timeframe for these changes. Step 1 of IM (Chapter 5) provides more detailed guidance on how to write these goals. In this subtask, the goals can be preliminary and further refined in an iterative manner as the planning team completes the remaining IM ADAPT tasks. After choosing an EBI to adapt in subsequent tasks, the team should report the expected degree of change and can further refine the goals for the adapted intervention if necessary.

Task 2: Discover EBIs That Potentially Match the Targets for Change *or* Determine Level of Evidence for a Selected EBI

The purpose of Task 2 is to help planners find interventions that already have an evidence base, and assess their potential application in the new situation. The planning team will complete subtask 2.1: search for EBIs OR (if starting with a selected EBI) evaluate the level of evidence of selected EBI and subtask 2.2: judge basic fit of the EBIs with the new population/setting, and organizational capacity or resources available for implementation. If searching for an EBI, completing these tasks will lead to the selection of one (or more) EBIs to carry forward to Task 3. Planners who already have an EBI in mind (as in the example below) and have reviewed the evidence base for the EBI, can go directly to subtask 2.2 to assess the EBI's basic fit. If planners would like to see other EBIs either because the basic fit was disappointing or they are curious to see what else has been tested, they can always return to subtask 2.1.

Search for EBIs OR (If Starting with a Selected EBI) Evaluate the Level of Evidence of Selected EBI

There are a number of ways to find EBIs including the program materials, protocols, and other documentation that form the EBIs. An EBI might be recommended or even required by a funder or a supervisor, suggested by a colleague, presented at a conference or meeting, identified in an online search of published evaluations of interventions, or on a website that provides information about specific interventions or systematic reviews of interventions. Website sources are usually freely available, unbiased, efficient, and easy to use. Below, we describe several websites that provide information about the sponsors/funders, content, standards of evidence, and features of each (Table 11.1). However the search begins, ultimately,

Table 11.1 Examples of Websites Offering Full EBIs, Evidence-based Approaches (EBAs) Based on Systematic Reviews, and Mixes of EBAs and EBIs with Varying Levels of Evidence and Access to Materials

1. Websites for EBIs with Guaranteed Access to Materials ("Full EBIs")

Evidence-based cancer control programs (formerly RTIPs):
https://ebccp.cancercontrol.cancer.gov/index.do
Publisher: U.S. Dept of Health and Human Services/National Cancer Institute/Division of Cancer Control & Population Sciences
Topics: Cancer screening, cancer control vaccinations, physical activity, nutrition, other cancer-related behaviors
Inclusion Criteria: Demonstrated psychosocial and/or behavioral outcomes evaluated in experimental or quasi-experimental studies published in a peer-reviewed journal in the last 10 years
Evidence Ratings: Evidence-based Cancer Control Programs (EBCCPs) score (research integrity, intervention impact, population reach, and effect size), and disseminability. Categories = 1–5 (Low to High). RE-AIM Score (reach, effectiveness, adoption, implementation, and maintenance) added 2012. Categories = percentage scores
Features: EBI descriptions, links to abstracts and articles, developers' contact information, implementation guides, links to *Community Guide* reviews, advanced search, RE-AIM notes section, program material order form, and link to related programs.

National registry of evidence-based programs and practices:
https://www.samhsa.gov/nrepp
Publisher: U.S. Dept of Health and Human Services/Substance Abuse and Mental Health Services Administration
Topics: Mental health, substance use
Inclusion Criteria: Programs evaluated in experimental or quasi-experimental studies with results published in peer-reviewed/professional journals, or documented in evaluation reports
Evidence Ratings: Based on study design/quality/confidence intervals (A–G), conceptual framework, intervention impact, implementation potential. Categories = Effective, Promising, Ineffective, Inconclusive
Features: EBI descriptions, Spanish language EBIs, downloadable full-text reports/manuscripts and supplementary materials, developers' contact information, general implementation advice/toolkit, user comments

2. EBAs Only (Based on Systematic Reviews)

AHRQ evidence-based practice center reports:
http://www.ahrq.gov/research/findings/evidence-based-reports/index.html
Publisher: U.S. Dept of Health and Human Services/Agency for Healthcare Research and Quality
Topics: Cancer screening, cancer control vaccinations, nutrition, other lifestyle behaviors, treatment, survivorship
Inclusion Criteria: Comparative effectiveness reviews, evidence reports, technical briefs, technology assessment program reports, U.S. Preventive Services Task Force evidence syntheses. Selection based on disease burden (severity, incidence, and prevalence of disease), potential impact, costs of the disease, availability of scientific data
Evidence Ratings: Based on strength of evidence. Categories = High, Moderate, Low, Insufficient
Features: Executive abstracts, and downloadable full text reports/manuscripts of systematic reviews, evidence summaries-General Approaches Only (Based on Systematic Reviews)

Cochrane:
http://www.cochrane.org/evidence
Publisher: Public and private sources/The Cochrane Collaboration
Topics: Screening, cancer control vaccinations, physical activity, nutrition, other lifestyle behaviors
Inclusion Criteria: Systematic reviews and meta-analyses (following the Cochrane protocol) of studies of defined quality testing the effectiveness of prevention services, programs and policies
Evidence Ratings: Many reviews now use the GRADE rating system
Features: Downloadable abstracts and reviews, evidence tables, resources in languages other than English, review methods (*Cochrane Handbook*)

Health evidence:
http://www.healthevidence.org/
Publisher: Canadian Govt Agencies/McMaster University
Topics: Screening, cancer control vaccinations, physical activity, nutrition, other lifestyle behaviors
Inclusion Criteria: Systematic reviews and meta-analyses of studies of defined quality testing the effectiveness of prevention programs and policies
Evidence Ratings: Quality assessment score, based on quality of methods and strength of evidence. Categories = Strong (8–10), Moderate (5–7), Weak (4 or less), designation for highly accessed interventions
Features: Review descriptions and downloadable abstracts, some links to downloadable reviews, some evidence tables, webinars, glossary

Table 11.1 (*Continued*)

The Community Guide:
https://www.thecommunityguide.org/
Publisher: U.S. Dept of Health and Human Services/Centers for Disease Control and Prevention
Topics: Screening, cancer control vaccinations, physical activity, nutrition, other lifestyle behaviors
Inclusion Criteria: Systematic reviews of studies of defined quality that test the effectiveness of prevention programs and policies for implementation in communities or primary healthcare settings
Evidence Ratings: Based on strength of evidence (study design/quality, intervention impact, number of studies, consistency of findings) and recommendations of the U.S. Community Preventive Services Task Force. Categories = Highly Recommended, Recommended, Recommended Against, Insufficient Evidence
Features: Downloadable reviews, evidence tables, logic models, lessons learned, research needs, links to RTIPS interventions, citations, general advice/toolkit about implementation, systematic review comparison tool, webinars for some reviews, similar intervention recommendations

3. Websites That Offer A Mix Of EBIs And Systematic Reviews (Without Guaranteed Access To EBI Materials)

Center for training and research translation:
http://www.centertrt.org/
Publisher: U.S. Centers for Disease Control and Prevention/University of North Carolina at Chapel Hill/Division of Nutrition, Physical Activity, and Obesity
Topics: Physical activity, nutrition, obesity prevention
Inclusion Criteria: Specific EBIs and general EBI strategies. Specific EBIs must be either "research tested interventions" (tested in one or more research studies, with demonstrated efficacy/effectiveness in improving one or more obesity-related outcomes, published in a peer-reviewed journal) or "practice-tested interventions" (practitioner-developed interventions not tested using more formal research methods that show promise based on underlying theory, approach, and an evaluation suggesting they improved one or more obesity-related outcomes) or "emerging interventions" (practitioner-developed interventions that meet the criteria for designation as practice-tested interventions except for direct evidence of effect on outcome)
Evidence Ratings: Based on study methods/quality, intervention impact, implementation potential, peer review. Categories = Research-based, Practice-based, Emerging
Features: EBI descriptions with core components identified, downloadable full-text reports/manuscripts, developers' contact information, implementation materials/guides for specific programs, general implementation advice/toolkit

Healthy people 2030:
www.healthypeople.gov
Publisher: U.S. Dept of Health and Human Services/Office of Disease Prevention and Health Promotion/Healthy People Team
Topics: Screening, cancer control vaccinations, physical activity, nutrition, other lifestyle/preventive behaviors
Inclusion Criteria: Specific EBIs (interventions, programs, services) and general EBI strategies with evidence of effectiveness, feasibility, reach, sustainability, and transferability
Evidence Ratings: Based on study methods/quality, intervention impact, number of studies (if part of a systematic review), and peer review. Categories = 1–4 (Low to High)
Features: Program descriptions, links and citations to full-text reports, general implementation advice/toolkits, similar intervention recommendations

National association of county and city health officials (NACCHO) model practices:
https://www.naccho.org/resources/model-practices
Publisher: National Association of County and City Health Officials
Topics: Screening, cancer control vaccinations, physical activity, nutrition, other lifestyle/preventive behaviors
Inclusion Criteria: Initiatives, programs, resources, and administrative practices and tools produced by local, state, and federal agencies, academic institutions, and other stakeholders that address local needs that have been evaluated, or present qualitative or quantitative evidence and have community collaboration, be innovative, responsive, and sustainable
Evidence Ratings: Based on strength of evidence. Categories = Model Practice, Promising Practice
Features: EBI descriptions (objectives, implementation costs and timeline, process and outcome evaluation, impact, innovation, and lessons learned), links to some EBI and local health department websites, general implementation advice/toolkit

(*continued*)

Table 11.1 (*Continued*)

National association of county and city health officials (NACCHO) toolbox:
http://www.naccho.org/toolbox/
Publisher: National Association of County and City Health Officials
Topics: Multiple lifestyle/preventive behaviors
Inclusion Criteria: Materials and resources (e.g., case examples, presentations, fact sheets, drills, evaluations, protocols, templates, reports, and training materials) produced by local, state, and federal agencies, academic institutions, and other stakeholders
Evidence Ratings: Based on user-generated ratings. Categories = 1–5 stars
Features: Downloadable toolkits, general implementation advice/toolkit about implementation

Trip (formerly turning research into practice):
https://www.tripdatabase.com/
Publisher: Public and private sources/TRIP
Topics: Screening, cancer control vaccinations, physical activity, nutrition and other lifestyle behaviors
Inclusion Criteria: Specific EBIs and general EBI strategies. Whether resources were part of a systematic review, evidence-based synopses, guidelines, primary research, controlled trials, ongoing systematic reviews, ongoing clinical trials, decision aids, etc.
Evidence Ratings: Color categories, based on strength of evidence: Secondary Evidence: systematic review, evidence-based synopses (green); Key Primary Research (blue); Clinical Q and A (teal); Primary Research Controlled Trials (red); Ongoing Systematic Reviews and Clinical Trials (yellow), Images, Videos, and others: Purple
Features: Links to all articles, and abstracts, general implementation advice/toolkit, advanced search and filter categories (most popular, latest, publication type), share on social media, access to blogs, images, and videos

U.S. centers for disease control and prevention (CDC) smoking and tobacco use:
http://www.cdc.gov/tobacco/
Publisher: U.S. Centers for Disease Control and Prevention/National Center for Chronic Disease Prevention and Health Promotion/Office on Smoking and Health
Topics: Smoking and tobacco use/control
Inclusion Criteria: Data, resources, practices, and programs focused on eliminating secondhand smoke exposure, promoting cessation, preventing initiation of tobacco use, eliminating disparities
Evidence Ratings: No identified ratings
Features: Some downloadable sample multimedia tools, infographics, fact sheets, documents, planning tools, data/statistics, recommended funding levels, best practices, links to related CDC websites, link to some resources for program development, surveillance and evaluation, General implementation advice/toolkit

the team will need to have one or more specific EBIs that can be evaluated for basic fit. While evidence-based approaches (EBAs) (e.g., one-on-one education, reducing structural barriers for increasing breast cancer screening as recommended by the *Guide to Community Preventive Services*) that provide guidance about what *types* of EBIs may be useful, the adaptation process described here is for adapting specific EBIs that have accompanying materials and protocols rather than generally recommended approaches. If the planners already have a selected EBI in mind, they can evaluate its evidence level. In doing so, they should conduct a literature search to identify evidence from reviews and meta-analyses, as well as from clinical guidelines, expert consensus papers, or practice-based evidence.

Levels of Evidence A question that arises when searching for an intervention to address needs in a given population and setting is: How much evidence is needed for an intervention to be considered "evidence-based"? All EBIs described as "evidence-based" do not have the same type or amount of evidence supporting their effectiveness. Ratings of the strength or quality of evidence are often presented as a pyramid, with systematic

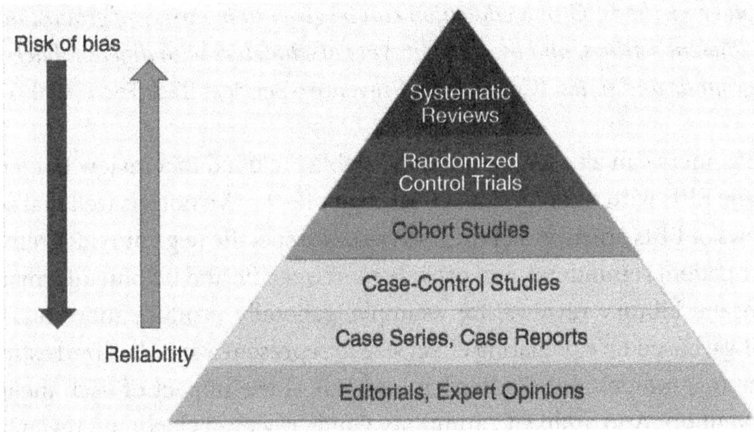

Figure 11.4 Pyramid of Evidence

reviews and meta-analyses at the top, and less rigorous sources—e.g., expert opinion—at the bottom. Figure 11.4 is one of many similar examples of this hierarchy. Resources for discussions about the quality of evidence can be found in the GRADE Handbook or the GRADE Working Group (Grading of Recommendations Assessment, Development, and Evaluation website, (http://www.gradeworkinggroup.org/) and the RE-AIM (Reach Effectiveness Adoption Implementation Maintenance website (http://www.reaim.org/).

In most "evidence-based-quality pyramids," systematic reviews are at the top because they typically assemble available published and unpublished evidence collected through professional searches, have explicit criteria for inclusion of studies in their analysis, include assessments of the quality of the individual studies that were included in the review, and use standardized methods for summarizing study results. Yet, challenges in understanding *summaries* of evidence remain. This is primarily because authors of reviews sometimes use broad eligibility criteria for selecting the studies included in the review. For example, the Guide to Community Preventive Services (*Community Guide*) often bases its selection of interventions to review on a *delivery vehicle*, e.g., using "local media," "group education," or "one-on-one" education to engender uptake of a particular cancer screening method. In looking more closely at the definition of group education in a *Community Guide* review, we see that several objectives and numerous types of change methods (e.g., modeling, and group discussion), doses, group size, and content were included in the recommendation that group education is effective for, say, screening for breast cancer. It also implies (through the vague description -see the excerpt below- provided by the authors) that planners will not find very much guidance on how to use *group education* as part of their health promotion intervention.

> *Group education is usually conducted by health professionals or by trained lay people who use presentations or other teaching aids in a lecture or interactive format, and often incorporate role modeling or*

other methods. Group education can be given to a variety of groups, in different settings, and by different types of educators with different backgrounds and styles. (Community Preventive Services Task Force, 2009)

Planners can also use the evidence table included in a review to identify specific EBIs with strong evidence for their effects. We note as well that some reviews of EBIs are in and of themselves more specific (e.g., provider reminders or patient reminders), and provide more specific and helpful information. Cochrane Library reviews, for example, generally produce more nuanced findings, based on calculating effect size to represent a standardized estimate of the magnitude (and confidence interval) of the impact of each included intervention. And, unlike Community Guide reviews, Cochrane reviews are updated regularly (https://www.cochranelibrary.com/home).

Moving down the evidence pyramid to randomized controlled trials (RCTs), we rely on the strength of random assignment and a control group to increase our confidence in findings that the intervention causes the effect on the outcomes measured (*internal validity*). High internal validity, however, does not mean that the intervention (even if implemented with fidelity) will have the same or similar effects across diverse cultural groups, settings, and times. One reason is that the RCT could have been conducted under ideal circumstances such as with a highly selected subset of the at-risk group, or using incentives for participants to engage in the intervention, or delivered by trained and closely supervised personnel hired specially for the trial. These and other elements distinguish an "efficacy trial" from a "pragmatic trial" with high *external validity* (generalizability) (Burlew et al., 2013; Glasgow, 2003; Lau, 2006). "Time" refers to such time-related aspects of a specific trial such as the then-current recommendations for screening or vaccination, and the stage on the adoption curve where it is easier or much more difficult to change behavior. Ideally, there will be several replications with increasing external validity to demonstrate that the intervention "works" across different populations, settings, and times. This was the case for the Smoke-free Homes (Take It Outside) intervention that was tested with usual 2-1-1 call center staff taking over intervention delivery from university staff and other pragmatic elements and with low-income callers who were either smokers themselves or living with smokers and who differed across the trials by race, ethnicity, rurality, and U.S. region (Bundy et al., 2019; Kegler et al., 2019; Mullen et al., 2016; Williams et al., 2016).

Although not as highly rated in most evidence hierarchies, policy and organizational change interventions based on non-randomized "quasi-experimental" designs may be more suitable for testing policy and multilevel interventions (see IM Step 6, Task 2, Chapter 10). This is explicitly recognized by Community Guide evidence criteria (Baron et al., 2009). And, although some health problems or behaviors have few EBIs of any design, a curated source such as the Center for Training and Research Translation with a rating of "emerging" or "practice-tested" (evidence derived from practice in the form of evaluation data or reports) (Table 11.1) might be the strongest evidence available for some physical activity, nutrition, and obesity prevention topics.

In searching for specific EBIs, we expect that planners will first look for interventions that were described through established and credible sources that compile lists of interventions with high standards for evidence of impact, such as Evidence-based Cancer Control Interventions or Canadian Best Practices Portal and that have strong impact scores and favorable RE-AIM or adaptability ratings (Table 11.1). Still considered evidence-based (but perhaps with somewhat less confidence), is an intervention with at least one peer-reviewed evaluation research study, showing a meaningful impact on a behavior or health outcome, that is unlikely to be the result of chance alone (moderate to small confidence interval). Planners should use the EBI with highest quality of evidence available—usually a specific intervention tested in at least one randomized trial with additional evidence from other trials of similar interventions from a systematic review.

Sources of EBIs Numerous websites (such as those listed in Table 11.1) offer EBIs and EBAs, and although not the only source, they are important and accessible to planners. In considering whether to use such web-based sources for information about EBIs, planners should consider six evaluation criteria: (adapted from Leeman et al., 2014; Leeman et al. 2014):

- Profit motive or other bias (Identify the website creator and sponsor)
- Alignment of the types of EBIs being disseminated (e.g., EBIs or EBAs, priority health conditions or behaviors) with objectives of planner(s)
- Level of rigor of the methods used to review the evidence
- Validity/strength of criteria applied by EBI developers to determine when an intervention was evidence-based and ready to be disseminated
- When the studies of which the evidence base was completed were conducted
- Quality and quantity of information/resources available to support implementation of the EBI

These criteria were used to select entries for Table 11.1 which presents websites in three categories according to the type of EBI they present:

1. **Websites that guarantee that developers of all of the listed EBIs will provide access to all materials and protocols ("full" or "packaged EBIs")**, e.g., Effective Interventions: HIV Prevention that Works (https://effectiveinterventions.cdc.gov/en/home.aspx). These websites save planners time by providing extensive information about the interventions and (usually) free access to materials.

2. **Websites that provide systematic reviews with evidence tables that give information about the specific interventions included in the review** as well as appraisals of the effectiveness of the overall group ("evidence-based *approaches*," *EBAs*), e.g., Cochrane Database of Systematic Reviews (https://www.cochranelibrary.com/cdsr/about-cdsr). Systematic reviews evaluate and summarize the findings across multiple studies to assess whether the EBA will produce similar results with differing intervention formats in multiple settings, populations, and contexts. Some details about the intervention, population, setting, and study design will be reported in an evidence table. If the review is a meta-analysis, it will also report the effect sizes (impact) of the individual research studies. Once an EBA looks as if it might fit with the problem in the new community, planners will have to select specific *EBIs* from the evidence table and they may then need to contact the intervention developers to obtain the materials.
3. **Websites that present a combination of specific EBIs (usually without guaranteed access to materials and protocols) and systematic reviews with or without evidence tables,** e.g., Canadian Best Practices Portal (http://cbpp-pcpe.phac-aspc.gc.ca/). This diverse category gives an overview of many types of EBIs and EBAs using a broader range of evidence quality, with labels such as "practice-based" and "promising." These EBIs might constitute the best evidence base for some health problems and health-promoting behaviors. Although locating specific EBIs and their corresponding materials on these sites can require more effort (compared to categories #1 and #2), these sites provide a useful overview of "what works."

During the search for EBIs, we recommend that planners first search category #1 websites for those focused on the health problem or behaviors that match the team's interests. If one or more of the EBIs on these websites is a potential fit (subtask 2), locating the corresponding materials will require less work from the team. If planners do not find a basic fit with a full EBI, however, or when they are curious about EBAs that might apply to their situation, looking at the systematic reviews listed on websites in category #2 will enlarge their range of possibilities. From the perspective of the strength of the evidence for an EBI, the ideal is to find a full EBI that is also included in an EBA from a systematic review. In the case of *The Community Guide*, for example, there is a link from the recommended cancer control EBAs, to the Evidence-based Cancer Prevention Programs website, where access to full EBIs is guaranteed; but this type of linkage is rare.

Yet another way to identify an EBI is through an online search, for example, in PubMed (https://ovidsp.ovid.com/), for evaluations of interventions or systematic reviews of intervention trials for the health problem or health-promoting behavior. For example, a planner could begin by typing in the advanced search box, "interventions to increase mammography screening in African American women." The search could be further restricted by language (e.g., English), type of publication (e.g., journal article), publication dates, whether it was tested in a RCT, and the age, sex, race/ethnicity of the study participants. The output would be a list of citations (authors, titles, and journal names and full citations), the abstracts of which could be scanned for information of interest. This strategy has the advantage of yielding the most up-to-date and relatively comprehensive information, but it can be a lot of work to read through the abstracts and then try to extract information that might be displayed on an EBI website. This description of a search could easily be adopted for systematic reviews and meta-analyses by adding the term "systematic review" to the search terms. Having the assistance of a trained librarian, especially one who can suggest filters (tested combinations of search terms), will help tailor the search to the planners' objectives.

Judge Basic Fit

The product of this subtask (judging basic fit) is a list of one or more EBIs that planners want to review further in Task 3. Table 11.2 includes the basic fit assessment criteria used in the Cancer Prevention and Control Research Network training program (https://cpcrn.org/training) (2021). A similar table in the IM ADAPT online tool adds several more criteria and allows the reader to assign two ratings to each criterion: (a) the importance of the criterion and (b) the degree to which an EBI appears to match the planner's new situation, based on Task 1.

EBI Fit—Health Problem, Behavior, and Environmental Conditions Table 11.2 is the most basic criterion. The key question which should be asked by implementation planners associated with this criterion is: "Does

Table 11.2 EBI Comparison Tool for CRC Screening[a]

			Does this EBI fit your context?				Does this EBI fit your context?		
Fit Criteria	**Findings**	**Evidence-Based Intervention 1**	**Yes**	**Some**	**No**	**Evidence-Based Intervention 2**	**Yes**	**Some**	**No**
Health Problem									
Objectives									
Priority population									
Setting									
Multi-level contributing factors									
Organization / Community Capacity and Resources									

[a] Figure adapted from (https://cpcrn.org/training) (2021).

the focus of the potential EBI match the targeted health problem (at the new site) and its causes—including behavioral or environmental conditions?" The answer to whether there is a "health problem-fit" is usually a simple "Yes" or "No." In the case of a "No" answer, planners may want to continue searching for EBIs that have lower levels of evidence or that address a similar problem or behavior. For example, a team that in the past was unable to find EBIs for COVID-19 vaccination might instead search for EBIs that address other vaccines for adults, with the idea of adapting one of these to COVID-19 vaccination.

EBI Fit—Determinant Objectives Proper specification (by planners) of the determinants to be addressed by an EBI is fundamental to the logic of the intervention. And, looking at determinants often helps identify additional EBIs that might be suitable. For example, planners interested in finding an EBI that could be used for a grant-funded project were unable to find one for their niche priority population of Vietnamese nail salon workers. When they considered important determinants, (e.g., attitudes, barriers to access), they found the same determinants in an EBI designed for a low-income Hispanic population in an urban area. Both groups were similarly constrained by (e.g., they shared determinants) low insurance coverage, long working hours, and provider gender and language. Thus in this case, although adaptation will be needed, adaptation of core content addressing determinants may be similar, indicating potential fit in this category.

EBI Fit—Communication Channels and Delivery Vehicles Alignment between the EBI's communication channels and delivery vehicles in the new group is another important criterion to judge the fit of EBIs. Interventions include both interpersonal and mediated communication channels, as well as delivery vehicles. For instance, an EBI may be delivered through a social media communication channel with social media delivery vehicles such as Facebook, Twitter, or others. When the interpersonal communication channel is used, the delivery vehicle can be healthcare providers, peer leaders, lay health workers, teachers, or others. Adapters may also examine the communication channels and delivery vehicles in consideration of methods of behavioral change and their practical applications, as these provide insights into how the intervention needs to be delivered. For example, self-efficacy, a determinant, could be targeted by a behavioral change method like goal setting. Thus, adapters need to evaluate if the EBI can be adapted to utilize communication channels and delivery vehicles that are appropriate for applying goal-setting-related practical applications.

EBI Fit—Priority Population/At-Risk Group While it may be preferable to select EBIs that have been used for a similar population and setting, this is often not possible. A planner should not outright reject an EBI that otherwise fits just because the at-risk group differs in some characteristics (such as ethnicity or race). Having similar determinants and delivery channels might be of greater importance in considering fit although it is highly likely that some adaptations (particularly of surface structure as described by Resnicow) will be needed (Castro et al., 2015; Resnicow et al., 1999). Thus, in some cases, rating the fit of this criterion as a "maybe" to be examined more closely in Step 3, is valid. Another possibility is the case that there are several EBIs that feature the same at-risk group but one or more do not address determinants that are important for the planner's priority population. Here, the planner would award a higher "fit score" to those with both surface identity- and determinants-fit.

EBI Fit—Organizational Capacity This criterion addresses the match of the resources necessary for implementing an EBI with the adopting organization's capacity. The key question associated with this criterion is, "Does the intervention fit with the organizational mission, strategic goals, and resources?" When a planning group recognizes a mismatch due to lack of capacity, it might consider whether training or technical support could help with the organizational capacity development. We strongly recommend that planners consider undertaking capacity development efforts, rather than deleting a component of an EBI out of convenience, simply because it does not match an organization's capacity. If, however, the EBI appears to match other criteria but there are changes that may be necessary to make it more feasible for the organization, planners may consider modifications to make the EBI delivery more feasible, keeping in mind that these sorts of adaptations may affect the EBI's feasibility and effectiveness.

Task 3: Assess Fit and Plan Adaptation

In the previous task, the team created a short list of potential EBIs. Task 3 helps planners make decisions about adaptations needed to an EBI which can inform the final selection of an EBI if planners have chosen more than one option. If starting with a selected EBI, planners Task 3 will result in a list of needed adaptations to improve fit. The specific subtasks include: subtask 3.1: use *EBI Mapping* (Walker et al., 2022) to describe and create a logic model of the existing intervention; subtask 3.2: compare the logic model of change to the logic model of the EBI—judge fit of behavioral and environmental targets, determinants addressed, methods and practical applications used, delivery fit, and design features including cultural elements; and subtask 3.3: judge implementation fit and make decisions about what should change considering core elements (core functions) and how to retain them. In subtask 3.1, planners create a logic model of the candidate EBI(s) through a process we call "EBI Mapping." Using EBI Mapping to create a logic model of the existing EBI (i.e., describing the mechanisms of action and logic of how the EBI was intended to work including the specific targets of the EBI) will facilitate a comparison of the EBI's logic model with the logic model of change created in Task 1. This comparison also happens in Task 3 (in a subsequent subtask). EBI Mapping uses intervention development tasks in reverse order. This approach facilitates detailed judgments about fit and enables consideration of adaptations that might be needed for each candidate (Szeszulski et al., 2022; Walker et al., 2022). Subtasks 3.2 and 3.3 assess the detailed fit between each EBI and the new situation, and help the team to decide how much change is needed for each, and ultimately, which is the most appropriate selection.

Use EBI Mapping to Describe and Create a Logic Model of the Existing Intervention

The materials, activities, and publication reports for each candidate EBI are the focus of the EBI mapping exercise, described in Figure 11.5.

Specify Who the Materials and Activities are for Planners should start by organizing the EBI materials (e.g., handouts, curriculum, apps, videos, manuals, guidelines, etc.) into smaller parts (which may include materials, activities or sets of materials/activities, and implementation manuals). Audiences include the at-risk population(s), environmental change agents, and implementers. Some EBIs will target all three; others, one or two (see Figure 11.6). As an illustration, in Figure 11.6 we analyzed an intervention that was designed to increase physical activity among breast cancer survivors. This intervention has a component for health care providers, one for patients in clinical settings, and a third directed toward community social

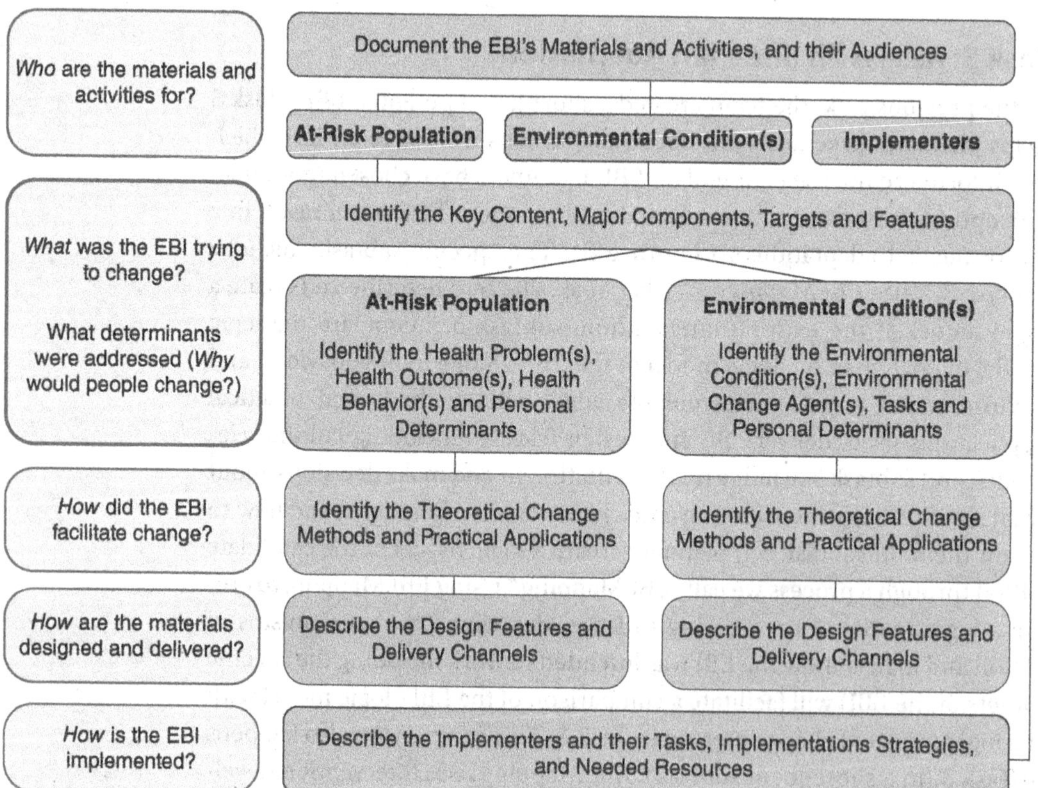

Figure 11.5 EBI Mapping. [a]Figure adapted from Walker et al. (2022)

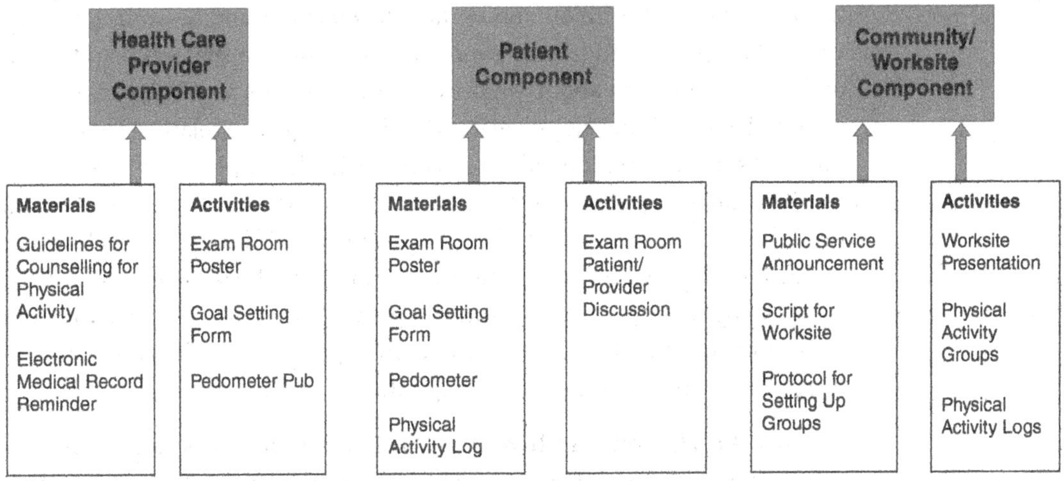

Figure 11.6 Three-Component EBI: Targeting Health Care Providers, Patients, and Community

support for physical activity at worksites. Nested under each of these major components, we encountered both materials and activities. For example, to stimulate patient-provider discussion, the healthcare provider component (environmental change agent) included a handout for patients with guidelines for physical activity in cancer survivors, a prompt in the electronic medical record to stimulate a discussion about the importance of physical activity for survivors, and a patient handout to support the discussion. In the patient component (at-risk population), there is the patient handout (also listed in the provider component), a goal-setting form, and an exam-room poster. Again, the materials were in support of one activity, the patient-provider discussion. This program also has a worksite component (implementer) with activities to form physical activity groups (supported by printed protocols) and a motivational session with a coach (supported by goal-setting forms).

Specify What the EBI Is Trying to Change and What Determinants are Addressed Next planners need to identify the health problem, health outcome(s), and health-promoting behaviors to be addressed by the EBI—for both the at-risk population and/or for individuals who can affect environmental change. For each audience, the behaviors should be broken into subbehaviors promoted by the EBI, aimed at achieving the health outcome. Subbehaviors (called performance objectives in IM, Step 2) are the specific actions that must be completed to accomplish the broader health behavior. For example, an EBI to encourage CRC screening (FIT test) may address subbehaviors including, asking the provider for a screening kit, reading the instructions, following the instructions correctly, and returning it to the clinic. The next action for the planning team is to figure out the personal determinants—factors such as attitudes and skills—that the EBI addresses to change the behaviors and subbehaviors. Planners should list only the health problems, health outcomes, health behaviors, and personal determinants that the EBI addresses ***explicitly*** based on the materials and avoid making assumptions about what the EBI developers would logically have included. For EBIs developed using IM, this task will be relatively easy since much of this information will already be available for planners to review. It can be difficult, however, to identify determinants that have not yet been described by the developers of the original EBI or if they used unclear and confusing terms. Clues can sometimes be found in the *measures* defined by EBI developers, or text of descriptive reports. Care must be taken, however, to confirm whether the measures actually represent determinants targeted by the intervention or are merely aspirational.

Identify the Theoretical Change Methods and Practical Applications In this task, the planning team describes the proposed mechanisms through which the change(s) were expected to occur in the EBI by specifying the *theoretical change methods. These are defined as general techniques or processes that have been proven to alter determinants of target behavior or environmental outcomes* (Kok et al., 2016). *Examples of change methods include tailoring, discussion, and cooperative learning among others* (Aronson, 2002; DiClemente & Graydon, 2020; Petty et al., 2009).

If the mechanisms or "functions" of the EBI (or in IM language-change methods) are not described in either the materials or published articles, a planner will need to infer what change methods were used and how they were applied (the EBI's practical applications of these methods). There are two ways to do this. One way is to look at the determinants and consider possible change methods that may have been used (based on the types of methods that are known to influence determinants—see methods tables in Chapter 7). Another way is to closely examine the materials and activities and determine the practical applications used. Practical applications are specific translations of methods for practical use that fit the priority population and context. These practical applications will likely include one or more methods. For example, in the logic model of change for a school-based sex education program, *Long Live Love*, one determinant was *attitude* (the students should describe the advantages of condom use and other safe-sex options), and *active learning* was one method selected to address this determinant. The practical applications that were employed in this context included inquiry teaching, group discussion, a quiz, and interviews (Kok et al., 2016) Sometimes it is easier to identify practical applications and change methods in EBI materials as compared to trying to identify determinants targeted. Additionally, in some cases, EBIs that target environmental conditions do not operate through an environmental change agent. In these cases, the methods directly target the environment, a process, or a condition that affects the behavior of the at-risk group. Chapter 7 described such methods focused on changing the environment environmental change methods such as those described should be identified here.

Describe How the Materials are Designed and Delivered Design features can be considered part of the "surface structure" of the EBI and can include: the look and feel of materials, cultural elements, readability, branding, and contact information. It is important to note that "surface" does not imply unimportance. Studies have demonstrated that materials that appeal to an audience because they are culturally relevant, include images and pictures with which they can identify, and are at the correct reading and comprehension level, are much more likely to have an impact (Ballard, 2021; Huang & Shen, 2016; Johnson and Delk, 2024; Rademakers & Heijimans, 2018; Johnson, 2024). Thus, it is important to describe the current design features and determine needed modifications. Planners can describe design features for a set of materials/activities or for individual ones depending on the characteristics of the EBI and if there are different design features across materials and activities. Delivery channels. materials and activities are especially important for planners to consider when thinking about the resources required for the EBI and the feasibility of adapting delivery. It is, for example, usually easier to adapt print, or other more readily modifiable materials, than video or illustrations.

Describe How the EBI Is Implemented Some EBIs clearly describe how they should be implemented specifying who the implementers were, what they had to do to implement, and what materials and activities (implementation strategies) were used to build implementation capacity and/or address and barriers to implementation. For example, some fields such as counseling expect program developers to document their interventions with manuals that will guide implementation—at least the training aspects—and they will specify the credentials of the counselors. In the case of many health promotion EBIs, however, the implementers, their tasks, and the resources needed to support them will not be clearly protocolized and implementation manuals may not exist. Since the process of intervention adaptation (including adaptation of implementation strategies) is intricate and is not amenable to "boilerplate" materials, guides, or processes. During the adaptation process, it is important to clearly understand how the EBI was implemented in the past and any lessons learned during its use and evaluation as well as what potential changes may be needed given the new population and setting. Planners should gather as much information as possible through interviews, surveys, and focus groups with intervention developers, implementers, and the intended beneficiaries of the intervention.

Compare the Logic Model of the EBI to the Logic Model of Change (From Task 1)

The planners now compare the logic model of the EBI with the logic model of change for the new population and setting. Specifically, they will assess the fit of behavioral and environmental targets, determinants addressed, methods and practical applications used, delivery fit, and design features, including cultural elements and determine what changes are needed to enhance fit.

Judge Fit of Behavioral and Environmental Outcomes The team will first determine if the EBI targets the risk behaviors and environmental changes they aim to address by reviewing both the EBI's logic model and comparing it to the logic model and change. The example guiding questions they will ask include: Does this EBI address the behavioral and environmental changes in the logic model of change and in the project goals for the new context? Which behaviors and environmental factors are addressed by the content of the EBI? Are the performance objectives (subbehaviors) addressed in the EBI necessary to carry out the behavior or to make changes in the environment in a new context? The planners also need to consider what adaptations need to be made to the EBI to improve its fit in the new context. Sample guiding questions include: To better fit the program goals, what adaptations would need to be made? What behaviors or environmental factors need to be added or removed? What performance objectives need to be added, modified or removed? Does the group need to break down behaviors into more detailed, smaller steps? How feasible are the changes in the new context? Do the proposed changes create the risk of damaging or eliminating the intervention's core elements in the new group?

Judge Fit of Determinants Addressed and Methods and Practical Applications Used The planning team now evaluates not only the fit of the determinants, change methods, and practical applications used in the EBI for the next context but also their alignment at a theoretical level. This includes determining whether the selected method is indeed well-matched with the targeted determinant and if the application accurately translates the method. The following guiding questions can be useful: "Is the selected method indeed a good fit for the targeted determinant?" "Is the application a correct translation of the method?" Does the EBI contain theory-based change methods that are likely to impact the target determinants in the next context? Does the EBI use practical applications that are likely to be feasible in the next context? To better fit, what modifications in determinants or change methods can be made? What determinants need to be added or removed to meet the needs of the next context? How feasible are these changes? Do they create the risk of damaging or eliminating the EBI's core elements?

When judging such fit, the planning team can examine the logic model of change and (looking at the EBI logic model) determine what coincides, what is missing in the existing EBI, and what is there that may not be needed. In other words, the planners decide (based on this comparison) what needs to be added, deleted, and/or modified. At this point planners may want to further review the EBI materials and their messages (e.g., messages about risk delivered through in-person role-playing) as they can inform the targeted determinant (risk awareness), change methods used (modeling), and practical applications (in-person role-playing). Importantly, adapters need to be cautious when making significant adaptations to change methods and determinants, as this can alter the core elements (function) of the EBI. In general, we recommend avoiding the deletion of change methods and remembering that the EBIs under consideration have been evaluated and judged to be effective. When a group chooses to add change methods to strengthen an intervention, it should ensure that the determinants addressed are important in the new community, and that the addition of methods to address them does not create excess burden for either participants or implementers.

Judge Fit of Delivery, Design Features Including Cultural Elements
The planning group assesses the delivery, design, and cultural aspects of the EBI in a new context. Delivery fit primarily concerns reaching the target users, like patients. Design fit and cultural relevance involve evaluating the EBI's design features (credibility, readability, graphics, etc.) with the needs of the new population and setting. This includes ensuring cultural congruence in language, activities, values, etc., depicted in the intervention. Collaboration with community partners and intended users is crucial, particularly for insights into cultural aspects such as language, family depictions, communication norms, spirituality, ethnic identity, and more. If these perspectives were not covered in the initial needs assessment, they should be explored at this stage. The planning team may use the following guiding questions: Will the EBI's delivery approach effectively reach the targeted groups? How will participants perceive the format and design of the EBI materials? Do language, content, readability, visuals, and layout align with the new population's expectations? Are the EBI materials current and relevant?

Importantly, planners will need to continue exercising caution when adjusting the delivery approach because some delivery channels are related to change methods, such as role modeling and the cultural credibility of a message. Having a program delivered by a peer may create greater receptivity to a message than would be achieved by another channel (e.g., healthcare provider). Conversely, if health professionals were the deliverers, their expertise might significantly enhance the credibility of the message and the participants' willingness to comply. Another area requiring caution is in altering design features such as graphics, pictures, music, and layouts. Planners should ensure that the content and change methods are maintained, so the intended influence on determinants is not lost. For instance, changing photographs in brochures into drawings or cartoon images might affect the impact of the method (e.g., modeling) since the audience may not identify with the person in the same way." Planners must also be careful not to introduce subtle changes in features like facial expressions. A new photograph with a frowning doctor instead of a smiling one could significantly alter the content and message.

Judge Implementation Fit and Make Decisions About What Should Change Considering Core Elements (Core Functions) and How to Retain Them

The planning team evaluates the implementation fit and determines necessary changes while retaining core elements. They first assess who will implement the adapted intervention and what materials they need, reviewing whether existing protocols and materials are suitable or require modifications. Planners should consult Step 5 in IM for planning implementation interventions for additional guidance.

Next, the team decides on changes concerning the core elements of the EBI. Core elements, also known as core functions or active ingredients, are likely crucial for the EBI's effectiveness. These typically include content (messages) and change methods (e.g., modeling, facilitation) targeting specific determinants. Altering these elements should be done with great caution and ideally in consultation with the original developers.

Some changes can be made with moderate caution. These include adding target behaviors or details to behaviors (performance objectives) for the at-risk group, health-promoting environmental conditions, behaviors of environmental agents, and strengthening weak or absent determinants and change methods in the original EBI. Deleting irrelevant behaviors or performance objectives for the new population or setting, or those not considered crucial for health outcomes, also requires moderate caution. However, planners should be wary of removing behaviors as most EBIs haven't been tested for the impact of such deletions on overall effectiveness. Thus, greater caution is advised when deleting recommended behaviors that don't align with the new community's goals. Other changes requiring less caution include modifying language and graphics to suit a new culture, simplifying reading levels or enhancing comprehensibility (provided the message stays the same), and adding details to behaviors of environmental agents and program components to better address behaviors.

Task 4: Adapt Intervention Components

After completing Task 3, the planning team will have selected an intervention to use and will have created an "adaptation to-do list" to guide this next step. Working from this list, the team will complete the following subtask 4.1: prepare design documents for the adaptations, subtask 4.2: create and pretest adapted materials, and subtask 4.3: produce final adapted materials and activities.

Prepare Design Documents for the Adapted Activities and Materials

As noted in Chapter 8 (IM Step 4) design documents are materials specifically created to facilitate the detailed communication of a team's intentions to those involved in writing or selecting content from available resources, as well as in designing graphics and other forms of communication. Table 11.3 provides an example of a simple template for preparing a

Table 11.3 Examples from the Design Document Template for Telephone Counseling Program

Change	Where	New Content or Content Edits
		Change Behavior: From Mammography to Appointment Keeping (At-Risk Group)
Add: Mammography Appointment Keeping	Throughout manual	Throughout, change "making an appointment" to "keeping an appointment."
		Change Determinants and Methods
Add: Foundational Conversation Script	At beginning of the counseling script	**Example: Active Listening** **Step 1: Ask** "Sometimes women tell us there are things that make it hard to go to their appointment. How is it for you?" **Step 2: Rephrase** "It sounds like you . . .. . . Does that sound right?" If woman is reluctant: Reluctant woman does not volunteer reasons or talks about worries/beliefs, you may explore her worries/beliefs "It sounds like you are little worried/reluctant. . ." If the woman volunteers a reason, rephrase reason. "It sounds like you . . . ." If the woman has not volunteered the reason, ask about the reason. "What is making you worried about your mammogram or worried about keeping the appointment?" Continue with Step 2 of Active Listening: Rephrase "It sounds like you . . .. Do I have that right?" Go to barriers and counsel as needed. After discussing worry barriers – continue to logistic barriers below "We've talked some about your worries about your mammogram. I would like to make sure that you don't have any other barriers that will keep you from your appointment."
Add: Role Model Story (Outcome Expectations)	In all barrier scripts.	**Example: Too Busy** If they state they are too busy to attend appointment: **Step 2. Rephrase (Reflect Barrier)** "It sounds like you have so many responsibilities that it feels hard to make time for your mammogram. Did I get that right?" **Step 3. Explore (Dig Deeper, Open the Door)** "Can you tell me more about what usually gets in the way?" **Step 4. Normalize & Validate (Empathy + Common Ground)** "You're not alone, many women in our community have said the same thing. Some of them told us that they are too busy taking care of others to take care of themselves. Others said that they are just too busy making a living or doing all the other work that we women do." **Step 5. Reframe with Positive Outcome Expectation (Modeling / Persuasion)** "But some women have told us that it's important to have a mammogram to make sure to stay healthy for all of those who depend on them."

(*continued*)

Table 11.3 (*Continued*)

Change	Where	New Content or Content Edits
		Change Delivery, Design Features, and Cultural Elements
Change: Initial Designation of Stage of Change	At beginning of the counseling script	**Example: Active Listening** "Ok, great. Let's talk about your upcoming appointment." **Active Listening Step 1: Question** "How confident are you that you will keep your mammogram appointment?" ** If NO barriers – PROBE "There have been women in our community who say they are confident in keeping their appointment, but miss because they are worried about something. Is there anything that concerns you?" ** If STILL NO BARRIERS, skip to LOGISTICAL BARRIERS (next page)
Add: Barriers from Local Needs Assessment	In all barrier scripts.	**Active Listening** **Step 1. Question/Explore** "Many women have different feelings about getting a mammogram. How do you feel about your upcoming appointment?" **Example: Afraid of Finding Cancer** If they identify fear of finding cancer as a barrier: **Step 2. Rephrase** "Many women have different feelings about getting a mammogram. How do you feel about your upcoming appointment?" "When we spoke to some women in our community, they said that they would rather not know if they have breast cancer. Some women said that as long as they feel fine, they don't want to look for trouble." One woman said "If it is not broke, don't fix it." "Other women say something else, which is very true: "If you have cancer, you'll find out eventually." And, we have to remember; 9 out of 10 times a mammogram does not find anything abnormal. Getting a mammogram does NOT mean you have cancer." **Step 3. Probe (Non-judgmentally Explore Beliefs / Source of Fear)** "Can you tell me more about what feels most frightening for you?" "Some women say they are afraid of the test itself, while others say they are afraid of what the results might mean. How is it for you?" **Step 4. Normalize & Validate** "You're not alone, many women in our community have shared the same worries." "It makes sense that you would feel that way. Waiting for results, or even thinking about cancer, can be scary." **Step 5. Reframe with Information + Positive Outcome Expectation** "The important thing to remember is that 9 out of 10 mammograms do not find anything abnormal." "And if something is found, catching it early usually means it can be treated more easily." "Getting your mammogram is a way to take control, rather than letting the worry control you."

Table 11.3 (*Continued*)

Change	Where	New Content or Content Edits
		Step 6. Encourage Self-Efficacy "Many women who felt scared at first told us that going through with the mammogram gave them peace of mind." "How confident do you feel about keeping your appointment, even with those worries?" **Step 7. Transition to Barriers/Logistics if Needed** "We've talked about your worries, which are important. I'd also like to make sure there aren't any other things, like transportation, timing, or other commitments, that might make it harder to keep your appointment."

document to guide creating of the new navigation component. The template links the planned change determinants (e.g., skill development, attitudes, outcome expectations, self-efficacy, perceived barriers) and methods (e.g., guided practice, modeling, and persuasive communication) to the location of the change in program materials (i.e., online navigation tracking platform) and activities. It also cues the team to write the messages that support the change. For example, if the change is to expand the focus on skill development (determinant) with guided practice (change method), a team would write the instructions for guided practice and note what communication methods would be necessary to accompany the text. If proposed changes include the *addition* of determinants and change methods (rather than simply enhancing them), we suggest preparing a "mini matrix" that pairs the new determinants with performance objectives to create change objectives (see IM Step 2). In this case, the planners are essentially "creating" new program components or activities and are following IM processes for doing so. To finalize the design document, the plan was shared with the planning team, and feedback was incorporated.

Create and Pretest Adapted Materials

Once the team has decided which parts of the intervention will be adapted, and what the new content will be, the next task is pretesting newly adapted or created materials and activities to ensure that the proposed changes are acceptable to the new priority population (see IM Step 4). See IM Step 4 for a description of the stages and processes for how to work with individuals or groups responsible for creating the images or other creative elements. While the focus of pretesting should be on newly created elements and heavily adapted ones, planners may also want to pretest unchanged intervention components to judge their acceptability and engagement with new participants. Soliciting the direct responses of participants and implementers to intervention materials is important to determine whether adaptation decisions made were appropriate and to make additional changes based on pretesting results. During this pretesting phase, individuals or groups respond to program ideas, materials, and components to identify needed corrections. Questions that planners may pose to participants include: What do you understand from this material? Tell me about the people depicted: are they like you? Do you find them believable? What would you be likely to do, after seeing this material? What do you especially like? What do you dislike?

If the planning group decides to make changes based on the pretesting results, they should ensure not to eliminate essential elements, especially change methods. However, the way those methods are operationalized (practical applications) could differ across priority populations or interventions.

Producing Final Adapted Materials and Activities

Chapter 8 describes how to produce or oversee the production of program materials. One caveat is to make sure not to make unintended changes when making planned adaptations, by clearly and rigorously documenting both the planned changes and the changes that are actually implemented.

Task 5: Plan for Implementation of the Adapted EBI

In this task, the planning team will plan implementation of the adapted EBI in a new priority setting. The subtasks include: subtask 5.1: use Implementation Mapping processes to identify implementers, implementation behaviors, and outcomes; subtask 5.2: assess needed changes to existing implementation strategies; subtask 5.3: develop implementation scope, sequence, and protocols; and subtask 5.4: plan logistics including budget, staffing, and materials.

Use Implementation Mapping Processes to Identify Implementers, Implementation Behaviors, and Outcomes

If available, the planning team can review the implementation protocol of the original EBI and then compare it to the implementation considerations for the new site. This comparison helps identify implementers, implementation behaviors, and outcomes necessary to establish a new implementation protocol tailored to the adapted EBI. To pinpoint implementers, the team may ask, "Who will deliver the adapted intervention?" To determine the required implementation behaviors, they could ask, "What behaviors do the implementers need to perform to deliver the adapted intervention?" and "Which implementation outcomes should be achieved?" For a more detailed explanation of the Implementation Mapping process, refer to Chapter 9.

Assess Needed Changes to Existing Implementation Strategies

The planning team begins with a thorough review of the existing implementation strategies of the original EBI. This review entails dissecting the strategies to understand their relevance to new contexts. It involves considering the logistical and contextual differences and similarities between the original setting and the new one, ensuring a deep understanding of how these variables may affect the effectiveness of the existing implementation strategy in a new context. The planning team can benefit from using insights from previous tasks. In particular, key findings from tasks such as the assets assessment (subtask 1.1), the capacity to implement (subtask 1.3), and evaluations of delivery fit and cultural congruence (subtasks 3.3 and 3.4) are especially informative. These elements collectively guide the team in determining the necessary adjustments. By integrating this information, the planning team can identify which components of the existing implementation strategies may be retained or need modification, ensuring that the adapted strategies are both effective and suitable for the new implementation setting.

Develop Implementation Scope, Sequence, and Protocols

The planning team specifies how much of the adapted intervention will be implemented, in what order, and over what period of time. All this information should be clearly written to provide explicit implementation instructions, enabling implementers to understand what to do, as well as when and how to do it. For more details, see Chapter 9.

Plan Logistics Including Budget, Staffing, and Materials

The planning team develops logistical plans that address the budget required for implementation efforts, staffing, and materials. The adapted intervention may necessitate various types of logistical planning and resources different from the original EBI. Therefore, the team should thoroughly evaluate the necessary logistical resources and develop comprehensive plans to secure them, thereby facilitating the successful implementation of the adapted intervention in a new setting.

Task 6: Test the Adapted Intervention

The purpose of this task is to evaluate whether an adapted EBI achieves the same results in the new setting with the made adaptations ("effect evaluation") and to assess how successfully the program was implemented, including its reach to the priority population ("process evaluation"). The findings from previous tasks, such as logic models and the explicit adaptation plan, will lay the groundwork for these subtasks. These include: subtask 6.1: reviewing the logic model of change, matrices, and implementation plan to guide process and effect evaluation; subtask 6.2: developing process evaluation questions and identifying measures; subtask 6.3: developing effect evaluation questions, identifying measures, and selecting a design; subtask 6.4: pilot testing and finalizing the evaluation plan; and subtask 6.5: planning when and how to report evaluation findings. In this chapter, our focus is on the evaluation of the adaptation. For detailed information, refer to Step 6 of IM (Chapter 10).

Review the Logic Model of Change, Matrices, and Implementation Plan to Guide Process and Effect Evaluation

The planning team initially reviews the logic model of change, matrices, and implementation plans from previous tasks to guide the development process and effect evaluation planning. The process evaluation focuses on the delivery of the adapted intervention, encompassing changes in determinants, the implementation context, the intervention's reach and fidelity, dosage, and the implementation of behavioral change methods. This evaluation is crucial to assess the program's reach, its delivery completeness and fidelity, and participant reactions. It also evaluates the reception of the original EBI elements by the target group.

Effect evaluation examines the EBI's impact on QOL, health indicators, behaviors, environmental conditions, and program objectives, including performance objectives and change objectives. This evaluation aims to understand how the modified intervention achieves its expected outcomes. Due to feasibility and time frame constraints, adapters typically do not evaluate all outcomes but focus on those effectively demonstrating the intervention's impact. The evaluation scope is often limited to the extent covered in the original EBI's evaluation, primarily addressing behavior or environmental conditions rather than health outcomes or QOL. The original EBI's scope, outcome indicators, and measures often serve as benchmarks for determining the evaluation's extent for the adapted version. Additionally, the interests of implementers and the implementation environment are considered when selecting effect evaluation measures.

Develop Process Evaluation Questions and Identify Measures

The planning team formulates process evaluation questions that focus primarily on the group receiving the adapted EBI, rather than on a comparison or control group. They need to identify measures that are well-suited to their specific context. In selecting these measures, the team should emphasize the adaptations made to both the intervention and implementation strategies. Often, the planning team may need to develop their own measures, as existing ones might not perfectly fit their context. Examples of such questions could include: How many people completed the adapted intervention? How many participants are not from the intended priority population? How many people dropped out of the adapted intervention? What is the fidelity level of the adapted intervention? What resources or contextual factors influence its delivery? To what degree are participants satisfied with the adapted intervention? What resources, facilities, and funding are necessary to support the intervention adequately? When developing or tailoring these measures, the planning team should strive to create ones with good reliability and validity.

Develop Effect Evaluation Questions, Identify Measures, and Select a Design

The planning team typically focuses on effect outcomes and measures that are feasible within the research project's timeframe and can adequately demonstrate the adapted intervention's effect. When standardized, validated measures for general health and QOL outcomes are available, the planning team can utilize them. When selecting these measures, they should consider those with sound reliability and validity. It is likely that they still need to develop additional effect questions and measures tailored to their evaluation context. They may consider the following example effect questions: "What specific improvements in QOL and health conditions have been observed after the adapted intervention?" "What improvements in behavior and environmental conditions are observed following the intervention?" and "How does the intervention influence personal determinants within the target population?" The team should also explore questions about factors proximal to the adapted intervention, which helps in understanding the causal logic behind the results. When considering the extent of the adaptation and the strength of the evidence supporting the original EBI, the team may opt for "shortcuts" in the logic model. If the adaptation is minimal and the original EBI has strong evidence linking determinants to behavioral and environmental changes, measuring determinants alone may be sufficient, albeit with caution.

In selecting a study design, the team should consider how indicators of the intervention's effects compare to pre- and post-program scenarios, and whether observed changes can be attributed to the intervention. Various designs (Brown et al., 2017a, 2017b; Curran et al., 2024), including hybrid designs, Sequential Multiple Assignment Randomized Implementation Trials (SMART) (Collins et al., 2007), SMART with adaptive randomization (SMART-AR) (Cheung et al., 2015), and MOST (Collins et al., 2007) implementation trials, are available. Hybrid designs can be particularly useful (Curran, 2022; Landes et al., 2020). For significant adaptations, a hybrid type 1 design might be chosen to evaluate effectiveness in a new context while exploring implementation outcomes. For minor adaptations, a hybrid type 3 design might focus more on implementation outcomes. If there's equal interest in evaluating both intervention and implementation outcomes, a hybrid type 2 design could be appropriate. For more details, refer to Chapter 10.

Pilot Test and Finalize the Evaluation Plan

The planning team pilot tests their evaluation plans, ideally with intended intervention users, implementers, and others, before finalizing them. The findings from the pilot tests offer the team an opportunity to learn the feasibility of these measures in the priority populations and contexts and to refine their plans and measures. The intended users of the measures and agents involved in the evaluation may perceive the selected measures as a poor fit for them. For instance, when the adapted intervention targets adults with attention issues, they may find it difficult to complete a long-form survey. If so, the planning team would be better off selecting a short-form survey. They might also require a quiet examination room to help participants maintain their focus while completing the survey. Some participants, especially implementers who are busy healthcare providers, may prefer completing outcome measures at their own pace using an asynchronous method, such as a web survey. Likewise, the planners can explore several planning methods, test them, and finalize them to promote a rigorous evaluation process. As a poor fit or conduct of measures can compromise the rigor of the evaluation process, this fine-tuning process is helpful for the planning team to rigorously evaluate the process and effect of the adapted intervention.

Plan When and How to Report Evaluation Findings

The planning team can plan and report their findings by utilizing established reporting standards. They should consider various reporting guidelines and select the one that best suits their particular context. Good examples of established templates include the Enhancing the QUAlity and Transparency Of Health Research (EQUATOR) Network (Altman et al., 2008; EQUATOR Network, 2025), the Consolidated Standards of Reporting Trials (CONSORT) (Hopewell et al., 2025; Moher et al., 2001), Case Report (CARE) guidelines (Riley et al., 2017), and the Standards for Reporting Qualitative Research (SRQR) (Dossett et al., 2021), among others, to enhance the clarity and openness of their evaluation reports.

CASE STUDY

A Case Study of Program Adaptation Using IM ADAPT to Increase Breast and Cervical Cancer Prevention and Early Detection Among Latinas

A planning team comprising UTHealth intervention researchers along with members from the community-based community health worker (CHW) organization, ProSalud, was formed to address the need to increase breast and cervical prevention and early detection among medically underserved Latinas in Houston. The team started by identifying a behavioral intervention called *Cultivando la Salud* (CLS), which was originally developed for migrant farmworkers using the IM program planning framework (Fernández et al., 2005). CLS is a CHW-delivered and community-based breast and cervical cancer screening behavioral intervention originally developed and tested among Mexican-American residing in home settings in farmworker communities in Texas, New Mexico, and California (Fernández et al., 2005).

This case study focuses on the application of IM ADAPT to adapt an EBI for a new urban setting and priority population while maintaining the integrity (theoretical grounding and evidence-based strategies) of the original intervention. In this case study, the planning team had already identified CLS as the EBI to be adapted. Task 1, however, is still needed to ensure a clear understanding of the needs in the new community and setting. Below, the process used is described in detail.

Task 1: Assess the Needs and Assets of the New Population and/or Setting and Develop a Logic Model of Change

Conduct a Needs and Assets Assessment and Develop a Logic Model of the Problem

To develop a logic model of the problem, the planning team, which comprised UTHealth researchers, ProSalud CHWs in the new urban setting, and the ProSalud CHW organization director, conducted a needs and assets assessment using a participatory approach. As part of this needs assessment, both planning team meetings and literature reviews were used. The planning team first decided to expand the priority population beyond the original CLS intervention to ensure that the adapted intervention would encompass all age groups recommended by the American Cancer Society (ACS) for breast and cervical cancer screening, as well as HPV vaccination guidelines. Consequently, the new intervention added HPV vaccination and prioritized medically un-and underinsured Latinas, 21 years old and older and residing in an urban setting, specifically in Houston, Texas. Breast and cervical cancer were specified as the QOL issues that can arise from the target health problem.

Through the needs assessment, behavioral and environmental factors that influence breast and cervical cancer screening and HPV vaccination were further identified. The behavioral factors identified include rarely/never undergoing mammography, Pap tests, and HPV vaccination. Several environmental factors were also noted, such as inconvenient clinic hours and lack of transportation, among others. Additionally, personal determinants that can contribute to these behavioral factors were pinpointed. These determinants included low perceived susceptibility to breast and cervical cancer (Daniel et al., 2023; Vamos et al., 2015) and; negative attitude toward Pap tests, mammograms, and HPV vaccination (Daley et al., 2006; Fernández et al., 2014; Morales-Campos et al., 2021). Figure 11.7 describes the final logic model of the problem.

Develop a Logic Model of Change

The planning team developed the logic model of change (Figure 11.8) based on the synthesis from planning team discussions, the logic model of the problem, literature review, materials from the original CLS intervention, and behavioral theory that guided the development of the original EBI (specifically,

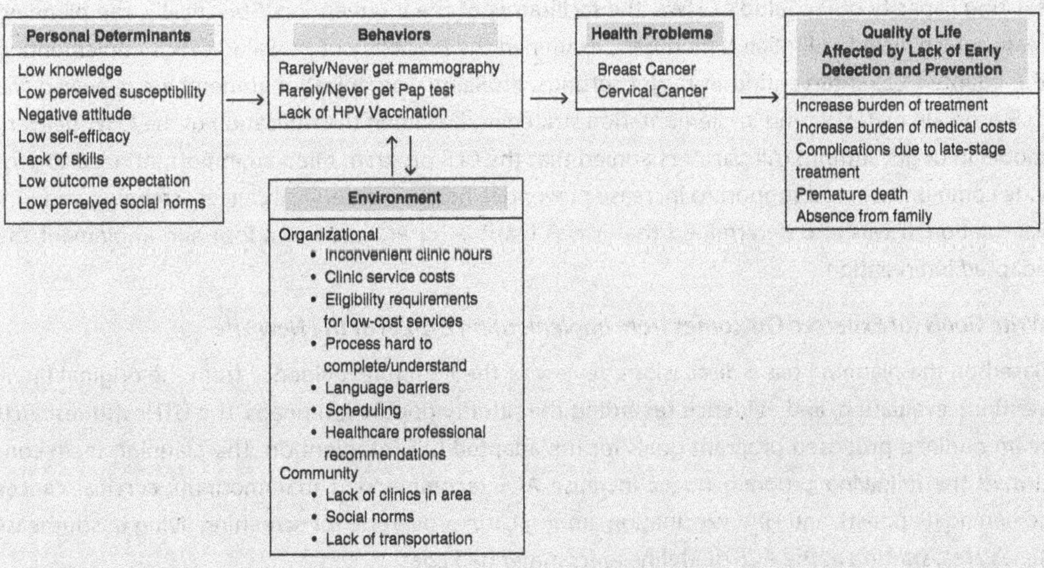

Figure 11.7 Logic Model of the Problem

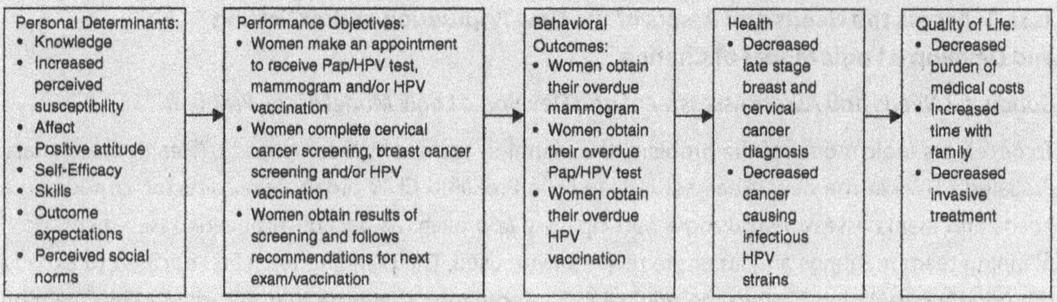

Figure 11.8 Logic Model of Change for All Outcomes

informed by Fishbein's Integrative Behavior Model (Fishbein et al., 2001)). The team specified health, QOL, and behavioral outcomes by drawing information from the original CLS intervention. For example, the logic model retained the behavioral outcomes from the original intervention and introduced a new target outcome: HPV vaccination, which was informed by the team's formative work.

To identify performance objectives, the team brainstormed, "What do people need to do to achieve the desired health outcomes, such as HPV vaccination?" Throughout the brainstorming, planning team members refined the performance objectives from the original intervention to align with the adapted intervention contexts, using insights from Fishbein's Integrated Behavior Model. Additionally, performance objectives focused on overcoming environmental and structural barriers to accessing affordable services in urban areas were included. Finally, findings from the literature review, planning group discussions, and program development materials from the original intervention to identify personal determinants were incorporated into the final logic model of change (Figure 11.8).

Assess Capacity to Implement

The planning team assessed the organizational capacity of ProSalud to implement the adapted intervention. The team aimed to assess whether the adaptation of the CLS program would fit within the existing capacity of ProSalud's CHWs, the facilitators of the intervention. Specifically, the planning team, which included ProSalud members, examined the feasibility of ProSalud CHWs implementing the adapted CLS intervention in target settings. ProSalud's organizational members reviewed the CLS program materials and implementation strategies, including the utilization of the CHW delivery model in target settings. All partners agreed that the CLS program filled an important need to provide community-based support to increase preventive breast and cervical cancer screening and HPV vaccination. It was also determined that it was feasible for ProSalud to adopt and implement the adapted intervention.

Write Goals for Expected Outcomes from Implementing the EBI at the New Site

Based on the planning team discussions, review of the literature, evidence from the original intervention's evaluation, and evidence regarding the priority population needs, the UTHealth research team outlined proposed program goals for the adapted CLS intervention. The planning team confirmed the following program goals: increase ACS recommended mammogram, cervical cancer screening (Pap test), and HPV vaccination among Latinas overdue for screening living in southeast Texas area, starting at the ACS guidelines-recommended ages.

Task 2: Discover EBIs That Potentially Match the Targets for Change and Assess the Level of Evidence and Fit or (If EBI Has Been Selected Already) Determine the Level of Evidence and Fit for a Selected EBI

Search for EBIs and Evaluate the Level of Evidence or Determine Level of Evidence of a Previously Selected EBI and Judge Basic Fit

The UTHealth research team and ProSalud started with identification of an agreement on the selection of the CLS EBI to adapt to the new urban setting and priority population. Because of the results of the EBIs implementation with Mexican-Americans residing in home settings in farmworker communities in Texas, New Mexico, and California, the UTHealth research team and ProSalud members determined the level of evidence to be strong enough to move forward with adaptation. They also agreed that the CLS EBI, once adapted for the new population and setting, would be a good fit.

Task 3: Assess Fit and Plan Adaptation

Use EBI Mapping to Describe and Create a Logic Model of the Existing Intervention

The original CLS intervention's materials and activities, as well as audience and setting for delivery, were documented in the original CLS logic model. EBI Mapping was used to create a logic model of the adapted program, SEMM.

Compare the Logic Model of Change to the Logic Model of the EBI; Judge Fit of Behavioral and Environmental Targets, Determinants Addressed, Methods and Practical Applications Used, Delivery Fit, and Design Features Including Cultural Elements

Because the logic model of change was developed based on the synthesis from planning team discussions, the logic model of the problem, literature review, materials from the original CLS intervention, and behavioral theory that guided the development of the original EBI, when comparing the logic model of change to the logic model of the EBI, it was determined that some changes in the program would be necessary to ensure fit for the new urban setting and priority population.

When assessing the behavioral and environmental targets, the planning team found that there were similar behavioral outcomes focused on participants completing needed cancer screenings. However, to ensure timely uptake of cervical screening, and align the intervention with the updated cervical cancer prevention guidelines at that time, the age for participation would need to be changed. The following new program objectives for cervical cancer prevention were included: (1) women obtain their overdue mammogram for women over 40 years of age; (2) women obtain their overdue cervical cancer screening (Pap test for women over 21 years of age and/or HPV test); and (3) women obtain their overdue HPV vaccination. Two performance objectives remained the same from the original program and an HPV screening was added to the cervical cancer screening-related performance objective, and an additional performance objective for HPV vaccination was incorporated. The adapted intervention's performance objectives included: (1) women make an appointment to receive a Pap test cervical cancer screening/mammogram/HPV vaccination; (2) women complete cervical/breast cancer screening/HPV vaccination; (3) women obtain results of the screening and follows recommendations for next exam; (4) women make an appointment to receive follow-up exams for abnormal screening results; and (5) women completes follow-up exams for abnormal screening results (Table 11.4).

The personal determinants that the original program addresses to change behaviors and subbehaviors were assessed. The fit of the determinants and change methods of the CLS intervention were

Table 11.4 Comparison of Original Program (CLS) and Adapted Program (SEMM): Health Goals, Priority Populations, Delivery Setting, Delivery Methods, and Materials (EBI Mapping)

Dimension	Cultivando la Salud (Original Intervention)	Salud en Mis Manos[a] (Adapted Intervention)
Priority population (Who)	Mexican-American, migrant farm workers, aged 50 and older	Un- and under-insured Latinas, 21 years old and older
Health outcomes	Cervical cancer early detection and prevention Breast cancer early detection and improved survival	Cervical cancer early detection and prevention. Breast cancer early detection and improved survival.
Behavioral outcomes	Increase mammogram screening Increase Pap test screening	Increase mammogram screening Increase Pap test screening Increase HPV test screening Increase HPV vaccination
Environmental and structural factors influencing health or behavior	Migrant farmworker health clinics provide access for the target population; Transportation barriers	Low access to affordable preventive healthcare; FQHCs and safetynet clinic complex eligibility process challenging for low literate women to complete to qualify for low-cost services; public hospitals have long wait times; transportation; childcare; work conflicts with clinic schedule
Delivery	One-on-one education by CHW	Group and one-on-one education by CHW One-on-one ongoing support by Health Coach Navigator (HCN)
Setting	Homes of migrant farmworkers	Community-based public places (e.g., community centers, small local businesses, health fairs) Telephone-based (CHW home office or organization office space)
Delivery materials and/methods	Flip book Video Referral to migrant farmworker clinic	Edited flip-book FQHC and safetynet clinic database to guide delivery of clinic referrals based on costs and location Plan of Action Activity Health coaching and navigation electronic guide (with coaching scripts) and tracking logs
Content (What)	Breast cancer screening Mammogram Cervical cancer screening Pap test	Breast cancer screening Mammogram Cervical cancer screening Pap test HPV test HPV vaccine How to qualify for financial coverage of medical care How to find a doctor/make appointments Goal setting to overcome complex barriers to accessing clinics

[a] Adapted CLS-Houston intervention strategies, and includes additional intervention strategies developed for delivery in urban and suburban settings.

compared to those of the new setting and priority population by comparing the logic models of the original CLS intervention with those created for the adapted intervention. Most determinants from the original program intervention were found relevant in the new priority population. However, new determinants were also incorporated, such as a negative attitude toward Pap tests, mammograms, and HPV vaccination and more emphasis on increasing perceived benefits regarding screening/HPV vaccination in the context of competing priorities for their time. In addition, self-efficacy and skills to make appointments and follow-up appointments to address the complex access barriers uninsured Latinas face in the new setting were included.

In consideration of the complex access barriers and eligibility requirements related to accessing low-cost services in the new setting and priority community, change methods and practical applications to increase participants' knowledge, skills and self-efficacy related to completing eligibility paperwork, and scheduling appointments were identified. Most change methods from the original CLS intervention such as modeling, persuasive communication, discussion, imagery and goal setting were incorporated in the adapted intervention. However, more emphasis on these methods was addressed by developing a new component—telephone-based health coach navigation. Health coach navigation sessions include a series of one-on-one goal setting and personal support sessions to address complex access barriers, as well as to provide persuasive communication and non-judgmental personal support to women in planning appointments in the context of other commonly reported competing priorities for their time (e.g., work, taking care of children, or other health priorities).

The planning team assessed the design features and delivery fit of the CLS intervention in the new setting and with regards to cultural fit with the new priority population. The original CLS intervention was delivered by a CHW in a one-on-one session using a large flip book. Because the delivery format was changed from one-on-one to a group format, there was a need to address individual participants' barriers through one-on-one follow-up support sessions. In addition, individualized follow-up support enabled more intensive support to navigate the complicated environmental factors in the urban community system and culture, thus a new delivery method, called health coach navigation calls, was introduced. From our planning sessions, we learned from CHWs that many women in urban settings face barriers to accessing medical care, including financial barriers, location, clinic hours, language, etc. The health coach navigation calls were designed to offer personal support, problem-solving, and empathetic listening as a way for the program to provide one-on-one barrier mitigation and personal support to help women overcome structural barriers in the urban setting. Lastly, the original video from the CLS intervention was removed due to its lack of relevance concerning the images, which reflected a rural setting, and included images of a more diverse age range of Latina women to better represent the younger ages of the priority groups targeted, especially for HPV vaccination.

Judge Implementation Fit and Make Decisions About What Should Change Considering Core Elements (Core Functions) and How to Retain Them

The planning team assessed the implementation fit of the CLS intervention in the new setting, including the CHW implementers' capacity to implement the intervention, as well as the acceptability of the implementation plan (i.e., reaching women door-to-door at their home residences). Through planning discussions with CHWs, the intervention implementers and the CHWs communicated that they felt reluctant to recruit women and deliver education door-to-door in Houston apartment complexes due to safety concerns. Therefore, the planning team changed the delivery plan from the original one-on-one, door-to-door intervention to delivery in community locations, with a focus on delivering the adapted behavioral education to groups. The planning team also developed community outreach and recruitment strategies that would require community organizations serving the priority population to partner with the community-based intervention (SEMM) to refer women to the SEMM program. Community partners also provided space for the CHWs to deliver the education session to women in community settings. To support women in overcoming complex structural barriers to accessing clinics, the team developed a health coach navigation implementation plan, designed to provide ongoing one-on-one telephone-based support to women after they completed the education session. The new community-based implementation plan required the development of new implementation materials and resources to support recruitment of women directly, as well as to promote engagement with community organizations to refer women to the SEMM program. Materials were developed to support community-wide outreach to develop a network of organizational partners throughout the community. The new SEMM program materials and resources also included new materials to support the health coach navigation program component, including a geographically specific clinic referral list, laptops, electronic forms to track patient navigation, and health coaching and navigation electronic protocol (with coaching messages and goal-setting steps), navigation tracking logs, and a CHW delivery manual.

The essential element of the CLS intervention, specifically content about breast and cervical cancer screenings, remained in the SEMM intervention. For SEMM, the planning team modified the information in response to changes in screening guidelines and also added information on the HPV vaccine and the new guidelines for HPV vaccination. The SEMM intervention also developed resources to support health coaching and navigation, providing clinic referrals based on required screenings, clinic financial coverage for uninsured or underinsured populations, and participants' preferred locations, as well as protocolized follow-up with women by a patient navigator to enroll women in the subsequent health coach navigation component of the program within two weeks of completing the education session. The new navigation component provided women the option of receiving ongoing personalized support to address personal barriers one-on-one to facilitate access to clinics for services.

Task 4: Adapt Intervention Components

Prepare Design Documents for the Adaptations

A subset of the planning team created the design document outlining what each of the new flipchart revisions should address (e.g., including updated guidelines for HPV vaccination). Additionally, the need for several educational images for inclusion in the newly adapted intervention was identified. The health coach navigation steps and tracking tools were also designed.

Create and Pretest Adapted Materials

The planning team conducted a case study for pretesting adapted materials to understand the strengths and challenges of the adapted materials. The case study included recruitment, scheduling eligible women for education sessions, education delivery in groups, and follow-up health navigation telephone support. Due to the rapid adaptation process used in this two-year funded project, further adaptations were based on feedback obtained from the CHWs. Continuous changes were made as the intervention was rolled out. During the delivery of the intervention, CHWs and CHW managers identified improvements, either in response to participants' questions during the education session or due to challenges in delivering the program. The experiences and observations of the CHW and CHW managers became the primary targets for gathering feedback and opportunities to refine the intervention. Through weekly debriefings with CHWs, the planning team determined the adaptation needs for material and programmatic tools (e.g., protocols). These observations also resulted in refinements to the recruitment tracking logs and callback schedule (initial HCN calls to participants, which were originally planned for two weeks post-education session, were shortened to two days). This change aimed to maintain a connection with women who responded more positively to a call with a shorter follow-up time.

Produce Final Adapted Materials and Activities

Throughout the pretesting and refinement processes, the planning group produced adapted materials covering breast cancer screening mammograms, cervical cancer screenings, Pap tests, HPV vaccines, how to qualify for financial coverage of medical care, how to find a doctor/make appointments, and goal setting and coach scripts to overcome complex barriers to accessing clinics.

Task 5: Plan for Implementation of the Adapted EBI

Use Implementation Mapping Processes to Identify Implementers, Implementation Behaviors, and Outcomes of the Adapted Intervention and Create/Adapt Strategies If Needed

Because the adaptation of the EBI was planned with the ProSalud community partners, the implementers were part of the planning process. To plan implementation behaviors program planners worked with ProSalud leadership and facilitated discussions with CHWs on the potential challenges and facilitators of implementing the program. New implementation support strategies included ongoing CHW meetings to support CHWs in overcoming implementation barriers. Weekly implementer meetings were planned to facilitate CHW implementation of the program. The meetings were designed to provide CHWs with implementation support, including facilitated discussions to share lessons learned and to identify and promote successful recruitment strategies. In addition, these meetings provided an opportunity for CHWs to share successes and problem solve challenges related to delivery of group education and the health coach navigation program components.

Develop Implementation Scope, Sequence, and Protocols

Because the health coach navigation component was new, and designed to provide women with ongoing support to overcome personal and structural barriers to accessing clinics, a new navigation protocol and tools were developed, To facilitate tracking of telephone-based navigation activities, health coach navigators used electronic tracking logs developed to record date and time of calls (or call attempts), specific support provided during navigation activities, as well as outcome of calls, including dates of completed screening or HPV vaccination(s). This tracking system was developed to assist the HCNs in tracking barriers identified, goals set, and support provided (to inform the next follow-up telephone call, if needed). Navigators were also able to provide women with appointment scheduling assistance, reminders, and follow-up calls post-appointment date to remind women to get their results and to provide support for additional clinical appointments, if needed.

Plan Logistics Including Budget, Staffing, and Materials

The budget for all phases of program adaptation, production of materials, staffing, and evaluation was planned by the UTHealth team with the ProSalud leadership. Intervention and implementation protocols were documented in a program Manual of Procedures, which also provided instructions for administrative tasks (e.g., keeping mileage and submitting timesheets) and logistics of planning SEMM delivery.

Task 6: Test the Adapted Intervention

Review the Logic Model of Change, Matrices, and Implementation Plan to Guide Process and Effect Evaluation

The logic model provided the road map for identifying indicators and measures for the evaluation. The primary outcomes planned for the SEMM intervention included completion of mammography, Pap test screening, and/or HPV vaccination (a secondary outcome, as it was added after the study began).

The behavioral determinants (e.g., self-efficacy, perceived pros and cons of screening, and perceived benefits, etc.) were also provided by the logic model for the adapted program (SEMM). Other potential mediating or moderating factors were identified to characterize screening patterns in our new priority population, such as demographic characteristics (e.g., age, country of origin, language preference, acculturation), as well as socioeconomic indicators, (e.g., employment status and education attainment), health care access (e.g., insurance, usual source of care, recent health concerns), and health history (e.g., previous history of screening behaviors, family history of cancer).

Evaluation of the adapted program included evaluation of the effectiveness of the adapted SEMM program on two different levels, (1) a programmatic level, focused on a process evaluation of the adaptation and resulting implementation of the adapted intervention, as well as (2) the primary outcome, the intervention's primary effect on increasing screening among participants.

Develop Process Evaluation Questions and Identify Measures

Metrics associated with activities planned and delivered were examined as part of the process evaluation plan. To determine the reach of the adapted SEMM intervention, after six months of implementation, the planning team examined reach defined in terms of number of eligible Latinas that completed the breast and cervical cancer screening/HPV vaccination needs assessment (eligibility) form, the number of eligible women reached (completed the CHW-delivered education session), and the number of cancer-specific screening referrals made. To assess the navigation program, program reach (percent of women who received at least one navigation call among participants who completed an education session), dose of the navigation program (number of navigation sessions completed), and types and numbers of referrals and/or navigation support provided were examined. To assess satisfaction with program delivery, a navigation satisfaction scale was identified, adapted, and utilized to collect satisfaction data on a six-month follow-up survey.

Develop Effect Evaluation Questions, Identify Measures, and Select a Design

The evaluation questions focused on examining the effect of the intervention on the behavioral outcomes (e.g., completion of a needed mammogram, Pap test or HPV vaccine acceptance), as well as subbehaviors identified as required to achieve the targeted outcome (e.g., appointments scheduled). Thus, an evaluation question for mammography was included, "What changes were made in making primary care doctor's appointments to get a mammogram referral?" To understand the mechanisms of change in regards to the effect of the intervention on the targeted behavioral determinants, evaluation questions were informed by the behavioral determinants documented on the logic model, with a strong focus on understanding whether there was a change in the newly identified and targeted determinants (e.g., change objective related to determinants such as self-efficacy and skills to schedule appointments).

To determine effectiveness of the adapted intervention on increasing screening a randomized study design was used with a SEMM intervention arm and a comparison arm (usual care included delivery of print education materials about breast and cervical cancer screening and HPV vaccination; this arm is also referred to as the delayed SEMM intervention). After CHWs completed the breast and cervical cancer and HPV vaccination needs assessment form, women who were identified as in need of a screening or HPV vaccine were invited to participate in the study designed to assess the effect of the adapted intervention on all outcomes. After CHWs read an informed consent form and explained the study (in Spanish or English), and the prospective participants signed the form, the participant was called by a bilingual research assistant who conducted baseline interviews in Spanish or English. The research assistant initiated a participant tracking form to document all contact information. After women were randomized to either a comparison arm (delayed SEMM program) or intervention group, data collectors immediately scheduled the participants' education session with a CHWs. Women in the comparison arm were delivered print education materials about breast and cervical cancer screening and HPV vaccination. At six months post-baseline, the data collectors conducted the follow-up survey with all participants and immediately invited the women in the comparison arm to attend the SEMM CHW-delivered education and navigation sessions.

As part of the effect evaluation, we planned descriptive analyses to characterize participants and examine any differences between the two randomized group arms across social and demographic variables (e.g., age, country of origin/ancestry, language preference, socioeconomic status, and access to health care). Chi-square tests were used to assess significant differences by categorical variables and t-tests by continuous variables (significance determined by $p < .05$). A logistic regression was used to evaluate the effect of the program on the dichotomized screening outcome (yes/no), while adjusting for potential imbalance by including in the model those significant variables identified in the descriptive analyses.

Pilot Test and Finalize the Evaluation Plan

Throughout the delivery of the program, we conducted weekly process monitoring of reach (both community partners and women reached to participate in the SEMM program), dose of navigation calls, and documented barriers and facilitators to implementation at weekly meetings with CHWs. These meetings informed ongoing adaptation to improve the program in the early phase of implementation. In the final evaluation plan, all outcomes were measured by self-report and collected through surveys implemented by bilingual, female data collectors who were not part of intervention delivery. The survey instrument was adapted from the original CLS study, which developed a 256-item baseline survey that included questions about mammography and Pap test screening history and knowledge and attitudes about screening, as well as general health and demographic characteristics.

Metrics related to intervention delivery were collected through program tracking forms. CHWs used recruitment forms to document women identified as needing a screening/HPV vaccine and enrolled to attend the education program). CHW group education session encounter forms to document education delivery activities were developed (e.g., number of women participants attending an education session, time spent delivering the education session, etc.). Navigators used navigation tracking logs to similarly document navigation activities (e.g., number of participants engaged in navigation, number of navigation calls made, barriers identified, etc.).

Plan When and How to Report Evaluation Findings

An important step to processing the results included processing the experience of the implementer. All evaluation results were discussed and interpreted with a project team, which included all the program implementers and evaluation subgroups. CHWs discussed challenges, opportunities, and informed adaptations. Ongoing discussions with implementers proved to be crucial for continuous program improvements, as well as to support satisfaction among the implementers. All results were reported back to program funders, as well as implementers.

Summary

In this chapter, we introduce the concept of using IM for the adaptation of EBIs to new populations and settings, referred to as IM ADAPT. EBIs encompass a wide range of strategies, such as policies, clinical guidelines, or health promotion interventions, proven effective through research. Adaptations can involve adding, deleting, or modifying various aspects of an EBI, including content, delivery format, or implementation strategies.

The chapter emphasizes the importance of adaptation as a more efficient and effective approach compared to creating entirely new interventions. Adapting EBIs can save time and resources, especially when working with diverse and underserved populations. Adaptations can improve engagement, acceptability, and health outcomes. The types and timing of adaptations are discussed, including planned adaptations made before or during implementation and spontaneous adaptations that occur without prior planning. The chapter introduces IM ADAPT as a tool primarily used for prospective planned adaptation. IM ADAPT allows planners to identify and plan for adaptations in both the EBI itself and its implementation strategies.

Addressing health equity through adaptation is a key theme, with the chapter emphasizing the importance of cultural adaptations and community engagement to serve diverse populations. Cultural adaptations involve modifying EBI content, activities, or language to align with cultural patterns, beliefs, and values. Engaging communities and key stakeholders ensures that adaptations are aligned with the needs and preferences of the local population.

The chapter discusses challenges in adaptation, including the need to identify and retain core elements of an EBI while balancing the desire for fit with the new context. Core elements are the essential components that make an EBI effective and should remain intact during adaptation. The chapter provides guidance on how to identify and prioritize core elements.

The IM ADAPT framework is described. It consists of six tasks that guide the adaptation process. These tasks involve assessing needs and assets, discovering EBIs, assessing fit and planning adaptations, adapting intervention components, planning for implementation, and testing the adapted intervention. The description of tasks is followed by an example. Overall, the chapter provides a comprehensive overview of the process of using IM ADAPT for the systematic adaptation of EBIs to new populations and settings, emphasizing the importance of cultural competence, community engagement, and retaining core elements.

Discussion Questions and Learning Activities

1. Explain the dilemma in the decision regarding adapting a program for a new setting and retaining fidelity to the original program to assure continuing effectiveness.
2. What is meant by the term core elements of an EBI?

3. Describe the sequence of activities for finding an EBI and what would you consider when deciding upon one.
4. Describe strengths and weaknesses of IM ADAPT as a systematic process for helping to improve fit of an EBI as it is used in a new site.

References

Aarons, G. A., Green, A. E., Palinkas, L. A., Self-Brown, S., Whitaker, D. J., Lutzker, J. R., Silovsky, J. F., Hecht, D. B., & Chaffin, M. J. (2012). Dynamic adaptation process to implement an evidence-based child maltreatment intervention. *Implementation Science, 7*(1), 1–9.

Altman, D. G., Simera, I., Hoey, J., Moher, D., & Schulz, K. (2008). EQUATOR: Reporting guidelines for health research. *The Lancet, 371*(9619), 1149–1150.

Alvidrez, J., Nápoles, A. M., Bernal, G., Lloyd, J., Cargill, V., Godette, D., Cooper, L., Horse Brave Heart, M. Y., Das, R., & Farhat, T. (2019). Building the evidence base to inform planned intervention adaptations by practitioners serving health disparity populations. *American Journal of Public Health, 109*(S1), S94–S101.

Aronson, E. (2002). Building empathy, compassion, and achievement in the jigsaw classroom. In J. Aronson (Ed.), *Improving academic achievement: Impact of psychological factors on education* (pp. 209–225). Academic Press. doi:10.1016/B978-012064455-1/50013-0

Austin, J. D., Rodriguez, S. A., Savas, L. S., Megdal, T., Ramondetta, L., & Fernandez, M. E. (2020). Using intervention mapping to develop a provider intervention to increase HPV vaccination in a federally qualified health center. *Frontiers in Public Health, 905*, 530596.

Ballard, A. M., Davis, A., & Hoffner, C. A. (2021). The Impact of Health Narratives on Persuasion in African American Women: A Systematic Review and Meta-Analysis. *Health Communication, 36*(5), 560–571. doi:10.1080/10410236.2020.1731936

Baron, R. C., Chattopadhyay, S. K., Coates, R. J., Habarta, N., Kalra, G. P., Kerner, J., Leeks, K. D., Melillo, S., Rimer, B. K., Wilson, K. M., & Community Preventive Services Task Force (CPSTF) (2009). *Increasing Cancer Screening: Group Education for Clients [for Breast, Cervical, and Colorectal Cancers]*. American Journal of Preventive Medicine, CPSTF Finding and Rationale Statement. doi:10.15620/cdc/164172

Barrera, M., Berkel, C., & Castro, F. G. (2017). Directions for the Advancement of Culturally Adapted Preventive Interventions: Local Adaptations, Engagement, and Sustainability. *Prevention Science, 18*, 640–648. doi:10.1007/s11121-016-0705-9

Bartholomew, L., Highfield, L., Hartman, M., Mullen, P., Leerlooijer, J., Ruiter, R., Fernández, M., & Kok Gund Parcel, G. (2016). Using intervention mapping to adapt evidence-based interventions. In *Planning health promotion programs. An intervention mapping approach* (4th ed., pp. 597–649). San Francisco, CA: Jossey-Bass.

Baumann, A. A., & Cabassa, L. J. (2020). Reframing implementation science to address inequities in healthcare delivery. *BMC Health Services Research, 20*(1), 1–9. doi:10.1186/s12913-020-4975-3

Baumann, A. A., Powell, B. J., Kohl, P. L., Tabak, R. G., Penalba, V., Proctor, E. K., Domenech-Rodriguez, M. M., & Cabassa, L. J. (2015). Cultural adaptation and implementation of evidence-based parent-training: A systematic review and critique of guiding evidence. *Children and Youth Services Review, 53*, 113–120.

Bernal, G., Jiménez-Chafey, M. I., & Domenech Rodríguez, M. M. (2009). Cultural adaptation of treatments: A resource for considering culture in evidence-based practice. *Professional Psychology: Research and Practice, 40*(4), 361.

Broder-Fingert, S., Kuhn, J., Sheldrick, R. C., Chu, A., Fortuna, L., Jordan, M., Rubin, D., & Feinberg, E. (2019). Using the multiphase optimization strategy (MOST) framework to test intervention delivery strategies: A study protocol. *Trials, 20*(1), 1–15.

Brown, B., Gabra, M. I., & Pellman, H. (2017a). Reasons for acceptance or refusal of human papillomavirus vaccine in a California pediatric practice. *Papillomavirus Research, 3*, 42–45.

Brown, C. H., Curran, G., Palinkas, L. A., Aarons, G. A., Wells, K. B., Jones, L., Collins, L. M., Duan, N., Mittman, B. S., & Wallace, A. (2017b). An overview of research and evaluation designs for dissemination and implementation. *Annual Review of Public Health, 38*, 1–22.

Brownson, R. C., Fielding, J. E., & Green, L. W. (2018). Building capacity for evidence-based public health: Reconciling the pulls of practice and the push of research. *Annual Review of Public Health, 39*, 27–53.

Bundy, Ł. T., Haardörfer, R., Kegler, M. C., Owolabi, S., Berg, C. J., Escoffery, C., Thompson, T., Mullen, P. D., Williams, R., Hovell, M., & Kahl, T. (2019). Disseminating a smoke free homes program to low-income households through 2-1-1: Results of a national impact evaluation. *Nicotine & Tobacco Research, 22*(4), 498–505. doi:10.1093/ntr/nty256

Burlew, A., Copeland, V., Ahuama-Jonas, C., & Calsyn, D. (2013). Does cultural adaptation have a role in substance abuse treatment? *Social Work in Public Health, 28*(3–4), 440–460. doi:10.1080/19371918.2013.774811

Cancer Prevention and Control Research Network. (2021). EBI Comparison Tool. Accessed March 6, 2023, https://cpcrn.org/training.

Card, J. J., Solomon, J., & Cunningham, S. D. (2011). How to adapt effective programs for use in new contexts. *Health Promotion Practice, 12*(1), 25–35. doi:10.1177/1524839909348592

Carvalho, M., Honeycutt, S., Escoffery, C., Glanz, K., Sabbs, D., & Kegler, M. (2013). Balancing fidelity and adaptation: Implementing evidence-based chronic disease prevention programs. *Journal of Public Health Management and Practice, 19*(4), 348–356. doi:10.1097/PHH.0b013e31826d80eb

Castro, F., & Yasui, M. (2017). Advances in EBI development for diverse populations: Towards a science of intervention adaptation. *Prevention Science, 18*(6), 623–629. doi:10.1007/s11121-017-0809-x

Castro, F. G., Barrera, M., & Martinez, C. R. (2004). The cultural adaptation of prevention interventions: Resolving tensions between fidelity and fit. *Prevention Science, 5*(1), 41–45.

Castro, Y., Fernández, M. E., Strong, L. L., Stewart, D. W., Krasny, S., Hernandez Robles, E., Heredia, N., Spears, C. A., Correa-Fernández, V., & Eakin, E. (2015). Adaptation of a counseling intervention to address multiple cancer risk factors among overweight/obese latino smokers. *Health Education & Behavior, 42*(1), 65–72.

Chambers, D. A., Glasgow, R. E., & Stange, K. C. (2013). The dynamic sustainability framework: Addressing the paradox of sustainment amid ongoing change. *Implementation Science, 8*(1), 117.

Chambers, D. A., & Norton, W. E. (2016). The adaptome: Advancing the science of intervention adaptation. *American Journal of Preventive Medicine, 51*(4), S124–S131.

Chen, E. K., Reid, M., Parker, S. J., & Pillemer, K. (2013). Tailoring evidence-based interventions for new populations: A method for program adaptation through community engagement. *Evaluation & the Health Professions, 36*(1), 73–92.

Cheung, Y. K., Chakraborty, B., & Davidson, K. W. (2015). Sequential multiple assignment randomized trial (SMART) with adaptive randomization for quality improvement in depression treatment program. *Biometrics, 71*(2), 450–459.

Cho, D., Basen-Engquist, K., Acquati, C., Pettaway, C., Ma, H., Markofski, M., Li, Y., Canfield, S. E., Gregg, J., & McNeill, L. H. (2020). Cultural adaptation of evidence-based lifestyle interventions for African American men with prostate cancer: A dyadic approach. *American Journal of Men's Health, 14*(6), 1557988320945449.

Collins, L. M., Murphy, S. A., & Strecher, V. (2007 May). The multiphase optimization strategy (MOST) and the sequential multiple assignment randomized trial (SMART): new methods for more potent eHealth interventions. *American Journal of Preventive Medicine, 32*(5 Suppl), S112–S118. doi:10.1016/j.amepre.2007.01.022

Curran, G. M., Landes, S. J., McBain, S. A., Pyne, J. M., Smith, J. D., Fernandez, M. E., Chambers, D. A., & Mittman, B. S. (2022 Dec). Reflections on 10 years of effectiveness-implementation hybrid studies. *Front Health Serv., 8*(2), 1053496. doi:10.3389/frhs.2022.1053496

Curran, G. M., and others. (2024). Design and analysis in dissemination and implementation research. In Ross C. Brownson, Graham A. Colditz, & Enola K. Proctor (Eds.), *Dissemination and implementation research in health: Translating science to practice, 3rd edn* (New York, 2023; online edn, Oxford Academic, 21 Mar. 2024). doi:10.1093/oso/9780197660690.003.0014

Daley, M. F., Liddon, N., Crane, L. A., Beaty, B. L., Barrow, J., Babbel, C., Markowitz, L. E., Dunne, E. F., Stokley, S., Dickinson, L. M., Berman, S., & Kempe, A. (2006). A national survey of pediatrician knowledge and attitudes regarding human papillomavirus vaccination. *Pediatrics, 118*(6), 2280–2289. doi:10.1542/peds.2006-1946

Damschroder, L. J., Aron, D. C., Keith, R. E., Kirsh, S. R., Alexander, J. A., & Lowery, J. C. (2009). Fostering implementation of health services research findings into practice: A consolidated framework for advancing implementation science. *Implementation Science, 4*(1), 1–15.

Damschroder, L. J., & Lowery, J. C. (2013). Evaluation of a large-scale weight management program using the consolidated framework for implementation research (CFIR). *Implementation Sci, **8**,* 51. doi:10.1186/1748-5908-8-51

Damschroder, L. J., Reardon, C. M., Widerquist, M. A. O., & Lowery, J. (2022). The updated consolidated framework for implementation research based on user feedback. *Implementation Science, 17*(1), 1–16.

Daniel, E. S., Nelson-George, T., Ramdeen-Mootoo, G., Nashwan, A. J., Seiwdass, P., & Victor, V. M. (2023). Knowledge, attitude, and intention to obtain HPV vaccination among undergraduate students in Saint Lucia.

DiClemente, C. C., & Graydon, M. M. (2020). 10 changing behavior using the transtheoretical model. In M. S. Hagger, L. D. Cameron, K. Hamilton, N. Hankonen, & T. Lintunen (Eds.), *The handbook of behavior change* (Vol. 136, pp. 136–149). Cambridge University Press. doi:10.1017/9781108677318.010

Dossett, L. A., Kaji, A. H., & Cochran, A. (2021). SRQR and COREQ reporting guidelines for qualitative studies. *JAMA Surgery, 156*(9), 875–876.

Durlak, J. A., & DuPre, E. P. (2008). Implementation matters: a review of research on the influence of implementation on program outcomes and the factors affecting implementation. *American journal of community psychology, 41*(3-4), 327–350. doi:10.1007/s10464-008-9165-0

Eisman, A. B., Kilbourne, A. M., Greene, D., Walton, M., & Cunningham, R. (2020). The user-program interaction: How teacher experience shapes the relationship between intervention packaging and fidelity to a state-adopted health curriculum. *Prevention Science, 21*, 820–829.

Ellis, D. M., Draheim, A. A., & Anderson, P. L. (2022). Culturally adapted digital mental health interventions for ethnic/racial minorities: A systematic review and meta-analysis. *Journal of Consulting and Clinical Psychology, 90*(10), 717.

EQUATOR Network. (2025, August 25). Comprehensive research reporting guidelines: EQUATOR Network overview. https://systematicliteraturereviews.com/equator-network/.

Escoffery, C., Lebow-Skelley, E., Udelson, H., Böing, E. A., Wood, R., Fernandez, M. E., & Mullen, P. D. (2019). A scoping study of frameworks for adapting public health evidence-based interventions. *Translational Behavioral Medicine, 9*(1), 1–10.

Escoffery, C., Mullen, P., Lebow-Skelley, E., Haardoerfer, R., Boing, E., Udelson, H., Reece, D., Wood, R., Hartman, M., & Fernandez, M. (2018). Systematic review of adaptations of public health evidence-based interventions. *Implementation Science, 13*(125). doi:10.1186/s13012-018-0815-09

Fernandez, M. E., Baumann, A. A., Beg, S. S. (2025). Cultural adaptations of interventions. In N. Schneiderman, T. A. Revenson, A. F. Abraído-Lanza, T. W. Smith, N. B. Anderson, M. H. Antoni, F. J. Penedo (Eds.), *APA handbook of health psychology, Vol. 3. Health psychology and public health* (pp. 127–153). American Psychological Association. doi:10.1037/0000396-008

Fernández, M. E., Gonzales, A., Tortolero-Luna, G., Partida, S., & Bartholomew, L. K. (2005). Using intervention mapping to develop a breast and cervical cancer screening program for Hispanic farmworkers: Cultivando La Salud. *Health promotion practice, 6*(4), 394–404. doi:10.1177/1524839905278810

Fernández, M. E., Melvin, C. L., Leeman, J., Ribisl, K. M., Allen, J. D., Kegler, M. C., Bastani, R., Ory, M. G., Risendal, B. C., & Hannon, P. A. (2014). The cancer prevention and control research network: An interactive systems approach to advancing cancer control implementation research and practice. *Cancer Epidemiology, Biomarkers & Prevention, 23*(11), 2512–2521.

Fishbein, M., Triandis, H. C., Kanfer, F. H., Becker, M., Middlestadt, S. E., & Eichler, A. (2001). Factors influencing behavior and behavior change. In A. S. Baum, T. A. Revenson, & J. E. Singer (Eds.), *Handbook of health psychology* (pp. 1–17). Mahwah, NJ: Lawrence Erlbaum.

Ginsburg, L. R., Hoben, M., Easterbrook, A., Andersen, E., Anderson, R. A., Cranley, L., Lanham, H. J., Norton, P. G., Weeks, L. E., & Estabrooks, C. A. (2020). Examining fidelity in the INFORM trial: A complex team-based behavioral intervention. *Implementation Science, 15*, 1–11.

Glasgow, R. E., Lichtenstein, E., & Marcus, A. C. (2003 Aug). Why don't we see more translation of health promotion research to practice? Rethinking the efficacy-to-effectiveness transition. *Am J Public Health.*, *93*(8), 1261–1267. doi:10.2105/ajph.93.8.1261

Hopewell, S., Chan, A. W., Collins, G. S., Hróbjartsson, A., Moher, D., Schulz, K. F., Tunn, R., Aggarwal, R., Berkwits, M., Berlin, J. A., Bhandari, N., Butcher, N. J., Campbell, M. K., Chidebe, R. C. W., Elbourne, D., Farmer, A., Fergusson, D. A., Golub, R. M., Goodman, S. N., Hoffmann, T. C., Ioannidis, J. P. A., Kahan, B. C., Knowles, R. L., Lamb, S. E., Lewis, S., Loder, E., Offringa, M., Ravaud, P., Richards, D. P., Rockhold, F.W., Schriger, D. L., Siegfried, N. L., Staniszewska, S., Taylor, R. S., Thabane, L., Torgerson, D., Vohra, S., White, I. R., Boutron, I. (2025). CONSORT 2025 statement: updated guideline for reporting randomised trials. *BMJ*, 389, e081123. doi: 10.1136/bmj-2024-081123

Huang, Y., & Shen, F. (2016). Effects of cultural tailoring on persuasion in cancer communication: A meta-analysis. *Journal of Communication*, *66*(4), 694–715. doi:10.1111/jcom.12243

Johnson O, Delk D. W. (2024). #Wematter: Creating culturally tailored health promotion content for Black and Latina college women on Instagram. *Digital Health*, doi:10.1177/20552076241241919

Kalver, E. H., McInnes, D. K., Yakovchenko, V., Hyde, J., Petrakis, B. A., & Kim, B. (2021). The CORE (Consensus on Relevant Elements) approach to determining initial core components of an innovation. *Frontiers in Health Services*, 1, 752177. doi:10.3389/frhs.2021.752177

Kegler, M., Haardoerfer, R., Melanson, T., Allen, L., Bundy, L., Kreuter, M., Williams, R., Hovell, M., & Mullen, P. D. (2019). Steps toward scalability: Illustrations from a smoke-free homes program. *Health Education & Behavior*, *46*(5), 773–781. doi:10.1177/1090198119848767

Kendall, P. C., & Frank, H. E. (2018). Implementing evidence-based treatment protocols: Flexibility within fidelity. *Clinical Psychology: Science and Practice*, *25*(4), e12271.

Kok, G., Gottlieb, N. H., Peters, G.-J. Y., Mullen, P. D., Parcel, G. S., Ruiter, R. A., Fernández, M. E., Markham, C., & Bartholomew, L. K. (2016). A taxonomy of behaviour change methods: An intervention mapping approach. *Health Psychology Review*, *10*(3), 297–312.

Koutoukidis, D. A., Lopes, S., Atkins, L., Croker, H., Knobf, M., Lanceley, A., & Beeken, R. J. (2018). Use of intervention mapping to adapt a health behavior change intervention for endometrial cancer survivors: The shape-up following cancer treatment program. *BMC Public Health*, *18*(1), 1–10. doi:10.1186/s12889-018-5329-5

Krivitsky, L. N., Parker, S. J., Pal, A., Meckler, L., Shengelia, R., & Reid, M. C. (2012). A systematic review of health promotion and disease prevention program adaptations: How are programs adapted? In E. Wethington & R. E. Dunifon (Eds.), *APA Bronfenbrenner series on the ecology of human development. Research for the public good: Applying the methods of translational research to improve human health and well-being* (pp. 73–99). American Psychological Association. doi:10.1037/13744-004

Kumpfer, K., Magalhães, C., & Xie, J. (2017). Cultural adaptation and implementation of family evidence-based interventions with diverse populations. *Prevention Science*, *18*(6), 649–659. doi:10.1007/s11121-016-0719-3

Kumpfer, K. L., Pinyuchon, M., de Melo, A. T., & Whiteside, H. O. (2008). Cultural adaptation process for international dissemination of the strengthening families program. *Evaluation & the Health Professions, 31*(2), 226–239.

Landais, L. L., van Wijk, E. C., & Harting, J. (2021). Smoking cessation in lower socioeconomic groups: Adaptation and pilot test of a rolling group intervention. *BioMed Research International, 2021*, 1–11.

Landes, S. J., McBain, S. A., & Curran, G. M. (2020). Reprint of: An introduction to effectiveness-implementation hybrid designs. *Psychiatry Research, 283*, 112630.

Lau, A. S. (2006). Making the case for selective and directed cultural adaptations of evidenceuc0u8208 based treatments: Examples from parent training. *Clinical Psychology: Science and Practice, 13*(4), 295–310.

Lee, S. J., Altschul, I., & Mowbray, C. T. (2008). Using planned adaptation to implement evidence-based programs with new populations. *American Journal of Community Psychology, 41*(3), 290–303.

Leeman, J., Calancie, L., Hartman, M. A. et al. (2015). What strategies are used to build practitioners' capacity to implement community-based interventions and are they effective?: a systematic review. *Implementation Science*, 10, 80. doi:10.1186/s13012-015-0272-7

Leeman, J., Teal, R., Jernigan, J., Reed, J. H., Farris, R., & Ammerman, A. (2014). What evidence and support do state-level public health practitioners need to address obesity prevention. *American journal of health promotion : AJHP, 28*(3), 189–196. doi:10.4278/ajhp.120518-QUAL-266

Marques, L., Valentine, S. E., Kaysen, D., Mackintosh, M. A., Dixon De Silva, L. E., Ahles, E. M., Youn, S. J., Shtasel, D. L., Simon, N. M., & Wiltsey Stirman, S. (2019). Provider fidelity and modifications to cognitive processing therapy in a diverse community health clinic: Associations with clinical change. *Journal of Consulting and Clinical Psychology, 87*(4), 357.

McCarthy, O. L., Mavodza, C., Chikwari, C. D., Dauya, E., Tembo, M., Hlabangana, P., Dembetembe, R., Mpakami, N., Bandason, T., Free, C., Smith, C., & Ferrand, R. A. (2022). Adapting an evidence-based contraceptive behavioural intervention delivered by mobile phone for young people in Zimbabwe. *BMC Health Services Research, 22*(1), 106. doi:10.1186/s12913-022-07501-9

Moher, D., Schulz, K. F., & Altman, D. G. (2001). The CONSORT statement: revised recommendations for improving the quality of reports of parallel-group randomised trials. *Lancet (London, England), 357*(9263), 1191–1194.

Moore, G., Campbell, M., Copeland, L., Craig, P., Movsisyan, A., Hoddinott, P., Littlecott, H., O'Cathain, A., Pfadenhauer, L., Rehfuess, E., Segrott, J., Hawe, P., Kee, F., Couturiaux, D., Hallingberg, B., & Evans, R. (2021). Adapting interventions to new contexts—the ADAPT guidance. *BMJ, 374*, n1679. doi:10.1136/bmj.n1679

Morales-Campos, D. Y., Snipes, S. A., Villarreal, E. K., Crocker, L. C., Guerrero, A., & Fernandez, M. E. (2021). Cervical cancer, human papillomavirus (HPV), and HPV vaccination: exploring gendered perspectives, knowledge, attitudes, and cultural taboos among Mexican American adults. *Ethnicity & health, 26*(2), 206–224. doi:10.1080/13557858.2018.1494821

Movsisyan, A., Arnold, L., Copeland, L., Evans, R., Littlecott, H., Moore, G., O'Cathain, A., Pfadenhauer, L., Segrott, J., & Rehfuess, E. (2021). Adapting evidence-informed population health interventions for new contexts: A scoping review of current practice. *Health Research Policy and Systems, 19*(1). doi:10.1186/s12961-020-00668-9

Mullen, P., Savas, L., Bundy, L., Haardörfer, R., Hovell, M., Fernández, M., Monroy, J., Williams, R., Kreuter, M., Jobe, D., & Kegler, M. (2016). Minimal intervention delivered by 2-1-1 information and referral specialists promotes smoke-free homes among 2-1-1 callers: A Texas generalization trial. *Tobacco Control, 25*, i10–i18. doi:10.1136/tobaccocontrol-2016-053045

National Cancer Institute (NCI). (n.d.) Using what works: Adapting evidence-based programs to fit your needs. http://cancercontrol.cancer.gov/usewhatworks/start.htm.

Pappaioanou, M., & Evans, C., Jr. (1998). Development of the guide to community preventive services: A U.S. Public health service initiative. *Journal of Public Health Management and Practice, 4*(2), 48–54. doi:10.1097/00124784-199803000-00007

Patel, V., Saxena, S., Lund, C., Thornicroft, G., Baingana, F., Bolton, P., Chisholm, D., Collins, P. Y., Cooper, J. L., Eaton, J., & Herrman, H. (2018). The Lancet Commission on global mental health and sustainable development. *The Lancet, 392*(10157), 1553–1598. doi:10.1016/S0140-6736(18)31612-X

Peters, G. J., de Bruin, M., & Crutzen, R. (2015). Everything should be as simple as possible, but no simpler: towards a protocol for accumulating evidence regarding the active content of health behaviour change interventions. *Health psychology review, 9*(1), 1–14. doi:10.1080/17437199.2013.848409

Petty, R. E., Barden, J., & Wheeler, S. C. (2009). The Elaboration Likelihood Model of persuasion: Developing health promotions for sustained behavioral change. In R. J. DiClemente, R. A. Crosby, & M. C. Kegler (Eds.), *Emerging theories in health promotion practice and research* (2nd ed., pp. 185–214). Jossey-Bass/Wiley.

Pot, M., Ruiter, R. A., Paulussen, T. W., Heuvelink, A., De Melker, H. E., Van Vliet, H. J., & Van Keulen, H. M. (2018). Systematically developing a web-based tailored intervention promoting HPV-vaccination acceptability among mothers of invited girls using intervention mapping. *Frontiers in Public Health, 6*, 226.

Rademakers, J., & Heijmans, M. (2018). Beyond Reading and Understanding: Health Literacy as the Capacity to Act. *International Journal of Environmental Research and Public Health, 15*(8), 1676. doi:10.3390/ijerph15081676

Ramanadhan, S., Mahtani, S. L., Kirk, S., Lee, M., Weese, M., Mita, C., & Brandt, H. M. (2022). Measuring capacity to use evidence-based interventions in community-based organizations: A comprehensive, scoping review. *Journal of Clinical and Translational Science*, 6, e92. doi:10.1017/cts.2022.426

Reed, A. K., Kohn, M. J., Stayman, S., Cole, A. M., Ko, C. W., Konnick, E. Q., Swanson, P. E., Zhang, Y., & Knerr, S. (2022). Patient navigation for hereditary colorectal cancer: Design of a randomized controlled trial to determine the effectiveness of pathways to genetic counseling. *Contemporary Clinical Trials, 116*, 106735.

Resnicow, K., Baranowski, T., Ahluwalia, J. S., & Braithwaite, R. L. (1999). Cultural sensitivity in public health: defined and demystified. *Ethnicity & disease, 9*(1), 10–21.

Riley, D. S., Barber, M. S., Kienle, G. S., Aronson, J. K., von Schoen-Angerer, T., Tugwell, P., Kiene, H., Helfand, M., Altman, D. G., & Sox, H. (2017). CARE guidelines for case reports: Explanation and elaboration document. *Journal of Clinical Epidemiology, 89*, 218–235.

Santiago, C. D., & Miranda, J. (2014). Progress in improving mental health services for racial-ethnic minority groups: A ten-year perspective. *Psychiatric Services, 65*(2), 180–185.

Savas, L. S., Atkinson, J. S., Figueroa-Solis, E., Valdes, A., Morales, P., Castle, P. E., & Fernandez, M. E. (2021). A lay health worker intervention to improve breast and cervical cancer screening among Latinas in El Paso, Texas: A randomized control trial. *Preventive Medicine, 145*, 106446.

Savas, L. S., Loomba, P., Shegog, R., Alaniz, A., Costa, C., Adlparvar, E., Allicock, M. A., Chenier, R., Goetz, M., & Markham, C. M. (2023). Using Implementation Mapping to increase uptake and use of Salud en Mis Manos: A breast and cervical cancer screening and HPV vaccination intervention for Latinas. *Frontiers in Public Health, 11*, 966553.

Scaccia, J. P., Cook, B. S., Lamont, A., Wandersman, A., Castellow, J., Katz, J., & Beidas, R. S. (2015). A practical implementation science heuristic for organizational readiness: R = MC^2. *Journal of community psychology, 43*(4), 484–501. doi:10.1002/jcop.21698

Schaalma, H., & Kok, G. (2009). Decoding health education interventions: The times are a-changin'. *Psychology and Health, 24*(1), 5–9.

Schoenwald, S. K., Sheidow, A. J., & Chapman, J. E. (2009). Clinical supervision in treatment transport: Effects on adherence and outcomes. *Journal of Consulting and Clinical Psychology, 77*(3), 410.

Serra, Y. A., Colón-López, V., Savas, L. S., Vernon, S. W., Fernández-Espada, N., Vélez, C., Ayala, A., & Fernández, M. E. (2017). Using intervention mapping to develop health education components to increase colorectal cancer screening in Puerto Rico. *Frontiers in Public Health, 5*, 324.

Smith, E., & Caldwell, L. (2007). Adapting evidence-based programs to new contexts: what needs to be changed? *The Journal of rural health : official journal of the American Rural Health Association and the National Rural Health Care Association, 23*(Suppl), 37–41. doi:10.1111/j.1748-0361.2007.00122.x

Szeszulski, J., Craig, D. W., Walker, T. J., Foster, M., Mullen, P. D., & Fernandez, M. E. (2022). Applying evidence-based intervention (EBI) mapping to identify the components and logic of colorectal cancer screening interventions. *Translational Behavioral Medicine, 12*(2), 304–323.

Vamos, C. A., Calvo, A. E., Daley, E. M., Giuliano, A. R., & López Castillo, H. (2015). Knowledge, behavioral, and sociocultural factors related to human papillomavirus infection and cervical cancer screening among inner-city women in Panama. *Journal of Community Health, 40*, 1047–1056.

van Daele, T., van Audenhove, C., Hermans, D., van den Bergh, O., & van den Broucke, S. (2012). Empowerment implementation: Enhancing fidelity and adaptation in a psycho-educational intervention. *Health Promotion International, 29*(2), 212–222.

Vroom, E. B., Massey, O. T., Akbari, Z., Bristol, S. C., Cook, B., Green, A. L., Levin, B. L., Tyson, D. M., & Johnson, M. E. (2022). Exploring perceptions of implementation practice capacity in community-based behavioral health organizations. *Journal of Community Psychology, 50*(3), 1700–1716.

Walker, T. J., Foster, M., Szeszulski, J., Craig, D. W., Mullen, P. D., & Fernández, M. E. (2022). Evidence-based intervention (EBI) mapping: A systematic approach to identify components and logic of evidence-based interventions. Under review. *BMC Public Health*, 2022 *22*(1), 1300.

Wandersman, A., Scheier, L. M. (2024). Strengthening the science and practice of implementation support: Evaluating the effectiveness of training and technical assistance centers. *Evaluation & the Health Professions*, 47(2):143-153. doi:10.1177/01632787241248768

Wandersman, A., Duffy, J., Flaspohler, P., Noonan, R., Lubell, K., Stillman, L., Blachman, M., Dunville, R., & Saul, J. (2008). Bridging the gap between prevention research and practice: The interactive systems framework for dissemination and implementation. *American Journal of Community Psychology, 41*(3–4), 171–181.

Watson, A. K., Hernandez, B. F., Kolodny-Goetz, J., Walker, T. J., Lamont, A., Imm, P., Wandersman, A., & Fernandez, M. E. (2022). Using implementation mapping to build organizational readiness. *Frontiers in Public Health, 10*, 904652.

Weiner, B. J., Lewis, C. C., Stanick, C., Powell, B. J., Dorsey, C. N., Clary, A. S., Boynton, M. H., & Halko, H. (2017). Psychometric assessment of three newly developed implementation outcome measures. *Implementation Science, 12*, 1–12.

Williams, N. (2006). The guide to community preventive services what works to promote health? *Occupational Medicine*, 57. doi:10.1093/occmed/kql098.

Williams, M. S., & Anyimukwu, C. (2020). The association between cardiovascular disease knowledge and risk factors among African American breast cancer survivors in the deep south. *Journal of Health Disparities Research and Practice, 13*(4), 7.

Williams, R. S., Stollings, J. H., Bundy, Ł., Haardörfer, R., Kreuter, M. W., Mullen, P. D., Hovell, M., Morris, M., & Kegler, M. C. (2016). Testing a minimal intervention to promote smoke-free homes among 2-1-1 callers: The North Carolina effectiveness trial. *PLoS One, 11*(11) doi:10.1371/journal.pone.0165086, e0165086.

Wiltsey Stirman, S., Baumann, A. A., & Miller, C. J. (2019). The FRAME: an expanded framework for reporting adaptations and modifications to evidence-based interventions. *Implementation Science, 14*, 58. doi:10.1186/s13012-019-0898-y

Wiltsey Stirman, S., Calloway, A., Toder, K., Miller, C. J., DeVito, A. K., Meisel, S. N., Xhezo, R., Evans, A. C., Beck, A. T., & Crits-Christoph, P. (2013a). Community mental health provider modifications to cognitive therapy: Implications for sustainability. *Psychiatric Services, 64*(10), 1056–1059.

Wiltsey Stirman, S., Kimberly, J., Cook, N., Calloway, A., Castro, F., & Charns, M. (2012). The sustainability of new programs and innovations: A review of the empirical literature and recommendations for future research. *Implementation Science, 7*, 17.

Wiltsey Stirman, S., Miller, C. J., Toder, K., & Calloway, A. (2013b). Development of a framework and coding system for modifications and adaptations of evidence—based interventions. *Implementation Science, 8*(1), 65.

Wingood, G. M., & DiClemente, R. J. (2008). The ADAPT-ITT model: a novel method of adapting evidence-based HIV Interventions. *Journal of acquired immune deficiency syndromes (1999), 47*(Suppl 1), S40–S46. doi:10.1097/QAI.0b013e3181605df1

Yapa, H., & Bärnighausen, T. (2018). Implementation science in resource-poor countries and communities. *Implementation Science, 13*(1), 154. doi:10.1186/s13012-018-0847-1

INDEX